Psychological Aspects of Cancer

Brian I. Carr • Jennifer Steel

Editors

Psychological Aspects of Cancer

A Guide to Emotional and
Psychological Consequences
of Cancer, Their Causes and Their
Management

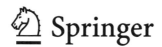 Springer

Editors
Brian I. Carr
Kimmel Cancer Center
Thomas Jefferson University
Philadelphia
Pennsylvania, USA

Jennifer Steel
Starzl Transplantation Institute
University of Pittsburgh
Pittsburgh
Pennsylvania, USA

ISBN 978-1-4614-4865-5   ISBN 978-1-4614-4866-2 (eBook)
DOI 10.1007/978-1-4614-4866-2
Springer New York Heidelberg Dordrecht London

Library of Congress Control Number: 2012951844

Printed on acid-free paper

Springer is part of Springer Science+Business Media (www.springer.com)

He used to say:
If I am not for myself, who will be
for me?
And if I am only for myself, what am I?
And if not now, then when?
–Hillel Mishna Avot 1:14

Who is wise? He who learns from every
person
–Ben Zoma Mishna Avot 4:1

For my daughters: Ophira and Feridey

Preface

The idea for this book of essays arose after several years during which the co-editors collaborated at the University of Pittsburgh on the medical oncology and psychological care of patients diagnosed with hepato-biliary cancer. Although the need for patient psychosocial support was evident, the time available in an ever-busy clinic was not conducive to the extended discussions that many patients and families wanted. The time pressures on staff in U.S. hospitals are increasing annually, in the name of system and business efficiencies. We noted a dichotomy between ideal total patient care in clinical practice and the realities of limited time per patient for employees of medical organizations. To some extent, patient-enabling Internet communication and services with health-care providers are beginning to be introduced with this dichotomy in mind. Still, the need for real-time, face-to-face contact and sufficient time with health professionals to hear and address their concerns are a patient priority.

He medical/psychological literature has exponentially expanded in the last decade with increasing documentation and sub-set characterization of various aspects of the quality of life of patients and their loved ones. Moreover, feedback from patients has resulted in a further proliferation of research that has extended to family and caregivers, who are rightly seen as important components of the patient environment, as well as subjects in need of study and care in their own right.

The arrival of unwelcome health-related news in the form of a cancer diagnosis would be expected to interrupt a person's self-perception and plans for his or her unfolding life story. Reflection on this interruption will likely result in fear and anxiety about the unknown quality and quantity of life that will now lie ahead. The major part of this book is taken up by considerations of the available resources in support of patient coping with his or her post-diagnosis new life structure as it is imagined and might become. Much of that is hypothesis and world-view driven, as seen in section C. Constructing a post diagnosis new life structure involves concepts of hope, meaning, and spirituality and their various impacts on coping, which in turn may change during the development and course of an individual's disease. All of this is concerned with the various cognitive and emotional aspects of coping with cancer and flows logically from the expected effects of disease on a person's thoughts, hopes, plans, and feelings. An emerging concept, however, is the idea of the potential reversibility of this process, in which thoughts and emotions might influence body function and disease development and its progression. For example, the concept that stress might be involved in and predisposing of cardiac ischemia and peptic dysfunction is very old. Evidence is emerging that these psychological and behavioral processes might also be involved in the development and/or progression of several chronic diseases, such as the inflammatory diseases and cancer. If mental processes can impact the immune and endocrine systems, then they might modulate the inflammatory and tumor growth processes that these systems mediate.

This book opens with two essays on the biological basis of emotion/mental-driven body processes and disease. The consequence of such considerations is that since thoughts and emotions can be modulated and changed with assistance from health-care professionals, then psychological counseling might be seen not only to help patients cope, but possibly to influence the disease itself. The book then proceeds to a section on genetic predispositions to cancer and the psychological considerations involved in screening and pre-emptive therapies and decision-making in cancer therapy. The third section deals with the philosophical and religious underpinnings of psychological factors involved in coping with disease state stressors and the roles of hope in coping. The fourth section is an acknowledgement that patients live in a social context, which often includes a partner and/or caregiver. The fifth section includes several essays on aspects and modalities of caregiving that are designed to help patients coping with their cancer and its aftermath, which increasingly extends for years. This is followed by a section with some considerations of approaches to dying and concerns of those who are left behind. The last section seeks to tie all this together and provide a resource chapter.

This book is not intended as a textbook, but as a set of essays for both health-care professionals and all people whose lives are directly or indirectly affected by cancer, to provide a sense of the activity and several new concepts in the rapidly expanding field of psychological support and psycho-social needs and context of the patient with cancer.

The book is presented in 7 sections: A. Biological basis; B. Prevention and decision-making; C. Theory in psychosocial oncology; D. The social context; E. Patient support; F. Advanced cancer: G. Wide-angle lens: resources and overview.

Puglia, Italy and Philadelphia, PA   Brian I. Carr

Contents

1 Psychoneuroimmunology and Cancer: Incidence, Progression, and Quality of Life 1
Christopher P. Fagundes, Monica E. Lindgren, and Janice K. Kiecolt-Glaser

2 Inflammation, Chronic Disease, and Cancer: Is Psychological Distress the Common Thread? 13
Feridey N. Carr and Elizabeth M. Sosa

3 Psychological Aspects of Hereditary Cancer Risk Counseling and Genetic Testing 31
Lisa G. Aspinwall, Jennifer M. Taber, Wendy Kohlmann, and Sancy A. Leachman

4 Mastectomy to Prevent Breast Cancer: Psychosocial Aspects of Women's Decision-Making 65
A. Fuchsia Howard, Lynda G. Balneaves, and Arminée Kazanjian

5 Decision Aids in Advanced Cancer 75
Natasha B. Leighl and Mary Ann O'Brien

6 Cancer Fatalism: Attitudes Toward Screening and Care 83
Miri Cohen

7 Positive Psychology Perspectives Across the Cancer Continuum: Meaning, Spirituality, and Growth 101
Crystal L. Park

8 Stress, Coping, and Hope 119
Susan Folkman

9 Religiousness and Spirituality in Coping with Cancer 129
Ingela C.V. Thuné-Boyle

10 Controversies in Psycho-Oncology 157
Michael Stefanek

11 **Psychosocial Interventions for Couples Coping with
    Cancer: A Systematic Review**.. 177
    Hoda Badr, Cindy L. Carmack, Kathrin Milbury,
    and Marisol Temech

12 **The Impact of Cancer and Its Therapies on Body Image
    and Sexuality** 199
    Susan V. Carr

13 **Cancer Caregivership** 213
    Youngmee Kim

14 **Psychosocial Interventions in Cancer** 221
    Catherine Benedict and Frank J. Penedo

15 **Quality of Life** 255
    John M. Salsman, Timothy Pearman, and David Cella

16 **Exercise for Cancer Patients: Treatment of Side Effects
    and Quality of Life**... 279
    Karen M. Mustian, Lisa K. Sprod, Michelle Janelsins,
    Luke Peppone, Jennifer Carroll, Supriya Mohile,
    and Oxana Palesh

17 **Use of the Classic Hallucinogen Psilocybin for Treatment
    of Existential Distress Associated with Cancer** 291
    Charles S. Grob, Anthony P. Bossis, and Roland R. Griffiths

18 **The Placebo and Nocebo Effects in Cancer Treatment**............ 309
    Franziska Schuricht and Yvonne Nestoriuc

19 **Psychological Factors and Survivorship: A Focus on
    Post-treatment Cancer Survivors**.. 327
    Ellen Burke Beckjord, Kerry A. Reynolds, and Ruth Rechis

20 **Complementary Mind–Body Therapies in Cancer**................... 347
    Daniel A. Monti and Andrew B. Newberg

21 **End-of-Life Communication in Cancer Care**............................ 361
    Wen-ying Sylvia Chou, Karley Abramson, and Lee Ellington

22 **The Intersection Between Cancer and Caregiver
    Survivorship** 371
    Jennifer Steel, Amanda M. Midboe, and Maureen L. Carney

23 **Resources for Cancer Patients** 385
    Carolyn Messner

24 **Bringing It All Together** 395
    Brian I. Carr

Index.. 407

Contributors

Karley Abramson, MPH University of Michigan School of Law, Ann Arbour, MI, USA

Lisa G. Aspinwall, PhD Department of Psychology, University of Utah, Salt Lake City, UT, USA

Hoda Badr, Ph.D Department of Ontological Sciences, Mount Sinai School of Medicine, New York, NY, USA

Lynda G. Balneaves, RN, PhD School of Nursing, The University of British Columbia, Vancouver, BC, Canada

Ellen Burke Beckjord, PhD, MPH Biobehavioral Medicine in Oncology Program, Department of Psychiatry, University of Pittsburgh Cancer Institute, University of Pittsburgh, Pittsburgh, PA, USA

Catherine Benedict, MS Department of Psychology, College of Arts & Sciences, University of Miami, Coral Gables, FL, USA

Anthony P. Bossis, PhD Department of Psychiatry, New York University School of Medicine, New York, NY, USA

Cindy L. Carmack, PhD Department of Behavioral Science, University of Texas M D Anderson Cancer Center, Houston, TX, USA

Maureen L. Carney, MD MB Kaiser Permanente, Sunnybrook Medical Office, Clackamas, OR, USA

Brian I. Carr, MD, FRCP, PhD IRCCS de Bellis Medical Center, Castellana Grotte, Puglia, Italy

Feridey N. Carr, PhD Department of Clinical Psychology, Alliant International University - Los Angeles, Alhambra, CA, USA

Susan V. Carr, MB.ChB, MPhil, MIPM, FFSRH Royal Womens Hospital, Melbourne, Australia

Jennifer Carroll, MD, MPH Department of Family Medicine, University of Rochester School of Medicine and Dentistry, Rochester, NY, USA

David Cella, PhD Department of Psychiatry and Behavioral Sciences, Robert H. Lurie Comprehensive Cancer Center, Institute for Healthcare Studies, Northwestern University Feinberg School of Medicine, Chicago, IL, USA

Department of Medical Social Sciences, Northwestern University Feinberg School of Medicine, Chicago, IL, USA

Division of Health and Biomedical Informatics in the Department of Preventive Medicine, Northwestern University Feinberg School of Medicine, Chicago, IL, USA

Wen-ying Sylvia Chou, PhD, MPH National Cancer Institute, Bethesda, MD, USA

Miri Cohen, PhD Department of Gerontology, School of Social Work, University of Haifa, Haifa, Israel

Lee Ellington, PhD University of Utah, Salt Lake City, UT, USA

Christopher P. Fagundes, PhD Institute for Behavioral Medicine Research, College of Medicine, The Ohio State University, Columbus, OH, USA

Susan Folkman, PhD Department of Medicine, University of California San Francisco, San Francisco, CA, USA

Roland R. Griffiths, PhD Department of Psychiatry, Johns Hopkins University School of Medicine, Baltimore, MD, USA

Department of Neuroscience, Johns Hopkins University School of Medicine, Baltimore, MD, USA

Charles S. Grob, MD Department of Psychiatry, Harbor-UCLA Medical Center, Torrance, CA, USA

A. Fuchsia Howard, RN, PhD School of Population and Public Health, Faculty of Medicine, The University of British Columbia, Vancouver, BC, Canada

Michelle Janelsins, PhD Department of Radiation Oncology, James P. Wilmot Cancer Center, University of Rochester School of Medicine and Dentistry, Rochester, NY, USA

Janice K. Kiecolt-Glaser, PhD Department of Psychiatry, Institute for Behavioral Medicine Research, College of Medicine, The Ohio State University, Columbus, OH, USA

Arminée Kazanjian, Dr. Soc chool of Population and Public Health, Faculty of Medicine, The University of British Columbia, Vancouver, BC, Canada

Youngmee Kim, PhD Department of Psychology, University of Miami, Coral Gables, FL, USA

Wendy Kohlmann, MS, CGC Huntsman Cancer Institute, High Risk Cancer Clinics, University of Utah, Salt Lake City, UT, USA

Sancy A. Leachman, MD, PhD Huntsman Cancer Institute, Salt Lake City, UT, USA

Department of Dermatology, Salt Lake City, UT, USA

Natasha B. Leighl, MD MMSc (Clin Epi), FRCPC Divison of Medical Oncology/Hematology, Princess Margaret Hospital, University of Toronto, Toronto, Canada

Monica E. Lindgren, BA Department of Psychology, Institute for Behavioral Medicine Research, College of Medicine, The Ohio State University, Columbus, OH, USA

Carolyn Messner, DSW, MSW, BCD, ACSW, FNAP, LCSW-R CancerCare, New York, NY, USA

Silberman School of Social Work at Hunter College, New York, NY, USA

Amanda M. Midboe, PhD Department of Psychiatry and Behavioral Sciences, Center for Health Care Evaluation, VA Palo Alto Health Care System, Stanford University School of Medicine, Stanford, CA, USA

Kathrin Milbury, PhD Department of Behavioral Science, University of Texas M D Anderson Cancer Center, Houston, TX, USA

Supriya Mohile, MD, MPH Department of Medicine, James P. Wilmot Cancer Center, University of Rochester School of Medicine and Dentistry, Rochester, NY, USA

Daniel A. Monti, MD Department of Psychiatry and Emergency Medicine, Myrna Brind Center of Integrative Medicine, Thomas Jefferson University and Hospital, Philadelphia, PA, USA

Karen M. Mustian, PhD, MPH, ACSM, FSBM Department of Radiation Oncology, Activity and Kinesiology (PEAK) Laboratory James P. Wilmot Cancer Center University of Rochester School of Medicine and Dentistry, Rochester, NY, USA

Yvonne Nestoriuc, PhD Clinical Psychology and Psychotherapy, Deparment of Psychology, Philipps University Marburg, Marburg, Germany

Mary Ann O'Brien, PhD Department of Family and Community Medicine, University of Toronto, Toronto, Canada

Oxana Palesh, PhD, MPH Department of Psychology, Stanford Cancer Institute, School of Medicine, Stanford University, Palo Alto, CA, USA

Crystal L. Park, PhD Department of Psychology, University of Connecticut, Storrs, CT, USA

Timothy Pearman, PhD Department of Medical Social Sciences, Robert H. Lurie Comprehensive Cancer Center, Northwestern University Feinberg School of Medicine, Chicago, IL, USA

Department of Psychiatry and Behavioral Sciences, Northwestern University Feinberg School of Medicine, Chicago, IL, USA

Frank J. Penedo, PhD Department of Medical Social Sciences, Northwestern University, IL, Chicago

Luke Peppone, PhD, MPH Department of Radiation Oncology, James P. Wilmot Cancer Center, University of Rochester School of Medicine and Dentistry, Rochester, NY, USA

Ruth Rechis, PhD Evaluation and Research, LIVESTRONG, Austin, TX, USA

Kerry A. Reynolds, PhD RAND Corporation, Santa Monica, CA, USA

John M. Salsman, PhD Department of Medical Social Sciences, Robert H. Lurie Comprehensive Cancer Center, Northwestern University Feinberg School of Medicine, Chicago, IL, USA

Franziska Schuricht Clinical Psychology and Psychotherapy, Department of Psychology, Philipps University Marburg, Marburg, Germany

Elizabeth M. Sosa, MA Department of Clinical Psychology, Alliant International University - Los Angeles, Alhambra, CA, USA

Lisa K. Sprod, PhD, ACSM Department of Radiation Oncology, James P. Wilmot Cancer Center, University of Rochester School of Medicine and Dentistry, Rochester, NY, USA

Michael Stefanek, PhD Office of the Vice President for Research, Indiana University, Bloomington, IN, USA

Jennifer Steel, PhD Division of Hepatobiliary and Pancreatic Surgery and Transplantation, Department of Surgery and Psychiatry, Center for Excellence in Behavioral Medicine, University of Pittsburgh School of Medicine, Pittsburgh, PA, USA

Jennifer M. Taber, MS Department of Psychology, University of Utah, Salt Lake City, UT, USA

Marisol Temech, BA Department of Oncological Sciences, Mount Sinai School of Medicine, New York, NY, USA

Ingela C.V. Thuné-Boyle, BSc (Hons.), MSc, PhD, CPsychol Research Department of Primary Care and Population Health, UCL Medical School (Royal Free Hospital Campus), London, UK

Psychoneuroimmunology and Cancer: Incidence, Progression, and Quality of Life

Christopher P. Fagundes, Monica E. Lindgren, and Janice K. Kiecolt-Glaser

Psychoneuroimmunology and Cancer

The notion that psychological factors affect cancer has been present throughout history [1]. The immune system plays a critical role in cancer incidence, progression, and quality of life; thus, the field of psychoneuroimmunology has been at the forefront of these investigations. Stress is an important factor that dysregulates immune function [2]. In this chapter, we first review evidence linking psychosocial factors to cancer incidence and progression. Then, we examine underlying biological mechanisms that may contribute to these links. Finally, we explore how dysregulated immune function contributes to cancer survivors' quality of life, particularly fatigue and depression.

C.P. Fagundes, Ph.D.
Institute for Behavioral Medicine Research,
The Ohio State University College of Medicine,
Columbus, OH, USA

M.E. Lindgren, B.A.
Department of Psychology, Institute for Behavioral
Medicine Research, The Ohio State University College
of Medicine, Columbus, OH, USA

J.K. Kiecolt-Glaser, Ph.D. (✉)
Department of Psychiatry, Institute for Behavioral
Medicine Research, The Ohio State University College
of Medicine, 460 Medical Center Drive, Room 130C,
Columbus, OH 43210-1228, USA
e-mail: janice.kiecolt-glaser@osumc.edu

Psychosocial Links to Cancer Incidence and Progression

Evidence suggests that psychological factors may be related to cancer incidence. A meta-analysis of 165 studies linked stress-related psychosocial factors with cancer incidence among those who were initially healthy [3]. For example, women who experienced stressful life events such as divorce, death of a husband, or death of a relative or close friend during a 5-year baseline period were more likely to be diagnosed with breast cancer during the next 15 years than those who did not experience these events [4]. In a prospective study of men and women aged 71 and over, those who were depressed over three separate time points were more likely to develop cancer than those who were not [5].

Although links between psychosocial factors and the onset of cancer exist, there is much stronger evidence that psychological factors play an important role in cancer progression and mortality [6, 7]. For example, metastatic breast cancer patients who reported no past traumatic events had longer disease-free intervals than those who experienced one or more traumatic events [8]. Early stage breast cancer patients who were more hopeless about their cancer were more likely to relapse within 5 years compared to those who were less hopeless [9]. In the same study, women who were more depressed were more likely to die within 5 years compared to those who were less depressed [9]. Hepatobiliary carcinoma patients

B.I. Carr and J. Steel (eds.), *Psychological Aspects of Cancer*,
DOI 10.1007/978-1-4614-4866-2_1, © Springer Science+Business Media, LLC 2013

who had higher levels of depressive symptoms at diagnosis had 6–9 months shorter survival than those who were less depressed [10]. A recent meta-analysis of 25 studies revealed that mortality rates are 39% higher among breast cancer patients diagnosed with major or minor depression compared to those not depressed [11].

Animal studies provide experimental evidence for relationships between stress and cancer, allowing for stronger causal inferences. Restraint is a common stressor in animals. Among rats who were exposed to a carcinogen, those who underwent a restraint stressor were more likely to develop a cancer tumor than those who were not restrained [12]. Furthermore, rats who were unable to escape restraint had earlier incidence of tumors, larger tumors, and lower survival time compared to rats who were able to escape [13].

In sum, there is considerable evidence that psychosocial factors play an important role in cancer. However, many well-designed studies have failed to find such links [11]. Given the many factors that contribute to cancer incidence and progression, this may not be surprising [14]. Accordingly, testing biologically plausible models that link psychosocial factors with cancer can help identify possible mechanisms underlying these associations [7].

Psychological Factors and Cancer Progression

One likely mechanism linking psychosocial outcomes to cancer progression is dysregulated immune function; stress can suppress cellular immune function and enhance inflammation [2]. The autonomic nervous system (ANS) and hypothalamic–pituitary–adrenal (HPA) axis compose the two major pathways by which stress dysregulates immune function. Lymphocytes, macrophages, and granulocytes have receptors for products secreted by the ANS and HPA axes [15]. Norepinephrine and epinephrine, catecholamines that are released by the sympathetic nervous system during stress, can promote tumor cell proliferation [16].

In the vast majority of cases, cancer becomes life threatening when it metastasizes. Metastasis occurs when cancer cells penetrate lymphatic and blood vessels, circulate through the blood stream, and then spread into other organs [16]. In order for metastasis to occur, blood vessels must grow new networks to the site of the tumor, a process known as angiogenesis.

Vascular endothelial growth factor (VGEF) is an important angiogenesis promoting agent that is first synthesized inside tumor cells and then secreted into surrounding tissue [17]. When VEGF binds to its receptor, a signal is transmitted into the endothelial cells, promoting endothelial cell growth [14]. This leads to the creation of new blood vessels that fuel the tumor. Catecholamines can modulate VEGF. For example, in several cell lines, both norepinephrine and epinephrine modulated the expression of VEGF [18, 19]. However, these effects were blocked by a beta-antagonist, an agent that inhibits sympathetic nervous system response [20].

Psychological factors can also modulate VEGF. Ovarian cancer patients who reported receiving more social support had lower levels of VEGF both in their serum and tumor tissues than those receiving less social support [21, 22]. Furthermore, colon cancer patients who were lonelier and/or depressed had higher levels of serum VEGF than those who were less lonely and/or depressed [23, 24].

When VEGF activates endothelial cells they produce matrix metalloproteinase (MMPs) enzymes, a family of matrix-degrading enzymes that contribute to angiogenesis by promoting endothelial cell migration [25]. Catecholamines stimulate secretion of MMPs by both tumor and stromal cells. Higher levels of stress and depression, as well as lower levels of social support, were associated with elevated MMP-9 among women with ovarian cancer [22]. Two in vitro studies provided additional support and mechanistic evidence. In one study, norepinephrine enhanced MMP production and increased the in vitro invasive potential of ovarian cancer cells by up to 189% [26]. These effects were blocked by beta-antagonists [26]. In another study, norepinephrine increased MMP-2 and MMP-9; the invasiveness of these cells were blocked using an MMP inhibitor and the beta-antagonist propranolol [20].

Proinflammatory cytokines such as interleukin 6 (IL-6) and IL-8 also promote angiogenesis. Norepinephrine stimulates the production of IL-6 and IL-8 in ovarian cancer and melanoma cell lines [18, 27]. Women with ovarian cancer who reported receiving less social support had higher serum IL-6 levels compared to those who received more social support [28]. This same association was also found at the site of the tumor [28].

Inflammation induces macrophages to shift from a phagocytic phenotype to a pro-tumor phenotype. Tumor associated macrophages (TAMs) promote tumor growth and invasion, and simultaneously downregulate adaptive immunity [29]. Excessive TAM proliferation is associated with poorer survival [30]. Using in vivo models of breast cancer tumors, pharmacologic activation of the sympathetic nervous system initiated the recruitment of additional TAMs to the primary tumor, while also promoting further pro-tumor macrophage differentiation [31]. The beta-blocker propranolol reversed the stressed-induced macrophage infiltration and inhibited tumor spread [31].

Cancer cells must resist anoikis, programmed cell death, in order to spread to other organs [32]. Anoikis is inhibited by beta-adrenergic activation of the cell adhesion enzyme, focal adhesion kinase (FAK; pFAKy397) [32]. Ovarian cancer patients with high levels of intratumoral norepinephrine also had elevated levels of pFAKy397 in their tumors [32]. Additionally, epinephrine reduced sensitivity to apoptosis in prostate and breast cancer cell lines [33].

Stress alters natural killer (NK) cell activity, an important antitumor defense [34]. Breast cancer survivors who reported greater distress during 18 months after surgery had poorer NK cell activity than those who were less distressed [35]. Furthermore, the survivors from this cohort who experienced faster emotional recovery following surgery showed greater improvements in NK cell activity compared to the women who recuperated

more slowly [36]. Men with localized prostate cancer who were more optimistic had greater NK cell cytotoxicity than those who were less optimistic [37].

Tumors can evade recognition and destruction by interfering with immune cell signaling. Accordingly, studies have considered the effect of stress on immune markers within the tumor microenvironment. Ovarian cancer patients who had more social support had greater NK cell activity in tumor infiltrating lymphocytes than those who had less support. Furthermore, those who were more distressed had poorer NK cell activity in tumor infiltrating lymphocytes than those who were less distressed [38, 39].

Gene Regulation

Biobehavioral factors are important in tumor gene expression [40]. Higher levels of depression and lower social support were associated with the upregulation of over 200 gene transcripts involved in tumor growth and progression [40]. Interestingly, ovarian tumors from women with higher levels of depression and lower levels of social support produced more norepinephrine compared to those with lower levels of depression and higher social support [40]. These findings suggest that psychosocial factors can impact cellular functioning, even at the molecular level.

Glucocorticoids

Glucocorticoids can impact cancer progression, as well as immunosurveillance. Glucocorticoids enhance tumor cell survival, downregulate the expression of DNA repair genes in breast cancer cells, and inhibit apoptosis following chemotherapy in breast cancer cells [41–43]. Additionally, cortisol can stimulate the growth of prostate and mammary cancer cells [44]. Prior to recurrence, breast cancer survivors who had higher levels of salivary cortisol were more likely to experience breast cancer reoccurrence compared to those who remained disease-free [45].

Circadian rhythm and cortisol production can be disrupted by psychological stress as well as sleep disturbances [46]. Long-term survival was shorter among breast cancer patients who had blunted circadian cortisol rhythms resulting from frequent nocturnal awakenings [46]. High plasma cortisol levels and depression were independently associated with suppressed immune responses to specific antigens in a separate sample of breast cancer patients [47]. Furthermore, diurnal cortisol disruption has been noted in breast cancer patients exhibiting greater functional disability, fatigue, and depression [48].

Oncoviruses

Viral infections can initiate tumorigenesis, and stress hormones influence the activity of various human tumor viruses [49]. Elevated antibody titers to a latent herpesvirus reflect poorer cellular immune system control over virus latency. Psychological stress and depression can drive latent virus reactivation or replication by impairing the ability of the cellular immune system to control viral latency [50]. For example, the heightened antibody titers to latent herpesviruses reported during academic exams, particularly EBV and HSV-1, appear to reflect alterations in the competence of the cellular immune response [51–53].

Human papilloma viruses (HPVs) establish infections in the stratified epithelium of the skin or mucous membranes and can cause genital warts. Almost all cervical cancers are caused by HPVs [54]. HPVs initiate tumor-supporting genetic and immunological changes when activated by glucocorticoids [49]. Stressful life events are a risk factor for increased progression of cervical dysplasia in HPV-positive women [55, 56].

Following infection with human immunodeficiency virus 1 (HIV1), catecholamines can accelerate AIDS-associated malignancies by increasing systemic susceptibility [49]. For example, people with heightened sympathetic nervous system activity are at increased risk for AIDS-associated B-cell lymphomas [57]. Catecholamines can also activate Kaposi sarcoma-associated herpesvirus by similar mechanisms to those that activate human T-cell lymphotropic viruses 1 and 2, two cancer-related viruses relevant to AIDS-patients [58, 59]. Stress hormones can thus impact a variety of cell-mediated immune responses affecting both the recognition of tumor viruses and the immunological defense against them.

In a study from our own lab that addressed the joint impact of social support and SES (indexed by education) in women who were dealing a potential or an actual breast cancer diagnosis, more highly educated women who had more support from friends had lower EBV antibody titers, reflecting better cellular immune function; however, for less educated women, friend support was not associated with EBV antibody titers [60]. This finding is health-relevant because recent research has highlighted links between herpesvirus reactivation and inflammation [61].

Quality of Life and Inflammation among Cancer Survivors

Thus far we have focused exclusively on how psychosocial factors interact with the immune system to contribute to cancer incidence and progression. However, over the past decade, some of the most promising work in the field of psychoneuroimmunology and cancer has focused on how the immune system interacts with the brain to contribute to cancer survivors' quality of life. Most of this work has focused on how inflammation contributes to sickness behaviors, fatigue, and depressive symptoms in breast cancer survivors.

Physically ill humans and animals exhibit sickness behaviors when exposed to an infection. Sickness behaviors are functional in that they help sick individuals restructure their perceptions and actions in order to conserve energy and resources [62]. Although feeling tired and lethargic is a normal and adaptive response to an acute infection, persistent low-grade inflammation has been linked to fatigue and depression [62]. Fatigue and depression can be side effects of long-term low-grade inflammation, representing a maladaptive version of inflammatory-induced sickness behaviors [62].

Proinflammatory cytokines can access the brain through a variety of key pathways including the leaky regions in the blood–brain barrier (e.g., circumventricular organs), cytokine-specific transport molecules expressed on brain endothelium, and vagal afferent fibers [63]. Proinflammatory cytokines act on the brain to facilitate sickness behaviors by reducing connectivity of brain areas associated with lethargy [64]. Furthermore, cytokines modify people's serotoninergic systems by increasing idoleamine 2,3 (IDO), reducing tryptophan production, and thus eventually serotonin levels [62]. In a separate pathway, proinflammatory cytokines can also influence HPA axis hormones that are associated with mood regulation, an indirect route [65].

Fatigue and Cancer Survivors

Fatigue is the most common problem among long-term cancer survivors [66], as well as the symptom that interferes most with daily life [67, 68]. Fatigue adversely affects overall quality of life, as well as many daily activities including mood, the sleep–wake cycle, and personal relationships [69–71]. Fatigue is a normal and expected response to chemotherapy and radiation [72]. However, fatigue persists many years beyond cancer treatment in a substantial number of cancer survivors [73]. Long-term fatigue among breast cancer survivors is particularly notable. For example, in a longitudinal study of 763 breast cancer survivors, 34% were fatigued 5–10 years after diagnosis, compared to 35% 1–5 years after diagnosis; 21% of the women were fatigued at both assessments, suggesting more severe or persistent fatigue among a significant proportion of cancer survivors [66]. Most studies addressing relationships between the immune system and fatigue have focused exclusively on breast cancer survivors.

In general, neither disease type nor treatment variables have demonstrated reliable associations with fatigue in cancer survivors. Specifically, type of cancer, disease stage at diagnosis, tumor size, number of nodes involved, presence and site of metastases, time since diagnosis, the type or extent of cancer treatment (including chemotherapy regime, dose, and cycles, and type of radiation), length of treatment, and time since treatment completion do not consistently predict the occurrence or severity of fatigue among survivors [73].

Bower and her colleagues have demonstrated that post-treatment breast cancer-related fatigue is associated with elevated inflammation. Breast cancer survivors with persistent post-treatment had higher levels of soluble inflammatory markers IL-1 receptor antagonist (IL-1ra), STNF-R11, and neopterin than breast cancer survivors who were not fatigued [70]. Interestingly, fatigue was not predicted by time since diagnosis or time since treatment. These findings were replicated in a subsequent study of fatigued and non-fatigued breast cancer survivors such that those who were fatigued had higher levels of soluble markers of proinflammatory cytokines than non-fatigued survivors (i.e., IL-1ra and soluble IL-6 receptor) [74].

Stress promotes inflammatory responses [2]. Fatigued cancer survivors show greater increased cytokine production when stressed compared to nonfatigued cancer survivors. Fatigued breast cancer survivors had greater increased LPS-stimulated IL-1β (beta) and IL-6 production from baseline to 30 min after the Trier Social Stress Task (TSST) than non-fatigued survivors [75]. Those who were fatigued also had greater increased CD4+ T lymphocytes compared to their non-fatigued counterparts [75].

In sum, fatigued breast cancer survivors show higher levels of resting and stress-induced stimulated proinflammatory cytokine levels compared to non-fatigued breast cancer survivors. However, less is known about whether inflammation is associated with fatigue in other types of cancer. Furthermore, little is known about the physiological mechanisms underlying persistent fatigue and inflammation.

Alterations in immune regulatory systems that are linked to inflammation may play an important role in fatigue [76]. Fatigued cancer survivors had 31% more circulating T-cells compared to non-fatigued cancer survivors. However, there were no alterations in circulating B-cell numbers [74].

Similarly, in another study, fatigued cancer survivors had elevated CD4+ T lymphocytes in contrast to nonfatigued cancer survivors [74]. Alterations in inflammatory markers may come from differences in the cellular immune response.

Autonomic nervous system functioning is linked to inflammation and may play a role in cancer related fatigue. Activation of the sympathetic branch of the autonomic nervous system enhances inflammation. As previously mentioned, stress heightens production of the catecholamines epinephrine and norepinephrine by the sympathetic nervous system. Norepinephrine induces nuclear factor-kappa B (NF-κB) transcription, which enhances proinflammatory cytokine production [77]. The parasympathetic branch of the autonomic nervous system works in opposition to the sympathetic branch. Higher parasympathetic activity can lower inflammation by inhibiting proinflammatory cytokine production [78]. Therefore, the combination of lower parasympathetic activity and higher sympathetic activity results in elevated inflammation.

In a recent study from our own lab, breast cancer survivors who reported more fatigue had significantly higher norepinephrine and lower heart rate variability (a measure of parasympathetic activity) than their less fatigued counterparts [79]. Fatigue was not related to treatment or disease variables including treatment type, cancer stage, time since diagnosis, and time since treatment [79]. Importantly, the relationship between HRV and cancer-related fatigue was sizeable. Based on research that has demonstrated characteristic age-related HRV decrements, the findings suggested a 20 year difference between fatigued and non-fatigued cancer survivors based on their HRV pattern, raising the possibility that fatigue may signify accelerated aging [79]. Given that both HRV and norepinephrine promote inflammatory responses, the findings may be tapping into the same physiological substrate that links proinflammatory cytokines to cancer-related fatigue and sickness behavior.

Cortisol acts to inhibit the release of proinflammatory cytokines. Cortisol peaks early in the morning and then decreases throughout the day [70]. In one study, breast cancer survivors had lower levels of morning serum cortisol than non-fatigued controls [70]. In another study, fatigued breast cancer survivors had flatter cortisol slopes across the day than non-fatigued survivors, as well as a rapid decline in cortisol levels in the evening among fatigued survivors [80]. Accordingly, these studies implicate both autonomic and HPA function in cancer-related fatigue and inflammation [79, 80].

Depression and Cancer Survivors

Cancer patients are three to five times more likely to experience major depression than non-cancer patients [81–83]. Major depression impairs cancer patients' quality of life as well as treatment adherence [81–83]. The immune system may play an important role in the etiology of cancer-related depression.

Although there is ample evidence that depressive symptoms can elevate inflammatory levels, there is also considerable evidence that proinflammatory cytokines contribute to depressive symptoms [65]. The association between inflammation and depressive symptoms has been found in a variety of different aging and diseased populations, including cancer survivors [84–87]. In a study of 114 patients with breast, lung, head and neck, or GI cancer, those who met criteria for clinical depression had higher levels of IL-6 compared to those that did not [88]. Another study of pancreatic, esophageal, and breast cancer patients demonstrated similar results [87].

Interferon, a proinflammatory cytokine, is used for the treatment of infectious diseases and some cancers. Between 20 and 50% of patients who receive interferon therapy develop significant depressive symptoms [87]. IFN-α-induced increases in IL-6 were positively related to increased depressive symptoms and anxiety over a 1-month period [89].

Experimental work provides additional evidence that inflammation induces depressive symptoms. Healthy volunteers who were injected with *Salmonella typhi* vaccine had increased post-vaccination levels of IL-6, IL-1ra, tumor necrosis factor-α (alpha) (TNF-α (alpha)), and negative mood compared to pre-vaccination levels compared to those injected with a placebo [90]. Antidepressants may be an effective strategy to minimize these negative consequences. In a double blind placebo-controlled trial, those who took a TNF-α (alpha) antagonist for the treatment of psoriasis had significant improvement in depressive symptoms compared with placebo-treated individuals [91].

Psychosocial Interventions and Biological Outcomes in Cancer

Many interventions have been developed to reduce cancer-related distress [92]. Given that depression and stress impact cancer biology, psychosocial interventions may impact cancer-related outcomes. Behavioral and psychosocial interventions for cancer patients have included cognitive-behavioral and stress management therapies, support groups, and psychoeducation [92].

Interventions that enhance social support, teach relaxation, and coping can improve neuroendocrine and cellular immune functioning. A 10-week, 10-session cognitive-behavioral stress management (CBSM) intervention reduced anxiety and depression, decreased social disruption, and increased benefit finding in women with stages I–III breast cancer who were recruited post-surgery [93]. Furthermore, compared to controls ($n=65$), women randomized to CBSM ($n=63$) had a significant decline in serum cortisol, greater Th1 cytokine production (interleukin-2 and interferon-y) and IL-2–IL-4 ratio after adjuvant treatment [93]. However, there were no group differences in CD4, CD8, CD56, CD56+CD3+, or CD19 cell counts [93]. Furthermore, there were no group differences for the ratio of interferon-y and IL-4 production [93].

A multicomponent biobehavioral intervention was designed to reduce emotional distress, improve health behaviors, and quality of life among 227 women who were treated for regional breast cancer. The baseline assessment occurred after surgery but before adjuvant therapy; the women participated in the intervention during adjuvant therapy. Those who received the intervention ($n=114$) perceived greater support and improved their dietary habits at the 4-month follow up compared to controls ($n=113$). Interestingly, among those who were assigned to the intervention group, T-cell proliferation remained stable or increased, while it declined in the controls [35]. However, there were no significant group differences in CD3, CD4, and CD8 counts [35].

Complementary and alternative-medicine interventions have also improved immunological function among cancer survivors. The standardized "healing touch" biotherapy (HT) is an alternative-medicine intervention designed to manipulate "energy fields" around the body to reduce symptom burden. In a randomized trial of 60 cervical cancer patients who were receiving chemotherapy and radiation, those who received HT ($n=21$) had higher level of NK cell cytotoxicity over the course of their treatment than those who did not ($n=39$) [94]. However, these changes did not parallel changes in NK cell number [94].

Caution should be exercised when interpreting psychosocial interventions that enhance immune function and cancer outcomes. As reviewed, there is evidence that psychosocial interventions may modulate immune function. However, many intervention studies have failed to show positive results [95]. Accordingly, more research is needed before definite conclusions are made.

Conclusion and Future Directions

Linkages between psychological factors and cancer have long been theorized, and researchers are now beginning to understand the mechanisms behind these links. Considerable work over the past decade has shown how psychological processes can impact pathways implicated in cancer progression. Furthermore, immune system dysregulation may have major implications for fatigue and depressive symptoms among cancer survivors.

Researchers have made great strides toward understanding how the brain and immune system interact to affect cancer survivors' quality of life and possibly morbidity and mortality. However, the vast majority of these studies have focused on a small proportion of cancer types. Cancer interacts with the immune system differently depending upon cancer type [96]. Furthermore, the ways in which people are psychologically affected by cancer differ based on a variety of factors including prognosis, treatment type, and pain—which are largely determined by cancer type (as well as stage) [97]. Accordingly, researchers should expand their investigations to encompass a wider range of cancers. Finally, cultural and socioeconomic factors play an important role in every aspect of the cancer experience [98, 99]; however, researchers have devoted little attention to this issue. For example, cultural and socioeconomic factors may exacerbate stress induced immune dysregulation [7]. Understanding how these factors interact to contribute to cancer outcomes is a critical direction for future research.

Acknowledgments The work on this chapter was supported in part by the following grants: National Institute on Aging (AG029562), National Cancer Institute (CA126857 and CA131029), and an American Cancer Society Postdoctoral Fellowship Grant PF-11-007-01-CPPB awarded to the first author.

References

1. Mukherjee S. The emperor of all maladies: a biography of cancer. New York: Scribner; 2010.
2. Glaser R, Kiecolt-Glaser JK. Stress-induced immune dysfunction: implications for health. Nat Rev Immunol. 2005;5:243–51.
3. Chida Y, Hamer M, Wardle J, Steptoe A. Do stress-related psychosocial factors contribute to cancer incidence and survival? Nat Clin Pract Oncol. 2008;5:466–75.
4. Lillberg K, Verkasalo PK, Kaprio J, Teppo L, Helenius H, Koskenvuo M. Stressful life events and risk of breast cancer in 10,808 women: a cohort study. Am J Epidemiol. 2003;157:415.
5. Penninx BWJH, Guralnik JM, Havlik RJ, et al. Chronically depressed mood and cancer risk in older persons. J Natl Cancer Inst. 1998;90:1888.
6. Ross K. Mapping pathways from stress to cancer progression. J Natl Cancer Inst. 2008;100:914.
7. Lutgendorf SK, Sood AK, Antoni MH. Host factors and cancer progression: biobehavioral signaling pathways and interventions. J Clin Oncol. 2010;28:4094.
8. Palesh O, Butler LD, Koopman C, Giese-Davis J, Carlson R, Spiegel D. Stress history and breast cancer recurrence. J Psychosom Res. 2007;63:233–9.
9. Watson M, Haviland J, Greer S, Davidson J, Bliss J. Influence of psychological response on survival in breast cancer: a population-based cohort study. Lancet. 1999;354:1331–6.
10. Steel JL, Geller DA, Gamblin TC, Olek MC, Carr BI. Depression, immunity, and survival in patients with hepatobiliary carcinoma. J Clin Oncol. 2007;25:2397.
11. Satin JR, Linden W, Phillips MJ. Depression as a predictor of disease progression and mortality in cancer patients. Cancer. 2009;115:5349–61.
12. Laconi E, Tomasi C, Curreli F, et al. Early exposure to restraint stress enhances chemical carcinogenesis in rat liver. Cancer Lett. 2000;161:215–20.
13. Visintainer MA. Tumor rejection in rats after inescapable or escapable shock. Science. 1982;216:437.
14. Fidler IJ. The pathogenesis of cancer metastasis: the 'seed and soil' hypothesis revisited. Nat Rev Cancer. 2003;3:453–8.
15. Padgett DA, Glaser R. How stress influences the immune response. Trends Immunol. 2003;24:444–8.
16. Costanzo ES, Sood AK, Lutgendorf SK. Biobehavioral influences on cancer progression. Immunol Allergy Clin North Am. 2011;31:109–32.
17. Saharinen P, Eklund L, Pulkki K, Bono P, Alitalo K. VEGF and angiopoietin signaling in tumor angiogenesis and metastasis. Trends Mol Med. 2011;17(7):347–62.
18. Yang EV, Kim SJ, Donovan EL, et al. Norepinephrine upregulates VEGF, IL-8, and IL-6 expression in human melanoma tumor cell lines: implications for stress-related enhancement of tumor progression. Brain Behav Immun. 2009;23:267–75.
19. Lutgendorf SK, Cole S, Costanzo E, et al. Stress-related mediators stimulate vascular endothelial growth factor secretion by two ovarian cancer cell lines. Clin Cancer Res. 2003;9:4514–21.
20. Yang EV, Sood AK, Chen M, et al. Norepinephrine up-regulates the expression of vascular endothelial growth factor, matrix metalloproteinase (MMP)-2, and MMP-9 in nasopharyngeal carcinoma tumor cells. Cancer Res. 2006;66:10357–64.
21. Lutgendorf SK, Johnsen EL, Cooper B, et al. Vascular endothelial growth factor and social support in patients with ovarian carcinoma. Cancer. 2002;95:808–15.
22. Lutgendorf SK, Lamkin DM, Jennings NB, et al. Biobehavioral influences on matrix metalloproteinase expression in ovarian carcinoma. Clin Cancer Res. 2008;14:6839–46.
23. Sharma A, Greenman J, Sharp DM, Walker LG, Monson JR. Vascular endothelial growth factor and psychosocial factors in colorectal cancer. Psychooncology. 2008;17:66–73.
24. Nausheen B, Carr NJ, Peveler RC, et al. Relationship between loneliness and proangiogenic cytokines in newly diagnosed tumors of colon and rectum. Psychosom Med. 2010;72:912–6.

25. Shih JY, Yuan A, Chen JJW, Yang PC. Tumor-associated macrophage: its role in cancer invasion and metastasis. J Cancer Molecules. 2006;2:101–6.
26. Sood AK, Bhatty R, Kamat AA, et al. Stress hormone-mediated invasion of ovarian cancer cells. Clin Cancer Res. 2006;12:369–75.
27. Nilsson MB, Armaiz-Pena G, Takahashi R, et al. Stress hormones regulate interleukin-6 expression by human ovarian carcinoma cells through a Src-dependent mechanism. J Biol Chem. 2007;282: 29919–26.
28. Costanzo ES, Lutgendorf SK, Sood AK, Anderson B, Sorosky J, Lubaroff DM. Psychosocial factors and interleukin-6 among women with advanced ovarian cancer. Cancer. 2005;104:305–13.
29. Sica A, Allavena P, Mantovani A. Cancer related inflammation: the macrophage connection. Cancer Lett. 2008;267:204–15.
30. Tsutsui S, Yasuda K, Suzuki K, Tahara K, Higashi H, Era S. Macrophage infiltration and its prognostic implications in breast cancer: the relationship with VEGF expression and microvessel density. Oncol Rep. 2005;14:425–31.
31. Sloan EK, Priceman SJ, Cox BF, et al. The sympathetic nervous system induces a metastatic switch in primary breast cancer. Cancer Res. 2010;70: 7042–52.
32. Sood AK, Armaiz-Pena GN, Halder J, et al. Adrenergic modulation of focal adhesion kinase protects human ovarian cancer cells from anoikis. J Clin Invest. 2010;120:1515–23.
33. Sastry KS, Karpova Y, Prokopovich S, et al. Epinephrine protects cancer cells from apoptosis via activation of cAMP-dependent protein kinase and BAD phosphorylation. J Biol Chem. 2007;282:14094–100.
34. Dunn GP, Bruce AT, Ikeda H, Old LJ, Schreiber RD. Cancer immunoediting: from immunosurveillance to tumor escape. Nat Immunol. 2002;3:991–8.
35. Andersen BL, Farrar WB, Golden-Kreutz DM, et al. Psychological, behavioral, and immune changes after a psychological intervention: a clinical trial. J Clin Oncol. 2004;22:3570–80.
36. Thornton LM, Andersen BL, Crespin TR, Carson WE. Individual trajectories in stress covary with immunity during recovery from cancer diagnosis and treatments. Brain Behav Immun. 2007;21:185–94.
37. Penedo FJ, Dahn JR, Kinsinger D, et al. Anger suppression mediates the relationship between optimism and natural killer cell cytotoxicity in men treated for localized prostate cancer. J Psychosom Res. 2006;60:423–7.
38. Lutgendorf SK, Sood AK, Anderson B, et al. Social support, psychological distress, and natural killer cell activity in ovarian cancer. J Clin Oncol. 2005;23: 7105–13.
39. Lutgendorf SK, Lamkin DM, DeGeest K, et al. Depressed and anxious mood and T-cell cytokine expressing populations in ovarian cancer patients. Brain Behav Immun. 2008;22:890–900.
40. Lutgendorf SK, DeGeest K, Sung CY, et al. Depression, social support, and beta-adrenergic transcription control in human ovarian cancer. Brain Behav Immun. 2009;23:176–83.
41. Antonova L, Mueller CR. Hydrocortisone down-regulates the tumor suppressor gene BRCA1 in mammary cells: a possible molecular link between stress and breast cancer. Genes Chromosomes Cancer. 2008;47:341–52.
42. Pang D, Kocherginsky M, Krausz T, Kim SY, Conzen SD. Dexamethasone decreases xenograft response to Paclitaxel through inhibition of tumor cell apoptosis. Cancer Biol Ther. 2006;5:933–40.
43. Flint MS, Kim G, Hood BL, Bateman NW, Stewart NA, Conrads TP. Stress hormones mediate drug resistance to paclitaxel in human breast cancer cells through a CDK-1-dependent pathway. Psychoneuroendocrinology. 2009;34:1533–41.
44. Zhao XY, Malloy PJ, Krishnan AV, et al. Glucocorticoids can promote androgen-independent growth of prostate cancer cells through a mutated androgen receptor. Nat Med. 2000;6:703–6.
45. Thornton LM, Andersen BL, Carson 3rd WE. Immune, endocrine, and behavioral precursors to breast cancer recurrence: a case-control analysis. Cancer Immunol Immunother. 2008;57:1471–81.
46. Sephton SE, Sapolsky RM, Kraemer HC, Spiegel D. Diurnal cortisol rhythm as a predictor of breast cancer survival. J Natl Cancer Inst. 2000;92:994–1000.
47. Sephton SE, Dhabhar FS, Keuroghlian AS, et al: Depression, cortisol, and suppressed cellmediated immunity in metastatic breast cancer. Brain Behav Immun 2009;23:1148–1155.
48. Weinrib AZ, Sephton SE, Degeest K, et al. Diurnal cortisol dysregulation, functional disability, and depression in women with ovarian cancer. Cancer. 2010;116:4410–9.
49. Antoni MH, Lutgendorf SK, Cole SW, et al. The influence of bio-behavioural factors on tumour biology: pathways and mechanisms. Nat Rev Cancer. 2006;6:240–8.
50. Glaser R, Kiecolt-Glaser JK. Stress-associated immune modulation and its implications for reactivation of latent herpesviruses. In: Glaser R, Jones J, editors. Human herpesvirus infections. New York: Dekker; 1994. p. 245–70.
51. Glaser R, Kiecolt-Glacer J, Stout J, Tarr K, Speicher C, Holliday J. Stress-related impairments in cellular immunity. Psychiatry Res. 1985;16:233–9.
52. Glaser R, Pearl D, Kiecolt-Glaser J, Malarkey W. Plasma cortisol levels and reactivation of latent Epstein-Barr virus in response to examination stress. Psychoneuroendocrinology. 1994;19:765–72.
53. Glaser R, Pearson G, Bonneau R, Esterling B, Atkinson C, Kiecolt-Glaser J. Stress and the memory T-cell response to the Epstein-Barr virus in healthy medical students. Health Psychol. 1993;12:435–42.
54. Zur Hausen H. Papillomaviruses in the causation of human cancers—a brief historical account. Virology. 2009;384:260–5.

55. Coker AL, Bond S, Madeleine MM, Luchok K, Pirisi L. Psychosocial stress and cervical neoplasia risk. Psychosom Med. 2003;65:644–51.

56. Pereira DB, Antoni MH, Danielson A, et al. Life stress and cervical squamous intraepithelial lesions in women with human papillomavirus and human immunodeficiency virus. Psychosom Med. 2003;65: 427–34.

57. Cole SW, Korin YD, Fahey JL, Zack JA. Norepinephrine accelerates HIV replication via protein kinase A-dependent effects on cytokine production. J Immunol. 1998;161:610–6.

58. Chang H, Dittmer DP, Shin YC, Hong Y, Jung JU. Role of Notch signal transduction in Kaposi's sarcoma-associated herpesvirus gene expression. J Virol. 2005;79:14371–82.

59. Turgeman H, Aboud M. Evidence that protein kinase A activity is required for the basal and tax-stimulated transcriptional activity of human T-cell leukemia virus type-I long terminal repeat. FEBS Lett. 1998;428:183–7.

60. Fagundes CP, Bennett BM, Alfano CM, et al. Social support and socioeconomic status interact to predict Epstein-Barr virus latency in women awaiting diagnosis or newly diagnosed with breast cancer. Health Psychol. 2012;31(1):11–9.

61. Stowe R, Peek M, Perez N, Yetman D, Cutchin M, Goodwin J. Herpesvirus reactivation and socioeconomic position: a community-based study. J Epidemiol Community Health. 2010;64:666.

62. Dantzer R, O'Connor JC, Freund GG, Johnson RW, Kelley KW. From inflammation to sickness and depression: when the immune system subjugates the brain. Nat Rev Neurosci. 2008;9:46–56.

63. Maier SF, Watkins LR. Cytokines for psychologists: implications of bidirectional immune-to-brain communication for understanding behavior, mood, and cognition. Psychol Rev. 1998;105:83–107.

64. Harrison NA, Brydon L, Walker C, Gray MA, Steptoe A, Critchley HD. Inflammation causes mood changes through alterations in subgenual cingulate activity and mesolimbic connectivity. Biol Psychiatry. 2009;66: 407–14.

65. Raison CL, Capuron L, Miller AH. Cytokines sing the blues: inflammation and the pathogenesis of depression. Trends Immunol. 2006;27:24–31.

66. Bower JE, Ganz PA, Desmond KA, et al. Fatigue in long-term breast carcinoma survivors: a longitudinal investigation. Cancer. 2006;106:751–8.

67. Ganz PA, Desmond KA, Leedham B, Rowland JH, Meyerowitz BE, Belin TR. Quality of life in long-term, disease-free survivors of breast cancer: a follow-up study. J Natl Cancer Inst. 2002;94:39–49.

68. Cleeland CS, Bennett GJ, Dantzer R, et al. Are the symptoms of cancer and cancer treatment due to a shared biologic mechanism? A cytokine-immunologic model of cancer symptoms. Cancer. 2003;97: 2919–25.

69. Collado-Hidalgo A, Bower JE, Ganz PA, Cole SW, Irwin MR. Inflammatory biomarkers for persistent fatigue in breast cancer survivors. Clin Cancer Res. 2006;12:2759–66.

70. Bower JE, Ganz PA, Aziz N, Fahey JL. Fatigue and proinflammatory cytokine activity in breast cancer survivors. Psychosom Med. 2002;64:604–11.

71. Lawrence DP, Kupelnick B, Miller K, Devine D, Lau J. Evidence report on the occurrence, assessment, and treatment of fatigue in cancer patients. J Natl Cancer Inst Monogr. 2004;32:40–50.

72. Smets E, Garssen B, Schuster-Uitterhoeve A, De Haes J. Fatigue in cancer patients. Br J Cancer. 1993;68:220.

73. Prue G, Rankin J, Allen J, Gracey J, Cramp F. Cancer-related fatigue: a critical appraisal. Eur J Cancer. 2006;42:846–63.

74. Bower JE, Ganz PA, Aziz N, Fahey JL, Cole SW. T-cell homeostasis in breast cancer survivors with persistent fatigue. J Natl Cancer Inst. 2003;95: 1165–8.

75. Bower JE, Ganz PA, Aziz N, Olmstead R, Irwin MR, Cole S. Inflammatory responses to psychological stress in fatigued breast cancer survivors: relationship to glucocorticoids. Brain Behav Immun. 2007;21: 251–8.

76. Bower JE. Cancer-related fatigue: links with inflammation in cancer patients and survivors. Brain Behav Immun. 2007;21:863–71.

77. Bierhaus A, Wolf J, Andrassy M, et al. A mechanism converting psychosocial stress into mononuclear cell activation. Proc Natl Acad Sci U S A. 2003;100: 1920–5.

78. Tracey KJ. Reflex control of immunity. Nat Rev Immunol. 2009;9:418–28.

79. Fagundes CP, Murray DM, Hwang BS, et al. Sympathetic and parasympathetic activity in cancer-related fatigue: more evidence for a physiological substrate in cancer survivors. Psychoneuroendocrinology. 2011;36(8):1137–47.

80. Bower JE, Ganz PA, Aziz N. Altered cortisol response to psychologic stress in breast cancer survivors with persistent fatigue. Psychosom Med. 2005;67:277–80.

81. Raison CL, Miller AH. Depression in cancer: new developments regarding diagnosis and treatment. Biol Psychiatry. 2003;54:283–94.

82. McDaniel JS, Musselman DL, Porter MR, Reed DA, Nemeroff CB. Depression in patients with cancer: diagnosis, biology, and treatment. Arch Gen Psychiatry. 1995;52:89.

83. Spiegel D, Giese-Davis J. Depression and cancer: mechanisms and disease progression. Biol Psychiatry. 2003;54:269–82.

84. Alesci S, Martinez PE, Kelkar S, et al. Major depression is associated with significant diurnal elevations in plasma interleukin-6 levels, a shift of its circadian rhythm, and loss of physiological complexity in its secretion: clinical implications. J Clin Endocrinol Metab. 2005;90:2522–30.

85. Miller GE, Stetler CA, Carney RM, Freedland KE, Banks WA. Clinical depression and inflammatory risk

markers for coronary heart disease. Am J Cardiol. 2002;90:1279–83.

86. Bouhuys AL, Flentge F, Oldehinkel AJ, van den Berg MD. Potential psychosocial mechanisms linking depression to immune function in elderly subjects. Psychiatry Res. 2004;127:237–45.

87. Musselman DL, Miller AH, Porter MR, et al. Higher than normal plasma interleukin-6 concentrations in cancer patients with depression: preliminary findings. Am J Psychiatry. 2001;158:1252–7.

88. Jehn CF, Kuehnhardt D, Bartholomae A, et al. Biomarkers of depression in cancer patients. Cancer. 2006;107:2723–9.

89. Bonaccorso S, Puzella A, Marino V, et al. Immunotherapy with interferon-alpha in patients affected by chronic hepatitis C induces an intercorrelated stimulation of the cytokine network and an increase in depressive and anxiety symptoms. Psychiatry Res. 2001;105:45–55.

90. Wright C, Strike P, Brydon L, Steptoe A. Acute inflammation and negative mood: mediation by cytokine activation. Brain Behav Immun. 2005;19:345–50.

91. Tyring S, Gottlieb A, Papp K, et al. Etanercept and clinical outcomes, fatigue, and depression in psoriasis: double-blind placebo-controlled randomised phase III trial. Lancet. 2006;367:29–35.

92. Jacobsen PB, Jim HS. Psychosocial interventions for anxiety and depression in adult cancer patients: achievements and challenges. CA Cancer J Clin. 2008;58:214–30.

93. Antoni MH, Lechner S, Diaz A, et al. Cognitive behavioral stress management effects on psychosocial and physiological adaptation in women undergoing treatment for breast cancer. Brain Behav Immun. 2009;23:580–91.

94. Lutgendorf SK, Mullen-Houser E, Russell D, et al. Preservation of immune function in cervical cancer patients during chemoradiation using a novel integrative approach. Brain Behav Immun. 2010;24:1231–40.

95. Moyer A, Sohl SJ, Knapp-Oliver SK, Schneider S. Characteristics and methodological quality of 25 years of research investigating psychosocial interventions for cancer patients. Cancer Treat Rev. 2009;35:475–84.

96. Reiche EMV, Nunes SOV, Morimoto HK. Stress, depression, the immune system, and cancer. Lancet Oncol. 2004;5:617–25.

97. Ciaramella A, Poli P. Assessment of depression among cancer patients: the role of pain, cancer type and treatment. Psychooncology. 2001;10:156–65.

98. Couzin J. Cancer research. Probing the roots of race and cancer. Science (New York, NY). 2007;315:592.

99. Zhang-Salomons J, Qian H, Holowaty E, Mackillop W. Associations between socioeconomic status and cancer survival: choice of SES indicator may affect results. Ann Epidemiol. 2006;16:521–8.

Inflammation, Chronic Disease, and Cancer: Is Psychological Distress the Common Thread?

Feridey N. Carr and Elizabeth M. Sosa

Inflammation, the hallmark feature of immunological response to invading microbes, has been implicated in a growing list of major diseases, including rheumatoid arthritis and lupus, inflammatory bowel disease, pulmonary and cardiovascular diseases, obesity, and diabetes mellitus. The focus on chronic inflammation has intensified since it has been linked with specific types of cancer, particularly those associated with viral infection or an inflammatory response. Although some chronic diseases have long been acknowledged to increase risk of malignancies, it is only within the past decade that chronic inflammation has been hypothesized to be a key factor in the development of cancer. While there is as of yet little evidence to suggest that psychological distress, particularly chronic stress and depression, directly affects the pathogenesis of tumors, there is an increasing amount of scholarship indicating that psychosocial factors directly contribute to the development and maintenance of chronic inflammation. In fact, it is possible that while depression may contribute and increase the levels of circulating proinflammatory cytokines, inflammation may itself act on the brain to induce depressive symptomatology. This chapter focuses on the primary

disease categories in which inflammation is a known contributor and discusses the mechanisms by which the inflammatory process interacts with carcinogenesis as well as psychological aspects of chronic inflammation. Some clinical considerations are offered for interventions targeting the anxio-depressive symptoms associated with major illness that may also disrupt the chronic inflammatory cycle and its resultant disease process.

Inflammation and Cancer

In 1863, Rudolf Virchow hypothesized that cancerous tumors originated at sites of chronic inflammation within the human body [1]. Virchow identified the role of inflammation in carcinogenesis when he noticed the presence of leucocytes in neoplastic tissue and suggested that the "limphoreticular infiltrate" reflected the origin of malignancies where inflammatory processes occurred [1]. Virchow's claim was not investigated for more than a century. Just recently, researchers have begun examining the hypothesized relationship and directing efforts to research the possible connection between chronic inflammation and cancer. Epidemiological studies have demonstrated that chronic inflammation predisposes individuals to a variety of cancers such as thyroid, bladder, cervical, prostate, esophageal, gastric, and colon [1, 2]. About 25% of all deaths from cancer worldwide are attributable to underlying infections and inflammatory

F.N. Carr, Ph.D. (✉) • E.M. Sosa, M.A.
Department of Clinical Psychology, California School
of Professional Psychology at Alliant International
University—Los Angeles, 1000S. Fremont Ave, Unit #5,
Alhambra, CA 91803, USA
e-mail: feridey.carr@gmail.com

B.I. Carr and J. Steel (eds.), *Psychological Aspects of Cancer*,
DOI 10.1007/978-1-4614-4866-2_2, © Springer Science+Business Media, LLC 2013

responses [3]. Chronic infection and inflammatory responses are known to have associations with the development of certain cancers, such as the human papilloma virus (HPV) and its relationship to cervical cancer, or the infection of hepatitis B and C viruses leading to hepatocellular carcinoma (HCC) [4]. Increased risk of tumor growth is associated with chronic inflammation caused by microbial infections and autoimmune diseases (e.g., inflammatory bowel disease and the risk of colon and colorectal cancers), as well as inflammatory conditions resulting from uncertain origins such as prostatitis, which can lead to prostate cancer [5–7]. Chronic inflammation contributes to a tumor promoting environment through various avenues that may include cellular transformation, the proliferation and survival of malignant cells, development of angiogenesis and metastasis, reduction of adaptive immune responses, and tumor response to chemotherapeutic drugs and hormones [7]. The inflammatory response and resultant tumors may be conceptualized as wounds that do not heal [8].

The role of chronic inflammation in the development of cancerous tissue easily becomes convoluted with many aspects that must be considered such as the contributions of various inflammatory cells, mediators, and signaling pathways in cancer genesis [7]. The inflammatory process involves the presence of inflammatory cells and inflammatory mediators which include chemokines and cytokines in tumor tissues, tissue remodeling and angiogenesis [7]. The prime endogenous promoters include transcription factors such as nuclear factor-kappB (NF-kB) and signal transducer activator of transcription-3 (Stat3) as well as major inflammatory cytokines, such as Interleukin Beta (IL-1 b), Interleukin 6 (IL-6), Interleukin 23 (IL-23) and tumor necrosis factor alpha (TNF-a) [9–12]. TNF-a was the first factor isolated as an anticancer cytokine but at dysregulated levels within the immune system, its presence mediates a variety of diseases [13]. TNF-a has also been demonstrated to be a major predictor of inflammation [14]. Several pro-inflammatory cytokines have been related to tumor growth, indicating that inflammation is associated with carcinogenesis [1, 15]. These

include IL-1, IL-6, IL-8, and IL-18. Interleukins are involved in different steps of tumor initiation and growth. Specifically, Negaard et al. demonstrated that individuals with hematological malignancies have increased bone marrow micro-vessel density as well as elevated levels of IL-6 and IL-8, possibly contributing to the malignant phenotype [16].

Chemokines are a family of proteins that play several roles in cancer progression, including angiogenesis, inflammation, and cell recruitment and migration. Chemokines also play a central role in leucocyte recruitment to sites of inflammation [1]. Most tumors produce chemokines that are one of two major groups, Alpha and Beta chemokines [1]. Evidence from murine models and human tumors propose that Beta chemokines contribute vastly to macrophage and lymphocyte infiltration in melanoma, carcinoma of the ovary, breast, and cervix, as well as in sarcomas and gliomas [1, 17, 18]. A key molecular link between inflammation and tumor promotion and progression is transcription factor NF-kB, which regulates TNF, interleukins, chemokines, and other molecular factors [9]. Although NF-kB is inactive in most cells, there is an activation state that is induced by a wide variety of inflammatory stimuli and carcinogens that, in turn, mediate tumorigenesis [19].

Inter-relationship Between Depression and Inflammation

The relationship between the brain and the peripheral organs, often referred to as the "mind-body" connection, is based on alterations in the endocrine and immune systems that lead to the chemical changes that occur in clinical depression. Pro-inflammatory cytokines, particularly IL-6, have been found to occur in greater quantities in depressed patients [20]. It has also been shown that about 45% of patients being treated medically with pro-inflammatory cytokine interferon-alpha (IFNa) developed symptoms of depression that was reversed once the treatment ended [21]. Inflammation is not only a contributing factor in depression but also in many domains of medical illness. Among patients diagnosed with major depression, there is evidence to suggest that relationships exist between severity and duration of depression and increased prevalence of other disease processes, such as cardiovascular disease, Type-2 diabetes, a variety of autoimmune diseases and cancer [22]. Major depressive disorders are also more prevalent in patients who suffer from illnesses that lead to chronic inflammation than healthy people [23]. While the presence of an inflammatory disease may initiate depressive symptoms in patients without preexisting psychological disorders, it is also the case that inflammation occurs in depressed patients who are not suffering from concurrent inflammatory disorders [24].

It is now known that the brain is not the "immune-privileged" organ that it was once presumed, as many thought it to be protected by the blood–brain barrier. Rather, the brain is very much influenced by the peripheral immune system where large molecules such as cytokines, chemokines and glucocorticoids originating in the peripheral organs can affect the neuronal pathways implicated in depression [20, 25]. Recently, it has been shown that symptoms of sickness (fatigue, decreased appetite, social withdrawal, disturbed sleep cycles, anhedonia and mild cognitive impairment), the normal bodily response to infection, are triggered by pro-inflammatory cytokines, including IL-1a and b, TNF-a and IL-6 [20]. These cytokines are responsible for developing the body's inflammatory (local and systemic) response to invading microbes. In doing so, they also impact neural circuitry within the brain, resulting in the behavioral symptoms of sickness. Such sickness behavior is remarkably similar to the symptoms of clinical depression. It is generally the role of anti-inflammatory cytokines to regulate the duration of these sickness symptoms, possibly by inhibiting pro-inflammatory cytokine production and interfering with pro-inflammatory cytokine signaling [26].

Despite the evidence to support the mechanism by which pro-inflammatory cytokines act on the brain, the directionality of the inflammation–depression relationship is as yet unclear.

As mentioned earlier, there is also research to suggest that depression may predispose people to developing illness. One study attempting to examine the directionality of the inflammation–depression relationship found that baseline depression scores of healthy (no medical illness) patients independently predicted change in IL-6. In contrast, IL-6 did not predict change in depression score [27]. The implication of those findings suggests that depression in previously healthy people may lead to inflammation and inflammation may be the mechanism through which depression potentiates chronic illness.

Rheumatic Disease

Rheumatic diseases, including rheumatoid arthritis (RA) and systemic lupus erythematosus (SLE) are autoimmune conditions that often involve periods of painful swelling and inflammation in the joints and muscles. The inflammatory stages of RA involve the infiltration by inflammatory cells of the synovial sublining, activating the production of pro-inflammatory cytokines, chemokines, and growth factors that results in synovial lining hyperplasia [28]. This process results in the hyper-activation of macrophage and fibroblast-like synoviocytes, which releases additional cytokines, chemokines, and growth factors [28]. This process leads to systemic inflammation and the production of enzymes that destroy the organized extracellular matrix [29]. IL-6, a cytokine that regulates the immune and inflammatory response, is thought to play pathologic roles in RA [30]. Increased IL-6 levels have been found in both serum and synovial fluid in patients with RA, and are also known to correlate with increased disease activity [31, 32]. Baecklund et al. examined disease activity and various secondary symptoms of rheumatic disease, as well as drug treatment to evaluate risk factors for the development of lymphoma, a cancer associated with RA [33]. In a nested case–control study with 41 patients and 113 controls, no association was found between any specific immunosuppressive drug and increased risk of lymphoma. However, a strong association was seen between disease activity and risk of developing lymphoma. In a similar study, Baecklund et al. investigated both RA patient cancer risk and the danger of anti-rheumatic treatment in lymphoma development [34]. After comparing 378 RA patients positive for malignant lymphoma history with 378 healthy controls, data revealed that individuals with severe disease activity were at increased risk of lymphoma. In addition, increased level of pro-inflammatory cytokines, not drug treatment, predicted lymphoma risk.

Although RA patients' increased risk for developing malignant lymphomas is not completely understood, there are several possible hypotheses that have emerged, including the role of immunosuppression, Epstein-Barr virus infection, and unregulated systemic inflammation [33–39]. In one systematic review and meta-analysis, Smitten et al. characterized the associated risk of four site-specific malignancies that included lymphoma, lung, colorectal, and breast cancer in patients with RA [40]. Results indicated that compared with the general population, RA patients have an approximately twofold increase in lymphoma risk and greater risk of Hodgkins than non-Hodgkins lymphoma. There was also data to suggest an increased risk of lung cancer but a decreased risk for colorectal and breast cancer.

The prevalence of psychological distress among patients with rheumatic diseases is a well known and highly documented phenomenon. Among patients with SLE, there is evidence to suggest a range of 16–65% of patients in active disease states who meet criteria for a psychological disorder [41, 42]. In particular, mood and anxiety disorders appear to be the most frequently occurring [41, 43]. One study showed that 69% of patients diagnosed with SLE were positive for a lifetime history of mood disorder and 52% for lifetime anxiety disorder [44]. Some research links psychological distress, particularly depression, with disease activity in SLE. Segui et al. evaluated patients for depression and anxiety during both active and inactive stages of their disease [42]. Forty percent of participants were diagnosed with a psychological disorder during

the acute phase, but only 10% met criteria a year later when the participants no longer displayed disease activity associated with SLE. However, it is often difficult to determine whether this phenomenon has biological influences or is a psychological adaptation to managing a chronic illness. In a study comparing depressive symptoms in patients with RA and patients diagnosed with osteoarthritis (a chronic non-inflammatory degenerative disease), those with the inflammatory disease were found to have significantly higher depressive symptoms [45]. The authors point out that while the two diseases are similar in terms of pain and functional impairments, the difference may be the neuroimmunobiological cytokine mechanism in inflammatory diseases, postulated to play a role in the development of depression. Psychological distress is associated with increased inflammation in both healthy individuals and RA patients [23, 46]. Depression could facilitate the development of inflammation by leading to poor health behaviors, hormonal dysregulation, and vulnerability to atherogenesis [47, 48]. Depression has also been specifically linked to increased levels of CRP and IL-6, as well as increased weight, which itself has been associated with the release of pro-inflammatory cytokines [49, 50].

While results suggest that some depressive symptoms are correlated with CRP and other biomarkers of inflammation, particularly among women with RA, the relationship may be at least partially explained by disease-related factors, such as increased pain among patients with higher levels of inflammation [51]. The proposition that inflammation leads to depression among RA patients may deserve closer evaluation in longitudinal studies. In addition to experiencing increased pain, patients with RA and SLE often have symptoms such as fatigue and sleep disturbance that may mimic or interact with depression. Results have indicated that depression is a stronger contributor to patient fatigue than self-reported disease activity [52]. Moreover, depression in patients with inflammatory disease predictor of mortality, affects quality of life, increases healthcare costs and contributes to disability [53].

Gastrointestinal Disease

Inflammatory bowel disease (IBD), including both Crohn's disease (CD) and ulcerative colitis (UC), is characterized by chronic inflammation and abnormal physiological immune response that flares and then remits throughout an individual's lifetime, often beginning in childhood. Current prevalence rates estimate that inflammatory bowel diseases affect 1.4 million people in the USA [54]. IBD is an example of a disease process where chronic inflammation is known to mediate the risk of cancer and involves both immune deregulation and autoimmunity. The precise mechanisms by which inflammation leads to tumor development are not yet clear; however, patients with IBD, both UC and CD, are at increased risk of developing colorectal cancer [55]. Ulcerative colitis is characterized by the inflammation of the mucosa of the colon and rectum. CD involves inflammation of the bowel wall and may include any part of the digestive tract from the mouth to the anus. Itskowitz and Yio highlight the various predisposing factors that contribute to the link between chronic inflammation and colorectal cancer (CRC) in IBD, explaining how risk of colorectal cancer in IBD increases with longer duration of colitis and with the extent of involvement of the large intestine [56]. There is also a positive association between the severity of colitis and the risk for colon cancer where the risk of colon cancer increases with the severity of disease. Rutter et al. examined risk factors for colorectal neoplasia in patients with UC using a case–control study. Sixty-eight participants were matched with two control patients from the same population on various factors [55]. Results revealed a highly significant correlation between colonoscopic and histological inflammation scores and the risk of colorectal neoplasia, demonstrating that the severity of colonic inflammation is an important determinant of colorectal neoplasia risk. Other studies have shown that IL-6 and STAT3 is activated in the intestinal mucosa in murine models of IBD and colitis-associated cancers [57, 58].

TNF-a concentration is also elevated in the serum and stool of IBD patients [59]. The increased level of TNF-a stimulates the production of other pro-inflammatory cytokines that further promotes the inflammatory process within the micro-environment [60]. Landi et al. examined the specific molecular elements that contribute to inflammatory responses in colorectal cancer and assessed the contributions of IL-6, IL-8, TNF-a, and peroxisome proliferator-activated receptor gamma (PPARG) genes toward the risk of colorectal cancer [61]. Results suggested that a polymorphism in the promoter of the IL-6 gene is associated with a significantly increased risk of colorectal cancer, whereas polymorphisms in the PPARG genes and IL-8 were related to significantly decreased risk. They concluded that IL-6 could be related to CRC through its role in affecting the low-grade inflammation status of the intestine.

The risk of colorectal cancer is much greater in a small subset of IBD patients who also have primary sclerosing cholangitis (PSC), a disorder characterized by inflammation, cholestasis, and fibrosis in the intra-hepatic and extra-hepatic biliary ducts [56, 62]. Shetty et al. compared patients with ulcerative colitis and co-occurring PSC with a random sample of UC controls without PSC and found that 25% of 132 UC patients with PSC developed colorectal cancer or dysplasia compared with 5.6% of 196 controls [63]. This study demonstrates that UC patients with PSC are at increased risk for developing colorectal cancer or dysplasia and therefore should be closely monitored by their physicians. Research also suggests that some anti-inflammatory medications can reduce the development of colorectal dysplasia and cancer [56, 64]. This last factor provides strong support for the relationship between chronic inflammation and resultant carcinoma and suggests that utilization of anti-inflammatory medications may reduce cancer risk.

Itskowitz and Yio suggest several possibilities that explain how inflammation may result in neoplastic transformation and progression in IBD [56]. One theory suggests that an increase in epithelial cell turnover occurs, perpetuating the molecular and DNA damage caused by heightened levels of pro-inflammatory cytokines and potentially exacerbating the carcinogenic process [56]. Another theory is that the oxidative stress accompanying chronic inflammation among patients with IBD creates an environment that is malignancy prone [65]. While more research is needed to better understand the link, there is mounting evidence demonstrating that chronic inflammatory processes foster an environment where carcinoma is more likely to occur.

Major depression has been shown to occur in 31% of patients diagnosed with CD, and in 27% of patients with UC [66]. Compared with patients diagnosed with erosive esophagitis, those with Crohn's disease (and thus chronic inflammation) have been found to have significantly higher rates of depression (25.4% vs. 8.2%). Depression was also found to be highest among patients with active disease states. Patients with functional gastrointestinal disorders such as irritable bowel syndrome have been shown to have even higher depressive symptoms than patients with organic disorders, such as IBD, as well as more severe depressogenic dysfunctional attitudes [67]. While there is little evidence that psychological distress is related to the onset of IBD, there is more consistent evidence that psychological factors such as depression, anxiety and chronic life stress contribute to disease course. This may be particularly true of daily life stress and depression among patients with UC and CD [68]. One study evaluating more than 450 patients with CD discovered that the odds of a patient presenting with an exacerbation of their illness increased 1.85 times for 1 standard deviation of perceived stress. After statistically controlling for the mood and anxiety components, the association between perceived stress and exacerbation of illness no longer existed [69].

An interesting theory surrounding the recent increase in reported cases of IBD suggests that lack of exposure to certain micro-organisms in industrialized societies may play a role in sensitizing modern immune systems. The theory implicates the over-sanitation of these societies in the rise of major depressive disorder, which may arise from a lack of contact with sources of anti-inflammatory, immunoregulatory signaling [70]. Due to a paucity of immune training, some predisposed individuals may be at greater risk of unnecessary inflammatory attacks on benign environmental and organic antigens. Increased levels of pro-inflammatory and depressogenic cytokines may lead to a higher prevalence of depressive disorders. This theory is often referred to as the "hygiene hypothesis" and though still in its infancy in terms of supporting evidence, the idea is rapidly gaining momentum. To this end, one randomized double-blind study was able to decrease anxiety in patients with chronic fatigue syndrome by introducing a probiotic [71]. Although these are certainly intriguing results, thus far there is little else in the clinical literature to suggest that intestinal microbiota may influence emotional state.

Patients with inflammatory bowel disease are viewed as a population at high risk for developing colorectal cancer, a leading cause of cancer-related mortality. One study evaluating the psychological implications of having such high-risk status found that among patients with IBD, those with higher perceived social support reported lower generalized distress [72]. Additionally, those with first degree relatives with both colorectal and non-colorectal cancers were found to have higher reported generalized distress. Although there is not yet much research connecting better psychological status with lower incidence of colorectal cancer, it is tempting to surmise whether psychological interventions could improve the course of irritable bowel disease and therefore decrease risk of related cancers.

Obesity and Type-2 Diabetes

The prevalence of obesity is increasing significantly in the USA and recent estimates demonstrate that nearly two-thirds of the population is currently either overweight or obese [73]. When abdominal obesity is accompanied by other metabolic risks such as insulin resistance, low HDL, and elevated triglycerides, individuals are at increased risk for developing Type-2 diabetes, hypertension, hyperlipidemia, and cardiovascular disease [74, 75]. Type-2 diabetes, hypertension and cardiovascular disease are all complications of disease processes that also involve chronic inflammatory mechanisms. Obesity is associated with a chronic, low-grade inflammation and can itself be viewed as an inflammatory condition since weight gain activates inflammatory pathways [76]. Studies have demonstrated that numerous inflammatory markers are highly correlated with the degree of obesity and insulin resistance [77, 78]. Serum levels of pro-inflammatory cytokines, including IL-6, TNF-a, and CRP are generally all elevated in individuals with obesity and insulin resistance [79].

It is clear that the adipocyte is an active participant in the generation of the inflammatory state in obesity. Adipocytes secrete several pro-inflammatory cytokines that promote inflammation, including IL-6 and TNF-a [80, 81]. Among patients with Type-2 diabetes, these cytokines can enhance insulin resistance directly in adipocytes, muscle, and hepatic cells [82, 83]. Hotamisligil et al. examined the expression pattern of TNF-a in adipose tissue and found that TNF-a plays a role in the abnormal regulation of this cytokine in the pathogenesis of obesity-related insulin resistance [84]. The increased levels of cytokines lead to hepatic production and the secretion of CRP, plasminogen activator inhibitor-1 (PAI-1), amyloid-A, alpha1-acid glycoprotein, and haptoglobin, which are all inflammatory markers that appear in the early stages of Type-2 diabetes and increase as the disease progresses [85]. Panagiotakos et al. evaluated the association between various markers of chronic inflammation in a population-based sample of 3,042 adults and found that compared with participants with normal body fat distribution, individuals with central fat exhibited 53% higher CRP levels, 20% higher TNF-a levels, 26% higher amyloid-A levels, 17% higher white blood cell counts, and 42% higher IL-6 levels [86]. They also found that all inflammatory biomarkers were related to body-mass index (BMI), waist, and waist-to-hip ratios. This study demonstrates a relationship between central adiposity and inflammation that can be associated with increased coronary disease risk. Some research

suggests that obesity stimulates inflammation through oxidative stress, which can result either from high levels of free radical production, a decrease in endogenous antioxidant defenses, or both [87–89]. The oxidative stress that is created activates the pro-inflammatory transcriptor factor, NF-kB, continuing to promote low-grade chronic inflammation [90, 91].

Several epidemiological studies have demonstrated that elevated weight and obesity, defined by a BMI higher than 25, results in significant increase for risk of cancer [92–94]. In a large population-based study, Calle et al. found that the relative risk of cancer-related deaths for men and women was 1.52 and 1.62, respectively [94]. The increase in risk was dependent on the type of cancer, with the largest observed risk being for HCC, the most common form of liver cancer. BMI, in both men and women, was also significantly associated with increased mortality due to cancer of the esophagus, colon and rectum, liver, gallbladder, pancreas, and kidney. Moreover, men with higher BMI were at increased risk of death from cancers of the stomach and prostate. Women showed increased risk for death from cancers of the breast, uterus, cervix, and ovary. Park et al. examined how obesity enhanced cancer risk and development by studying HCC in mice [95]. Results revealed that dietary and genetic obesity promoted the growth of tumors associated with the liver. There was a direct association between obesity-promoted HCC development and enhanced production of the tumor promoting cytokines IL-6 and TNF, both of which cause hepatic inflammation and activate the oncogenic transcription factor STAT3. Such data suggests that inflammatory mechanisms may mediate the association between obesity and cancer development.

The link between depression and obesity is a well-researched one with copious studies supporting it [96–98]. Both obesity and depression are public health problems with high prevalence rates and carry multiple health implications [99]. Evidence suggests that depressed individuals have about an 18% increased risk of becoming obese [96]. An examination of the association between obesity and depression revealed that large waist circumference and class III obesity

(BMI >40 kg/m^2) were associated with higher prevalence of depression among female participants only [100]. In a systematic review and meta-analysis of longitudinal studies examining the relationship between depression, weight, and obesity, results suggested a reciprocal relationship between depression and obesity [101]. In a separate review, Taylor and MacQueen examined the role of adipokines (cytokines that are secreted by adipose tissue) in mediating the relationship between obesity and depression [102]. Data revealed that obesity was generally accompanied by the presence of pro-inflammatory cytokines as well as elevated levels of adipokines. Such inflammation increases the risk for individuals with obesity to develop functional bowel disorders such as irritable bowel syndrome, as well as colorectal cancer [103, 104]. Given that sweeping behavioral changes are often necessary to avoid the extensive tissue damage that may result in uncontrolled Type-2 diabetes, targeting possible depression in patients with obesity and/or diabetes appears to be an important area for clinical intervention. In fact, assessing overweight or prediabetic patients for depression may also be a crucial step in prevention of serious medical illness.

Pulmonary and Cardiovascular Disease

Pulmonary disease, in particular chronic obstructive pulmonary disease (COPD), deserves special mention due to the fact that it is a progressive illness initiated and exacerbated by inflammatory processes. The illness involves a significant and generally progressive limitation in airflow of the lungs after long term exposure to irritants and resultant inflammation [105]. COPD is a disease noted for its chronic inflammation in both stable phases and during periods where it becomes exacerbated. It is often associated with comorbidities including cardiovascular disease, diabetes, and hypertension, illnesses involving chronic inflammatory mechanisms. COPD is an important risk factor for atherosclerosis, the beginning stage of heart disease [106, 107]. Several studies have demonstrated that even minimal reductions

in expiratory flow volume elevate the risk of ischemic heart disease, stroke, and sudden cardiac death two- to threefold, independently of other risk factors [106–108]. Even though the mechanisms responsible for this link continue to be examined, persistent low-grade systemic inflammation is believed to play a significant role in the development of clot formation [109]. CRP specifically has been implicated in the pathogenesis of plaque formation [110–112]. Examined data from participants evaluated in the Third National Health and Nutritional Examination Survey to determine whether CRP and other systemic inflammatory markers are present in patients with chronic airflow obstruction and whether they may be associated with cardiac injury [113]. Results indicated that individuals with severe airflow obstruction had circulating leukocyte, platelet, and fibrinogen levels that were higher than in individuals without airflow obstruction. They also discovered that these individuals were more likely to have an elevated circulating CRP level. This data suggests that low-grade systemic inflammation was present in participants with moderate to severe obstruction and was associated with increased risk of cardiac injury.

One of the hallmarks of COPD is a chronic inflammation of the lower airway. COPD increases the risk of lung cancer up to 4.5-fold among long-term smokers [113–115]. Cigarette smokers develop some degree of lung inflammation but individuals with COPD develop a greater degree that progresses with advanced disease [116]. Cigarette smoke induces the release of several pro-inflammatory cytokines and growth factors including IL-1, IL-8, TGF-beta, and G-CSF through an oxidative pathway [117]. The activation of epithelial growth factor receptor (EGFR) is elevated in bronchial biopsies from smokers with or without COPD compared to nonsmokers [118, 119]. The increased activation of EGFR has been identified to be an early abnormality found in smokers at high risk for developing lung cancer [120]. Moreover, NF-kB is activated by inflammatory processes and by oxidative stress. Since NF-kB is highly activated in both COPD and lung cancer, it is possible that it may provide the molecular association between inflammation and the pathogenesis of tumor in the lung [121].

Among patients with COPD, depression occurs with such a high prevalence that such psychological distress cannot be easily attributed to behavioral factors. In a recent study, prevalence of depression in a Japanese male sample of patients with COPD ranged from just under 30–40%, depending on the screening tool [122]. Severity of COPD also significantly predicted depressive symptoms in participants. In one study investigating whether depression was associated with systemic inflammation in COPD by using a range of biomarkers and several depression and fatigue scales, it was found that TNF-a was correlated with depression score. Patients with a higher TNF-a level had higher mean depression scores. A slightly weaker correlation occurred between TNF-a and fatigue [123]. As COPD results from inflammation and/or changes in immunological repair mechanisms, a "spill-over" of inflammatory mediators into circulation often results in greater systemic inflammation [124]. Systemic inflammation may aggravate any comorbid diseases, such as ischemic heart disease, lung cancer, diabetes and depression. Such co-occurring health problems may increase the severity of COPD, resulting in frequent hospitalizations, increased healthcare costs and disability. Psychological comorbidities, such as major depression and anxiety, affect the patient's ability to adhere to their physicians' recommendations and to cope personally with COPD.

Hypertension is a major risk factor for the development of cardiovascular disease, the prevalence of which is dramatically higher in women with a chronic inflammatory disease, such as SLE. In fact, some studies have shown that up to 74% of their patient samples have significant hypertension [125, 126]. It is likely than the pathogenesis of hypertension involves inflammatory mechanisms, including metabolic factors as well as pro-inflammatory cytokines. The inflammatory process involves adipose tissue, which produces cytokines (leptin and adiponectin) [127]. Blood pressure has been found to correlate with circulating inflammatory cytokines, such as IL-6, TNF-a,

and CRP [128]. One study found that the concentration level of circulating IL-6 and adhesion molecules could be modified by decreasing blood pressure in hypertensive subjects. After successfully treating the high blood pressure of participants, the circulating IL-6 was found to be significantly lower [129]. Relationships between inflammation and autonomic function have also been observed: in a sample of cardiac patients, heart-rate variability (HRV) was demonstrated to be negatively correlated with inflammatory biomarkers, CRP and IL-6 [130].

Hypertension is a significant risk factor for the development of certain types of malignancies [131–133]. In a study of health records evaluating almost 364,000 men, data revealed a direct relationship between higher blood pressure and increased risk of renal-cell carcinoma [134]. Another association was found to occur between obesity and hypertension and higher risk of renal-cell carcinoma. Importantly, after the 6th-year follow-up, the cancer risk rose further with increasing blood pressure and decreased with lowered blood pressure. In a systematic review of articles published between January 1966 and January 2000 examining the relationship between hypertension and malignancy, Grossman et al. suggested that individuals with hypertension experienced an increased rate of global cancer mortality, particularly with regard to renal-cell carcinoma [135].

Evidence suggests that depression and anger suppression (as opposed to anger expression) are strong predictors of hypertension [136]. Other types of psychological distress that are known to relate to higher blood pressure and poorer cardiovascular outcomes include loss of social support, cultural alienation, and difficulty coping with stressful events [137]. In the USA, historically underserved populations are especially likely to have overlapping psychological distress and higher rates of hypertension, particularly among the urban American Indian and African American communities [138, 139]. Recent research demonstrates that this pattern is also true among newly urbanized peoples, such as urban black South African community. Among a sample of urban black South Africans with hypertension, psychological distress

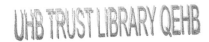

was associated with higher blood pressure as well as left ventricular hypertrophy [140]. It is interesting to note that depression among historically neglected communities is linked not only to hypertension, but also to cardiovascular disease, obesity, and chronic inflammatory diseases.

Despite increased media attention focused on prevention of cardiovascular disease (CVD), it continues to be the leading cause of death in the USA and the second most common cause of death worldwide [141]. Researchers have recently begun to examine the role of inflammation in atherogenesis and thrombosis and found that inflammatory processes play a role in all stages of atherothrombosis, known to be the underlying cause of approximately 80% of all sudden cardiac deaths [142]. The molecular process involves a response to oxidized low-density lipoprotein cholesterol, injury, or infection whereby leukocytes bind monocytes to the site of a developing lesion. The monocytes become macrophages, forming foam cells and initiating fatty streaks [143]. The macrophages are the main atherosclerotic inflammatory cells that induce a micro-environment that facilitates inflammation. At this stage, activation of macrophages, T lymphocytes, and smooth muscle cells (SMCs) leads to the release of additional mediators, including adhesion molecules, cytokines, chemokines, and growth factors, all of which play important roles in atherogenesis [143, 144]. In a study of carotid artery intima-media thickness (IMT) in hypertensive older adults, researchers found that inflammation, as measured by CRP, was one of the few predictors of arterial IMT [145]. In fact, new therapies aimed at preventing and treating atherosclerosis have targeted cytokine-based inflammatory mechanisms precisely because of the role of chronic inflammation in the development of atherosclerotic plaques [146].

Several studies have shown that elevations in CRP predict future risk of coronary episodes [147, 148]. Specifically, Pasceri et al. examined the effects of CRP on the expression of adhesion molecules in both human umbilical vein and coronary artery endothelial cells and found that CRP induces adhesion molecule expression in human endothelial cells in the presence of serum [149].

These findings support the hypothesis that CRP may play a direct role in promoting the inflammatory component of atherosclerosis. Sakkinen et al. evaluated the relationship between CRP and the development of myocardial infarction (MI) over a 20-year period in men in the Honolulu Heart Program and found that the odds of MI increased not only in the first few years of follow-up, but also as far as 20 years into the follow-up period, indicating that inflammation continues to affect the atherosclerotic process throughout all stages [150]. IL-6 is understood to be the principle pro-coagulant cytokine and can increase plasma concentrations of fibrinogen, plasminogen activator inhibitor type 1 and CRP, thereby amplifying inflammatory and pro-coagulant responses [149, 151].

Recent attention has focused on the role of mood disturbance among cardiac patients recovering from acute MI as results have suggested that depression contributes to adverse outcomes following cardiac events [152, 153]. In addition to other complications of cardiovascular disease, depression is known to increase the risk of mortality among this population [154]. In fact, the rate of mortality among depressed patients with cardiovascular disease is twice that of their non-depressed peers. Depression has also been demonstrated to have a predictive role in the development of coronary heart disease (CHD) in healthy individuals [155]. The risk of developing CHD has been shown to be about 60% greater in depressed but otherwise healthy patients. Depression is associated with poor health behaviors, higher life stress, passive coping styles as well as behavioral risk factors such as smoking, high fat diets, sedentary lifestyle and lack of adherence to medical advice [154]. Depression also plays a role in the development of local and systemic inflammation, which is associated with CHD [156]. Following episodes of cardiac arrest and cardiopulmonary resuscitation (CPR), survivors often suffer global cerebral ischemia after periods of brain blood flow deprivation. The levels of pro-inflammatory cytokines have been shown to increase dramatically following cerebral ischemia and this often results in the transportation of circulating immune cells across the blood–brain barrier [157]. Data indicate that the prevalence of depression rises considerably following the occurrence of cerebral ischemia, further exacerbating neuro-inflammation.

Treatment Considerations

Building on the past decade's examination of the psychological contributors to inflammation and consequent disease and cancer, an interesting question is whether psychological intervention may disrupt chronic inflammation and its resultant disease process. A few promising studies have attempted to shed light on the answer by targeting depressive symptoms in patients diagnosed with cancer. In one randomized clinical trial, newly diagnosed breast cancer patients with clinically significant symptoms of depression were assigned to one of two groups: one received the psychological intervention and the other only an assessment. Participants who received the psychological intervention demonstrated significantly reduced levels of depression, pain, fatigue, and pro-inflammatory biomarkers [158]. Interestingly, the effect of the intervention was mediated by its effect on depressive symptoms. In another randomized clinical trial, both depressed and nondepressed women post coronary artery bypass graft (CABG) surgery were assigned to either home-based cognitive behavioral therapy (CBT) or no intervention [159]. Depressed post-CABG women demonstrated decreased natural killer cell cytotoxicity (NKCC) as well as a higher frequency of infectious illness in the first 6 months after CABG. Depressed women who received the intervention demonstrated an increase in NKCC ($D=0.67$) and a decrease in IL-6 ($D=0.61$), CRP ($D=0.85$), and postoperative infectious illnesses ($D=0.93$). These results indicate that psychological status is related to impaired immunological functioning and increased rates of preventable illness.

Another angle examined in recent years has been the pharmacological treatment of depression, particularly with regard to selective serotonin-reuptake inhibitors (SSRIs) and tricylics. Researchers have found that activation of the serotonin 5-hydroxytryptamine (5-HT) 2A receptor, known for its role in brain neurotransmission, results in inhibition of TNF-a mediated inflammation [160]. One clinical trial that involved SSRI treatment of patients with major depression demonstrated a significant decrease in TNF-a and CRP [161]. The changes reflected similar decreases in self-reported depression symptoms. Similarly, other studies found that among patients with major depression treated with an SSRI, IL-6, IL-1 b and TNF-a levels were significantly lower post treatment [162, 163]. It has been demonstrated that the presence of serotonin is required for expression of the inflammatory markers IL-6 and TNF-a. However, it is interesting to note that lower serotonin levels increase, and higher levels decrease, the expression of pro-inflammatory cytokines [164]. The inverted U-shaped trend suggests that serotonin, and therefore mood state in general, is significant in influencing the inflammatory mechanism [160].

Conclusion and Future Directions

A current major debate among health care providers centers on the nature of the role of chronic inflammation in the pathogenesis of cancer. While it appears likely that the inflammatory mechanism is a major contributor toward a tumor-promoting environment that may also involve cellular transformation, the proliferation and survival of malignant cells, development of angiogenesis and metastasis, and reduction of adaptive immune response, direct causation between inflammation and tumor has not yet been established. Due to the rapid expansion of clinical and scientific literature on the topic, it is possible that more decisive evidence will be discovered within the next 5 years. Of perhaps equal interest (though perhaps to slightly different parties) is the interaction between psychological distress and chronic inflammation. While the directionality of this relationship remains unclear, and there is even evidence supporting bi-directionality, data suggests that psychological factors such as major depression, anxiety, chronic and daily life stress and anger suppression may trigger an inflammatory response. Unregulated, and often aggravated by the contribution of behavioral factors (dietary obesity, smoking, sedentary lifestyle), such immunological response often develops into chronic disease, some of which have been discussed in this chapter. Although there is no evidence to support a direct effect of psychological distress on the development of malignancies, psychosocial factors should be a target of critical importance in clinical settings as they are often modifiable and such intervention may alter or even prevent the course of chronic diseases associated with cancer development. Much of the literature discussed in this chapter indicated that illnesses such as rheumatic disease, gastrointestinal disease, obesity and Type-2 diabetes, and pulmonary and cardiovascular disease all have increased risk cancer development associated with chronic inflammation. The obvious and necessary question that follows is whether, and to what extent, reduction of psychological distress could improve the course of certain inflammatory diseases (or diseases where inflammation is a major feature) and therefore decrease risk of cancer.

The interaction between psychological distress and chronic disease is most acute in the health disparities among historically underserved populations in the USA, particularly among some American Indian/Alaska Natives (AI/AN), African American and Hispanic communities. Various risk factors contribute to such health disparities including ethnicity, social economic status, age, gender, literacy, transportation, and availability of services [165]. Compared with non-Hispanic Whites, AI/AN, Hispanics, Asians, and Pacific Islanders have much higher rates of cancer [166]. National data revealed increased long-term rates of renal-cell, HCC, thyroid, melanoma, bladder and pancreatic carcinomas as well as increased mortality rates from melanoma, esophageal, pancreatic, and liver cancers [166]. Ethnic and racial minority groups in the USA, particularly non-Hispanic Blacks, have a higher prevalence of CVD risk factors. Racial discrimination contributes to disparities in health-related domains, as new studies have linked self-reported

experiences of discrimination to adverse cardiovascular health outcomes and hypertension and have been more pronounced for African Americans [167, 168]. In fact, among a sample of older African American adults, experiences of discrimination have been associated with increased levels of pro-inflammatory cytokines [169]. Understanding the role of psychosocial factors can provide important targets for clinical assessment, connection with resources and interventions. Clinical literature examining health disparities within the context of the interaction between psychological distress and chronic disease is a relatively new but rapidly expanding field and warrants more efforts in this promising direction.

References

1. Balkwill F, Mantovani A. Inflammation and cancer: back to Virchow? Lancet. 2001;357:539–45.
2. Philip M, Rowley DA, Schreiber H. Inflammation as a tumor promoter in cancer induction. Semin Cancer Biol. 2004;14:433–9.
3. Hussain SP, Harris CC. Inflammation and cancer: an ancient link with novel potentials. Int J Cancer. 2007;121(11):2373–80.
4. Rakoff-Nahoum S. Why cancer and inflammation? Yale J Biol Med. 2006;79(3–4):123–30.
5. Gulumian M. The role of oxidative stress in diseases caused by mineral dusts and fibres: current status and future of prophylaxis and treatment. Mol Cell Biochem. 1999;196:69–77.
6. Ekbom A, Helmick C, Zack M, Adami H-O. Ulcerative colitis and colorectal cancer. N Engl J Med. 1990;323:1228–33.
7. Mantovani A, Paola A, Sica A, Balkwill F. Cancer-related inflammation. Nature. 2008;454:436–44.
8. Dvorak HF. Tumors: wounds that do not heal. Similarities between tumor stroma generation and wound healing. N Engl J Med. 1986;315:1650–9.
9. Karin M. Nuclear factor-kappaB in cancer development and progression. Nature. 2006;441:431–6.
10. Yu H, Kortylewski M, Pardoll D. Crosstalk between cancer and immune cells: role of STAT3 in the tumour microenvironment. Nat Rev Immunol. 2007;7: 41–51.
11. Voronov E, Shouval DS, Krelin Y, Cagnano E, Benharroch D, Iwakura Y, et al. IL-1 is required for tumor invasiveness and angiogenesis. Proc Natl Acad Sci U S A. 2003;100:2645–50.
12. Langowski JL, Zhang X, Wu L, Mattson JD, Chen T, Smith K, et al. IL-23 promotes tumour incidence and growth. Nature. 2006;442:461–5.

13. Aggarwal BB. Signalling pathways of the TNF superfamily: a double-edged sword. Nat Rev Immunol. 2003;3(9):745–56.
14. Balkwill F. Tumor necrosis factor or tumor promoting factor? Cytokine Growth Factor Rev. 2002;13(2):135–41.
15. Ariztia EV, Lee CJ, Gogoi R, Fishman DA. The tumor microenvironment: key to early detection. Crit Rev Clin Lab Sci. 2006;43:393–425.
16. Negaard HF, Iversen N, Bowitz-Lothe IM, et al. Increased bone marrow microvascular density in haematological malignancies is associated with differential regulation of angiogenic factors. Leukemia. 2009;23(1):162–9.
17. Kulbe H, Levinson NR, Balkwill F, Wilson JL. The chemokine network in cancer—much more than directing cell movement. Int J Dev Biol. 2004;48(5–6):489–96.
18. Mantovani A, Bottazzi B, Colotta F, Sozzani S, Ruco L. The origin and function of tumor-associated macrophages. Immunol Today. 1992;13:265–70.
19. Aggarwal BB, Shishodia S, Sandur SK, Pandey MK, Sethi G. Inflammation and cancer: how hot is the link? Biocehem Pharmacol. 2006;72:1605–21.
20. Dantzer R, O'Connor J, Freund G, Johnson R, Kelley K. From inflammation to sickness and depression: when the immune system subjugates the brain. Nat Rev Neurosci. 2008;9(1):46–57.
21. Quan N, Banks WA. Brain-immune communication pathways. Brain Behav Immun. 2007;21(6):727–35.
22. Murray CJ, Lopez AD. Global mortality, disability, and the contribution of risk factors: Global Burden of Disease Study. Lancet. 1997;349(9063):1436–42.
23. Steptoe A, Hamer M, Chida Y. The effects of acute psychological stress on circulating inflammatory factors in humans: a review and meta-analysis. Brain Behav Immun. 2007;21(7):901–12.
24. Leonard BE. The concept of depression as a dysfunction of the immune system. Curr Immunol Rev. 2010;6(3):205–12.
25. Godbout JP, Berg BM, Krzyszton C, Johnson RW. Alpha-tocopherol attenuates NFkappaB activation and pro-inflammatory cytokine production in brain and improves recovery from lipopolysaccharide-induced sickness behavior. J Neuroimmunol. 2005;169(1–2):97–105.
26. Heyen JR, Ye S, Finck BN, Johnson RW. Interleukin (IL)-10 inhibits IL-6 production in microglia by preventing activation of NF-kappaB. Brain Res Mol Brain Res. 2000;77(1):138–47.
27. Stewart JC, Rand KL, Muldoon MF, Kamarck TW. A prospective evaluation of the directionality of the depression-inflammation relationship. Brain Behav Immun. 2009;23(7):936–44.
28. Brown KD, Claudio E, Siebenlist U. The roles of the classical and alternative nuclear factor-kappaB pathways: potential implications for autoimmunity and rheumatoid arthritis. Arthritis Res Ther. 2008;10(4):212.
29. Amos N, Lauder S, Evans A, Feldmann M, Bondeson J. Adenoviral gene transfer into osteoarthritis synovial cells using the endogenous inhibitor Ikappa B alpha reveals that most, but not all, inflammatory and destructive mediators are NF-kappa B dependent. Rheumatology. 2006;45:1201–9.
30. Nishimoto N, Kishimoto T, Yoshizaki K. Anti-interleukin 6 receptor antibody treatment in rheumatic disease. Ann Rheum Dis. 2000;59:121–7.
31. Guerne PA, Zuraw BL, Vaughan JH, Carson DA, Lotz M. Synovium as a source of interleukin 6 in vitro: contribution to local and systemic manifestations of arthritis. J Clin Invest. 1989;83:585–92.
32. Madhok R, Crilly A, Watson J, Capell HA. Serum interleukin 6 levels in rheumatoid arthritis: correlations with clinical and laboratory indices of disease activity. Ann Rheum Dis. 1993;52:232–4.
33. Baecklund E, Ekbom A, Sparen P, Feltelius N, Klareskog L. Disease activity and risk of lymphoma in patients with rheumatoid arthritis: nested case-control study. Br Med J. 1998;317:180–1.
34. Baeklund E, Iliadou A, Askling J, Ekbom A, Backlin C, Granath F, et al. Association of chronic inflammation, not its treatment, with increased lymphoma risk in rheumatoid arthritis. Arthritis Rheum. 2006;54(3):692–701.
35. Jones M, Symmons D, Finn J, et al. Does exposure to immunosuppressive therapy increase the 10 year malignancy and mortality risks in rheumatoid arthritis? A matched cohort study. Br J Rheumatol. 1996;35:738–45.
36. Asten P, Barrett J, Symmons D. Risk of developing certain malignancies is related to duration of immunosuppressive drug exposure in patients with rheumatic diseases. J Rheumatol. 1999;26:1705–14.
37. van de Rijn M, Cleary M, Variakojis D, et al. Epstein-Barr virus clonality in lymphomas occurring in patients with rheumatoid arthritis. Arthritis Rheum. 1996;39:638–42.
38. Dawson T, Starkbaum G, Wood B, et al. Epstein-Barr virus, methotrexate, and lymphoma in patients with rheumatoid arthritis and primary Sjogren's syndrome: case series. J Rheumatol. 2001;28:47–53.
39. Wolfe F. Inflammatory activity, but not methotrexate or prednisone use predicts non-Hodgkins lymphoma in rheumatoid arthritis: a 25-year study of 1,767 RA patients. Arthritis Rheum. 1998;41:S188.
40. Smitten AL, Simon TA, Hochberg MC, Suissa S. A meta-analysis of the incidence of malignancy in adult patients with rheumatoid arthritis. Arthritis Res Ther. 2008;10(2):R45.
41. Bachen EA, Chesney MA, Criswell LA. Prevalence of mood and anxiety disorders in women with systemic lupus erythematosus. Arthritis Rheum. 2009;61(6):822–9.
42. Seguí J, Ramos-Casals M, García-Carrasco M, et al. Psychiatric and psychosocial disorders in patients with systemic lupus erythematosus: a longitudinal study of active and inactive stages of the disease. Lupus. 2000;9(8):584–8.

43. Waterloo K, Omdal R, Husby G, Mellgren SI. Emotional status in systemic lupus erythematosus. Scand J Rheumatol. 1998;27(6):410–4.

44. Nery FG, Borba EF, Viana VS, et al. Prevalence of depressive and anxiety disorders in systemic lupus erythematosus and their association with anti-ribosomal P antibodies. Prog Neuropsychopharmacol Biol Psychiatry. 2008;32(3):695–700.

45. Mella LF, Bértolo MB, Dalgalarrondo P. Depressive symptoms in rheumatoid arthritis. Rev Bras Psiquiatr. 2010;32(3):257–63.

46. Davis MC, Zautra AJ, Younger J, Motivala SJ, Attrep J, Irwin MR. Chronic stress and regulation of cellular markers of inflammation in rheumatoid arthritis: implications for fatigue. Brain Behav Immun. 2008;22(1):24–32.

47. Carney RM, Freedland KE, Miller GE, Jaffe AS. Depression as a risk factor for cardiac mortality and morbidity: a review of potential mechanisms. J Psychosom Res. 2002;53(4):897–902.

48. Raison CL, Capuron L, Miller AH. Cytokines sing the blues: inflammation and the pathogenesis of depression. Trends Immunol. 2006;27(1):24–31.

49. Miller GE, Stetler CA, Carney RM, Freedland KE, Banks WA. Clinical depression and inflammatory risk markers for coronary heart disease. Am J Cardiol. 2002;90(12):1279–83.

50. Miller GE, Freedland KE, Carney RM, Stetler CA, Banks WA. Pathways linking depression, adiposity, and inflammatory markers in healthy young adults. Brain Behav Immun. 2003;17(4):276–85.

51. Low CA, Cunningham AL, Kao AH, Krishnaswami S, Kuller LH, Wasko MC. Association between C-reactive protein and depressive symptoms in women with rheumatoid arthritis. Biol Psychol. 2009;81(2): 131–4.

52. Carr, FN, Nicassio, PM, Ishimori, ML, Moldovan, I, Katsaros, E, Torralba, K. Depression predicts patient-reported fatigue in systemic lupus erythematosus (SLE). In: Society for Behavioral Medicine Annual Meeting. Washington, DC; April 2011.

53. Bruce TO. Comorbid depression in rheumatoid arthritis: pathophysiology and clinical implications. Curr Psychiatry Rep. 2008;10(3):258–64.

54. Kiebles JL, Doerfler B, Keefer L. Preliminary evidence supporting a framework of psychological adjustment to inflammatory bowel disease. Inflamm Bowel Dis. 2010;16(10):1685–95.

55. Rutter M, Saunders B, Wilkinson K, et al. Severity of inflammation is a risk factor for colorectal neoplasia in ulcerative colitis. Gastroenterology. 2004;126(2): 451–9.

56. Itzkowitz SH, Yio X. Inflammation and Cancer IV. Colorectal cancer in inflammatory bowel disease: the role of inflammation. Am J Physiol Gastrointest Liver Physiol. 2004;287(1):G7–17.

57. Mitsuyama K, Matsumoto S, Rose-John S, et al. STAT3 activation via interleukin 6 trans-signalling contributes to ileitis in SAMP1/Yit mice. Gut. 2006;55:1263–9.

58. Becker C, Fantini MC, Schramm C, et al. TGF-beta suppresses tumor progression in colon cancer by inhibition of IL-6 trans-signaling. Immunity. 2004;21:491–501.

59. Braegger CP, Nicholls S, Murch SH, Steohens S, MacDonald TT. Tumour necrosis factor alpha in stool as a marker of intestinal inflammation. Lancet. 1992;339(8785):89–91.

60. Theiss AL, Jenkins AK, Okoro NI, Klapproth JMA, Merlin D, Sitaraman SV. Prohibitin inhibits tumor necrosis factor alpha-induced nuclear factor-kappa b nuclear translocation via the novel mechanism of decreasing importin-α3 expression. Mol Biol Cell. 2009;20(20):4412–23.

61. Landi S, Moreno V, Gioia-Patricola L, Guino E, Navarro M, de Oca J, et al. Association of common polymorphisms in inflammatory genes interleukin (IL)6, IL8, tumor necrosis factor NFKB1, and peroxisome proliferator-activated receptor with colorectal cancer. Cancer Res. 2003;63(13):3560–6.

62. Jayaram H, Satsangi J, Chapman RW. Increased colorectal neoplasia in chronic ulcerative colitis complicated by primary sclerosing cholangitis: fact or fiction? Gut. 2001;48:430–4.

63. Shetty K, Rybicki L, Brzezinski A, Carey WD, Lashner BA. The risk for cancer or dysplasia in ulcerative colitis patients with primary sclerosing cholangitis. Am J Gastroenterol. 1999;94(6):1643–9.

64. Smalley WE, DuBois RN. Colorectal cancer and nonsteroidal anti-inflammatory drugs. Adv Pharmacol. 1997;39:1–20.

65. Hussain SP, Hofseth LJ, Harris CC. Radical causes of cancer. Nat Rev Cancer. 2003;276:276–85.

66. Farrokhyar F, Marshall JK, Easterbrook B, Irvine EJ. Functional gastrointestinal disorders and mood disorders in patients with inactive inflammatory bowel disease: prevalence and impact on health. Inflamm Bowel Dis. 2006;12(1):38–46.

67. Kovács Z, Kovács F. Depressive and anxiety symptoms, dysfunctional attitudes and social aspects in irritable bowel syndrome and inflammatory bowel disease. Int J Psychiatry Med. 2007;37(3):245–55.

68. Maunder RG, Levenstein S. The role of stress in the development and clinical course of inflammatory bowel disease: epidemiological evidence. Curr Mol Med. 2008;8(4):247–52.

69. Cámara RJ, Schoepfer AM, Pittet V, Begré S, von Känel R; the Swiss Inflammatory Bowel Disease Cohort Study (SIBDCS) Group. Mood and nonmood components of perceived stress and exacerbation of crohn's disease. Inflamm Bowel Dis. 2011. doi:10.1002/ibd.21623.

70. Raison CL, Lowry CA, Rook GA. Inflammation, sanitation, and consternation: loss of contact with coevolved, tolerogenic microorganisms and the pathophysiology and treatment of major depression. Arch Gen Psychiatry. 2010;67(12):1211–24.

71. Rao AV, Bested AC, Beaulne TM, et al. A randomized, double-blind, placebo-controlled pilot study of a probiotic in emotional symptoms of chronic fatigue syndrome. Gut Pathog. 2009;1(1):6.

72. Rini C, Jandorf L, Valdimarsdottir H, Brown K, Itzkowitz SH. Distress among inflammatory bowel disease patients at high risk for colorectal cancer: a preliminary investigation of the effects of family history of cancer, disease duration, and perceived social support. Psychooncology. 2008;17(4):354–62.
73. Flegal KM, Carroll MD, Ogden CL, Johnson CL. Prevalence and trends in obesity among US adults, 1999–2000. JAMA. 2002;288:1723–7.
74. Lakka HM, Laaksonen DE, Lakka TA, et al. The metabolic syndrome and total and cardiovascular disease mortality in middle-aged men. JAMA. 2002;288:2709–16.
75. Laaksonen DE, Lakka HM, Niskanen LK, Kaplan GA, Salonen JT, Lakka TA. Metabolic syndrome and development of diabetes mellitus: application and validation of recently suggested definitions of the metabolic syndrome in a prospective cohort study. Am J Epidemiol. 2002;156:1070–7.
76. Shoelson SE, Herrero L, Naaz A. Obesity, inflammation, and insulin resistance. Gastroenterology. 2007;132(6):2169–80.
77. Festa A, D'Agostino Jr R, Howard G, Mykkanen L, Tracy RP, Haffner SM. Chronic subclinical inflammation as part of the insulin resistance syndrome: the insulin resistance atherosclerosis study (IRAS). Circulation. 2000;102:42–7.
78. Pickup JC, Crook MA. Is type II diabetes mellitus a disease of the innate immune system? Diabetologia. 1998;41:1241–8.
79. Kern PA, Ranganathan S, Li C, Wood L, Ranganathan G. Adipose tissue tumor necrosis factor and interleukin-6 expression in human obesity and insulin resistance. Am J Physiol Endocrinol Metab. 2001;280:E745–51.
80. Rajala MW, Sherer PE. Minireview: the adipocyte—at the crossroads of energy homeostasis, inflammation, and atherosclerosis. Endocrinology. 2003;144:3765–73.
81. Fain JN, Madan AK, Hiler ML, Cheema P, Bahouth SW. Comparison of the release of adipokines by adipose tissue, adipose tissue matrix, and adipocytes from visceral and subcutaneous abdominal adipose tissues of obese humans. Endocrinology. 2004;145:2273–82.
82. Bilan PJ, Samokhvalov V, Koshkina A, Schertzer JD, Samaan MC, Klip A. Direct and macrophage-mediated actions of fatty acids causing insulin resistance in muscle cells. Arch Physiol Biochem. 2009;115: 176–90.
83. Hotamisligil GS. Inflammation and metabolic disorders. Nature. 2006;444:860–7.
84. Hotamisligil GS, Arner P, Caro JF, Atkinson RL, Spiegelman BM. Increased adipose tissue expression of tumor necrosis factor-alpha in human obesity and insulin resistance. J Clin Invest. 1995;95:2409–15.
85. Fernandez-Real JM, Pickup JC. Innate immunity, insulin resistance and type 2 diabetes. Trends Endocrinol Metab. 2008;19:10–6.
86. Panagiotakos DB, Pitsavos C, Yannakoulia M, Chrysohoou C, Stefanidis C. The implication of obesity and central fat on markers of chronic inflammation: the attica study. Artherosclerosis. 2005;183:308–15.
87. Solinas G, Naugler W, Galimi F, Lee MS, Karin M. Saturated fatty acids inhibit induction of insulin gene transcription by JNK-mediated phosphorylation of insulin-receptor substrates. Proc Natl Acad Sci U S A. 2006;103:16454–9.
88. Lamb RE, Goldstein BJ. Modulating an oxidative-inflammatory cascade: potential new treatment strategy for improving glucose metabolism, insulin resistance, and vascular function. Int J Clin Pract. 2008;62:1087–95.
89. West IC. Radicals and oxidative stress in diabetes. Diabet Med. 2000;17:171–80.
90. Esposito K, Nappo F, Marfella R, et al. Inflammatory cytokine concentrations are acutely increased by hyperglycemia in humans: role of oxidative stress. Circulation. 2002;106:2067–72.
91. Evans JL, Goldfine ID, Maddux BA, Grodsky GM. Oxidative stress and stress-activated signaling pathways: a unifying hypothesis of type 2 diabetes. Endocr Rev. 2002;23:599–622.
92. Bianchini F, Kaaks R, Vainio H. Overweight, obesity, and cancer risk. Lancet Oncol. 2002;3:565–74.
93. Calle EE, Kaaks R. Overweight, obesity and cancer: epidemiological evidence and proposed mechanisms. Nat Rev Cancer. 2004;4:579–91.
94. Calle EE, Rodriguez C, Walker-Thurmond K, Thun MJ. Overweight, obesity, and mortality from cancer in a prospectively studied cohort of U.S. adults. N Engl J Med. 2003;348:1625–38.
95. Park EJ, Lee JH, Yu GY, et al. Dietary and genetic obesity promote liver inflammation and tumorigenesis by enhancing IL-6 and TNF expression. Cell. 2010;140(2):197–208.
96. de Wit LM, van Straten A, van Herten M, Penninx BW, Cuijpers P. Depression and body mass index, a u-shaped association. BMC Public Health. 2009;9:14.
97. Faith MS, Matz PE, Jorge MA. Obesity-depression associations in the population. J Psychosom Res. 2002;53(4):935–42.
98. Scott KM, McGee MA, Wells JE, Oakley Browne MA. Obesity and mental disorders in the adult general population. J Psychosom Res. 2008;64(1):97–105.
99. Penninx BW, Beekman AT, Honig A, et al. Depression and cardiac mortality: results from a community-based longitudinal study. Arch Gen Psychiatry. 2001;58(3):221–7.
100. Keddie AM. Associations between severe obesity and depression: results from the National Health and Nutrition Examination Survey, 2005–2006. Prev Chronic Dis. 2011;8(3). http://www.cdc.gov/pcd/issues/2011/may/10_0151.htm. Accessed 10 May 2011.
101. Luppino FS, de Wit LM, Bouvy PF, et al. Overweight, obesity, and depression: a systematic review and meta-analysis of longitudinal studies. Arch Gen Psychiatry. 2010;67(3):220–9.
102. Taylor VH, MacQueen GM. The role of adipokines in understanding the associations between obesity and depression. J Obes. 2010. doi:10.1155/2010/748048

103. Talley NJ. Definitions, epidemiology, and impact of chronic constipation. Rev Gastroenterol Disord. 2004;4 Suppl 2:S3–10.
104. John BJ, Abulafi AM, Poullis A, Mendall MA. Chronic subclinical bowel inflammation may explain increased risk of colorectal cancer in obese people. Gut. 2007;56(7):1034–5.
105. Barbu C, Iordache M, Man MG. Inflammation in COPD: pathogenesis, local and systemic effects. Rom J Morphol Embryol. 2011;52(1):21–7.
106. Schunemann HJ, Dorn J, Grant BJ, et al. Pulmonary function is a long-term predictor of mortality in the general population: 29-year follow-up of the Buffalo Health Study. Chest. 2000;118:656–64.
107. Bang KM, Gergen PJ, Kramer R, et al. The effect of pulmonary impairment on all-cause mortality in a national cohort. Chest. 1993;103:536–40.
108. Engstrom G, Lind P, Hedblad B, et al. Lung function and cardiovascular risk: relationship with inflammation-sensitive plasma proteins. Circulation. 2002;106(20):2555–60.
109. Ross R. Atherosclerosis: an inflammatory disease. N Engl J Med. 1999;340:115–26.
110. Hashimoto H, Kitagawa K, Hougaku H, et al. C-reactive protein is an independent predictor of the rate of increase in early carotid atherosclerosis. Circulation. 2001;104(1):63–7.
111. Koenig W, Sund M, Frohlich M, et al. C-reactive protein, a sensitive marker of inflammation, predicts future risk of coronary heart disease in initially healthy middle-aged men: results from the MONICA (Monitoring Trends and Determinants in Cardiovascular Disease) Augsburg Cohort Study, 1984 to 1992. Circulation. 1999;99:237–42.
112. Sin DD, Man SF. Why are patients with chronic obstructive pulmonary disease at increased risk of cardiovascular diseases? The potential role of systemic inflammation in chronic obstructive pulmonary disease. Circulation. 2003;107:1514–19.
113. Sin DD, Man SF. Systemic inflammation and mortality in chronic obstructive pulmonary disease. Can J Physiol Pharmacol. 2007;85:141–7.
114. Mannino DM. Epidemiology and global impact of chronic obstructive pulmonary disease. Semin Respir Crit Care Med. 2005;26:204–10.
115. Punturieri A, Szabo E, Croxton TL, Shapiro SD, Dubinett SM. Lung cancer and chronic obstructive pulmonary disease: needs and opportunities for integrated research. J Natl Cancer Inst. 2009;101:554–9.
116. Hogg JC, Chu F, Utokaparch S, et al. The nature of small-airway obstruction in chronic obstructive pulmonary disease. N Engl J Med. 2004;350:2645–53.
117. Hogg JC. Pathophysiology of airflow limitation in chronic obstructive pulmonary disease. Lancet. 2004;364:709–21.
118. O'Donnell RA, Richter A, Ward J, et al. Expression of ErbB receptors and mucins in the airways of long-term current smokers. Thorax. 2004;59:1032–40.
119. Kurie JM, Shin HJ, Lee JS, et al. Increased epidermal growth factor receptor expression in metaplastic bronchial epithelium. Clin Cancer Res. 1996;2: 1787–93.
120. Franklin WA, Veve R, Hirsch FR, Helfrich BA, Bunn Jr PA. Epidermal growth factor receptor family in lung cancer and premalignancy. Semin Oncol. 2002;29:3–14.
121. Karin M. NF-kappaB as a critical link between inflammation and cancer. Cold Spring Harb Perspect Biol. 2009;1(5):a000141.
122. Hayashi Y, Senjyu H, Iguchi A, et al. Prevalence of depressive symptoms in Japanese male patients with chronic obstructive pulmonary disease. Psychiatry Clin Neurosci. 2011;65(1):82–8.
123. Al-shair K, Kolsum U, Dockry R, Morris J, Singh D, Vestbo J. Biomarkers of systemic inflammation and depression and fatigue in moderate clinically stable COPD. Respir Res. 2011;12:3.
124. Barnes PJ, Celli BR. Systemic manifestations and comorbidities of COPD. Eur Respir J. 2009;33(5): 1165–85.
125. Al-Herz A, Ensworth S, Shojania K, Esdaile JM. Cardiovascular risk factor screening in systemic lupus erythematosus. J Rheumatol. 2003;30(3): 493–6.
126. Petri M. Detection of coronary artery disease and the role of traditional risk factors in the Hopkins Lupus Cohort. Lupus. 2000;9(3):170–5.
127. Lyon CJ, Law RE, Hsueh WA. Minireview: adiposity, inflammation, and atherogenesis. Endocrinology. 2003;144(6):2195–200.
128. Bautista LE, Vera LM, Arenas IA, Gamarra G. Independent association between inflammatory markers (C-reactive protein, interleukin-6, and TNF-alpha) and essential hypertension. J Hum Hypertens. 2005;19(2):149–54.
129. Vázquez-Oliva G, Fernández-Real JM, Zamora A, Vilaseca M, Badimón L. Lowering of blood pressure leads to decreased circulating interleukin-6 in hypertensive subjects. J Hum Hypertens. 2005;19(6): 457–62.
130. Frasure-Smith N, Lespérance F, Irwin MR, Talajic M, Pollock BG. The relationships among heart rate variability, inflammatory markers and depression in coronary heart disease patients. Brain Behav Immun. 2009;23(8):1140–7.
131. Dyer AR, Stamler J, Berkson DM, Lindberg HA, Stevens E. High blood-pressure: a risk factor for cancer mortality? Lancet. 1975;1:1051–6.
132. Raynor Jr WR, Shekelle RB, Rossof AH, Maliza C, Paul O. High blood pressure and 17-year cancer mortality in the Western Electric Health Study. Am J Epidemiol. 1981;113:371–7.
133. Buck C, Donner A. Cancer incidence in hypertensives. Cancer. 1987;59:1386–90.
134. Chow WH, Gridley G, Fraumeni JF, Jarvholm B. Obesity, hypertension, and the risk of kidney cancer in men. N Engl J Med. 2000;343:1305–11.
135. Grossman E, Messerli FH, Boyko V, Goldbourt U. Is there an association between hypertension and cancer mortality? Am J Med. 2002;112:479–86.
136. Ohira T. Psychological distress and cardiovascular disease: the Circulatory Risk in Communities Study (CIRCS). J Epidemiol. 2010;20(3):185–91.

137. Malan L, Schutte AE, Malan NT, et al. Specific coping strategies of Africans during urbanization: comparing cardiovascular responses and perception of health data. Biol Psychol. 2006;72(3):305–10.
138. Reid JL, Morton DJ, Wingard DL, Garrett MD, von Muhlen D, Slymen D. Obesity and other cardiovascular disease risk factors and their association with osteoarthritis in Southern California American Indians, 2002–2006. Ethn Dis. 2010;20(4):416–22.
139. Heard E, Whitfield KE, Edwards CL, Bruce MA, Beech BM. Mediating effects of social support on the relationship among perceived stress, depression, and hypertension in African Americans. J Natl Med Assoc. 2011;103(2):116–22.
140. Mashele N, Van Rooyen JM, Malan L, Potgieter JC. Cardiovascular function and psychological distress in urbanised black South Africans: the SABPA study. Cardiovasc J Afr. 2010;21(4):206–11.
141. Roger VL, Go AS, Lloyd-Jones DM, et al. Heart disease and stroke statistics–2011 update: a report from the American Heart Association. Circulation. 2011;123(4):e18–209.
142. Albert CM, Ma J, Rifai N, et al. Prospective study of C-reactive protein, homocysteine, and plasma lipid levels as predictors of sudden cardiac death. Circulation. 2002;105:2595–9.
143. Willerson JT, Ridker PM. Inflammation as a cardiovascular risk factors. Circulation. 2004;109:II2–110.
144. Libby P, Ridker PM. Novel inflammatory markers of coronary risk. Theory versus practice. Circulation. 1999;100:1148–50.
145. Amer MS, Elawam AE, Khater MS, Omar OH, Mabrouk RA, Taha HM. Association of high-sensitivity C-reactive protein with carotid artery intima-media thickness in hypertensive older adults. J Am Soc Hypertens. 2011;5(5):395–400.
146. Little PJ, Chait A, Bobik A. Cellular and cytokine-based inflammatory processes as novel therapeutic targets for the prevention and treatment of atherosclerosis. Pharmacol Ther. 2011;131(3):255–68.
147. Ridker PM, Cushman M, Stampfer MJ, Tracy RP, Hennekens CH. Inflammation, aspirin, and risks of cardiovascular disease in apparently healthy men. N Engl J Med. 1997;336:973–9.
148. Ridker PM, Glynn RJ, Hennekens CH. C-reactive protein adds to the predictive value of total and HDL cholesterol in determining risk of first myocardial infarction. Circulation. 1998;97:2007–11.
149. Pasceri P, Willerson JT, Yeh ET. Direct proinflammatory effect of C-reactive protein on human endothelial cells. Circulation. 2000;102: 2165–8.
150. Sakkinen P, Abbott RD, Curb JD, et al. C-reactive protein and myocardial infarction. J Clin Epidemiol. 2002;55:445–51.
151. Willerson JT. Systemic and local inflammation in patients with unstable atherosclerotic plaques. Prog Cardiovasc Dis. 2002;44:469–78.
152. Frasure-Smith N, Lespérance F, Talajic M. Depression following myocardial infarction: impact on 6-month survival. JAMA. 1993;270(15):1819–25.
153. Welin C, Lappas G, Wilhelmsen L. Independent importance of psychosocial factors for prognosis after myocardial infarction. J Intern Med. 2000;247(6):629–39.
154. Barth J, Schumacher M, Herrmann-Lingen C. Depression as a risk factor for mortality in patients with coronary heart disease: a meta-analysis. Psychosom Med. 2004;66(6):802–13.
155. Rugulies R. Depression as a predictor for coronary heart disease. a review and meta-analysis. Am J Prev Med. 2002;23(1):51–61.
156. Appels A, Bär FW, Bär J, Bruggeman C, de Baets M. Inflammation, depressive symptomtology, and coronary artery disease. Psychosom Med. 2000;62(5):601–5.
157. Norman GJ, Zhang N, Morris JS, Karelina K, Berntson GG, DeVries AC. Social interaction modulates autonomic, inflammatory, and depressive-like responses to cardiac arrest and cardiopulmonary resuscitation. Proc Natl Acad Sci U S A. 2010;107(37):16342–7.
158. Thornton LM, Andersen BL, Schuler TA, Carson 3rd WE. A psychological intervention reduces inflammatory markers by alleviating depressive symptoms: secondary analysis of a randomized controlled trial. Psychosom Med. 2009;71(7):715–24.
159. Doering LV, Cross R, Vredevoe D, Martinez-Maza O, Cowan MJ. Infection, depression, and immunity in women after coronary artery bypass: a pilot study of cognitive behavioral therapy. Altern Ther Health Med. 2007;13(3):18–21.
160. Yu B, Becnel J, Zerfaoui M, Rohatgi R, Boulares AH, Nichols CD. Serotonin 5-hydroxytryptamine(2A) receptor activation suppresses tumor necrosis factor-alpha-induced inflammation with extraordinary potency. J Pharmacol Exp Ther. 2008;327(2):316–23.
161. Tuglu C, Kara SH, Caliyurt O, Vardar E, Abay E. Increased serum tumor necrosis factor-alpha levels and treatment response in major depressive disorder. Psychopharmacology (Berl). 2003;170(4):429–33.
162. Basterzi AD, Aydemir C, Kisa C, et al. IL-6 levels decrease with SSRI treatment in patients with major depression. Hum Psychopharmacol. 2005;20(7):473–6.
163. Leo R, Di Lorenzo G, Tesauro M, et al. Association between enhanced soluble CD40 ligand and proinflammatory and prothrombotic states in major depressive disorder: pilot observations on the effects of selective serotonin reuptake inhibitor therapy. J Clin Psychiatry. 2006;67(11):1760–6.
164. Kubera M, Maes M, Kenis G, Kim YK, Lasoń W. Effects of serotonin and serotonergic agonists and antagonists on the production of tumor necrosis factor alpha and interleukin-6. Psychiatry Res. 2005; 134(3):251–8.
165. Smedley BD, Stith AY, Nelson AR. Unequal treatment: confronting racial and ethnic disparities in health care. Washington, DC: The National Academies Press; 2002.
166. Ward E, Jemal A, Cokkinides V, et al. Cancer disparities by race/ethnicity and socioeconomic status. CA Cancer J Clin. 2004;54(2):78–93.

167. Roberts CB, Vines AI, Kaufman JS, James SA. Cross-sectional association between perceived discrimination and hypertension in African-American men and women: the pitt county study. Am J Epidemiol. 2008;167:624–32.

168. Lewis TT, Barnes LL, Bienias JL, Lackland DT, Evans DA, Mendes de Leon CF. Perceived discrimination and blood pressure in older African American and White adults. J Gerontol A Biol Sci Med Sci. 2009;64A:1002–8.

169. Lewis TT, Aiello AE, Leurgans S, Kelly J, Barnes LL. Self-reported experiences of everyday discrimination are associated with elevated C-reactive protein levels in older African-American adults. Brain Behav Immun. 2010;24(3):438–43.

Psychological Aspects of Hereditary Cancer Risk Counseling and Genetic Testing

3

Lisa G. Aspinwall, Jennifer M. Taber,
Wendy Kohlmann, and Sancy A. Leachman

Cancer is a common disease with many underlying etiologies. Most cancers are sporadic occurrences related to aging, environmental exposures or the interactions of low-penetrance genes. However, approximately 5% of cancers occur due to an inherited cancer predisposition syndrome [1]. Families with hereditary cancer syndromes are generally characterized by multiple occurrences of cancer on the same side of the family, individuals with multiple primary cancers, and an earlier than average age of cancer onset.

Hereditary cancer risk counseling (HCRC) is the process of identifying families at risk for hereditary cancer syndromes with the ultimate goal of minimizing cancer-related morbidity and mortality. This is typically achieved when members of families known to have a hereditary cancer syndrome are recommended to engage in earlier and more frequent screening and other risk-reducing strategies. In addition to improved medical management, HCRC and genetic testing are intended to have important psychological

benefits, such as reducing uncertainty about cancer risk, increasing perceived control over cancer risk, and providing information about children's cancer risk [2–4].

The purpose of this chapter is to describe the major elements of hereditary cancer risk counseling and to review both behavioral and psychological antecedents and outcomes of genetic counseling and test reporting for such cancer syndromes as hereditary breast and ovarian cancer (HBOC) and hereditary colon cancer (Lynch syndrome and FAP). We will examine potential moderators of these effects, including recent efforts to understand multiple trajectories of psychological outcomes following counseling and testing, and their implications for both research design and clinical application. It is important to note that this chapter is not intended to present an exhaustive review, but instead a selective consideration of research on the major cancer syndromes for which genetic counseling and testing have been extensively studied. We also highlight newer areas of inquiry, such as genetic testing for hereditary melanoma. Throughout this chapter, we will examine ways in which hereditary cancer risk counseling and genetic testing may be seen as powerful tools that may be used in an ongoing effort to manage hereditary cancer risk, rather than as isolated or new stressors. Consistent with this view, we present a model that integrates new research on the antecedents and consequences of hereditary cancer risk counseling and genetic testing with an analysis of the key elements of different cancer syndromes and their management.

L.G. Aspinwall, Ph.D. (✉) • J.M. Taber, M.S.
Department of Psychology, University of Utah,
380 South 1530 East, Room 502, Salt Lake City,
UT 84112, USA
e-mail: lisa.aspinwall@psych.utah.edu

W. Kohlmann, M.S., CGC
High Risk Cancer Clinics, Huntsman Cancer Institute,
University of Utah, Salt Lake City, UT 84112, USA

S.A. Leachman, M.D., Ph.D.
Department of Dermatology, Huntsman Cancer Institute,
University of Utah, Salt Lake City, UT 84112, USA

B.I. Carr and J. Steel (eds.), *Psychological Aspects of Cancer*,
DOI 10.1007/978-1-4614-4866-2_3, © Springer Science+Business Media, LLC 2013

We conclude with a discussion of methodological issues involving participant recruitment, self-selection into testing and research participation, and underrepresentation of ethnic minority respondents. These issues may inform the interpretation of results to date concerning psychological outcomes and may also guide the design of future studies.

Components of Hereditary Cancer Risk Counseling

Table 3.1 outlines the essential components of hereditary cancer risk counseling. The recommendations outlined by the National Society of Genetic Counselors and the American Society of Clinical Oncology for providing hereditary cancer risk counseling have served as the basis for clinical practice, as well as many research studies [5, 6]. As shown in Table 3.1, these recommendations specifically include educating patients about their cancer risk, reviewing basic genetics and inheritance patterns and management options, and exploring the psychological implications of this information for the individual and his or her family.

During HCRC, a genetic counselor conducts a detailed review of the medical and family history in order to evaluate whether a hereditary cancer syndrome may have caused the clustering of cancers reported in a family. In addition to reviewing the medical facts of the cancer history (i.e., etiology, treatment), this initial intake is also an opportune time to determine the patient's motivations for seeking additional information, his or her perceived risk, current attitudes towards and access to cancer screening services, and sources of social support. Assessment of psychological status, access to health care, and support resources helps providers to anticipate patients' potential reactions to cancer risk information and identify those who may be at risk for negative emotional outcomes or those in need of additional resources to access recommended management procedures.

As shown in Table 3.1, hereditary cancer risk counseling includes the assessment and provision of detailed risk information, including personal risk for developing cancer, likelihood of harboring a genetic mutation, and risks for other family members. In addition, patients are informed of the options available for managing their cancer risk, and the effectiveness of these approaches for reducing cancer or ensuring detection of cancer at an earlier, more treatable stage. Table 3.2 summarizes the general population prevalence, causative gene or genes, lifetime cancer risks (often for multiple cancers), and management recommendations for each of the major hereditary cancer syndromes. Of the more than 50 hereditary cancer syndromes that have been identified [7], hereditary breast and ovarian cancer (HBOC) and Lynch syndrome (formerly referred to as hereditary nonpolyposis colorectal cancer, HNPCC) are the two most common and well-studied conditions.

Hereditary cancer risk counseling is recommended prior to having genetic testing in order for the patient to be able to give informed consent for the testing [6]. As shown in Table 3.1, the process of obtaining informed consent during HCRC includes discussion of the reason that the test is being offered; possible results from testing (e.g., positive, negative or a variant of uncertain significance); options for estimating cancer risk if testing is declined; implications of test results for family members; accuracy of the test; cost of the test; possibility of negative psychological outcomes such as increased depression, anxiety or guilt; the possibility of insurance discrimination; and management options [6]. Discussion of these topics allows the patient to weigh the pros and cons of deciding for or against genetic testing.

Ideally, genetic testing is performed first in a family member with a personal history of the type of cancer for which the family is being evaluated. Throughout this review, we refer to family members with a history of the particular hereditary cancer as *affected* family members and to those without a personal history as *unaffected* family members. Further, family members who test positive for a mutation are often referred to as *carriers* in this review, and individuals testing negative for a family mutation are often referred to as *noncarriers*. Beginning the testing with an

Table 3.1 Components of hereditary cancer risk counseling

Component	Description
Review of patient history	A detailed review of the patients' personal and family history is needed to distinguish between familial clusters of cancer due to sporadic occurrence, shared environmental/lifestyle factors, or low-penetrance genes compared to those families that may have a hereditary cancer syndrome. Ideally, medical records, particularly pathology reports, are obtained to confirm reported cancers in the family.
Psychological assessment	Evaluation of psychosocial factors will allow the clinician to understand the patient's motivation for seeking cancer risk assessment and level of understanding of medical information, and to anticipate whether cancer risk assessment may lead to negative psychological consequences. Psychological assessment includes evaluation of the following: • Motivations for seeking counseling, such as planning medical management, determining risk for family members, and/or relief from uncertainty • Beliefs about the cause(s) of cancer and their estimated cancer risk • Cultural and familial beliefs about cancer and its inheritance • Socioeconomic factors such as health insurance status and concerns about potential discrimination • Potential psychological responses to cancer risk information • Attitudes about efficacy of screening and risk-reducing options • Coping resources that the patient may utilize
Cancer risk assessment	Cancer risk estimates can be made based on personal and family history information, computer-based models (e.g., Gail model, CancerGene), and from the results of genetic testing. During hereditary cancer risk counseling, several different types of risk information may be presented: • Risk for developing particular types of cancer • Risk of harboring a genetic mutation that may cause an increased cancer risk • Risk of passing a genetic mutation on to family members • How risk may be modified by certain behavioral, screening or surgical approaches

Pre-genetic testing	When appropriate based on personal and family history, genetic testing may be offered to the patient. Prior to genetic testing, the following should be discussed:
	• Purpose of the genetic test
	• Implications of a positive, negative and variation of uncertain significance (VUS) result
	  • How results may affect management
	  • Implications for family members' cancer risk
	  • Possibility of health or life insurance discrimination
	  • Potential psychological responses, such as increased distress, cancer worry, or survivor guilt
	• Likelihood that a mutation will be identified based on the strength of the pattern of cancer in the family and sensitivity of the testing technology
	• Accuracy of the test
	• Cost of the test

Post-genetic testing	When genetic testing is pursued, disclosure of genetic test results also includes a discussion of the following: • Impact of the result on cancer risk • Implications for screening and management • The need to inform other relatives about the outcome of genetic testing, implications of their risk and the options available to them • Prevention and testing options for minors (as applicable)
Surveillance/treatment/ follow-up	Individuals should receive screening, prevention and treatment options that are tailored based on their test result, family history, and personal medical history. They will need to be scheduled for appropriate interventions, and offered referrals to appropriate resources and screening interventions (e.g., other medical specialists, support groups, online resources). Hereditary cancer syndromes typically affect cancer risk throughout the lifespan and ongoing screening and follow-up are usually necessary.

affected person maximizes the likelihood of detecting the causative mutation if there is one present in the family. Testing the first person in the family involves comprehensive analysis of the gene or genes associated with the syndrome in order to try to identify a mutation. This testing often costs $1,000–$2,000 per gene being analyzed. There are three possible outcomes from genetic testing: positive, negative, and variant of uncertain significance. A positive result means that a deleterious mutation was identified. This result confirms the diagnosis of a hereditary cancer syndrome in the individual and provides a likely explanation for the increased number of cancers seen in the individual's family. Other relatives, including unaffected family members, can then be tested for the specific mutation previously identified at a much reduced cost (typically $300–$475). The purpose of this testing is to determine if they have inherited the familial mutation and are also at an increased risk for the cancers associated with the hereditary syndrome. If they have not inherited the mutation, unaffected family members could be spared from unnecessary anxiety and screening procedures.

A negative result in the initial individual being evaluated means that no mutation was identified; however, this result cannot rule out the possibility of a hereditary predisposition to cancer in the family. Because current technologies may miss some types of mutations and there may be other hereditary causes of cancer risk yet to be identified, families with strong cancer histories should be counseled that a negative result indicates that the cause of the cancer in their family remains unknown and that screening to promote early detection is still recommended. Because no definitive explanation of the cause of the cancer risk in the family is provided, this type of result is often referred to as "uninformative" in this review.

A third possible outcome from genetic testing is finding a variant of uncertain significance (VUS). This is a result in which a genetic alteration is identified, but there are not sufficient data to determine whether this alteration is associated with cancer or if it is simply a benign alteration due to normal human genetic variation. While

variants of uncertain significance are often eventually reclassified as deleterious mutations or as normal results as additional research is conducted, the initial disclosure of a VUS can be frustrating and confusing for the patient. Furthermore, prior to reclassification, this result should not be used to guide medical management.

Behavioral Outcomes of Cancer Genetic Counseling and Testing

Table 3.2 summarizes the management recommendations for each of the major cancer syndromes we will review in this chapter. In the following sections, we review major behavioral outcomes of cancer genetic testing, including more frequent screening and uptake of prophylactic surgery (as applicable). We also highlight the potential of genetic counseling for hereditary melanoma to promote potentially life-saving improvements in both screening and primary prevention behaviors in high-risk individuals.

Hereditary Breast and Ovarian Cancer

As shown in Table 3.2, female *BRCA1/2* mutation carriers are advised to have careful breast surveillance with monthly self-breast exams, biannual clinical breast exams, and breast imaging beginning at age 25 or to consider prophylactic mastectomy. Prophylactic removal of the ovaries and fallopian tubes (prophylactic oophorectomy) is recommended between 35 and 40 years of age. Prophylactic mastectomy is associated with a 90% reduction in breast cancer risk, and oophorectomy is associated with an 85–90% reduction in ovarian cancer risk and a 50% reduction in breast cancer risk if performed before the onset of menopause [8, 9]. While risk-reducing mastectomy significantly reduces the risk for developing breast cancer, the survival benefit in choosing risk-reducing mastectomy over annual breast screening is small. Thus, either screening or surgery is considered an appropriate course of management, and women choosing either

Table 3.2 Features of common hereditary cancer syndromes and corresponding management recommendations

Condition	Genes	Population prevalence of gene mutations	Inheritance	Lifetime cancer risks		Management recommendations
Hereditary breast/ovarian cancer (HBOC)	BRCA1 BRCA2	1/400	Autosomal Dominant	*BRCA1* Breast Ovarian *BRCA2* Breast Ovarian	50–80% 40% 50–80% 10–20%	Breast • Annual mammogram and breast MRI beginning at age 25 • Consideration of prophylactic mastectomy Ovarian • Prophylactic removal of the ovaries and fallopian tubes between 35 and 40 years of age
Lynch syndrome (previously known as Hereditary Nonpolyposis Colorectal Cancer [HNPCC])	MLH1 MSH2 MSH6 PMS2	1/400	Autosomal Dominant	Colon Endometrium Stomach Ovary Urinary tract Small bowel Brain	50–80% 25–60% 6–13% 4–12% 1–4% 3–6% 1–3%	Colon • Colonoscopy every 1–2 years beginning at age 25 Endometrium • Consider prophylactic hysterectomy after completion of childbearing Other • Upper endoscopy examinations every 1–3 years beginning at age 30 • Annual urine cytology
Familial adenomatous polyposis (FAP)	APC	1/3,000	Autosomal Dominant	Colon Duodenum Pancreas Thyroid	Approaches 100% without prophylactic removal of the colon 4–12% 2% 1–2%	Colon • Colonoscopy beginning at age 10 • Colectomy when polyps become too numerous to monitor Duodenum • Upper endoscopy exams every 1–3 years beginning at age 25 Thyroid • Annual physical exam of the thyroid
Hereditary melanoma	CDKN2A (also called *p16*)	1/2,500	Autosomal Dominant	Melanoma Pancreatic	67% 17%	Skin • Dermatology exams every 6–12 months beginning at age 10–12 • Monthly skin self-exams • Minimize UVR exposure Pancreas • Pancreatic cancer screening is still considered investigational. Options include endoscopic ultrasound and MRI.

(continued)

Table 3.2 (continued)

Condition	Genes	Population prevalence of gene mutations	Inheritance	Lifetime cancer risks	Management recommendations
Li–Fraumeni syndrome (LFS)	*p53*	1/20,000	Autosomal Dominant	50% risk for developing cancer by age 30, and a 90% lifetime cancer risk. Common LFS-related cancers include the following: • Breast • Soft tissue and osteosarcomas • Brain tumors • Adrenocortical tumors • Gastrointestinal cancers	Breast • Clinical breast exams every 6–12 months beginning at age 20 • Annual mammograms and breast MRI beginning at age 20 Other • At this time there are limited data on the best screening approaches for other cancers. Brain MRI and total MRI are being considered as possible approaches
Von Hippel–Lindau	*VHL*	1/40,000	Autosomal Dominant	High risk for developing many different benign and malignant tumors including: • Retinal angiomas • Cerebellar and spinal hemangioblastomas • Renal carcinoma • Pheochromocytoma • Pancreatic tumors	Eye • Annual eye exams beginning in infancy Brain/spine • MRI of brain and spine every 2 years beginning in adolescence Abdominal tumors • MRI of the abdomen every 2 years beginning in adolescence • Annual blood work

approach can be considered adherent [10]. In contrast, because no effective screening for ovarian cancer currently exists, there is a significant survival benefit in choosing oophorectomy.

Mammography. Typically, mammography rates increase among *BRCA1/2* mutation carriers following counseling and testing [11]. A review of nine studies found that 59–92% of carriers received a mammogram in the year following testing, while only 30–53% of noncarriers did so in the same time frame [11]. Only two of these studies showed increased mammography rates among noncarriers. In an early prospective study by Lerman and colleagues [12], over half of the participants had a mammogram in the year prior to testing (68% of 84 carriers, 55% of 83 noncarriers, and 67% of 49 test decliners). One year following testing, rates decreased to 44% for noncarriers and 54% for decliners, but remained stable among carriers (68%). However, because noncarriers were advised to undergo mammograms every 1–2 years between ages 40 and 49 and annually starting at age 50, noncarriers' mammography rates varied by age such that 70% of noncarrier women 50 and older had received a mammogram within the 1-year time frame. Interestingly, 30% of noncarrier women under age 40 also received a mammogram, despite the lack of a physician recommendation. In a large prospective study, carriers ($n = 91$) and noncarriers ($n = 170$) reported equivalent rates of mammography at baseline. However, after 1 year significantly more carriers (92%) than noncarriers (30%) had received a mammogram [13], with 100% of carriers over 50 having received a mammogram and only 41% of noncarriers over 50 having received one, despite a recommendation of annual mammograms for all women over 50 regardless of risk. Thus, rates of mammography are consistently higher for carriers and for older women. These age-related compliance issues may be due in part to variable recommendations for mammography screening for women at general population breast cancer risk.

Breast self-examination and clinical breast examination. Although some studies report prospective increases in the performance of breast self-examination among mutation carriers [14], rates of clinical and self breast examinations are generally high prior to testing and remain high among both carriers (upwards of 90%) and noncarriers (77–89%) following testing ([11]; see also [13]).

Ovarian cancer screening. Even though ovarian cancer screening has not been shown to be effective, carriers are more likely to undergo both transvaginal ultrasound and CA-125 than noncarriers [15]. Rates of CA-125 screening ranged from 21 to 32% in carriers and 5–6% in noncarriers, and rates of transvaginal ultrasound ranged from 15 to 59% among carriers and 5–8% among noncarriers [11]. Three years following testing, 75% of *BRCA1/2* mutation carriers in one study had at least one transvaginal ultrasound [16].

Prophylactic mastectomy. Uptake of risk-reducing mastectomy has increased over time, with early studies showing an uptake of 0–15% among unaffected mutation carriers and more recent studies reporting rates of 20–37% (see [17] for review). A review of eight studies found that rates of prophylactic mastectomy among carriers ranged from 0 to 51% in the year post-testing [11]. A study that followed 374 women who had *BRCA1/2* mutation testing for an average of 5 years found that 37% of carriers underwent mastectomy following testing, as did a small proportion of participants with uninformative results (6.8%) [17]. As expected, no noncarriers in this study underwent mastectomy. In this study, an additional 24 carriers had risk-reducing mastectomy (potentially in conjunction with treatment of a breast cancer) prior to undergoing genetic counseling and testing. Therefore, 47% of carriers overall had undergone risk-reducing mastectomy either before or after testing.

Several factors have characterized individuals who choose to undergo mastectomy. First, carriers with cancer are typically more likely to undergo mastectomy than unaffected carriers [15] because of the role of mastectomy in breast cancer treatment. Second, rates of mastectomy following *BRCA1/2* genetic testing may be higher in countries other than the USA, where concerns about financial and insurance discrimination are lower [15]. Older women (but see [17]) and women with children are more likely to undergo mastectomy due to lower concern about consequences that may influence reproductive decisions [15, 16]. Additionally, women who had had their ovaries removed and for whom it had been greater than 10 years since their cancer diagnosis were less likely to elect mastectomy [17]. The authors suggest that women who undergo oophorectomy prior to menopause reduce their breast cancer risk significantly, which reduces the overall benefit of a mastectomy.

Prophylactic oophorectomy. Uptake of oophorectomy is often higher than mastectomy uptake, 13–65% [11], because there are strong recommendations for removal of the ovaries and fallopian tubes as no effective screening approach for ovarian cancer is available [10]. One study of 91 *BRCA1/2* mutation carriers found that women who underwent oophorectomy were more likely to have had children than those who did not and were somewhat older; no women without children underwent oophorectomy [13]. Of note, some high-risk women undergo prophylactic surgery due to their familial history prior to the identification of a genetic mutation. Once a genetic mutation is identified, some of these women will subsequently test negative for the mutation (53% of 80 women who underwent prophylactic surgery in one study [14]). Therefore, hereditary cancer risk counseling is not only beneficial for identifying those at high risk, but also for identifying noncarriers who have not inherited the causative mutation and can be spared unnecessary procedures.

Changes in other health behaviors. There are limited data on changes in other cancer-relevant health behaviors. Watson et al. [13] assessed health behavior changes following *BRCA1/2* genetic testing, and found that 52% of female carriers, 43% of female noncarriers, 44% of male carriers, and 44% of male noncarriers reported having done something else to help them stay healthy and/or avoid cancer. Specifically, for both carriers and noncarriers, approximately 30% reported changes in diet, approximately 15% reported increased exercise, and around 5–10% reported smoking cessation. Thus, these findings suggest that hereditary cancer risk counseling and genetic testing may motivate improvements in cancer-relevant health behaviors among both carriers and noncarriers.

Patients receiving test results that are uninformative or indicate a variant of uncertain significance. It is important to note that the reviews we have described thus far did not generally assess behavioral outcomes among individuals who received uninformative results. Such women have family histories of breast and/or ovarian cancer, but either no identifiable mutation or a variant of uncertain significance. For these individuals, counselors derive empiric risk estimates from an individual's personal and family history which are used to determine management recommendations. Schwartz et al. [17] examined the rate of prophylactic surgery in women who received uninformative *BRCA1/2* test results. They found that 6.8% and 13.3% had risk-reducing mastectomy and oophorectomy, respectively, after receiving an uninformative test result. The mastectomies consisted of prophylactic removal of the contralateral breast in women who already had breast cancer, which may have been an appropriate option for them to consider despite the uninformative test result due to early age of onset or family history. Rates of mammography screening among affected women who had remaining breast tissue did not differ significantly between women receiving positive versus uninformative results (92% vs. 89%). However, women with *BRCA1/2* mutations were much more likely to have breast MRI than those with uninformative results (51% vs. 27%) [17].

Hereditary Colon Cancer

Lynch syndrome (previously known as hereditary nonpolyposis colorectal cancer, or HNPCC) and familial adenomatous polyposis (FAP) are the two most common causes of hereditary colorectal cancer. As shown in Table 3.2, Lynch syndrome is associated with an increased risk for multiple cancers, especially colorectal and endometrial cancer [18]. Individuals with mutations in the Lynch syndrome genes are recommended to begin annual screening at age 25. Individuals with Lynch syndrome who have a colonoscopy every 1–2 years have substantially reduced mortality [19], though the effectiveness of approaches for screening for other Lynch-related cancers is less well established [20].

FAP is characterized by the development of numerous precancerous colonic polyps, and without surgery to remove the colon, the risk for progression of these polyps to colorectal cancer approaches 100%. As shown in Table 3.2, individuals with FAP are also at increased risk for developing cancers in the beginning of the small intestine (duodenum), stomach, and thyroid. Other rare manifestations of FAP include the development of fibrous tumors called desmoids. While benign, these tumors can grow aggressively and be associated with significant morbidity and mortality. Infants and young children are also at increased risk for developing hepatoblastoma, a rare form of liver cancer. Unlike most hereditary cancer syndromes which present in adulthood, FAP is associated with a risk for cancer early in life, and genetic testing is recommended for at-risk children by age 10 [18]. Individuals with FAP are recommended to begin having colonoscopies at age 10 and to have prophylactic colectomy when the polyps become too numerous to manage endoscopically. Removal of the colon rarely requires a colostomy because usually the rectum can be left intact or an internal pouch can be formed from the distal end of the small intestine (ileoanal pouch). Annual surveillance of the rectum or ileoanal pouch is still necessary. Upper endoscopy exams beginning between 20 and 25 years of age are also recommended to monitor polyp development in the stomach and duodenum.

Colonoscopy. A review of multiple studies found that between 58 and 100% of Lynch syndrome mutation carriers underwent colonoscopy in the 2 years following testing, compared to only 0–40.5% of noncarriers ([11]; see also [15, 21]). These rates are consistent with recommendations made to carriers and noncarriers, respectively. These numbers represented increases from baseline for carriers in five out of six studies reviewed. In one study, rates of colonoscopy among 22 carriers, 49 noncarriers, and 27 test decliners ranged from 6 to 36% pretesting and did not differ among groups. Following genetic testing, colonoscopy rates among carriers increased from 36 to 73% 1 year following testing, but were much lower and unchanged from baseline among both noncarriers (16%) and those who declined testing (22%) [22]. In this study, respondents (regardless of mutation status) who at 1 month following testing reported at least a moderate amount of control over developing colon cancer were more likely to undergo colonoscopy than those who reported little or no control. Stoffel [21] found that both having a close relative with early-onset colorectal cancer and having had hereditary cancer risk counseling predicted adherence to colon cancer screening among individuals with Lynch syndrome.

Uptake of FAP testing and screening adherence. Douma et al. [23] reviewed all papers published between 1986 and 2007 (17 total) regarding behavioral and psychological outcomes in FAP. Uptake of testing was high, ranging from 62 to 97%, and adults undergoing testing indicated concerns about their own and their children's future health as primary motivating factors. FAP differs from hereditary breast/ovarian cancer and Lynch syndrome in that it is appropriate to test children. Prior genetic testing to identify the mutation in the family and provider recommendation were the most significant factors associated with parents electing to have their children undergo genetic testing for FAP. Lack of provider recommendation and cost were found to be significant barriers to the uptake of FAP genetic testing for minors [24].

There are limited data on screening outcomes after receiving a diagnosis of FAP [23]. Management of individuals with FAP is difficult for researchers to track in that it typically involves an initial evaluation to determine the extent of polyposis, a decision to proceed with prophylactic surgery, and then continued screening of remaining at-risk organs and tissues. Recommendations for patients vary considerably based on the extent of polyposis and whether and what type of surgery has been performed. One study of 150 members of FAP families [25] found that only 54% of individuals who had a diagnosis of FAP were compliant with management recommendations. Factors that predicted increased adherence to screening were having the diagnosis confirmed by the identification of a mutation, having insurance coverage, provider recommendation for screening, and perceiving a higher than average risk for colon cancer. Further, a 2002 study [26] found that 42% of noncarriers were not reassured by testing negative for the mutation that had caused FAP in the family and intended to continue screening. Similar lack of confidence in genetic results has not been reported with other syndromes. FAP differs from other hereditary cancer syndromes in that a clinical diagnosis can often be easily made by doing a colonoscopy to evaluate the presence or absence of polyps. Individuals with a family history of FAP may be interested in having a colonoscopy to confirm the results of genetic testing. Other syndromes are not associated with any type of easily evaluated, premalignant features, so FAP is the only syndrome with a readily available clinical option for validating test results.

Hereditary Melanoma

Genetic testing for hereditary melanoma is just entering clinical practice, with the first formal recommendation for its use published in 2009 [27]. Of all melanomas, 5–10% have a familial clustering, and 20–40% of these are associated with a pathogenic mutation in $CDKN2A/p16$ (or simply $p16$), a tumor suppressor that regulates cell cycle and senescence. As shown in Table 3.2, recommendations to $p16$ mutation carriers include not only monthly skin self-examinations (SSEs) and annual or semiannual professional total body skin examinations (TBSEs), but also recommen-

dations to minimize ultraviolet radiation (UVR) exposure. This recommendation stems from the finding that the penetrance of $p16$ mutations shows striking geographic variation which correlates with regional levels of UVR intensity, ranging from 58% in the UK to 76% in the USA and 91% in Australia [28]. Thus, members of high-risk families are counseled to avoid UVR exposure, to wear sunscreen of at least SPF 30, and to wear protective clothing. For this reason, the study of behavioral adherence among melanoma-prone families has the potential to elucidate how genetic counseling and testing may influence daily prevention behaviors.

Sun-protection behaviors. In general, in melanoma-prone families, family members with a history of melanoma report much greater adherence to prevention and screening recommendations than do family members who have yet to develop the disease (see [29] for review). For example, unaffected members of high-risk families have reported frequent sunbathing, tanning bed use, and sunburns [30, 31]. In our own prospective study of 60 adults (including 33 mutation carriers) from two large Utah $p16$ kindreds, unaffected carriers reported much less frequent use of sunscreen (30.7% of the time versus 55.6%), protective clothing (48.2% vs. 69.4%), and UVR avoidance (staying in the shade and avoiding peak exposure, 57.3% vs. 73.6%) than their affected counterparts, and were much less likely to indicate that these behaviors were part of their daily routine [29]. Genetic counseling and test reporting increased intentions to practice all three methods of photoprotection in the next 6 months, and a 1-month follow-up yielded evidence of a marginally significant increase in all three photoprotective behaviors. Additionally, more than one-third of unaffected carriers reported having adopted a new photoprotective behavior since receiving test results. Follow-up data at the 2-year mark suggested continued improvements in the use of photoprotective clothing, and significant increases in the degrees to which respondents reported that all three prevention behaviors (especially protective clothing use and UVR avoidance) were part of their daily routine [32].

Skin self-examinations. As was the case for sun-protection behaviors, pretesting adherence among unaffected family members was highly variable and frequently poor—nearly two-thirds reported conducting skin self-examinations less frequently than the recommendation of one per month [33]. At the 1-month follow-up, all unaffected carriers reported conducting one or more skin exams since the counseling session, and 54.6% of them reported either having adopted a new screening behavior or modifying their existing practice to be more frequent and/or more thorough. Of particular importance, the reported thoroughness of these exams also showed improvement. Participants were asked to complete a checklist of 11 body sites examined during SSE, ranging from scalp to bottoms of feet. At baseline, unaffected carriers averaged 5.46 body sites; at the 1-month follow-up, these reports had improved to an average of 8.82 body sites. Results from the 2-year follow-up indicated that these gains in thoroughness were sustained, resulting in SSEs that were nearly as thorough as those reported by affected family members [32].

Clinical total body skin examinations. We also examined the impact of genetic counseling and test reporting on intentions to receive a professional total body skin exam and on receipt of these exams at follow-up. Intentions to obtain TBSEs increased significantly in all groups immediately following counseling and test reporting. At the 2-year follow-up, dramatic improvement in the proportion of unaffected carriers receiving a TBSE in the past year was reported—from 21.4 to 66.7% [32]. Similarly high rates of TBSE adherence in the year following test reporting among *p16* mutation carriers have been reported by Kasparian et al. [34].

Therefore, although these findings await replication in a larger sample of members of high-risk families, they suggest that melanoma genetic testing is successful in promoting improvements in daily sun-protection behaviors, the frequency and thoroughness of monthly skin self-examinations, and compliance to recommendations regarding annual professional total body skin examinations. Furthermore, unaffected family members who received positive genetic test results reported levels of prevention and screening behavior that were comparable to the high level of adherence reported by family members with a melanoma history. These results suggest that melanoma genetic testing may successfully alert high-risk patients prior to disease onset, facilitating early detection and perhaps even prevention.

Pancreatic cancer screening. As shown in Table 3.2, it is important to note that *p16* mutations also confer an up to 17% lifetime risk of pancreatic cancer [35], and little is known about the impact of pancreatic cancer risk counseling on the uptake of screening recommendations. In contrast to melanoma, pancreatic cancer offers little prospect of successful prevention or early detection. Therefore, both the psychological and behavioral impact of this information remains an important future direction for research on *p16* counseling and testing (see [36] and [37] for discussion).

Psychological Outcomes of Cancer Genetic Counseling and Testing

As we have reviewed, evidence to date supports the idea that hereditary cancer risk counseling and testing promote potentially life-saving improvements in cancer screening and other recommended behaviors. Such tests also offer the potential psychological benefits of reducing uncertainty about cancer risk and providing useful health information for oneself and one's offspring [2–4]. However, since the advent of such testing, researchers have been concerned that these advances in personalized medicine may come with a psychological cost, namely inducing or exacerbating anxiety, depression, or cancer worry [38–40]. In the following sections, we will review what is known from both quantitative and qualitative research about negative and positive psychological outcomes of cancer genetic testing, describe multiple measures that have been designed to capture these outcomes, and present an emerging view that cancer genetic counseling and testing may be best conceptualized not as a new stressor with which people must cope, but rather as powerful tools to be used in an ongoing and often long-standing effort to understand and manage familial cancer risk [3, 4]. We conclude this section with the presentation of an integrative model for understanding the antecedents and consequences of hereditary cancer risk counseling and genetic testing.

Psychological Distress and Other Potential Negative Outcomes of Cancer Genetic Counseling and Testing

A large body of literature has examined distress and other negative responses reported by patients waiting for a genetic test result and at various time intervals after learning results (typically up to 1 year of follow-up; for reviews, see [2, 41–43]). In general, research has found little evidence for sustained increases in distress after receiving a positive genetic test result for cancer susceptibility (i.e., HBOC or Lynch syndrome) up to 3 years after genetic testing [2, 41, 42]. Instead, depression and anxiety decrease over time among both carriers and noncarriers of genetic mutations, although these decreases tend to be greater and to occur more quickly among noncarriers [39, 41]. Two recent papers suggest that melanoma genetic testing similarly does not increase anxiety, depression, or cancer worry, but rather seems to result in either short- or longer-term decreases in psychological distress [34, 37].

Though psychosocial issues in FAP families appear to be relatively understudied, elevated reports of anxiety and depression following FAP testing are a potential exception to this pattern of low distress. In Douma et al.'s [23] review, two of the three studies examining psychological outcomes found evidence of clinical levels of anxiety and/or depression following genetic testing, with particularly elevated rates of anxiety among adult mutation carriers with low self-esteem or low optimism [44].

Understanding short-term increases in psychological distress following positive test results.

Despite this general consensus, some researchers have found slight to moderate short-term increases in distress among individuals testing positive for genetic mutations [43, 45–47], particularly among unaffected participants [2, 48] and those with high levels of baseline (pretesting) anxiety [49]. However, distress returned to baseline 1 year following testing [46] or was comparable to distress among noncarriers [50]. A recent study of *BRCA1/2* testing by Beran and colleagues [45] illustrates some of the psychological and methodological complexities of understanding adaptation to genetic test results. The researchers examined prospective changes in depression, anxiety, positive and negative mood, and cancer-specific distress from baseline to 1, 6, and 12 months following receipt of test results among 155 women (38 mutation carriers), of whom more than half had a personal history of breast or ovarian cancer. Across nearly all psychological outcomes (except anxiety), mutation carriers' reports of depression, mood, and cancer-specific distress showed a curvilinear pattern, such that distress increased significantly at 1 and 6 months before either returning to or approaching baseline. For cancer-specific distress, carriers' reports remained elevated compared to noncarriers, but the authors suggested that this difference was due to the sharp decline in cancer-specific distress among noncarriers. These findings suggest that researchers' decisions about the optimal timing of assessments of psychological outcome and clinicians' decisions about the timing of efforts to support counselees in managing their results should be sensitive to potential short-term increases in the year following test reporting. The authors explained, "For mutation carriers, the immediate months after test receipt often involve decisions about prophylactic options and communication of results to family and friends; these activities, accompanied by one's own emotional and cognitive processing of the result, may explain the heightened distress observed during this period" (p. 114).

Understanding variability in responses to positive genetic test results. Although group means for depression and anxiety among mutation carriers may be within normal limits in most studies, it is important to examine variability in responding. For example, in the study just described [45], the authors noted that although group means were within normal limits, depression scores on the CES-D exceeded the clinical cutoff for more than one-third of the *BRCA1/2* mutation carriers at both 1 and 6 months following test reporting. Continued examination of the individual differences, socioeconomic factors (income, education), coping factors, and relationship and familial support factors that may contribute to these different outcomes at different times is essential both to understanding psychological adjustment to genetic counseling and testing and to designing effective tailored programs to address the psychological needs of different groups of patients.

One particularly interesting approach to understanding differences in psychological adaptation to genetic test results comes from a recent study by Ho et al. [51]. Drawing on the different trajectories of psychological adaptation identified in the bereavement literature [52], Ho et al. [51] examined trajectories of depression and anxiety 2 weeks, 4 months, and 1 year following testing in 76 Hong Kong Chinese adults who underwent genetic testing for Lynch syndrome. Of particular interest, only a few participants (4.3%) reported a "recovery pattern" defined by short-term increases in anxiety that subsided in the year following testing. Consistent with research showing low levels of distress, the most frequently reported pattern was a resilient pattern (67%) in which participants who were not particularly anxious or depressed before testing remained this way in the year following testing. However, a small subset of participants who were depressed or anxious prior to testing (7–9%), reported high distress at all follow-up assessments, suggesting that testing itself did not cause or exacerbate anxiety or depression. A fourth subset of patients (13–16%) showed delayed reaction trajectories in which depression and anxiety were low immediately following testing, but increased by 1 year. These findings regarding distinct trajectories of psychological outcomes highlight the need to use appropriate timing for follow-up assessments. Further, knowing that at least a subset of respondents may

experience increased distress up to 1 year following test reporting may promote the development of follow-up or booster interventions to support such individuals. As this work proceeds, it will be important to develop research studies with sufficient power to examine socioeconomic, individual difference, and social support factors that may predict the different trajectories, as such knowledge is essential to the design of early interventions to provide additional support to individuals at risk for either continued or delayed distress.

As a final illustration of what researchers and clinicians may gain from considering variability in psychological outcomes, Hadley et al. [53] prospectively examined depressive symptoms among 134 Lynch syndrome mutation carriers as a function of performance of a colonoscopy in the 6 months following testing. At baseline, 22% of respondents had clinically significant depression levels on the CES-D, which dropped slightly to 16% at the 6-month follow-up; interestingly, baseline depression was not associated with depression at 6 months. Following testing, 52% of carriers underwent colonoscopy in the relatively short follow-up period of 6 months, compared to only 31% of carriers in the year prior to testing, with a total of 69% having undergone colonoscopy in this 18-month period. Regression analyses controlling for multiple psychological and demographic variables indicated that carriers who did not undergo a colonoscopy post-testing were six times more likely to have clinically significant depression levels than those who did undergo colonoscopy, while baseline depression scores were not associated with colonoscopy uptake. These results provide evidence that engaging in preventive screening behaviors may serve to decrease negative psychological responses to undesired genetic test results. While genetic testing serves to reduce uncertainty about risk, the authors suggest that undergoing colonoscopy may serve as a coping strategy that serves to reduce uncertainty about cancer status [53].

Understanding responses to uninformative or variant of uncertain significance test results. One important subgroup of patients at risk for increased distress is those who receive test results that are either uninformative or indicate a variant of uncertain significance (VUS). Although a recent review found that women receiving uninformative *BRCA1/2* results reported small decreases in cancer-specific distress at both short- and long-term follow-up assessments comparable to those reported by noncarriers [43], individuals who received inconclusive results and who did not have a personal cancer history reported greater decreases in distress than those with a cancer history, suggesting that they may have interpreted inconclusive test results as negative test results [43]. In contrast, participants receiving uninformative *BRCA1/2* negative results who expected to receive positive test results reported greater testing-related distress [54]. In this large prospective study, women who received a VUS had higher anxiety and depression at 1 and 6 months following testing, as well as greater testing-related distress in the following year, than women who received other kinds of uninformative results [54].

Responses to the finding of a VUS likely depends on the patient's interpretation of this information. A retrospective interview study of 24 women found that 73% misinterpreted their VUS as a genetic predisposition for cancer, and 29% recalled having been given a pathogenic result as opposed to an uncertain result. Nearly half of the participants who interpreted the VUS as pathogenic underwent prophylactic surgery [55].

Understanding testing-specific forms of distress. In addition to general psychological distress (i.e., depression, anxiety), researchers have also examined types of worry or concern that are specific to the testing context. Paramount among these are concerns about passing elevated cancer risk to one's children and being subject to health and life insurance discrimination [14, 56–58]. In one study of *BRCA1/2* testing, approximately 20% of carriers reported that they often worried about insurance discrimination [14]. Further, nearly 40% of affected carriers and approximately 25% of unaffected carriers reported that they often felt guilt about passing on the mutation [14]. Similarly, 60% of affected carriers and 35% of

unaffected carriers reported fear of their children developing cancer. Interestingly, the proportion of mutation carriers reporting fears with regard to their children's risk greatly exceeded the proportion of carriers (less than 20%) who reported fears about their own cancer development. Our own studies of *p16* genetic testing for melanoma revealed similar concerns about children's cancer risk, which were especially elevated 1 month following counseling and test reporting [37]. Similar to psychological distress, such negative responses tend to be short-lived, and may be the result of heightened cognitive processing regarding one's test result and future plans [45, 57]. Despite these potential short-term negative outcomes, there is no evidence that mutation carriers regret having undergone either *BRCA1/2* or *p16* genetic testing [14, 37].

Understanding Both Positive and Negative Outcomes of Cancer Genetic Testing

As the preceding sections suggest, reports of sustained psychological distress following hereditary cancer risk counseling and testing are rare. In comparison with the large number of studies and measures assessing potential increases in distress, the assessment of positive psychological responses and potential benefits of genetic counseling and test reporting has received less attention. For example, in the widely used Multidimensional Impact of Cancer Risk Assessment [MICRA] developed in a large sample of women undergoing *BRCA1/2* testing [56], the positive experiences subscale is comprised of four items (two assessing feelings of happiness and relief, two assessing satisfaction with family communication), compared to six for distress and nine for uncertainty. Some of the standalone MICRA items capture important positive outcomes, such as whether respondents have "a clear understanding of my choices for cancer prevention or early detection," and for affected family members, whether "the genetic test result has made it easier to cope with my cancer." These two latter items received high scores from carriers in our melanoma genetic testing study both 1 and 6 months after test reporting [37]. The high endorsement of these items suggests that there are important psychological benefits of cancer genetic testing and that expanding existing measurement options to capture these benefits would be worthwhile.

We continue our review with evidence from qualitative studies of the perceived advantages and disadvantages of having undergone counseling and testing for HBOC, Lynch syndrome, and hereditary melanoma. Then we review the methods and findings of studies utilizing diverse measures to capture some of these specific positive and negative outcomes of hereditary cancer risk counseling and testing, including emotional benefits, both positive and negative effects on the self-concept, and feelings of mastery and self-efficacy with respect to managing cancer risk.

Qualitative Accounts of the Costs and Benefits of Hereditary Cancer Risk Counseling and Testing

Hereditary breast and ovarian cancer. Several studies provide retrospective assessments of patients' perceived advantages and disadvantages of having undergone HBOC genetic testing. For example, Lim et al. [59] interviewed 47 women (23 carriers, 24 noncarriers) without a history of breast or ovarian cancer. Participants had undergone counseling and testing 1–70 months earlier (median = 13 months). In terms of perceived advantages, particularly for carriers, two predominant themes were identified — (1) that knowledge is powerful (concerns about being at high risk had been validated by the test; removal of uncertainty concerning cancer risk had produced a sense of control; and knowledge afforded an "opportunity to prepare emotionally and mentally"), reported by 73.9% of carriers; and (2) that counseling and testing had provided increased access to and more favorable attitudes toward screening programs and surgical options, reported by 56.5% of carriers. One carrier said, "I can do something about it and have more control" (p. 123), while another noted, "Knowing allows me to do something positive." Another noted, "Now I know it is a priority

and have a more positive attitude toward screening." Most carriers reported no disadvantages. Participants who reported disadvantages described intrusive thoughts about cancer risk and loss of innocence. The authors note that of the minority of women reporting these concerns, all were less than 48 years old and had received their results less than 13 months ago.

Almost all noncarriers reported perceived advantages of genetic testing, primarily peace of mind ("Now I don't think I am next in line.") and feeling normal ("I now feel like part of the normal population"). Noncarriers also expressed relief that they had not passed the mutation onto their children. Only one noncarrier, who subsequently underwent prophylactic surgery, reported no perceived advantages. Most noncarriers indicated no disadvantages of having undergone testing, with the exception of one participant who reported concerns about becoming complacent about breast cancer risk.

Similar results were obtained by Claes et al. [60] in an interview study of 41 women (20 carriers, 21 noncarriers) who had undergone genetic testing for HBOC 1 year earlier. All respondents reported at least one advantage, and the two most frequent responses were "instrumental advantages" consisting of the increases in perceived control or knowledge about health behavior options (75% of carriers) and "certainty/reduction of uncertainty" (40% of carriers; 23.8% of noncarriers). The most common advantage noted by noncarriers was reassurance and relief (71.4%). Of particular note, 70% of carriers and 25% of noncarriers reported at least one disadvantage, with wide variation in the particular disadvantages reported (e.g., uncertainty, survivor guilt, feelings of hopelessness, increased anxiety, increased risk perceptions). Participants also reported a variety of changes in specific domains, particularly in body image ("different experience of breasts," consequences of preventive surgery), emotions (experience of personal growth, increased anxiety), and relationships with relatives (more or less closeness and support).

Lynch syndrome. Claes et al. [61] interviewed 72 participants following testing for Lynch syndrome. Consistent with the above findings, participants reported both advantages and disadvantages of testing. All but one carrier and two noncarriers reported at least one advantage, and again, the two most frequently cited advantages by carriers were instrumental advantages (89%) and reduction of uncertainty (33%). For noncarriers, the most frequently cited advantages were reassurance (50%), learning that children were not at risk (39%), and decreased need for screening (33%). In contrast to the above studies of HBOC, more than half of the carriers, as well as 17% of noncarriers, reported at least one disadvantage of knowing their results. For carriers, the major disadvantages reported were the burden of regular medical examinations (22%) and psychological burdens (19%); for noncarriers, they involved difficulties arising from having different results compared to their relatives (i.e., survivor guilt, feelings of exclusion, relatives' negative reaction to the disclosure of a favorable test result). As in the HBOC studies reported above, participants reported some degree of change in different life domains, such as body image (especially the perception of physical symptoms and whether or not they were interpreted as signs of potential cancer), and both heightened worry and personal growth.

Hereditary melanoma. The availability of preventive options to reduce melanoma risk through daily reduction of UVR exposure makes possible a different set of perceived costs and benefits of melanoma genetic test reporting and counseling. We were particularly interested in whether this information would increase perceived control over melanoma risk, or alternatively, whether the heightened vigilance created by having to confront one's elevated risk each time one steps outside would increase distress. To investigate these possibilities as well as other perceived advantages or disadvantages of receiving test results, we asked respondents at three times in the year following counseling and test reporting to describe any benefits or limitations of having received their test results [37]. The results were striking—nearly all participants (approximately 95%) at each assessment listed one or more positive aspects of learning their genetic test results, while only 15.9% overall (11.9% at 1 month, 8.1% at 6 months, and 3.3% at 1 year) listed a negative aspect at any assessment. Similar to findings from interviews with patients who have undergone testing for HBOC or Lynch syndrome, all participants who listed a disadvantage also listed one or more benefits.

Participants described benefits in three major thematic areas: emotional, informational, and behavioral. Perceived emotional benefits were reported by 71.4% of noncarriers and 26.1% of carriers. Noncarriers were especially likely to report feelings of relief for themselves and their children that they did not carry the mutation, while carriers reported decreased fatalism and guilt concerning melanoma risk. For example, one noncarrier wrote, "I grew up thinking I was doomed to get melanoma. Knowing that I am negative for the *p16* gene has brought me much relief." One carrier noted, "I feel that there are choices and options for the better about taking steps to prevent melanoma. It is not hopeless." For another carrier, a positive test result provided an explanation for prior cancer ("I don't feel quite so guilty about having had melanoma, as I did when I thought it was all due to my sun exposure.")

For mutation carriers, the primary perceived benefits were informational and behavioral: 78.3% reported increased knowledge about melanoma risk and its management, and 65.2% reported improvement in health behaviors or plans to increase their practice of photoprotection and screening for themselves and their families. The informational benefits reported by carriers conveyed a strong sense of perceived control and empowerment. One carrier wrote, "The more information the better. The more I know, the more I'll be able to take precautionary measures and get skin checkups," while another wrote, "I like being informed and have the chance to prepare for the challenges that come in life. Prevention is half the battle!" Reported improvements in prevention and screening behaviors conveyed the same sentiment: "I think more about what I'm doing in the sun and take more measures to protect myself and my family. I also feel more in control of what happens to me by the knowledge

I have," and "Having the test results be positive has increased my vigilance. And it has made me more aware of increased risk to my children." A majority of noncarriers (95.2%) also reported increased knowledge about melanoma risk and its management, with a smaller proportion (38.1%) reporting improved prevention and screening behaviors.

As illustrated above, participants' reported improvements in photoprotection and screening frequently included their children. Given the potential role of early childhood and adolescent sun exposure in the etiology of melanoma, early implementation of prevention behaviors may be especially important [62]. Further, members of these high-risk families expressed considerable interest in genetic testing for their minor children [62]. Specifically, when surveyed immediately following counseling and test reporting as well as 2 years later, the vast majority (86.9%) wanted melanoma genetic testing for their minor children [62], with 69.8% expressing the belief that having this knowledge would allow families to implement better prevention and screening behaviors. The following written comments from participants in response to questions concerning whether, when, and why children should be tested illustrate these possibilities [32]:

- Maybe testing for their parents to know from birth to start preventive steps and then more education as the child matures to take responsibility for themselves to watch for changes, etc.
- They could be informed at early age to watch more diligently and more forcefully counseled against those crazy TANS!!!
- I feel the more aware we are the more we can support each other. Like entire family using sunscreen, wearing hats, etc.
- Better to take precautions at a young age before any real serious damage is done… Forknowledge is forewarned is forprepared [sic].

These findings suggest some potentially interesting possibilities for future study—that high-risk families both desire and report using genetic counseling information to improve prevention and screening for minor children [37, 62] and that reports of individual behavior change may underestimate this kind of family-wide change in cancer-relevant behaviors.

Finally, reports of disadvantages of receiving test results were rare (15.9% of respondents overall) and included reports of discouragement ("A little discouraging, but I would rather know"), frustration ("Just that there is no genetic way of fixing it yet—it ticks me off."), and insurance concerns. Only one participant, a noncarrier, reported decreased vigilance as a disadvantage of receiving test results.

Summary. These qualitative studies indicate that hereditary cancer risk counseling and testing have both positive and negative outcomes, but rarely exclusively negative ones. Among the consistent benefits reported by mutation carriers are increased knowledge about risk and appropriate management and increases in perceived control over cancer risk. Depending on the particular cancer syndromes, these advantages may come with costs, such as altered body image, concern for family members, and feelings of being burdened by the demands of accelerated screening. We turn now to quantitative assessments of these and other costs and benefits.

Quantitative Assessment of Positive and Negative Outcomes of Hereditary Cancer Risk Counseling and Testing

In this next section, we review several instruments that have been designed to assess specific responses to genetic counseling and testing with regard to their ability to capture the costs and benefits reported by participants in qualitative studies. Our review emphasizes measurement issues because the increased use of standardized measures in future research will facilitate comparisons of the psychological impact of hereditary cancer risk counseling and testing for different cancer syndromes, for different groups of patients, and with different counseling protocols. As we will see, some of the measures are likely applicable to testing for all or most genetic risks, while others are necessarily specialized to capture particular aspects of specific cancer syndromes.

Feelings of relief and other positive experiences. As noted earlier, potential negative outcomes of genetic counseling and testing have received far greater research attention than potential positive outcomes. As expected, noncarriers report greater relief and happiness than carriers on the positive experiences subscale of the MICRA [14, 37, 56]; however, positive experiences involving family supportiveness and communication are reported equally by both carriers and noncarriers [37, 56]. In our studies of melanoma genetic testing, we supplemented the MICRA items concerning happiness and relief with the items concerning a sense of peace and acceptance about one's test results. Unlike happiness and relief, these items were endorsed at equally high levels by affected carriers, unaffected carriers, and noncarriers. Thus, expanding the range of positive emotional experiences that may follow counseling and testing may provide a more detailed picture of potential emotional outcomes.

Reductions in uncertainty regarding cancer risk. The potential for cancer genetic testing to reduce uncertainty (or alternately, to increase certainty) for both carriers and noncarriers is frequently mentioned as a benefit in qualitative studies; however, this concept has yet to be fully captured by existing inventories. The Psychological Adaptation to Genetic Information Scale (PAGIS, [63]) includes a certainty subscale consisting of items assessing counselees' understanding of how they came to have a particular gene alteration, the health risks their relatives face, the chances of passing the gene alteration to one's children, and the ability to explain to other people the meaning of having a particular gene alteration. However, these items seem to capture more about knowledge arising from and personal understanding of the genetic explanations and management recommendations provided during the counseling session than about the psychological effects of reduced uncertainty (or increased certainty) concerning cancer risk itself.

Perceived personal control, self-efficacy, and mastery with respect to cancer risk. Control perceptions can be assessed as either increases or decreases in perceived control following a positive or negative test result. The MICRA assesses decreases in perceived control, with an item in the distress subscale assessing feelings of loss of control. Three other inventories assess perceptions of improved control following counseling and test reporting. The Perceived Personal Control measure (PPC; [64]) captures multiple aspects of understanding and managing familial cancer risk. Sample items are, "I feel I know the meaning of the problem for my family's future," "I feel I have the tools to make decisions that will influence my future," and "I feel I can make decisions that will change my family's future." Originally conceptualized as three subscales (cognitive control, decision control, and behavior control), the scale was recently found to form a single reliable factor [65]. The PAGIS self-efficacy subscale assesses perceptions of self-efficacy for managing the effects of having a disease-causing genetic mutation or genetic disorder. Sample items are, "I am confident that I can work out any problems having this gene might cause," and "I believe that there are things I can do to avoid the problems that may arise from having this gene." The third inventory that assesses mastery perceptions following genetic counseling and testing was specifically developed with both focus groups and large-scale surveys of people who had undergone *BRCA1/2* testing and testing for hereditary colorectal cancer [58, 66, 67]. In this framework, mastery perceptions are described as an element of the self-concept, and thus this work will be described more fully in the next section.

Impact of cancer genetic counseling on the self-concept. A particularly rich set of studies by Esplen and colleagues [58, 66, 67] has identified multiple ways in which cancer genetic counseling and the receipt of a positive test result may influence the self-views of high-risk patients. Individual interviews and focus groups were conducted with both affected and unaffected patients who had undergone counseling and testing to assess how that experience changed how they thought about themselves. Based on these interviews and focus groups, Esplen and colleagues developed specific scales to assess the impact of cancer genetic testing for *BRCA1/2*, FAP, and Lynch syndrome. The scales were then subjected both to factor analysis and convergent and divergent validation with other related concepts.

The resulting *BRCA* Self-Concept Scale consists of three factors: *stigma* (e.g., "I feel isolated because of my test result," "I feel labeled," "I feel burdened with this information"), *vulnerability* (e.g., "I distrust my body," "I feel like a walking time bomb," "I am worried that cancer will be found when I go for screening"), and *mastery* (e.g., "I know my body well," "I am in control of my health," "I am hopeful about myself in the future"). Higher scores indicate a more negative impact of genetic test results on self-concept. In the two large samples of women attending high-risk breast cancer clinics in which the scale was validated, mean reported impact was greatest for vulnerability (3.85 on a scale ranging from 1 = strongly disagree to 7 = strongly agree), intermediate for stigma (2.72), and least for the negative impact on perceptions of mastery (1.46). Importantly, if one were to reverse score the mastery subscale so that higher scores indicated greater mastery, the resulting mean would indicate perceptions of mastery near the maximum value of the scale.

The self-concept scales developed for FAP [66] and Lynch syndrome [67] illustrate the importance of understanding how the specific demands of different cancer syndromes influence the self-concept. For example, the FAP self-concept scale [66] includes diminished feelings of physical and sexual attractiveness, as well as concerns about bowel control in addition to the stigma, self-esteem, and mastery items described above; concerns about bowel control and gastrointestinal symptoms such as pain and bleeding are also a major component of the Lynch syndrome self-concept scale [67]. Importantly, given the focus on women in most studies of *BRCA1/2* outcomes, the validation study of the FAP self-concept scale included a large number of men with a diagnosis of FAP, and scores on the subscales, as well as the total impact on the self-concept, were similar for men and women.

As suggested by Esplen and colleagues [58, 66], these scales will likely have a multitude of potentially important uses in both research and practice. First, the scales may be used to identify patients who may benefit not only from longer-term follow-up, but also from different forms of counseling. For example, the psychosocial support needs of a patient who feels stigmatized and isolated are likely to be different from one whose concerns center on cancer fear and body image or low perceived mastery and diminished hope for the future. The particular impacts assessed by the three subscales may also suggest specific interventions—for example, support groups to assist those who feel isolated and stigmatized. Second, an important goal for future research is to examine how these specific impacts of genetic testing are related to subsequent decision making about screening and prevention options. For example, Esplen et al. [58] note that feelings of stigma and vulnerability may increase anxiety and thereby interfere with screening attendance. Conversely, a resulting sense of empowerment or mastery through genetic knowledge may promote health behaviors to manage risk. Third, the scales may be used to examine the cancer-related self-concept of members of high-risk families prior to testing. Esplen et al. [58] advance the interesting prediction that the pretesting self-concept may differ based on whether patients have experienced multiple losses due to cancer in the family or have observed survival among affected family members. Finally, these authors suggest that the scales may be used to examine family members who receive negative test results and have difficulty incorporating this new and unexpected information into the self-concept. Examining how feelings of cancer vulnerability may persist in such patients may be useful in understanding and assisting those who have difficulty disengaging from the intensive surveillance programs they may have lived with for many years (see also [68]).

The scale development efforts undertaken by Esplen and colleagues highlight several issues of importance for understanding psychological outcomes of hereditary cancer risk counseling and testing. First, all three disease-specific self-concept scales include both positive (mastery, self-esteem) and negative impacts (vulnerability, stigma, diminished physical and sexual attractiveness) on the self-concept among mutation carriers following counseling and testing, and patients appear to endorse (on average) low perceptions of stigma, intermediate perceptions of vulnerability, and high levels of mastery. Second, the specific impacts on self-views are different for different hereditary cancers, likely due to the different recommendations concerning prophylactic surgery and the implications of such surgery for sexual behavior and body image. As genetic testing becomes available for more hereditary cancers, it will be important to understand which aspects of different cancer syndromes (e.g., age of onset, involvement of reproductive system, availability of preventive options, etc.) have different effects on the self-concept. Third, this more nuanced view of the impact of the hereditary cancer risk counseling and testing on the self-concept suggests important areas in which to focus intervention efforts to reduce negative changes and promote feelings of mastery and self-esteem. Finally, research in this area might benefit from integration with recent efforts to understand the impact of cancer on the self-concept using such notions as illness centrality, or the degree to which one's illness (or risk for it) has become part of one's personal identity [69, 70].

Using Measures of Posttraumatic Growth and Benefit Finding to Understand Positive Changes Following Genetic Counseling and Testing

Another recent development is the application of measures and methods from the study of posttraumatic growth and other changes in life following adversity to understanding psychological outcomes of genetic testing. In a study of 108 women who had undergone *BRCA1/2* testing, Low et al. [71] surveyed participants regarding both posttraumatic growth and approach-oriented forms of coping following receipt of test results. Overall, reports of posttraumatic growth were highly variable, and 83.3% of women endorsed at least one positive life change to at least a small degree. Reports of posttraumatic growth (often called benefit finding) were greatest among affected carriers, who reported greater posttrau-

matic growth on all five subscales (personal strength, appreciation of life, interpersonal relationships, new possibilities in life, and spiritual change) of the Posttraumatic Growth Inventory (PTGI, [72]) than either unaffected carriers or both affected and unaffected noncarriers. As predicted by theories of posttraumatic growth, reports of benefit finding on the PTGI were positively correlated with both reported test-related distress and approach-oriented coping. Interestingly, the greater reports of benefit finding among affected carriers were mediated by their greater reported use of approach-oriented coping. The authors suggested that these benefits may accrue from taking an active approach to some of the challenges women likely experience following testing, such as disclosing results to family members and making prophylactic treatment decisions. Handling these challenges actively may yield increased support from family members and an increased sense of control related to medical management options. These findings, although based on retrospective accounts of benefit finding and coping, do suggest that for women with a history of breast or ovarian cancer who employ active approach-oriented coping methods, genetic testing may lead to positive perceived psychological and interpersonal changes. As this work proceeds, it will be important to examine why unaffected carriers did not report similar perceived benefits or growth, or alternatively, whether the personal experience of cancer diagnosis and resulting distress are necessary to trigger benefit finding.

An Integrative Model for Understanding Multiple Determinants of the Psychological and Behavioral Impact of Hereditary Cancer Risk Counseling and Genetic Testing

Having illustrated through quantitative and qualitative data that there are multiple positive and negative psychological outcomes of cancer genetic counseling and testing as well as different potential trajectories of outcomes, the next steps for future research are to try to understand the

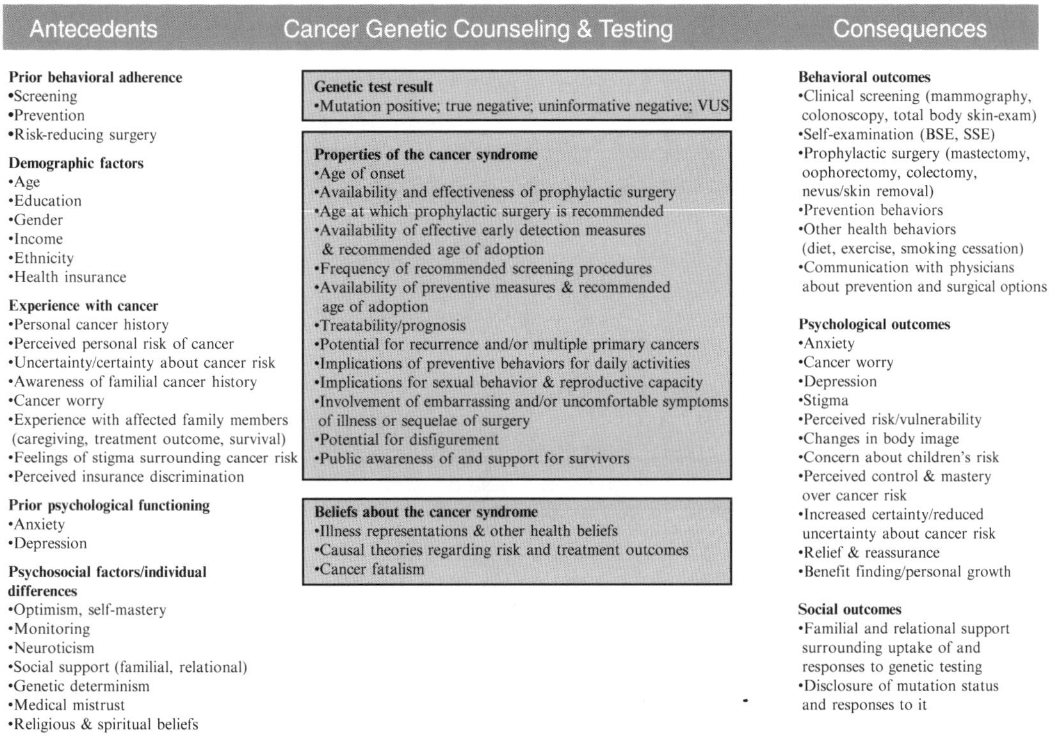

Antecedents	Cancer Genetic Counseling & Testing	Consequences

Antecedents

Prior behavioral adherence
•Screening
•Prevention
•Risk-reducing surgery

Demographic factors
•Age
•Education
•Gender
•Income
•Ethnicity
•Health insurance

Experience with cancer
•Personal cancer history
•Perceived personal risk of cancer
•Uncertainty/certainty about cancer risk
•Awareness of familial cancer history
•Cancer worry
•Experience with affected family members
 (caregiving, treatment outcome, survival)
•Feelings of stigma surrounding cancer risk
•Perceived insurance discrimination

Prior psychological functioning
•Anxiety
•Depression

Psychosocial factors/individual differences
•Optimism, self-mastery
•Monitoring
•Neuroticism
•Social support (familial, relational)
•Genetic determinism
•Medical mistrust
•Religious & spiritual beliefs

Cancer Genetic Counseling & Testing

Genetic test result
•Mutation positive; true negative; uninformative negative; VUS

Properties of the cancer syndrome
•Age of onset
•Availability and effectiveness of prophylactic surgery
•Age at which prophylactic surgery is recommended
•Availability of effective early detection measures
 & recommended age of adoption
•Frequency of recommended screening procedures
•Availability of preventive measures & recommended
 age of adoption
•Treatability/prognosis
•Potential for recurrence and/or multiple primary cancers
•Implications of preventive behaviors for daily activities
•Implications for sexual behavior & reproductive capacity
•Involvement of embarrassing and/or uncomfortable symptoms
 of illness or sequelae of surgery
•Potential for disfigurement
•Public awareness of and support for survivors

Beliefs about the cancer syndrome
•Illness representations & other health beliefs
•Causal theories regarding risk and treatment outcomes
•Cancer fatalism

Consequences

Behavioral outcomes
•Clinical screening (mammography,
 colonoscopy, total body skin-exam)
•Self-examination (BSE, SSE)
•Prophylactic surgery (mastectomy,
 oophorectomy, colectomy,
 nevus/skin removal)
•Prevention behaviors
•Other health behaviors
 (diet, exercise, smoking cessation)
•Communication with physicians
 about prevention and surgical options

Psychological outcomes
•Anxiety
•Cancer worry
•Depression
•Stigma
•Perceived risk/vulnerability
•Changes in body image
•Concern about children's risk
•Perceived control & mastery
 over cancer risk
•Increased certainty/reduced
 uncertainty about cancer risk
•Relief & reassurance
•Benefit finding/personal growth

Social outcomes
•Familial and relational support
 surrounding uptake of and
 responses to genetic testing
•Disclosure of mutation status
 and responses to it

Fig. 3.1 A model for understanding the antecedents and consequences of responses to hereditary cancer risk counseling and genetic testing for different cancer syndromes

multiplicity of factors that may influence these outcomes. Figure 3.1 presents a list of potentially impactful antecedent factors and properties of the cancer syndromes themselves in conjunction with an expanded set of behavioral and psychological outcomes identified by our review. We will describe each part of the model in turn and then illustrate how recent work on multiple "life trajectories" among young women who obtained testing for *BRCA1/2* [73] illustrates what might be gained from a more detailed understanding of some of these antecedent factors.

Potential predictors of responses to genetic testing. Figure 3.1 presents the detailed list of potential antecedent factors, including prior risk perceptions and associated cancer worry and uncertainty, adherence to screening and prevention recommendations, and experience with cancer in the family. The inclusion of these factors highlights the recognition that, rather than conceptualizing perceived risk, uncertainty, and distress as outcomes of genetic testing, baseline levels of these factors may profitably be seen as important elements of patients' motivations for seeking counseling and testing that may influence their responses to such testing. That is, as we have suggested throughout this chapter, the information provided by hereditary cancer risk counseling and genetic test reporting are inputs to already ongoing efforts to understand and manage familial cancer risk. Understanding these antecedent factors should improve efforts to better understand and support patients who may experience different outcomes. Thus, researchers should ask for which patients and for what cancer syndromes will counseling and test reporting reduce distress and uncertainty, and for which do these interventions have the potential to maintain or exacerbate distress.

As suggested by our discussion of different trajectories, baseline anxiety and depression have received attention as potential moderators of responses to hereditary cancer risk counseling and testing, and there has been some limited examination of other individual differences that may influence responses to testing, such as optimism [44] and monitoring [74]. It remains a challenge for future research to recruit and retain sufficient sample sizes to allow a prospective examination of how individual differences are related to specific outcomes of genetic testing, especially as participants should optimally be stratified by mutation status and personal cancer history. However, such efforts will be important to understanding whether and how hereditary cancer risk counseling protocols might be tailored to people with different beliefs about the future and preferences for health information. Similarly, understanding how religious and spiritual beliefs predict uptake of and responses to genetic testing represents an important avenue for future research (see, e.g., [75–78]).

Important properties of the cancer syndrome. As this figure highlights, the particular psychological outcomes one might expect from hereditary cancer risk counseling and testing may depend on properties of the cancer syndrome itself, particularly the management options available for different cancer syndromes, as well as developmental concerns such as age of onset and age at which either prophylactic surgery or other prevention and screening options are recommended. For example, age of onset and age at which prophylactic surgery is recommended distinguish FAP from other syndromes, whereas hereditary melanoma is distinguished by the availability of preventive measures that should be implemented as early as possible to reduce cumulative UVR exposure. As *p16* counseling and testing for minors become more widely implemented, it will be important to understand both the prospective medical and psychosocial outcomes of proactively managing UVR exposure in young members of high-risk families. Further, the particular management recommendations required by different cancers pose different adaptational challenges—as illustrated in Fig. 3.1, the presence of embarrassing, uncomfortable symptoms and treatments that have implications for sexual behavior and body image pose unique, ongoing challenges [58, 66, 67].

Another property of hereditary cancer syndromes that has yet to be fully examined for its psychological impact is vulnerability to multiple primary cancers and to more than one kind of cancer. For example, melanoma may develop anywhere on the body where there is skin (not necessarily in existing nevi, not necessarily in sun-exposed areas). Further, the successful excision and treatment of one melanoma does not reduce vulnerability to future melanomas. Thus, there is no single prophylactic surgery that could prevent all melanoma—lifelong vigilance is required. These distinctions may have important consequences for understanding the impact of genetic testing on survivorship issues for different forms of hereditary cancer, as a positive genetic test result makes one's risks for new cancers or different cancers an ever-present, lifelong possibility.

Last, cancer syndromes differ in the residual risks that apply to noncarriers of the particular mutation. In general, testing negative for a familial mutation returns a person's risk to general population status. However, there may be cases in which a patient's personal history may still indicate an elevated risk even when a mutation is not identified, such as a patient who previously had colon polyps but is a noncarrier of a Lynch syndrome mutation, or a patient with such phenotypic risk factors for melanoma as dysplastic nevi who is a noncarrier of a *p16* mutation. The ways in which such patients synthesize clinical and genetic information may influence risk perceptions, cancer worry, and adherence to screening following counseling about a negative test result.

Multiple, potentially interrelated psychological and behavioral outcomes. Throughout the chapter, we have emphasized that members of high-risk families report both positive and negative psychological outcomes of genetic testing—for example, increased vulnerability to cancer, but also increased perceptions of self-efficacy to manage cancer risk. Thus, continued attention to measurement of both kinds of outcomes should be a priority for future research. Further, research that examines how these positive and negative outcomes are functionally related (for example, the idea that some distress is necessary to promote benefit finding and personal growth [72]; see also [79, 80]) would enrich our understanding of how participants incorporate the information provided by counseling and testing into their ongoing efforts to manage familial cancer risk.

We emphasize also that the psychological and behavioral outcomes of cancer genetic counseling and testing should not be seen as independent of one another, in that many of the recommendations, particularly those involving prophylactic surgery, may affect important psychosocial outcomes (see, e.g., [81, 82]). Further, there are also important reciprocal relations to consider, as several authors have theorized that psychological outcomes, such as anxiety and depression, may influence adherence to screening recommendations. Specifically, anxiety among carriers may lead to avoidance of screening [58], and carriers may elect accelerated screening or prophylactic surgery to reduce anxiety and cancer worry (see, e.g., [53, 73]). Persistent anxiety and cancer worry may also account for overutilization of screening among noncarriers. Note that these outcomes may depend in important ways on the management options available for different cancer syndromes.

Importantly, the list of behavioral outcomes to consider in conjunction with psychological outcomes includes other changes made to promote health in general, such as changes in diet, exercise, smoking, and stress management. Assessment of these behaviors may extend to family-wide changes, including the encouragement of relatives to improve prevention and screening efforts [37, 83, 84]. Finally, another set of important behavioral outcomes to assess involves patient communication with physicians about their prevention or surgical options following genetic testing [85]. Such discussions may be important predictors of medical management decisions, given the ability of physician recommendations to influence patient choices.

Familial and relational processes involved in discussing and managing hereditary cancer risk. Finally, multiple authors have noted potentially important relationships involving social responses to disclosure of mutation status and family support and communication processes to psychological outcomes [86]. As many authors have noted, genetic testing poses unique challenges to the understanding of familial communication and support, especially as multiple family members receive different test results [87, 88]. Further, spouses and partners are also affected. This recognition has led to many interesting studies of the dynamics of family communication [89, 90], and of the impact on the index patient of factors such as spousal anxiety that may influence how the patient manages the implications of a positive *BRCA1/2* test [91].

Future directions for integrative analyses of the antecedents and consequences of genetic testing. Researchers are just starting to pinpoint the particular concerns and experiences with familial and personal cancer that patients may bring to the counseling setting that may create different outcome trajectories. A particularly interesting recent study illustrates the ways in which these different concerns and experiences give rise to different uses of counseling and testing to inform patients' efforts to understand and manage cancer risk. Hamilton et al. [73] retrospectively assessed the events leading up to and following *BRCA1/2* testing among 44 female *BRCA1/2* mutation carriers aged 18–39, approximately half of whom had a history of breast cancer. The researchers found that women typically described one of four major "life trajectories" of genetic testing. One subset of women was "acutely aware" of the risk in their family and essentially grew up aware that they had the potential for increased breast cancer risk. Women in this trajectory who did not elect to undergo prophylactic surgery often felt a high amount of distress and anxiety between clinical screenings, often prompting them to undergo risk-reducing surgery. A second subset of women was motivated to undergo genetic testing because of the death of their mother due to breast cancer, and often perceived mastectomy to be less anxiety-provoking than not electing surgery. A third subset of women was notified of their risk by a health care provider and saw the decision to undergo genetic testing as less emotionally laden than women in the first two trajectories and perceived that actions could be taken in order to take control of their health. Finally, a fourth subset of women was prompted to undergo testing due to a personal diagnosis of breast cancer. For these women, treating breast cancer was the primary concern and genetic testing was of secondary importance—as such, some women often chose aggressive treatment strategies, such as bilateral mastectomy, prior to genetic testing.

This study highlights the diverse, complicated, and often emotional decisions—and the varying personal experiences—that young women with familial breast cancer risk bring to the counseling setting. This study also emphasizes the need to examine an individual's personal and familial experiences with breast cancer prior to testing as this can bring to light potentially important predictors of subsequent behavioral and emotional outcomes of genetic testing. Hamilton et al. [73] note, "A pedigree denoting family history of cancer is a two-dimensional iconic representation of risk; a life trajectory is a multidimensional description of the processes of knowing one's risk" (p. 150). Further, we note that almost all of the factors identified as potential antecedents in Fig. 3.1 may be brought to bear in understanding these women's experiences and decisions to undergo genetic testing. This example also highlights the ways in which decisions about specific clinical management options (prophylactic surgery, screening) may be influenced by emotional outcomes arising from perceived risk. Continued attention to these diverse trajectories of cancer experience, risk perceptions, emotional experiences, and behavioral outcomes is likely to yield important information about the decision-making process surrounding hereditary risk counseling and testing, as well as how counseling and testing may best be tailored to assist people in managing cancer risk.

Methodological Issues and Future Directions

Although this is not an exhaustive review, we wish to highlight some methodological issues that have potentially great implications for understanding the conclusions we have presented here concerning the psychological and behavioral outcomes of hereditary cancer risk counseling and testing. Some of these issues, such as differences between family members who accept or decline

counseling and testing, may be inherent in the study of testing uptake, whereas others, such as the greater inclusion of ethnic minority respondents and increased attention to rare syndromes that predispose an individual to multiple cancers, represent important priorities for future research.

Recruitment and Other Procedural Differences Between Research and Clinical Settings

The recruitment strategy employed in studies of cancer genetic testing may have a large impact on the inferences one can draw about testing uptake and corresponding psychological and behavioral outcomes. Participants in studies of genetic testing outcomes typically come from one of two sources—members of high-risk families (often from existing cancer registries) recruited as part of a research study or adults who have presented themselves to a high-risk cancer clinic (clinical populations). Systematic differences may exist based on the source of recruitment. As suggested by Lerman and colleagues [39], distress following testing may be lower in research populations than clinical populations who self-refer for genetic testing. Additionally, in the context of research studies, genetic testing uptake rates following counseling may also be underestimated compared to adults who self-refer, as these latter participants have already demonstrated considerable interest in learning their results by contacting the clinic on their own [39]. Further, because research studies often provide counseling and testing free of charge, they may not provide an accurate assessment of the relation of socioeconomic status (SES) to uptake. On the other hand, one could argue that recruitment from research populations may extend genetic counseling and testing studies to a larger number of participants, including those who had not previously considered it for multiple reasons, including lack of knowledge, lower perceived risk, and barriers such as cost. Finally, in research settings, participants may have access to more resources and validated materials, and the materials they receive may be culturally tailored [92], resulting in a more optimal genetic testing experience [39].

Differences Between Acceptors and Decliners of Cancer Genetic Counseling and Testing

For obvious ethical reasons, one cannot randomly assign family members to undergo genetic counseling and testing. That participants must "opt in" to participate in genetic counseling research invites a host of confounding variables that accompany such self-selection (see [93] for discussion). There are potentially important demographic and psychosocial differences between members of high-risk families who present themselves for genetic testing or who chose to be tested when invited to undergo genetic testing as part of a research study and those who decline. The antecedent factors listed in Fig. 3.1 may influence genetic testing uptake as well as genetic testing and counseling outcomes. A frequent finding is that family members with greater perceived risk of developing a given disease and greater worry about developing the disease are more likely to be interested in and to elect genetic testing [3]. These findings are consistent with the idea that genetic counseling and testing are perceived as tools to manage heightened cancer risk, but they also raise the possibility that these benefits may be limited to participants with high prior perceived risk and cancer worry.

Further, it is likely that there are other important demographic and psychosocial differences between acceptors and decliners that may influence our understanding of psychological and behavioral outcomes. For example, in addition to having greater cancer risk perceptions and higher cancer worry, women who presented themselves for *BRCA1/2* counseling were younger and more likely to be married, had a higher level of education and greater household income, were more likely to be Jewish (*BRCA1/2* has high penetrance in Ashkenazi Jewish adults), had a higher risk of carrying the mutation, were more likely to have seen a gynecologist more than twice in the past year, and were more likely to have discussed genetic testing with their physician [94]. Women who elected to undergo *BRCA1/2* testing reported greater perceived benefits of testing, reported that gaining information for their family members was more important, and were less likely to be concerned about life insurance discrimination than those who declined [95]. Additionally, women who declined HBOC genetic counseling were more likely to anticipate negative emotional reactions to testing than women who underwent counseling [96].

Among 119 high-risk Australian adults invited to receive melanoma genetic testing as part of a research study, the 25 acceptors had higher perceived melanoma risk, greater melanoma-specific distress on the Impact of Events Scale, and lower fatalism about the lethality of melanoma and the corresponding value of early detection [34]. Additionally, acceptors also reported greater perceived benefits of genetic testing, such as its potential to increase certainty about cancer risk, improve planning for the future, provide information about children's risk, and provide information that would help patients reduce their own risk. Acceptors were also more likely to be married—perhaps due to greater support or encouragement to undergo genetic testing (see also [97])—and to have a greater number of affected family members [34]. In contrast, a Dutch study found that participants who reported high levels of worry about melanoma or pancreatic cancer were likely to decline to learn their results following counseling [36].

As these examples suggest, participants who elect testing and research participation may differ in a number of attitudes and beliefs relevant to understanding the outcomes of testing, as well as prior psychological distress and medical utilization. However, it would be premature to conclude that people who decline genetic testing are necessarily more anxious or fearful than those who accept. As reviewed above, the current evidence is conflicting, with multiple studies suggesting that family members who are most concerned about their cancer risk are more likely to uptake testing and counseling [3]. Further, some evidence suggests that there may be distinct sets of beliefs (e.g., that factors other than genes and heredity are important contributors to their cancer risk, or that a genetic test will not have an impact on their health behaviors sufficient to warrant the test) and emotional concerns (e.g., fear) that predict declining genetic testing [98]. Thus, family members who decline testing often have heterogeneous reasons, and it will be important to continue to qualify research conclusions based on what can be learned about the multiple differences between acceptors and decliners.

Racial and Ethnic Disparities in Genetic Testing Knowledge and Uptake

Another critical issue for both research and clinical application involves the underrepresentation of racial and ethnic minorities in cancer genetics research. There are important racial and ethnic disparities in genetic testing knowledge and uptake and a relative paucity of research on the psychological and behavioral outcomes of genetic testing among ethnic minority individuals. These health disparities do not reflect differences in cancer burden among different USA ethnic groups—in fact, African Americans have higher risk of colon cancer, and African American men are at higher risk for prostate cancer. There are also biological differences between cancers occurring in different ethnic groups and differences in outcomes that extend beyond disparities in access to care that are not fully understood. For example, white women are more likely to get breast cancer after age 45, but the rate of breast cancer is greater in African American women prior to age 45, and mortality is higher for African American women at any age [99]. Racial disparities in the uptake of genetic testing for HBOC have been well described [100]. Specifically, White adults are more likely to self-refer for BRCA1/2 genetic testing than African American adults [94], and in one study less than 50% of African American women who underwent counseling for *BRCA1/2* mutations underwent genetic testing [97]. Racial disparities have not yet been examined in the context of genetic testing for Lynch syndrome and are more difficult to study in melanoma where risk is overwhelmingly higher among Whites.

There are several potential explanations for disparities in uptake [94]. The first is knowledge—African American and Hispanic adults are less likely to have heard of genetic testing than White adults [101–103]. According to a 2005 NIH survey of nearly 30,000 adults, nearly 50% of White adults were aware of genetic testing, while slightly fewer than one-third of African American adults and only 20% of Hispanic adults were aware of genetic testing for cancer risk ([102]; see similar findings in [104]). These racial differences are only partly explained by other demographic factors such as SES, education, or insurance status [102]. However, length of residency in the USA and education account for a large portion of the difference in knowledge between Whites and Hispanics, while region of residency in the USA (i.e., knowledge in the West is greater than knowledge in the South) explains additional variance in the difference between Whites and African American adults [102].

Because sociodemographic factors do not entirely account for the difference in genetic testing awareness, a second potential explanation for racial disparities in genetic testing uptake involves culturally determined attitudes about genetic testing. Research increasingly suggests that ethnic minorities' mistrust of the health care system or of individual physicians contributes to differential engagement in the health care system. Medical mistrust has been most extensively studied in the areas of research participation, HIV prevention, general mistrust of the health care system, trust in physicians, utilization of medical services, adherence to medical recommendations, and cancer screening rates [105–112]. Armstrong and colleagues [94] suggest that medical mistrust may similarly contribute to disparities in genetic test uptake. Specific to genetic testing, African Americans are "more likely to report that the government would use genetic tests to label groups as inferior, and less likely to endorse the potential health benefits of testing" ([101], p. 363; see also [104]). Similarly, Latinas high in medical mistrust report fewer perceived benefits to genetic testing, greater barriers, and greater concerns about abuses of genetic testing [113]. In contrast, some researchers reported an unexpected finding that African American women had more positive attitudes toward genetic testing for HBOC than White women, as well as less knowledge [114].

To reduce such disparities, researchers have developed culturally tailored genetic counseling that addresses specific cultural attitudes and beliefs that may differ among ethnic groups. Culturally tailored counseling typically includes questions during the counseling session about spirituality and religious values, temporal orientation, and communalism. Conflicting data exist as to whether culturally tailored genetic counseling for HBOC results in greater uptake of *BRCA1/2* testing or more favorable outcomes among African American women than does standard genetic counseling [97, 115]. Thus, at present, it is unclear whether a failure to address specific cultural beliefs plays a significant role in contributing to racial disparities in testing uptake. Further, culturally tailored counseling does not seem to address issues surrounding medical mistrust, and it is possible that there may be other culturally determined beliefs that may be predictive of testing uptake and should be addressed.

A third potential explanation for the disparities in genetic testing uptake is that African Americans are seeing a subset of physicians with lower rates of both ordering genetic tests and referring patients for genetic testing [94], as physicians with primarily ethnic minority patients are less likely to have ordered genetic tests or referred patients to genetic testing services than physicians with a lower proportion of ethnic minority patients [116].

Finally, while research is beginning to address these multiple explanations for ethnic disparities in genetic testing knowledge and uptake, it is important to note that African Americans and Whites have received the most attention from researchers. Very few studies focus on the knowledge of, interest in, and actual uptake of genetic testing among Latinos or Asian-Americans. Latinas may be particularly important to study, as their knowledge of genetic testing is even lower than that of African American women, and Latinas have reported greater perceived disadvantages (such as anticipating feeling ashamed if they tested positive) of cancer genetic testing than African American women, although ethnicity did not predict these attitudes above and beyond the sociodemographic characteristics of income, education, language preference, and years in the USA [104]. Furthermore, medical mistrust and a prefer-

ence for speaking Spanish predicted greater perceived disadvantages of genetic testing above and beyond ethnicity, sociodemographic factors, and genetic testing awareness.

Extending the Study of Psychological and Behavioral Outcomes to Rare Hereditary Cancer Syndromes

Finally, as previously noted, over 50 hereditary cancer syndromes have been identified. Each one of these conditions is associated with its own unique cancer risks, with some being highly penetrant. For many of these syndromes, there are limited data indicating the optimal approaches for managing the cancer risk to direct patient decision making. There are also correspondingly limited data on psychological and behavioral outcomes of counseling and genetic testing.

Li–Fraumeni syndrome (LFS) and Von Hippel–Lindau (VHL) are two examples of highly penetrant, rare hereditary cancer syndromes. As shown in Table 3.2, these syndromes have quite different properties from the major cancer syndromes for which genetic testing outcomes have been extensively studied. Specifically, these syndromes are associated with the development of cancer in early childhood and a very high-risk for cancer development in multiple parts of the body rather than one or two predominant cancer risks. Due to the rarity of these syndromes, there are little validated data on the effectiveness of screening and preventive approaches available for patients and families receiving these types of diagnoses.

Li–Fraumeni syndrome. Li–Fraumeni syndrome is caused by mutations in the *p53* gene, which confers a 50% risk of developing cancer by age 30 and a 90% lifetime cancer risk. Individuals with LFS are at risk for cancers throughout the body and the most common cancers seen are brain, breast, osteosarcomas, soft tissue sarcomas, lung, hematologic, and adrenocortical [7]. Because the entire body is at high risk for cancer development, screening to ensure early detection is extremely difficult, and to date there is only one small study showing improved survival from an aggressive screening protocol [117]. Due to lack of clear preventive strategies, rates of genetic testing among families with LFS have been low, with three studies reporting uptake rates of approximately 39–55% [118–120]. Low self-efficacy in dealing with a positive *p53* test result has been shown to be associated with greater cancer worry and greater decisional conflict about having *p53* testing [121]. The issues of self-efficacy for managing positive results may be particularly important in LFS families because of the lack of clear options for mitigating cancer risk. A study of a Dutch cohort of LFS families did not find significant differences in distress between those testing positive or negative or those deciding not to be tested. However, as with other hereditary syndromes, those with low levels of social support were more likely to have clinically significant levels of distress regardless of the outcome of testing [120]. It is important to note that the few studies looking at the outcomes of genetic testing in families with LFS have only looked at short-term outcomes, and it is possible that there may be adverse long-term effects of living with elevated risk for multiple cancers and uncertainty regarding the efficacy of cancer screening recommendations.

Von Hippel–Lindau. Von Hippel–Lindau is another rare hereditary cancer syndrome caused by mutations in the *vhl* gene. Individuals with this condition develop multiple benign and malignant tumors beginning in adolescence. The retina, cerebellum, spine, kidneys, pancreas, and adrenal glands are the primary organs affected, and as is the case with LFS, rigorous screening is required to evaluate all at-risk areas, and there are no effective risk-reducing options. A study of 171 individuals who had previously undergone genetic testing for VHL found that overall 40% of participants experienced clinically significant levels of VHL-related distress. Carriers reported the most distress (50% of carriers), but 36% of noncarriers also reported significant distress. Noncarriers' reportedly high distress may be due to concern for affected family members' health, the burdens of

being a caregiver for affected family members, or feelings of guilt for being spared [122].

The model we have presented highlights multiple aspects of the risk for cancer, including age of onset and risk for multiple cancers, in conjunction with the availability of effective screening options, as key determinants of the psychological and behavioral outcomes of genetic testing. Understanding how members of families with these rare syndromes cope with heightened uncertainty, high penetrance, and limited early detection options represents an important goal for future research and clinical application.

Conclusion

To ask how people cope with the knowledge of increased cancer risk following genetic testing misses the point that many members of high-risk families have grown up with this risk and are already keenly aware of it based on their experience with multiple family members. Instead, an emerging view is that predictive genetic testing for hereditary cancer risk may best be seen as an important step in an ongoing process of managing both psychological and behavioral aspects of familial cancer risk [3]. Consistent with this view, we presented an organizing framework for future research on antecedents and consequences of hereditary cancer risk counseling and testing for different cancer syndromes. This framework situates hereditary cancer risk counseling and testing as tools to be used by patients and their families in an ongoing process of managing familial cancer risk and psychological concerns arising from awareness of this risk.

Our review demonstrated that hereditary cancer risk counseling and testing have a powerful impact on screening adherence, other risk-reducing behaviors such as prophylactic surgery, and in the case of hereditary melanoma, primary prevention behaviors such as reduction of UVR exposure. These findings suggest that hereditary cancer risk counseling and testing may play a role not only in potentially life-saving early detection efforts, but also in proactive efforts to reduce one's risk of developing cancer [4]. As shown in our program of research on familial melanoma, these efforts extend beyond individual patients to family members, particularly minor children [37, 62].

With regard to psychological outcomes, our review suggests that early concerns that cancer genetic testing would induce enduring general psychological distress are not generally supported by research. However, there is increasing recognition that there may be multiple different trajectories of outcomes and particular subgroups of patients who may be vulnerable to increased depression and/or anxiety. Being able to predict in advance who these patients will be in order to offer them additional support will allow for more targeted and successful intervention efforts.

Moving beyond depression, anxiety, and cancer worry, studies of other psychological outcomes indicate that patients often report both costs and benefits of hereditary risk counseling and testing. Qualitative data from structured interviews and open-ended questions on survey instruments suggest considerable benefits, some of which may not yet be adequately captured by standardized measures. Work on benefit finding and posttraumatic growth following other major life events, including adaptation to cancer, may prove useful here. As suggested by this review, it is important to understand how these different positive and negative outcomes of receiving positive test results may be related to the subsequent practice of screening behavior and the adoption of other recommended health behaviors to manage risk.

Finally, the ultimate goal in achieving an integrated view of both the costs and benefits of cancer risk counseling and testing is to understand how best to support individuals from high-risk families and to manage their personal and familial cancer risk. This understanding in turn will help maximize the potential benefits of personalized medicine for cancer prevention through early detection and treatment. Examining these processes among members of various ethnic minorities and among families facing risks for rare hereditary cancer syndromes remain priorities for future research.

Acknowledgments The authors were supported in part in the preparation of this chapter by Award Number R01CA158322 from the National Cancer Institute. The content is solely the responsibility of the authors and does not necessarily represent the official views of the National Cancer Institute or the National Institutes of Health. The authors acknowledge the use of core facilities supported by The National Institutes of Health 5P30CA420-14 awarded to Huntsman Cancer Institute from National Cancer Institute (NCI) Cancer Center Support Grants, the genetic counseling core facility supported by the Huntsman Cancer Foundation, and The National Institutes of Health Office of the Director 1KL2RR025763-01 National Center for Research Resources awarded to the University of Utah. We thank Marjan Champine and Tammy Stump for helpful comments on an earlier version of this manuscript and Angela Newman for assistance with its preparation.

References

1. Scheuner MT, McNeel TS, Freedman AN. Population prevalence of familial cancer and common hereditary cancer syndromes. The 2005 California Health Survey Interview. Genet Med. 2010;12(11):726–35.
2. Croyle RT, Smith KR, Botkin JR, Baty B, Nash J. Psychological responses to *BRCA1* mutation testing: preliminary findings. Health Psychol. 1997;16:63–72.
3. Gooding HC, Organista K, Burack J, Biesecker Bowles B. Genetic susceptibility testing from a stress coping perspective. Soc Sci Med. 2006;62:1880–90.
4. Aspinwall LG. Future-oriented thinking, proactive coping, and the management of potential threats to health and well-being. In: Folkman S, editor. The Oxford handbook of stress, health, and coping. New York: Oxford University Press; 2011. p. 334–65.
5. Trepanier A, Ahrens M, McKinnon W, Peters J, Stopfer J, Crumet Campbell S, Manley S, Culver JO, Acton R, Larsen-Haidle J, Correia LA, Bennett R, Pettersen B, Ferlita TD, Costalas JW, Hunt K, Donlon S, Skrzynia C, Farrell C, Callif-Daley F, Vockley CW. Genetic cancer risk assessment and counseling: recommendation of the National Society of Genetic Counselors. J Genet Couns. 2004;13: 83–114.
6. Robson ME, Storm CD, Weitzel J, et al. American Society of Clinical Oncology policy statement update: genetic testing for cancer susceptibility. J Clin Oncol. 2003;21(12):2397–406.
7. Lindor NM, McMaster ML, Lindor CJ, Greene MH, et al. Concise handbook of familial cancer susceptibility syndromes-second edition. J Natl Cancer Inst Monogr. 2008;38:1–93.
8. Rebbeck TR, Kauff ND, Domcheck SM. Meta-analysis of risk reduction estimates associated with risk-reducing salpingo-oophorectomy in *BRCA1* or

BRCA2 mutation carriers. J Natl Cancer Inst. 2009;101(2):80–7.

9. Kauff ND, Domceh SM, Friebel TM, et al. Risk-reducing salpingo-oophorectomy for the prevention of BRCA1 and BRCA2 associated breast and gynecological cancer: a multicenter prospective study. J Clin Oncol. 2008;26(8):1331–7.

10. Kurian AW, Sigal BM, Plevritis SK. Survival analysis of cancer risk reduction strategies for BRCA1/2 mutation carriers. J Clin Oncol. 2009;28:222–31.

11. Heshka JT, Palleschi C, Howeley H, Wilson B. Wells PS. A systematic review of perceived risks, psychological and behavioral impacts of genetic testing. Genet Med. 2008;10: 19–32.

12. Lerman C, Hughes C, Croyle RT, Main D, Durham C, Snyder C, Bonney A, Lynch JF, Narod SA, Lynch HT. Prophylactic surgery decisions and surveillance practices one year following BRCA1/2 testing. Prev Med. 2000;31(1):75–80.

13. Watson M, Foster C, Eeles R, Eccles D, Ashley S, Davidson R, Mackay J, Morrison PJ, Hopwood P, Evans DG. Psychosocial impact of breast/ovarian (BRCA1/2) cancer-predictive genetic testing in a UK multi-centre clinical cohort. Br J Cancer. 2004;91(10):1787–94.

14. Lynch HT, Snyder C, Lynch JF, Karatoprakli P, Trowonou A, Metcalfe K, Narod SA, Gong G. Patient responses to the disclosure of BRCA mutation tests in hereditary breast-ovarian cancer families. Cancer Genet Cytogenet. 2006;165:91–7.

15. Beery TA, Williams JK. Risk reduction and health promotion behaviors following genetic testing for adult-onset disorders. Genet Test. 2007;11:111–23.

16. Foster C, Watson M, Eeles R, et al. Predictive genetic testing for BRCA1/2 in a UK clinical cohort: three-year follow-up. Br J Cancer. 2007;96:718–24.

17. Schwartz MD, Isaacs C, Graves KD, Poggi E, Peshkin BN, Gell C, Finch C, Kelly S, Taylor KL, Perley L. Long-term outcomes of BRCA1/BRCA2 testing: risk reduction and surveillance. Cancer. 2012;118(2):510–7.

18. Jasperson KW, Tuohy TM, Neklason DW, Burt RW. Hereditary and familial colon cancer. Gastroenterology. 2010;138(6):2044–58.

19. Jarvinen HJ, Renkonen-Sinisalo L, Aktan-Colln K, et al. Ten years after mutation testing for Lynch syndrome: cancer incidence and outcome in mutation positive and mutation negative family members. J Clin Oncol. 2009;27(28):4793–7.

20. Kohlmann W, Gruber SB. Lynch syndrome. In: Pagon RA, Rirk TD, Dolan CR, Stephens K, editors. GeneReviews. Seattle: University of Washington; 2011. Seattle; 1993–2004.

21. Stoffel EM, Mercado RC, Kohlmann W, Ford B, et al. Prevalence and predictors of appropriate colorectal cancer surveillance in Lynch syndrome. Am J Gastroenterol. 2010;105(8):1851–60.

22. Hughes Halbert C, Lynch H, Lynch J, Main D, Kucharski S, Rustgi AK, Lerman C. Colon cancer screening practices following genetic testing for hereditary nonpolyposis colon cancer (HNPCC) mutations. Arch Intern Med. 2004;164:1881–7.

23. Douma KFL, Aaronson NK, Vasen HFA, Bleiker EMA. Psychosocial issues in genetic testing for familial adenomatous polyposis: a review of the literature. Psychooncology. 2008;17:737–45.

24. Levine FR, Coxworth JE, Stevenson DA, Tuohy T, Burt RW, Kinney AY. Parental attitudes, beliefs, and perceptions about genetic testing for FAP and colorectal cancer surveillance in minors. J Genet Couns. 2010;19(3):269–79.

25. Kinney AY, Hicken B, Simonsen SE, Venne V, Lowstuter K, et al. Colorectal cancer surveillance behaviors among members of typical and attenuated FAP families. Am J Gastroenterol. 2007;102(1): 153–62.

26. Michie S, Weinman J, Miller J, Collins V, Halliday J, Marteau TM. Predictive genetic testing: high risk expectations in the face of low risk information. J Behav Med. 2002;25:33–50.

27. Leachman SA, Carucci J, Kohlmann W, et al. Selection criteria for genetic assessment of patients with familial melanoma. J Am Acad Dermatol. 2009;61:677.e1–e14.

28. Bishop D, Demenais F, Goldstein A, Bergman W, Bishop J, Bressac-de Paillerets B, et al. Geographical variation in the penetrance of CDKN2A mutations for melanoma. J Natl Cancer Inst. 2002;94:894–903.

29. Aspinwall LG, Leaf SL, Kohlmann W, Dola ER, Leachman SA. Patterns of photoprotection following CDKN2A/p16 genetic test reporting and counseling. J Am Acad Dermatol. 2009;60:745–57.

30. Bergenmar M, Brandberg Y. Sunbathing and sun-protection behaviors and attitudes of young Swedish adults with hereditary risk for malignant melanoma. Cancer Nurs. 2001;24:341–50.

31. Brandberg Y, Jonell R, Broberg M, Sjoden P-O, Rosdahl I. Sun-related behaviour in individuals with dysplastic naevus syndrome. Acta Derm Venereol (Stockh). 1996;76:381–4.

32. Aspinwall LG, Taber JM, Leachman SA. Genetic testing and the proactive management of familial cancer risk. In: Directions in stress and coping research in chronic illness. Society for Behavioral Medicine, Seattle; April, 2010. Abstract available in Ann Behav Med, 39 (Suppl), s126.

33. Aspinwall LG, Leaf SL, Dola ER, Kohlmann W, Leachman SA. CDKN2A/p16 genetic test reporting improves early detection intentions and practices in high-risk melanoma families. Cancer Epidemiol Biomarkers Prev. 2008;17:1510–9.

34. Kasparian N, Meiser B, Butow P, Simpson J, Mann G. Genetic testing for melanoma risk: a prospective cohort study of uptake and outcomes among Australian families. Genet Med. 2009;11:265–78.

35. Vasen HF, Gruis NA, Frants RR, van Der Velden PA, Hille ET, Bergman W. Risk of developing pancreatic cancer in families with familial atypical multiple

mole melanoma associated with a specific 19 deletion of p16 (p16-Leiden). Int J Cancer. 2000;87: 809–11.

36. de Snoo F, Riedijk S, Tibben A, et al. Genetic testing in familial melanoma: uptake and implications. Psychooncology. 2008;17:790–6.

37. Aspinwall LG, Taber JM, Leaf SL, Kohlmann W, Leachman SA. Genetic testing for hereditary melanoma and pancreatic cancer: a longitudinal study of psychological outcome. Psycho-oncology. 2011. doi: 10.1002/pon.2080

38. Horowitz MJ, Field NP, Zanko A, Donnelly EF, Epstein C, Longo F. Psychological impact of news of genetic risk for Huntington disease. Am J Med Genet. 2001;103:188–92.

39. Lerman C, Croyle RT, Tercyak KP, Hamann HA. Genetic testing: psychological aspects and implications. J Consult Clin Psychol. 2002;70:784–97.

40. Marteau TM, Croyle RT. The new genetics: psychological responses to genetic testing. BMJ. 1998;316:693–6.

41. Broadstock M, Michie S, Marteau T. Psychological consequences of predictive genetic testing: a systematic review. Eur J Hum Genet. 2000;8:731–8.

42. Collins VR, Meiser B, Ukomunne OC, Gaff C, St John DJ, Halliday JL. The impact of predictive genetic testing for hereditary nonpolyposis colorectal cancer: three years after testing. Genet Med. 2007;9:290–7.

43. Hamilton JG, Lobel M, Moyer A. Emotional distress following genetic testing for hereditary breast and ovarian cancer: a meta-analytic review. Health Psychol. 2009;28:510–8.

44. Michie S, Bobrow M, Marteau T. Predictive genetic testing in children and adults: a study of emotional impact. J Med Genet. 2001;38:519–26.

45. Beran TM, Stanton AL, Kwan L, Seldon J, Bower JE, Vodermaier A, Ganz PA. The trajectory of psychological impact in BRCA1/2 genetic testing: does time heal? Ann Behav Med. 2008;36:107–16.

46. Meiser B, Collins V, Warren R, Gaff C, St John DJB, Young M-A, Harrop K, Brown J, Halliday J. Psychological impact of genetic testing for hereditary non-polyposis colorectal cancer. Clin Genet. 2004;66:502–11.

47. Van Roosmalen MS, Stalmeier PFM, Verhoef LCG, Hoekstra-Weebers JEHM, Oosterwijk JC, Hoogerbrogge N, Moog U, van Daal WAJ. Impact of BRCA1/2 testing and disclosure of a positive result on women affected and unaffected with breast or ovarian cancer. Am J Med Genet A. 2004; 124A:346–55.

48. Gritz ER, Peterson SK, Vernon SW, Marani SK, Baile WF, Watts BG, Amos CI, Frazier ML, Lynch PM. Psychological impact of genetic testing for hereditary nonpolyposis colorectal cancer. J Clin Oncol. 2005;23:1902–10.

49. Lodder L, Frets PG, Trijsburg RW, Meijers-Hiejboer J, Klijn JGM, Diuvenvoorden HJ, Tibben A, Wagner A, van der Meer CA, van den Ouweland AMW, Niermeijer MF. Psychological impact of receiving a BRCA1/BRCA2 test result. Am J Med Genet. 2001;98:15–24.

50. Smith AW, Dougall AL, Posluszny DM, Somers TJ, Rubinstein WS, Baum A. Psychological distress and quality of life associated with genetic testing for breast cancer risk. Psychooncology. 2008;17:767–73.

51. Ho SMY, Ho JWC, Bonanno GA, Chu ATW, Chan EMS. Hopefulness predicts resilience after hereditary colorectal cancer genetic testing: a prospective outcome trajectories study. BMC Cancer. 2010; 10:279.

52. Bonanno GA, Wortman CB, Lehman DR, Tweed RG, Haring M, Sonnega J, Carr D, Nesse RM. Resilience to loss and chronic grief: a prospective study from preloss to 18-months postloss. J Pers Soc Psychol. 2002;83(5):1150–64.

53. Hadley DW, Ashida S, Jenkins JF, Calzone KA, Kirsch IR, Koehlya LM. Colonoscopy use following mutation detection in Lynch syndrome: exploring a role for cancer screening in adaptation. Clin Genet. 2011;79:321–8.

54. O'Neill SC, Rini C, Goldsmith RE, Valdimarsdottir H, Cohen LH. Distress among women receiving uninformative BRCA1/2 results: 12-month outcomes. Psychooncology. 2009;18:1088–96.

55. Vos J, Otten W, van Asperen C, Jansen A, Menko F, Tibben A. The counsellees' view of an unclassified variant in BRCA1/2: recall, interpretation, and impact on life. Psychooncology. 2008;17:822–30.

56. Cella D, Hughes C, Peterman A, Chang C-H, Keshkin BN, Schwartz MD, Wenzel L, Lemke A, Marcus A, Lerman C. A brief assessment of concerns associated with genetic testing for cancer: the Multidimensional Impact of Cancer Risk Assessment (MICRA) questionnaire. Health Psychol. 2002;21: 564–72.

57. Hooker GW, Leventhal K-G, DeMarco T, Peshkin BN, Finch C, Wahl E, Rispoli Joines J, Brown K, Valdimarsdottir H, Schwartz MD. Longitudinal changes in patient distress following interactive decision aid use among BRCA1/2 carriers: a randomized trial. Med Decis Making. 2011;31(3):412–21.

58. Esplen MJ, Stuckless N, Hunter J, Liede A, Metcalfe K, Glendon G, Narod S, Kutler K, Scott J, Irwin E. The BRCA Self-Concept Scale: a new instrument to measure self-concept in BRCA1/2 mutation carriers. Psychooncology. 2009;18:1216–29.

59. Lim J, Macluran M, Price M, Bennett B, Butow P, kConFab Psychosocial Group. Short- and long-term impact of receiving genetic mutation results in women at increased risk for hereditary breast cancer. J Genet Couns. 2004;13(2):115–33.

60. Claes E, Evers-Kiebooms G, Denayer L, Decruyenaere M, Boogaerets A, Philippe K, Legius E. Predictive genetic testing for hereditary breast and ovarian cancer: psychological distress and illness representations 1 year following disclosure. J Genet Couns. 2005;14(5):349–63.

61. Claes E, Denayer L, Evers-Kiebooms G, Boogaerts A, Philippe K, Tejpar S, Devriendt K, Legius E. Predictive testing for hereditary nonpolyposis colorectal cancer: subjective perception regarding colorectal and endometrial cancer, distress, and health-related behavior at one year post-test. Genet Test. 2005;9:54–65.

62. Taber JM, Aspinwall LG, Kohlmann W, Dow R, Leachman SA. Parental preferences for CDKN2A/p16 testing of minors. Genet Med. 2010;12(12): 823–38.

63. Read CY, Perry DJ, Duffy ME. Design and psychometric evaluation of the Psychological Adaptation to Genetic Information Scale. J Nurs Scholarsh. 2005;37(3):203–8.

64. Berkenstadt M, Shiloh S, Barkai G, Katznelson MB, Goldman B. Perceived personal control (PPC): a new concept in measuring outcome of genetic counseling. Am J Med Genet. 1999;82(1):53–9.

65. Smets EM, Pieterse AH, Aalfs CM, Ausems MG, van Dulmen AM. The perceived personal control (PPC) questionnaire as an outcome of genetic counseling: reliability and validity of the instrument. Am J Med Genet A. 2006;140(8):843–50.

66. Esplen MJ, Stuckless N, Berk T, Butler K, Gallinger S. The FAP self-concept scale (adult form). Fam Cancer. 2009;8(1):39–50.

67. Petersen HV, Domanska K, Bendahl P-O, Wong J, Carlsson C, Bernstein I, Esplen MJ, Nilbert M. Validation of a self-concept scale for Lynch Syndrome in different nationalities. J Genet Counsel. 2011;20:308–13.

68. Kelly K, Leventhal H, Andrykowski M, Toppmeyer D, Much J, Dermody J, Marvin M, Baran J, Schwalb M. Using the common sense model to understand perceived cancer risk in individuals testing for BRCA1/2 mutations. Psychooncology. 2005;14:34–48.

69. Helgeson VS. Survivor centrality among breast cancer survivors: implications for well-being. Psychooncology. 2011;20:517–24.

70. Wiebe DJ, Berg CA, Palmer DL, Korbel C, Beveridge RM. Illness and the self: examining adjustment among adolescents with diabetes. Paper presented: Society of Behavioral Medicine, Washington, DC; 2002.

71. Low CA, Bower JE, Kwan L, Seldon J. Benefit finding in response to BRCA1/2 testing. Ann Behav Med. 2008;35:61–9.

72. Tedeschi RG, Calhoun LG. The posttraumatic growth inventory: measuring the positive legacy of trauma. J Trauma Stress. 1996;9:455–71.

73. Hamilton R, Williams JK, Bowers BJ, Calzone K. Life trajectories, genetic testing, and risk reduction decisions in 18–29 year old women at risk for hereditary breast and ovarian cancer. J Genet Counsel. 2009;18:147–59.

74. Shiloh S, Koehly L, Jenkins J, Martin J, Hadley D. Monitoring coping style moderates emotional reactions to genetic testing for hereditary nonpolyposis colorectal cancer: a longitudinal study. Psychooncology. 2008;17:746–55.

75. Leaf SL, Aspinwall LG, Leachman SA. God and agency in the era of molecular medicine: religious beliefs predict sun-protection behaviors following melanoma genetic test reporting. Arch Psychol Relig. 2010;32:87–112.

76. Aspinwall LG, Leaf SL, Leachman SA. Meaning and agency in the context of genetic testing for familial cancer. In: Wong PTP, editor. The human quest for meaning: Theories, research, and applications. 2nd ed. New York: Routledge; 2012; 457–94.

77. Kinney AY, Coxworth JE, Simonson SE, Fanning JB. Religiosity, spirituality, and psychological distress in African-Americans at risk for having a hereditary cancer predisposing gene mutation. Am J Med Genet C Semin Med Genet. 2009;151C:13–21.

78. Schwartz MD, Hughes C, Roth J, Main D, Peshkin BN, Isaacs C, et al. Spiritual faith and genetic testing decisions among high-risk breast cancer probands. Cancer Epidemiol Biomarkers Prev. 2000;9(4):381–5.

79. Aspinwall LG, Tedeschi RG. The value of Positive Psychology for Health Psychology: progress and pitfalls in examining the relation of positive phenomena to health. Ann Behav Med. 2010;39:4–15.

80. Aspinwall LG, Tedeschi RG. Of babies and bathwater: a reply to Coyne and Tennen's views on positive psychology and health. Ann Behav Med. 2010;39:27–34.

81. van Oostrom I, Meijers-Heijboer H, Lodder LN, Duivenvoorden HJ, van Gool AR, Seynaeve C, van der Meer CA, Klijn JGM, van Geel BN, Burger CW, Wladimiroff JW, Tibben A. Long-term psychological impact of carrying a BRCA1/2 mutation and prophylactic surgery: a 5-year follow-up study. J Clin Oncol. 2003;21(20):3867–74.

82. Tercyak KP, Peshkin BN, Brogan BM, DeMarco T, Pennanen MF, Willey SC, Magnant CM, Rogers S, Isaacs C, Schwartz MC. Quality of life after contralateral prophylactic mastectomy in newly diagnosed high-risk breast cancer patients who underwent BRCA1/2 gene testing. J Clin Oncol. 2007;25: 285–91.

83. Hay J, Ostroff J, Martin A, Serle N, Soma S, Mujumdar U, Berwick M. Skin cancer risk discussions in melanoma-affected families. J Cancer Educ. 2005;20:240–6.

84. Hay J, Shuk E, Zapolska J, Ostroff J, Lischewski J, Brady MS, Berwick M. Family communication patterns after melanoma diagnosis. J Fam Commun. 2009;9:209–32.

85. Kinney AY, Simonsen SE, Baty BJ, et al. Risk reduction and provider communication following genetic counseling and BRCA1 mutation testing in an African-American kindred. J Genet Couns. 2006;15(4):293–305.

86. Gaff CL, Clarke AJ, Atkinson P, Sivell S, Elwyn G, Iredale R, Thornton H, Dundon J, Shaw C, Edwards A. Process and outcome in communication of genetic information within families: a systematic review. Eur J Hum Genet. 2007;15:999–1011.

87. Peterson SK, Watts BG, Koehly LM, Vernon SW, Baile WF, Kohlmann WK, Gritz ER. How families

communicate about HNPCC genetic testing: findings from a qualitative study. Am J Med Genet C Semin Med Genet. 2003;119C(1):78–86 [Special Issue: Genetic Testing and the Family].
88. Hamann HA, Smith TW, Smith KR, Croyle RT, Ruiz JM, Kircher JC, Botkin JR. Interpersonal responses among sibling dyads testing for *BRCA1/BRCA2* gene mutations. Health Psychol. 2008;27(1):100–9.
89. Peters JA, Vadaparampil ST, Kramer J, Moser RP, Court LJ, Loud J, Greene MH. Familial testicular cancer: interest in genetic testing among high-risk family members. Genet Med. 2006;8(12):760–70.
90. Peters JA. Unpacking the blockers: understanding perceptions and social constraints of health communication in hereditary breast ovarian cancer (HBOC) susceptibility families. J Genet Couns. 2011;20(5): 450–64.
91. Wylie JE, Smith KR, Botkin JR. Effects of spouses on distress experienced by BRCA1 mutation carriers over time. Am J Med Genet C Semin Med Genet. 2003;119C(1):35–44.
92. Kinney AY, Bloor LE, Mandal D, Simonsen SE, Baty BJ, Holubkov R, Seggar K, Neuhausen S, Smith K. The impact of receiving genetic test results on general and cancer-specific psychologic distress among members of an African-American kindred with a *BRCA1* mutation. Cancer. 2005;104(11): 2508–16.
93. Marteau TM, French DP, Griffin SJ, Prevost AT, Sutton S, Watkinson C, Attwood S, Hollands GJ. Effects of communicating DNA-based disease risk estimates on risk-reducing behaviours. Cochrane Database Syst Rev. 2010;(10):CD007275.
94. Armstrong K, Micco E, Carney A, Stopfer J, Putt M. Racial differences in the use of *BRCA1/2* testing among women with a family history of breast or ovarian cancer. JAMA. 2005;293:1729–36.
95. Armstrong K, Calzone K, Stopfer J, Fitzgerald G, Coyne J, Weber B. Factors associated with decisions about clinical *BRCA1/2* testing. Cancer Epidemiol Biomarkers Prev. 2000;9:1251–4.
96. Thompson HS, Valdimarsdottir HB, Duteau-buck C, Guevarra J, Bovbjerg DH, Richmond-Avellaneda C, Amarel D, Godfrey D, Brown K, Offit K. Psychosocial predictors of *BRCA* counseling and testing decisions among urban African-American women. Cancer Epidemiol Biomarkers Prev. 2002;11:1579–85.
97. Halbert CH, Kessler L, Stopfer JE, Domchek S, Wileyto EP. Low rates of acceptance of *BRCA1* and *BRCA2* test results among African American women at increased risk for hereditary breast-ovarian cancer. Genet Med. 2006;8(9):576–82.
98. Riedijk SR, de Snoo RA, van Dijk S, Bergman W, van Haeringen A, Silberg S, van Elderen TM, Tibben A. Hereditary melanoma and predictive genetic testing: why not? Psychooncology. 2005;14(9):738–45.
99. American Cancer Society. Cancer facts & figures 2008. Atlanta: American Cancer Society; 2008.

http://www.cancer.org/acs/groups/content/@nho/documents/document/2008cafffinalsecuredpdf.pdf
100. Hall MJ, Olopade OI. Disparities in genetic testing: thinking outside the *BRCA* box. J Clin Oncol. 2006;24(14):2197–203.
101. Peters N, Rose A, Armstrong K. The association between race and attitudes about predictive genetic testing. Cancer Epidemiol Biomarkers Prev. 2004; 13(3):361–5.
102. Pagan JA, Su D, Li L, Armstrong K, Asch DA. Racial and ethnic disparities in awareness of genetic testing for cancer risk. Am J Prev Med. 2009;37(6): 524–30.
103. Armstrong K, Weber B, Ubel PA, Guerra C, Schwartz JS. Interest in BRCA1/2 testing in a primary care population. Prev Med. 2002;34(6):590–5.
104. Thompson HS, Valdimarsdottir HB, Jandorf L, Redd W. Perceived disadvantages and concerns about abuses of genetic testing for cancer risk: differences across African American, Latina and Caucasian women. Patient Educ Couns. 2003;51:217–27.
105. Harris Y, Gorelick PH, Samuels P, Bempong I, et al. Why African Americans may not be participating in clinical trials. J Natl Med Assoc. 1996;88(1):630–4.
106. Whetten K, Reif S, Whetten R, Murphy-McMillan LK. Trauma, mental health, distrust, and stigma among HIV-positive persons: implications for effective care. Psychosom Med. 2008;70:531–8.
107. Halbert CH, Weathers B, Delmoor E, Mahler B, Coyne J, Thompson HS, Have TT, Vaughn D, Malkowicz S, Bruce LD. Racial differences in medical mistrust among men diagnosed with prostate cancer. Cancer. 2009;115(11):2553–61.
108. Halbert CH, Armstrong K, Gandy Jr OH, Shaker L. Racial differences in trust in health care providers. Arch Intern Med. 2006;166:896–901.
109. Hammond WP, Matthews D, Mohottig D, Agyemang A, Corbie-Smith G. Masculinity, medical mistrust, and preventive health services delays among community-dwelling African-American men. J Gen Intern Med. 2010;25(12):1300–8.
110. Gonzalez JS, Penedo FJ, Llabre MM, Duran RE, Antoni MH, Schneiderman N, Horne R. Physical symptoms, beliefs about medications, negative mood, and long-term HIV medication adherence. Ann Behav Med. 2007;34(1):46–55.
111. Purnell JQ, Katz ML, Andersen BL, Palesh O, Figueroa-Moseley C, Jean-Pierre P, Bennett N. Social and cultural factors are related to perceived colorectal cancer screening benefits and intentions in African Americans. J Behav Med. 2010;33:24–34.
112. Dovidio JF, Penner LA, Albrecht TL, Norton WE, Gaertner SL, Shelton JN. Disparities and distrust: the implications of psychological processes for understanding racial disparities in health and health care. Soc Sci Med. 2008;67(3):478–86.
113. Sussner KM, Thompson HS, Valdimarsdottir HB, Redd WH, Jandorf L. Acculturation and familiarity with, attitudes towards and beliefs about genetic

testing for cancer risk within Latinas in East Harlem, New York City. J Genet Counsel. 2009;18:60–71.

114. Hughes C, Gomez-Caminero A, Benkendorf J, Kerner J, Isaacs C, Barter J, Lerman C. Ethnic differences in knowledge and attitudes about *BRCA1* testing in women at increased risk. Patient Educ Couns. 1997;32:51–62.

115. Charles S, Kessler L, Stopfer JE, Domchek S, Halbert CH. Satisfaction with genetic counseling for BRCA1 and BRCA2 mutations among African American women. Patient Educ Couns. 2006;63: 196–204.

116. Shields AE, Burke W, Levy DE. Differential use of available genetic tests among primary care physicians in the United States: results of a national survey. Genet Med. 2008;10(6):404–14.

117. Villani A, Tabori U, Schiffman J, et al. Biochemical and imaging surveillance in germline TP53 mutation carriers with Li-Fraumeni syndrome: a prospective observational study. Lancet Oncol. 2011;12(6): 559–67.

118. Patenaude AF, Schneider KA, Kieffer SA, et al. Acceptance of invitations for p53 and BRCA1 predisposition testing: factors influencing potential utilization of cancer genetic testing. Psychooncology. 1996;5:241–50.

119. Peterson SK, Pentz RD, Blanco AM, et al. Evaluation of a decision aid for families considering p53 genetic counseling and testing. Genet Med. 2006;8(4): 226–33.

120. Lammens CRM, Aaronson NK, Wagner A, et al. Genetic testing in Li-Fraumeni syndrome: uptake and psychosocial consequences. J Clin Oncol. 2010;28(18):3008–14.

121. Peterson SK, Pentz RD, Marani S, et al. Psychological functioning in persons considering genetic counseling and testing for Li-Fraumeni syndrome. Psychooncology. 2008;17:783–9.

122. Lammens CRM, Bleiker EMA, Verhoef S, et al. Psychosocial impact of von Hippel-Lindau disease: levels and sources of distress. Clin Genet. 2010; 77:483–92.

Mastectomy to Prevent Breast Cancer: Psychosocial Aspects of Women's Decision-Making

4

A. Fuchsia Howard, Lynda G. Balneaves, and Arminée Kazanjian

Introduction

The advent of genetic testing to determine whether a woman carries a genetic mutation (*BRCA1* or *BRCA2*) that predisposes her to hereditary breast and ovarian cancer has created the situation wherein women are faced with the decision of whether or not to undergo mastectomy to prevent breast cancer. This difficult decision varies from patient to patient and is profoundly shaped by social and psychological factors.

Women found to carry a BRCA1/2 mutation have a markedly increased probability of developing cancer. To manage their 45–87 % lifetime risk of breast cancer [1–3], *BRCA1/2* carriers have the option of ongoing breast cancer screening or risk-reducing mastectomy (RRM). In the majority of western counties, breast cancer screening (i.e., clinical breast exam, breast self exam, mammography, MRI, breast ultrasound) is recommended to *BRCA1/2* mutation carriers as a means of identifying cancers at an early stage when the prognosis of treatment is good, thus reducing the risk of dying from cancer. The most effective means of preventing breast cancer, however, is through RRM. RRM is the surgical removal of healthy breast tissue prior to the development of cancer, generally offered with the option of reconstructive surgery. This reduces a woman's risk of developing breast cancer by 95 % [4]. Given the significant impact of RRM on women'sbodies and their lives, it is considered a very personal decision that only a woman can make. Rather thanrecommend RRM, in Canada, the USA, and many European countries, it is generally framed as an optionfor women to discuss with a health care professional [5–7]. Although some women choose to do nothing, the majority of BRCA1/2 carriers face choosing between ongoing breast cancer screening and RRM. An understanding of how women make this difficult and complex decision is foundational to supporting women and guiding the development of decision support interventions.

Diversity in the uptake of RRM as well as the timing of this decision are important considerations. Perceived risk, decisional conflict and uncertainty, as well as psychological considerations and the family context are key aspects of this decision-making process. The degree of patient involvement in RRM decision-making is also influential. These psychosocial factors have important implications for the provision of decision support. In this chapter we review research pertaining to these issues.

A.F. Howard, R.N., Ph.D. (✉) • A. Kazanjian, Dr. Soc
School of Population and Public Health, Faculty of Medicine, The University of British Columbia, Vancouver, BC, Canada
e-mail: fuchsia.howard@ubc.ca

L.G. Balneaves, R.N., Ph.D.
School of Nursing, The University of British Columbia, Vancouver, BC, Canada

B.I. Carr and J. Steel (eds.), *Psychological Aspects of Cancer*,
DOI 10.1007/978-1-4614-4866-2_4, © Springer Science+Business Media, LLC 2013

Diversity in the Uptake and Timing of Decision-Making

Women's decisions about whether or not to undergo RRM appear to be shaped by their broader social and cultural context. Marked international differences in women's uptake of RRM have been documented and attributed to health care providers' recommendations and cultural variations [8, 9]. When compared across nine countries of residence, the uptake of RRM among *BRCA1/2* carriers was relatively minimal, ranging from 2.7 % in Poland to 36.3 % in the USA [8]. In contrast, at least 50 % of *BRCA1/2* carriers in Denmark and the Netherlands undergo RRM [10, 11]. Variation in attitudes towards RRM among health care professionals has also been documented. Geneticists in the Canadian city of Montreal were found to discuss RRM with *BRCA1/2* carriers more often than geneticists in Marseilles, France or Manchester, England [12]. The authors of this study suggested these differences could be attributed to wider cultural differences, for example in conceptualizations of health, prevention and risk management, paternalism and autonomy, and femininity. They also highlighted cultural differences among physicians in the interpretation of new scientific evidence as well as the adoption of scientific innovation. Physicians in places where there is leadership in genetic testing research will likely introduce new ideas and recommendations related to these technological innovations more rapidly into clinical practice [12]. Others have commented that it is difficult to determine whether geographic differences in RRM are due to differences in culturally based preferences and values of patients or to surgeon's partiality for surgery [9]. Regardless, the broader social and cultural context is clearly influential.

Not only is there diversity in women's uptake of RRM, but there also appears to be variation in the timing of decision-making. Most women are presented the option of RRM when they receive their genetic test results and the majority who undergo RRM do so within the first year or two [13]. For example, in a study of 211 *BRCA1/2* carriers in England, 59 % of *BRCA1* and 83 % of *BRCA2* carriers underwent RRM within 2 years of receiving a genetic test result [14]. Decisions made shortly following receipt of genetic test results are likely made quickly and do not involve extensive information processing or consultations with a range of individuals [15]. Some women have characterized their decision to undergo RRM as easy and a "no brainer" when considering their cancer risk [15, 16]. RRM may represent a strategy for coping with fear, anxiety and distress associated with their high-risk status. Some women who make RRM decisions shortly following receipt of genetic testing appear to have engaged in decision-making about RRM long before genetic testing based on their awareness of cancer in their family [15].

There is, however, a subgroup of women who delay this decision and undergo RRM years after receiving their genetic test results [13, 14, 17, 18]. Recent research has described some women's decision-making processes about RRM as dynamic, prolonged and changing over time [19, 20]. These women need more time to achieve a level of comfort with their RRM decisions that they are then able to follow through with [19]. Women in one study constructed the 'right time' to decide about RRM to be when they had taken enough time to deliberate, better medical and surgical options were available, and the health care system could meet their needs. The 'right time' was also once they had considered RRM in the context of their lives, coped with their emotions, and sorted through issues and conflicts within themselves, with their family, and with health care professionals [20]. Some women postponed deciding about RRM until important events occurred, such as marriage, or key phases of their lives were completed, such as childbearing [20]. Extending the decision-making process as a means of coping with emotions has also been reported by women deciding about breast cancer treatment [21]. Clearly, not all women decide about RRM in the same timeframe, rather, the timing of women's decisions appears to be influenced by social and emotional factors in the context of their lives.

Perceived Risk, Decisional Conflict and Uncertainty

Information given to women found to carry a *BRCA1/2* mutation often contains novel concepts, technical terms, statistics, and medical jargon. Women face the challenge of interpreting and personalizing complex information in the context of preexisting beliefs and strong emotions, as well as decisional conflict and uncertainty. These women often struggle to understand their future breast cancer risk and how their risk changes across the lifespan. The majority of carriers either overestimate or underestimate their cancer risk and interpret it as an absolute—either they will or they will not develop cancer [22]. Genetic test results and objective risk estimates have little influence on women's perceived cancer risk because individuals tend to base their estimates on long-standing beliefs and previous life experiences, often including cancer in their family [23, 24]. Women may reframe objective cancer risk estimates in a way that allows them to maintain their preexisting emotional, experiential, and relational sense of cancer risk [23]. Women's perceived levels of breast cancer risk have important implications: heightened perceived cancer risk is associated with both increased anxiety among genetic mutation carriers [25] and with women's use of RRM [26].

It has been assumed that many women experience substantial decisional conflict when faced with the option of RRM [27, 28]. Decisional conflict occurs when the following exist: scientific uncertainty about the benefits and harms of treatment options, choices with large potential for gains and losses, value trade-offs in selecting a particular course of action, and potential regrets associated with a selected option [29]. In a study in Netherlands, women with the strongest feelings of anticipated regret, that is the amount of regret they thought they would have if they were diagnosed with breast cancer after rejecting the option of RRM, were more inclined toward RRM than women who expected to have less intense feelings of regret [30]. The authors suggested that the impact of anticipated regret on women's

decisions may represent women's attempts to cope with uncertainty. Tan and colleagues [31] found that the two most important reasons for women to postpone RRM were uncertainty about proceeding with surgery and the need for more risk information. The lack of conclusive information about the risk of breast cancer and the personal implications of RRM can be particularly problematic [19, 32, 33]. In an attempt to resolve their uncertainty about the potential impact of RRM on their lives women have reported spending significant time reviewing information, vacillating from one position to the other, and seeking additional sources of information, including stories from other women and additional medical opinions [15, 19]. Further research is needed to understand the impact of diverse opinions and advice on women's decisional conflict and uncertainty, as well as how women resolve conflict when differing opinions are garnered.

Psychological Considerations Associated with RRM

A positive *BRCA1/2* test result and subsequent discussions about the option of RRM can evoke strong emotions of anxiety, distress, fear and worry. Psychological distress is long standing for many women because of personal experiences of a previous cancer diagnosis and treatment, having witnessed family members living with cancer, or caring for affected relatives [15, 16, 23]. Women generally experience emotional distress shortly following receipt of their positive genetic test results, but their distress subsides within a year [34]. However, a subgroup of women experience prolonged emotional distress [35–37]. This is more common among women who have a history of depression, lost a relative to hereditary cancer, experienced past traumatic events, grew up in a "cancer family" (i.e., long standing family history of cancer) and have small children [38]. There is also evidence from one study that although most women's distress decreases the year following genetic testing, some experience a significant increase in anxiety and depression 5 years later [39]. It is possible that genetic testing alters levels of distress only temporarily, but that other factors, particularly RRM decisions, influence the intensity of distress long term.

Heightened levels of distress can interfere with a woman's capacity to absorb, interpret and remember information about RRM. Emotions are often the first automatic reaction to information and can guide subsequent information processing, judgment and interpretations [40, 41]. This is particularly salient because women are often distressed shortly after receiving their genetic test results, at which point they often consult health care professionals about their options. The majority of research with *BRCA1/2* mutation carriers suggests a positive relationship between distress, anxiety and decisions to undergo RRM in the year following genetic testing [17, 26, 42–44]. Women have reported perceiving their breasts as "time bombs" and RRM represented a strategy for managing distress and anxiety about developing cancer [45]. In contrast, other women have reported that the option of RRM is too emotionally overwhelming to consider and, thus, best avoided [15].

There is evidence that women also consider how surgery will affect their self-identity and self-concept while making decisions about RRM. A woman who identifies as a 'mutation carrier' might experience an increased sense of vulnerability and mortality associated with cancer and a loss of control over one's health [46, 47]. This could lead to further psychological distress, feelings of helplessness, and poor self-efficacy, interfering with a woman's ability to make RRM decisions. For many women, the decision about RRM also involves considering what the loss of their breasts will mean to them as a woman. Some women do not consider the loss of their breasts as significant [15, 16]. Others have reported questioning their ability to adapt to the functional consequences of RRM, including not being able to breastfeed and loss of breast sensitivity and related pleasure, and the effect this could have on their role as a mother or intimate partner [15]. Women's concerns about whether RRM, with or without reconstruction, will be disfiguring, negatively affect their body image and sexuality, and contribute to feelings of a loss of femininity and womanhood are also influential [15, 16, 48–51]. When considering RRM, some women reflect on their willingness,

readiness or ability to face these challenges to their self-concept [15]. At times women resist changes in their self-concept and decide against RRM as a way to reinforce current perceptions of themselves (e.g., a woman with two breasts), while at other times, RRM may facilitate changes in self-concept that women are willing and able to accept (e.g., a woman who does not attach much significance to her breasts). In other words, accommodating shifts in self-concept, particularly related to womanhood, appears to be an integral part of the RRM decision-making process.

Family Matters

The family context, particularly family experiences of cancer and family roles and responsibilities, create resources and demands that appear to strongly influence women's RRM decisions. Women draw on their family members' experiences of having had cancer and breast surgery. In general, women who carry *BRCA1/2* mutations and are aware of a family history of breast cancer, particularly from a young age, are more likely to undergo RRM [13, 17, 18, 52]. Women also rely heavily on the RRM experiences of their siblings and other family members who are *BRCA1/2* mutation carriers to guide their own decisions about RRM [19]. Women who witnessed family members cope with complications associated with breast surgery or reconstruction might be fearful of developing similar complications and avoid RRM, whereas women whose family members have had good surgical outcomes might be motivated to undergo RRM.

For some women, decisions about RRM are interwoven with their desire to fulfill their obligations to support and care for their family [15, 51]. RRM is perceived by some women as providing the best chance of survival. This then enables them to fulfill their obligations to their family and prevent family members from having to become caregivers in the event of a cancer diagnosis [51, 53]. In contrast, other women have reported deciding against RRM because of the long convalescence required following surgery and the effect this would have on their ability to provide practical and economic support to their family [51]. In countries such as the USA, where health insurance coverage for these procedures varies significantly and individuals without insurance coverage have to pay out-of-pocket [54], the financial burden might have substantial implications for a woman and her family and act as a barrier to RRM. Research in this area is currently needed. Concerns about the significant time and financial costs of travel and childcare associated with undergoing RRM can also be significant for women living in rural areas [15].

Many women involve family members in the decision-making process because this is in accordance with their family norms. Moreover, women often perceived that their overall health and the function of their bodies have implications for their intimate relationship status and the lives of others, particularly spouses [15, 50]. Although many family members are supportive of women who are faced with the choice of RRM, other family members complicate the decision-making process by avoiding discussions about RRM, or disagreeing or negatively reacting to a woman's decision [15, 55]. Wanting to remain sensitive to family members' concerns, some women have described postponing their decisions about RRM until conflicts with family members were resolved [15]. Women have reported that their attempts to balance the needs of others with their own needs occasionally constrains their RRM decision-making [15, 51, 56].

Patient Involvement

In contrast to decisions about surgery to treat breast cancer wherein shared decision-making is considered the goal [57], decisions about RRM are made primarily by women, with some input from health care professionals. This is largely the result of RRM being framed as optional rather than recommended and of the predominant nondirective approach used by health care practitioners during genetic counseling. The underlying assumption of a nondirective approach is that by providing patients with the appropriate information in a neutral and nondirective manner, they will be able to reach a decision that reflects their

own values and is consistent with their preferences [58, 59]. Although a nondirective approach is appropriate for many women, for some, this complicates the decision-making process regarding RRM because they want more direction from health care professionals [15].

Some researchers consider nondirective decision support inadequate and have advocated for incorporating a shared decision-making approach in such circumstances [60, 61]. Shared decision-making requires at least two participants (the patient and the physician) be involved, the sharing of information between both parties, the building of a consensus about the preferred treatment, and agreement on the final decision [57]. Research on treatment decision-making among breast cancer patients demonstrates marked variation in patient's desire for involvement in treatment decisions, ranging from wanting an active or shared role to preferring a passive role or to delegate the decision to their physician [62–65]. Among these patients, achieving a match between actual and preferred involvement is critical because this correspondence is a strong predictor of patient satisfaction, which in turn, is a key determinant of psychological well-being and quality care [66–69]. Whether a nondirective or a shared decision-making approach is more appropriate for decisions about RRM remains to be seen. Alternatively, shared decision-making could complement a nondirective approach by providing guidance about how to engage patients in determining or negotiating the degree of desired involvement of health care professionals [60]. If shared decision-making is integrated into the provision of RRM decision support, it will be important to asses each woman's preferred level of involvement and her desire for family involvement.

Decision Support and Interventions

Decisions about RRM vary substantially from patient to patient and are shaped by women's social and psychological contexts. This challenges health care professionals to move beyond the current emphasis on cognitive processing of probabilities, risks and benefits as the primary focus when delivering decision support. Decision support and interventions are required that focus on perceived risk, decisional conflict, and uncertainty, as well as a woman's emotional well-being, her self-identity, and her relationships.

Considering how women's perceived risk, decisional conflict, and uncertainty shape decisions about RRM can motivate, but also prolong and complicate, the decision-making process, efforts to address these issues are likely to be beneficial. Appropriate strategies may include various means of communicating different types of information, individualizing this information where possible, and assisting women to explore their preferences and values associated with the risks and benefits [70]. A decision aid for RRM has demonstrated effectiveness in decreasing decisional conflict [27]. However, this decision aid did not reduce psychological distress. Moreover, not all decisional conflict or uncertainty can be reduced because women are faced with broad ranges of probabilities about their likelihood of developing breast cancer and there are numerous unanswered questions about how and when cancer might develop. Thus, it is imperative that women are assisted to manage this inherent uncertainty. Providing psychological support and interventions aimed at coping with uncertainty might also help women with RRM decisions.

Incorporating standard psychological assessments and supports into genetic counseling is warranted to detect and manage psychological distress and to help women considering RRM come to an informed decision [17, 45, 58]. Patient assessment tools to screen for psychological distress among BRCA1/2 carriers are currently under development and testing [71, 72]. Tools to assess the degree to which a woman's self-identity is threatened by RRM decisions include the recently developed self-concept scale [73]. In addition, counseling strategies are needed that will help women reflect on their feelings about the effects of RRM on femininity, sexuality and body image may be helpful [70]. In the meantime, offering psychological consultations to women who are trying to make decisions about RRM may be appropriate. In the study by Patenaude et al. [74], all women considering RRM believed psycho-

logical consultation would aid their decision-making. Tan et al. [31] also reported that 70 out of 73 women accepted an optional psychological consultation prior to RR surgery, and that additional psychological support was given to 31 % of participants prior to and 14 % after RRM. This indicates a high level of acceptability of psychological consultations. Yet, this may be a controversial recommendation among health care professionals who are concerned that incorporating routine psychological assessments and consultations into decision support is paternalistic.

Research provides evidence that acknowledging family influences in RRM decisions is warranted. Tools to assist women with mobilizing support and resources, communicating with family members about hereditary breast cancer risk management, and working through family conflict may be useful [56]. Family interventions may also be important for some, and specialist staff with expertise in family dynamics may be required for such interventions. Family members might benefit from educational and psychosocial support that involves the provision of information, clarification of misconceptions, exploration of the impact of RRM on the family, and the promotion of family coping and adjustment to the decision-making process [74].

Researchers have only recently developed interventions to support RRM decision-making and further work is needed to evaluate and compare these different approaches [19, 75, 76]. Moreover, efforts towards developing novel decision support interventions that take into account individual differences and changes that occur over time and across different social and psychological contexts will be as useful next step.

Conclusion

A woman's decision about RRM is much more complex than interpreting the statistical risk of developing breast cancer. Women's decisions appear to grounded in broader social and cultural contexts and vary regarding when decisions are made. Women's perceived risk of developing breast cancer, as well as decisional conflict and uncertainty, appear to be significant and add to the complexity of these decisions. Emotional distress and self-identity also factor into women's decisions and can act as motivators to engage or disengage in decision-making. Considering the role that family members play, women's decision-making ought to be conceptualized as a relational endeavor. Supporting women to make decisions that align with their values and beliefs and optimizes quality of life while also acknowledging the substantial risk of breast cancer is no simple task. Decision support and interventions that are available when women want and need support and that address perceived risk, uncertainty, emotional and relational aspects of women's decision-making are likely to be beneficial [15, 20]. It will be important in future research to develop, evaluate and compare different approaches to supporting women who are faced with the option of RRM.

The era of 'new genetics' has presented the challenge of translating genetic technologies and information into improved health and well-being. If we are to realize the full benefits of technological advances in science, then as our understanding of biological processes and risks evolves, so too must our understanding of human behavior related to those advances. In other words, to maximize health outcomes, not only must we personalize health care services based on patients' genetic profiles, but we must also personalize health care services based on patients' psychosocial profiles. Cancer care is no exception.

References

1. Antoniou A, Pharoah PD, Narod S, et al. Average risks of breast and ovarian cancer associated with BRCA1 or BRCA2 mutations detected in case series unselected for family history: A combined analysis of 22 studies. Am J Hum Genet. 2003;72:1117–30.
2. Evans DG, Shenton A, Woodward E, Lalloo F, Howell A, Maher ER. Penetrance estimates for BRCA1 and BRCA2 based on genetic testing in a clinical cancer genetics service setting: Risks of breast/ovarian cancer quoted should reflect the cancer burden in the family. BMC Cancer. 2008;8:155.
3. Ford D, Easton DF, Stratton M, et al. Genetic heterogeneity and penetrance analysis of the BRCA1 and BRCA2 genes in breast cancer families. the breast cancer linkage consortium. Am J Hum Genet. 1998;62:676–89.
4. Rebbeck TR, Friebel T, Lynch HT, et al. Bilateral prophylactic mastectomy reduces breast cancer risk in BRCA1 and BRCA2 mutation carriers: The PROSE study group. J Clin Oncol. 2004;22:1055–62.
5. Horsman D, Wilson BJ, Avard D, et al. Clinical management recommendations for surveillance and risk-reduction strategies for hereditary breast and ovarian cancer among individuals carrying a deleterious BRCA1 or BRCA2 mutation. J Obstet Gynaecol Can. 2007;29:45–60.
6. Nelson HD, Huffman LH, Fu R, Harris EL. U.S. Preventive Services Task Force. Genetic risk assessment and BRCA mutation testing for breast and ovarian cancer susceptibility: Systematic evidence review for the U.S. preventive services task force. Ann Intern Med. 2005;143:362–79.
7. National Comprehensive Cancer Network. NCCN clinical practice guidelines in oncology. Genetic/Familial high-risk assessment: Breast and ovarian. NCCN; 2009;V.I. Available from: http://www.nccn.org.
8. Metcalfe KA, Birenbaum-Carmeli D, Lubinski J, et al. International variation in rates of uptake of preventive options in BRCA1 and BRCA2 mutation carriers. Int J Cancer. 2008;122:2017–22.
9. Julian-Reynier CM, Bouchard LJ, Evans DG, et al. Women's attitudes toward preventive strategies for hereditary breast or ovarian carcinoma differ from one country to another: Differences among english, french, and canadian women. Cancer. 2001;92:959–68.
10. Skytte A. Risk-reducing mastectomy and salpingo-oophorectomy in unaffected BRCA mutation carriers: Uptake and timing*. Clin Genet. 2010;77:342–9.
11. Meijers-Heijboer EJ, Verhoog LC, Brekelmans CT, et al. Presymptomatic DNA testing and prophylactic surgery in families with a BRCA1 or BRCA2 mutation. Lancet. 2000;355:2015–20.
12. Bouchard L, Blancquaert I, Eisinger F, et al. Prevention and genetic testing for breast cancer: Variations in medical decisions. Soc Sci Med. 2004;58:1085–96.
13. Friebel TM, Domchek SM, Neuhausen SL, et al. Bilateral prophylactic oophorectomy and bilateral prophylactic mastectomy in a prospective cohort of unaffected BRCA1 and BRCA2 mutation carriers. Clin Breast Cancer. 2007;7:875–82.
14. Evans DG, Lalloo F, Ashcroft L, et al. Uptake of risk-reducing surgery in unaffected women at high risk of breast and ovarian cancer is risk, age, and time dependent. Cancer Epidemiol Biomarkers Prev. 2009;18: 2318–24.
15. Howard A, Balneaves LG, Bottorff JL, Rodney P. Preserving the self: The process of decision making about hereditary breast and ovarian cancer risk reduction. Qual Health Res. 2011;21:502.
16. McQuirter M, Castiglia LL, Loiselle CG, Wong N. Decision-making process of women carrying a BRCA1 or BRCA2 mutation who have chosen prophylactic mastectomy. Onc Nurs Society. 2010;37: 313–20.

17. Antill Y, Reynolds J, Young MA, et al. Risk-reducing surgery in women with familial susceptibility for breast and/or ovarian cancer. Eur J Cancer. 2006;42: 621–8.

18. Bradbury AR, Ibe CN, Dignam JJ, et al. Uptake and timing of bilateral prophylactic salpingo-oophorectomy among BRCA1 and BRCA2 mutation carriers. Genet Med. 2008;10:161–6.

19. McCullum M, Bottorff JL, Kelly M, Kieffer SA, Balneaves LG. Time to decide about risk-reducing mastectomy: A case series of BRCA1/2 gene mutation carriers. BMC Womens Health. 2007;7:3.

20. Howard AF, Bottorff JL, Balneaves LG, Kim-Sing C. Women's constructions of the 'right time' to consider decisions about risk-reducing mastectomy and risk-reducing oophorectomy. BMC Womens Health. 2010;10:24.

21. Pierce PF. Deciding on breast cancer treatment: A description of decision behavior. Nurs Res. 1993;42:22–2.

22. Hamilton R. Genetics: Breast cancer as an exemplar. Nurs Clin North Am. 2009;44:327–38.

23. d'Agincourt-Canning L. The effect of experiential knowledge on construction of risk perception in hereditary breast/ovarian cancer. J Genet Couns. 2005;14:55–69.

24. Kenen R. Ardern-Jones A, Eeles R. Family stories and the use of heuristics: Women from suspected hereditary breast and ovarian cancer (HBOC) families. Sociol Health Illn. 2003;25:838–65.

25. Rantala J, Platten U, Lindgren G, et al. Risk perception after genetic counseling in patients with increased risk of cancer. Hered Cancer Clin Pract. 2009;7:15.

26. Howard AF, Balneaves LG, Bottorff JL. Women's decision making about risk-reducing strategies in the context of hereditary breast and ovarian cancer: A systematic review. J Genet Couns. 2009;18(6): 578–97.

27. Metcalfe KA, Poll A, O'Connor A, et al. Development and testing of a decision aid for breast cancer prevention for women with a BRCA1 or BRCA2 mutation. Clin Genet. 2007;72:208–17.

28. Schwartz MD, Valdimarsdottir HB, DeMarco TA, et al. Randomized trial of a decision aid for BRCA1/ BRCA2 mutation carriers: Impact on measures of decision making and satisfaction. Health Psychol. 2009;28:11–9.

29. O'Connor AM, Wennberg JE, Legare F, et al. Toward the 'tipping point': Decision aids and informed patient choice. Health Aff (Millwood). 2007;26:716–25.

30. van Dijk S, van Roosmalen MS, Otten W, Stalmeier PF. Decision making regarding prophylactic mastectomy: Stability of preferences and the impact of anticipated feelings of regret. J Clin Oncol. 2008;26: 2358–63.

31. Tan MB, Bleiker EM, Menke-Pluymers MB, et al. Standard psychological consultations and follow up for women at increased risk of hereditary breast cancer considering prophylactic mastectomy. Hered Cancer Clin Pract. 2009;7:6–8P.

32. Meiser B, Butow P, Friedlander M, et al. Intention to undergo prophylactic bilateral mastectomy in women at increased risk of developing hereditary breast cancer. J Clin Oncol. 2000;18:2250–7.

33. Metcalfe KA, Liede A, Hoodfar E, Scott A, Foulkes WD, Narod SA. An evaluation of needs of female BRCA1 and BRCA2 carriers undergoing genetic counselling. J Med Genet. 2000;37:866–74.

34. Hamilton JG, Lobel M, Moyer A. Emotional distress following genetic testing for hereditary breast and ovarian cancer: A meta-analytic review. Health Psychol. 2009;28:510–8.

35. Coyne JC, Kruus L, Racioppo M, Calzone KA, Armstrong K. What do ratings of cancer-specific distress mean among women at high risk of breast and ovarian cancer? Am J Med Genet A. 2003;116:222–8.

36. Mikkelsen EM, Sunde L, Johansen C, Johnsen SP. Psychosocial consequences of genetic counseling: A population-based follow-up study. Breast J. 2009;15: 61–8.

37. Smith AW, Dougall AL, Posluszny DM, Somers TJ, Rubinstein WS, Baum A. Psychological distress and quality of life associated with genetic testing for breast cancer risk. Psychooncology. 2008;17:767–73.

38. Meiser B. Psychological impact of genetic testing for cancer susceptibility: An update of the literature. Psychooncology. 2005;14:1060–74.

39. van Oostrom I, Meijers-Heijboer H, Lodder LN, et al. Long-term psychological impact of carrying a BRCA1/2 mutation and prophylactic surgery: A 5-year follow-up study. J Clin Oncol. 2003;21:3867–74.

40. Reyna VF. A theory of medical decision making and health: Fuzzy trace theory. Med Decis Making. 2008;28:850–65.

41. Zajonc RB. Feeling and thinking: Preferences need no inferences. Am Psychol. 1980;35:151.

42. Claes E, Evers-Kiebooms G, Decruyenaere M, et al. Surveillance behavior and prophylactic surgery after predictive testing for hereditary breast/ovarian cancer. Behav Med. 2005;31:93–105.

43. Lodder LN, Frets PG, Trijsburg RW, et al. One year follow-up of women opting for presymptomatic testing for BRCA1 and BRCA2: Emotional impact of the test outcome and decisions on risk management (surveillance or prophylactic surgery). Breast Cancer Res Treat. 2002;73:97–112.

44. Unic I, Verhoef LC, Stalmeier PF, van Daal WA. Prophylactic mastectomy or screening in women suspected to have the BRCA1/2 mutation: A prospective pilot study of women's treatment choices and medical and decision-analytic recommendations. Med Decis Making. 2000;20:251–62.

45. Brain K, Gravell C, France E, Fiander A, Gray J. An exploratory qualitative study of women's perceptions of risk management options for familial ovarian cancer: Implications for informed decision making. Gynecol Oncol. 2004;92:905–13.

46. Lim J, Macluran M, Price M, Bennett B, Butow P. kConFab Psychosocial Group. Short- and long-term impact of receiving genetic mutation results in women

at increased risk for hereditary breast cancer. J Genet Couns. 2004;13:115–33.

47. D'Agincourt-Canning L. A gift or a yoke? Women's and men's responses to genetic risk information from BRCA1 and BRCA2 testing. Clin Genet. 2006;70:462–72.

48. Helms RL, O'Hea EL, Corso M. Body image issues in women with breast cancer. Psychol Health Med. 2008;13:313–25.

49. Hamilton R, Williams JK, Skirton H, Bowers BJ. Living with genetic test results for hereditary breast and ovarian cancer. J Nurs Scholarsh. 2009;41:276–83.

50. Staton AD, Kurian AW, Cobb K, Mills MA, Ford JM. Cancer risk reduction and reproductive concerns in female BRCA1/2 mutation carriers. Fam Cancer. 2008;7:179–86.

51. Hallowell N. 'You don't want to lose your ovaries because you think 'I might become a man''. Women's perceptions of prophylactic surgery as a cancer risk management option. Psychooncology. 1998;7:263–75.

52. Metcalfe KA, Foulkes WD, Kim-Sing C, et al. Family history as a predictor of uptake of cancer preventive procedures by women with a BRCA1 or BRCA2 mutation. Clin Genet. 2008;73:474–9.

53. Hatcher MB, Fallowfield LJ. A qualitative study looking at the psychosocial implications of bilateral prophylactic mastectomy. Breast. 2003;12:1–9.

54. Kuerer HM, Hwang ES, Anthony JP, et al. Current national health insurance coverage policies for breast and ovarian cancer prophylactic surgery. Ann Surg Oncol. 2000;7:325–32.

55. Douglas HA, Hamilton RJ, Grubs RE. The effect of BRCA gene testing on family relationships: A thematic analysis of qualitative interviews. J Genet Couns. 2009;18(5):418–35.

56. Etchegary H, Miller F, deLaat S, Wilson B, Carroll J, Cappelli M. Decision-making about inherited cancer risk: Exploring dimensions of genetic responsibility. J Genet Couns. 2009;18:252–64.

57. Charles C, Gafni A, Whelan T. Shared decision-making in the medical encounter: What does it mean?(or it takes at least two to tango). Soc Sci Med. 1997;44:681–92.

58. Schwartz MD, Peshkin BN, Tercyak KP, Taylor KL, Valdimarsdottir H. Decision making and decision support for hereditary breast-ovarian cancer susceptibility. Health Psychol. 2005;24:S78–84.

59. Sharpe NF, Carter RF. Genetic Testing: Care, Consent, and Liability. Hoboken, NJ: Wiley; 2006.

60. Elwyn G, Gray J, Clarke A. Shared decision making and non-directiveness in genetic counselling. J Med Genet. 2000;37:135–8.

61. Smets E, van Zwieten M, Michie S. Comparing genetic counseling with non-genetic health care interactions: Two of a kind? Patient Educ Couns. 2007;68:225–34.

62. Levinson W, Kao A, Kuby A, Thisted RA. Not all patients want to participate in decision making. J Gen Intern Med. 2005;20:531–5.

63. Janz NK, Wren PA, Copeland LA, Lowery JC, Goldfarb SL, Wilkins EG. Patient-physician concordance: Preferences, perceptions, and factors influencing the breast cancer surgical decision. J Clin Oncol. 2004;22:3091.

64. Sabo B, St-Jacques N, Rayson D. The decision-making experience among women diagnosed with stage I and II breast cancer. Breast Cancer Res Treat. 2007;102:51–9.

65. Beaver K, Luker KA, Owens RG, Leinster SJ, Degner LF, Sloan JA. Treatment decision making in women newly diagnosed with breast cancer. Cancer Nurs. 1996;19:8.

66. Hack TF, Degner LF, Watson P, Sinha L. Do patients benefit from participating in medical decision making? longitudinal follow-up of women with breast cancer. Psychooncology. 2006;15:9–19.

67. Katz SJ, Hawley ST. From policy to patients and back: Surgical treatment decision making for patients with breast cancer. Health Aff. 2007;26:761.

68. Lantz PM, Janz NK, Fagerlin A, et al. Satisfaction with surgery outcomes and the decision process in a Population-Based sample of women with breast cancer. Health Serv Res. 2005;40:745–68.

69. Keating NL, Guadagnoli E, Landrum MB, Borbas C, Weeks JC. Treatment decision making in early-stage breast cancer: Should surgeons match patients' desired level of involvement? J Clin Oncol. 2002; 20:1473.

70. MacDonald DJ, Sarna L, Weitzel JN, Ferrell B. Women's perceptions of the personal and family impact of genetic cancer risk assessment: Focus group findings. J Genet Couns. 2010;19:148–60.

71. van Dooren S, Duivenvoorden HJ, Passchier J, et al. The distress thermometer assessed in women at risk of developing hereditary breast cancer. Psychooncology 2009;18:1080–87.

72. Esplen MJ, Cappelli M, Rayson D, et al. Psychosocial health service implications for genetic testing: A clinical and training needs assessment. Canadian Institute of Health Research Operating Grant. Retrieved December 6, 2009, from: http://www.cihr-irsc.gc.ca/e/28776.html#Oustanding

73. Esplen MJ, Stuckless N, Hunter J, et al. The BRCA self-concept scale: A new instrument to measure self-concept in BRCA1/2 mutation carriers. Psychooncology 2009;18:1216–29.

74. Patenaude AF, Orozco S, Li X, et al. Support needs and acceptability of psychological and peer consultation: Attitudes of 108 women who had undergone or were considering prophylactic mastectomy. Psychooncology 2008;17:831–43.

75. Esplen MJ, Hunter J, Leszcz M, et al. A multicenter study of supportive-expressive group therapy for women with BRCA1/BRCA2 mutations. Cancer. 2004;101:2327–40.

76. McKinnon W, Naud S, Ashikaga T, Colletti R, Wood M. Results of an intervention for individuals and families with BRCA mutations: A model for providing medical updates and psychosocial support following genetic testing. J Genet Couns. 2007;16:433–56.

Decision Aids in Advanced Cancer

5

Natasha B. Leighl and Mary Ann O'Brien

Decisions in Advanced Cancer

Treatment decision-making in advanced cancer remains a challenge. When the goal of treatment is not cure, both patients and their physicians may be reluctant to discuss frank details of limited prognosis, palliative goals of therapy, and initiate planning for end-of-life care. Decisions in advanced cancer are increasingly complex. The number of palliative systemic (i.e., drug therapy) and other options and available lines of treatment are rapidly growing. But most systemic and other treatments in advanced cancer are associated with only modest survival and quality of life benefits. However, whether an individual patient will benefit from treatment is uncertain, while at least some toxicity from treatment is almost guaranteed [1].

N.B. Leighl, M.D., M.M.Sc (Clin Epi), F.R.C.P.C (✉)
Divison of Medical Oncology/Hematology,
Princess Margaret Hospital, University of Toronto,
5-105 610 University Ave, Toronto, ON,
Canada M5G 2M9
e-mail: Natasha.Leighl@uhn.on.ca

M.A. O'Brien, Ph.D
Department of Family and Community Medicine,
University of Toronto, 500 University Avenue, 5th floor,
Toronto, ON, Canada M5G 1V7
e-mail: maryann.obrien@utoronto.ca

Informed Consent: What Do Advanced Cancer Patients Know?

Many studies suggest that the majority of patients do wish to discuss prognosis in advanced disease [2–4]. They also wish to be active participants in decision-making about their treatment and medical care, although this varies in the literature from 40 to 73 % desiring shared decision-making with their physician [2]. However, many are not equipped to make informed decisions about their care [5, 6]. Informed consent to treatment requires certain elements. These include a discussion of prognosis with and without treatment, a review of risks and benefits, and of alternative options. In a series of consultations with advanced oncology outpatients, Gattellari et al. documented that only 58 % were informed about life expectancy, 36 % discussed the impact of therapy on their quality of life, and only 44 % discussed supportive care alone, (i.e., no chemotherapy) as an alternative option [6]. In one British study, 26 of 37 advanced cancer outpatients were given either vague or no information on the impact of palliative chemotherapy on their survival [7]. While the quality of information on the internet is improving, often patient information materials are not in a useful format to help patients make informed decisions, or do not apply to their situation [8, 9].

In order to make informed choices about treatment in advanced cancer, patients and their families need to understand their prognosis, the impact of treatment and palliative goals of care, and

B.I. Carr and J. Steel (eds.), *Psychological Aspects of Cancer*,
DOI 10.1007/978-1-4614-4866-2_5, © Springer Science+Business Media, LLC 2013

options. Even when such information is given to patients, there may still be issues of misunderstanding. Studies have demonstrated that as many as one third of cancer patients misunderstand the information received [10, 11]. This misunderstanding may be related to physician and patient communication techniques, information overload, as well as patient anxiety and even denial. A study of 244 Australian cancer patients revealed that less than 20 % correctly estimated the chance of treatment achieving cure, prolonging life or palliating symptoms [11]. Denial and clarity of information were predictive of patient understanding. In addition, the information physicians give patients may be incorrect. Studies have shown that both physicians and patients may overestimate life expectancy and benefits of treatment [4, 12, 13]. Physicians may also often underestimate patients' desires for information and decision involvement in advanced cancer, and as few as 37 % would share realistic survival estimates with their advanced cancer patients [2, 4, 13–15].

Patient treatment decisions appear based on what they understand, or misunderstand, about their prognosis and options [16–18]. Weeks et al. studied 916 patients in hospital with advanced non-small cell lung cancer or colon cancer, and found that although doctors were accurate in their predictions of patient life expectancy, the majority of patients, 82 %, overestimated their life expectancy, and nearly 60 % were overly optimistic [16]. Those who were overly optimistic were nearly three times more likely to choose aggressive treatment over supportive care alone. However, their survival was not improved over those patients who chose supportive care alone.

Decision Aids as Decision-Making Support Tools

Many tools have been developed in order to enhance patient understanding, their decision involvement, and to increase the quality of decisions made. These include information booklets, question prompt lists, anxiety reduction techniques, communication training for both patients

and physicians, and decision aids (DAs) [2, 4, 19]. DAs are defined as "interventions designed to help people make specific and difficult choices among options by providing information on the options and outcomes relevant to the person's health status" [20]. In addition to information about options and outcomes, DAs provide support to patients in clarifying their values for those different health outcomes and treatment options, to facilitate decision-making.

Systematic reviews of randomized trials of DAs, including a recent review of 34 trials of DAs in cancer, have demonstrated that use of patient DAs results in higher knowledge scores, lower decisional conflict scores, and in some trials, increased patient participation in decision-making [19]. In general, no significant increases in anxiety are seen, and greater satisfaction with decision-making has been demonstrated in some trials with the use of DAs. The majority of DAs developed for decision-making in oncology address decisions about cancer screening, adjuvant therapy, and primary treatment in the setting of curable cancer. The development of DAs in the setting of incurable cancer has remained more challenging, where prognosis and goals of therapy clearly differ from decisions about potentially curative therapy. Balancing the potential benefits and toxicities of palliative therapy is complex, particularly when patients and families are unwilling to accept the goals of therapy. Patients with advanced cancer have greater need for emotional support, symptom control, as well as greater needs for accurate information and the opportunity to be involved in decisions about their care.

Decision Aids in Advanced Cancer

To date, at least nine studies have been published describing the development of DAs for patients with metastatic cancer, and one for locally advanced lung cancer [1, 3, 21–30]. One has been evaluated through a randomized trial, with 3 other randomized trials of DAs in advanced cancer ongoing [30, 31]. These are further described in Table 5.1.

Table 5.1 Randomized trials of decision aids in advanced cancer

First Author	Cancer Type	Study Design	Treatment options	Status/Outcomes
Leighl [30]	Metastatic colorectal cancer	RCT N=207	First-line chemotherapy + SC v. SC alone	Completed - DA significantly improved patient understanding; no increase in anxiety, no difference in decisional conflict, satisfaction, decisions, decision involvement
Oostendorp [31]	Advanced colorectal, breast or ovarian cancer	RCT N=170	Second-line chemotherapy + SC v. SC alone	Ongoing Primary outcome: patient well-being
Leighl [personal communication]	Advanced breast cancer	RCT	First-line chemo-therapy + SC v. SC alone	Closed for poor accrual 2007
Meropol	Advanced solid tumors	RCT N=720	Not reported	Accrual completed NCT 00244868 Primary outcomes: satisfaction with patient-physician communication, decisional conflict, treatment options expectations
Tyson	Stage III or IV non-small cell lung cancer	RCT N not reported	Not reported	Ongoing NCT00579215
Yun [34]	Advanced cancer patients' caregivers	RCT N=444	Discuss terminal prognosis versus controlling cancer pain (control)	Completed DA did not change frequency of discussion of terminal prognosis but did decrease caregiver decisional conflict over 6 months, depression at 1 month
Volandes	Advanced solid tumours (some restrictions on lines of therapy) with less than 1 year prognosis	RCT N=150	CPR versus no CPR at end of life	Ongoing NCT01241929 Primary outcome: Preferences for CPR

RCT: randomized controlled trial; SC: supportive care

In advanced ovarian cancer, Elit and colleagues developed a decision board to elicit patient preferences for different treatment options [21]. In the board, two chemotherapy options were described for patients with suboptimally debulked ovarian cancer, including potential side effects and disease outcomes. Although currently only one of the treatment options described is still widely used, the board was used to provide prognostic information to 98 % of patients, which was previously uncommon. It was further shown to be a reliable, valid method of sharing information about advanced ovarian cancer with patients.

A number of DAs have been developed for patients with advanced lung cancer, given the poor prognosis of this disease and modest outcomes with treatment. Fiset et al. developed a DA for patients with metastatic non–small-cell lung cancer considering supportive care (including palliative radiotherapy) with or without first-line chemotherapy, a workbook and an audiotape for patients to take home after the oncology consultation [22]. The aid improved patient knowledge of options and outcomes, and reduced decisional conflict. Most physicians and patients reviewing the aid found it acceptable, although as many as 20 % of patients were upset by the prognostic information. For patients with locally advanced (Stage III inoperable) non-small cell lung cancer, Brundage and colleagues developed a DA to help patients decide between palliative or short course radiotherapy (5 fractions) and radical chemoradiation (30 fractions, concurrent vinorelbine/cisplatin) [23]. After initial development in surrogate patients [24], they tested the aid in patients considering a treatment decision. The aid describes the different treatment options and side effects associated with each treatment choice, including the impact on physical and social functioning. Structured interviews were then conducted to complete trade-off exercises, clarifying the patient's values for median, 1- and 3-year survival with each treatment option. While feasible and considered useful by patients to complete, implementation in clinic has been hampered by the lack of resources to conduct in depth, structured interviews in a busy outpatient clinical setting. Another DA has been developed for patients with metastatic non-small cell lung cancer, with a booklet that physicians can use in the consultation to review prognostic information, treatment options and decision-making between supportive care (including palliative radiotherapy) with or with first-line palliative platinum-based chemotherapy [25]. Patients can then take the booklet and an accompanying audiotape home for further review before a final decision is made. While the aid improved patient knowledge using a pre–post test design, all advanced cancer patients surveyed reported that they believed metastatic lung cancer was curable, despite explicit statements to the contrary within the DA. Patients also identified that the prognostic estimates and treatment gains were not sufficiently hope-giving, although evidence-based, and that maintaining and promoting hope was an important element of the decision-making process.

For metastatic prostate cancer, one DA consisted of a letter that 159 patients took home, reviewing two potential first-line hormonal treatment options — surgical castration versus therapy with a luteinizing hormone-releasing hormone [26]. Patients were encouraged to discuss treatment choices with their families, and after selecting an approach, they completed a decision questionnaire prior to starting treatment. Over 90 % were satisfied with their treatment decision at 3 months' follow up. In another study, Chadwick et al. reported on 51 patients with advanced prostate cancer considering medical or surgical orchidectomy for first-line hormonal treatment, who were offered a structured interview to assist them with decision-making [27]. In the interview, patients reviewed the treatments involved, their benefits, and adverse effects. Treatment convenience and the physician's recommendation were identified as the major determinants of treatment decisions.

At least two DAs have been developed in breast cancer. These include a booklet that oncologists use with patients during the consultation, that patients then take home with an accompanying audiotape or CD, for those considering supportive care with or without first-line chemotherapy for metastatic breast cancer [28]. Twenty-four women with advanced breast cancer reviewed the aid and would recommend it to others making a similar decision. A subsequent randomized trial was halted early because of poor accrual. Among accrual barriers were the perceptions of a few oncologists that supportive care alone without first-line chemotherapy in advanced breast cancer was not a valid treatment option. Sepucha and colleagues developed a DVD and booklet for women with advanced breast cancer considering palliative chemotherapy in addition to supportive care [29]. The aid was acceptable and did not increase distress, with an increase in the concordance of patient and provider goals of treatment over time, (from 50 % at baseline, to up to 74 % at 3 months, not statistically significant).

For patients with metastatic colorectal cancer considering supportive care with or without palliative first-line chemotherapy, a DA has been developed to facilitate decision-making and to improve patient understanding about disease and treatment options [1, 30]. Evidence from randomized trials and individual patient meta-analyses describing the potential benefits and toxicities of different standard treatment options, including supportive care alone, was incorporated and illustrated using graphic formats, with a values clarification exercise. The aid, in the format of a take-home booklet and audiotape, was highly acceptable to patients, and in a pilot study of 27 patients, significantly improved knowledge about prognosis and treatment outcomes, without increasing anxiety [1]. A randomized trial using the DA was successfully completed, randomizing 207 Australian and Canadian patients with advanced colorectal cancer considering supportive care with or without first-line systemic therapy, to use of the DA in decision-making or usual care [30]. Oncologists used the booklet in the initial discussion about therapy, and outcomes included the impact of the DA on patient understanding, decision quality, anxiety, decisions made and quality of life. Patients randomized to receive the DA demonstrated significantly greater understanding of prognosis, treatment options, and benefits and toxicities of treatment ($p < 0.001$). In particular, an additional 28 % that received the DA correctly understood the palliative goals of therapy, compared to an additional 13 % in the control arm. Decisional conflict, treatment decisions, achievement of involvement preferences, and decision and consultation satisfaction were similar between the two groups. Anxiety was also similar between the groups, and decreased over time. Most patients were confident enough to make a decision in the first consultation, (although knowledge did continue to increase about prognosis and treatment options over time), and 74 % chose chemotherapy, 7 % supportive without chemotherapy, and another 10 % a watch and wait strategy. Those with higher levels of understanding were more likely to make definitive decisions for or against chemotherapy, while those selecting a watch-and-wait strategy showed the lowest levels of understanding.

Smith et al. have recently published a pilot trial of information aids for patients with incurable breast, colorectal, lung and hormone-refractory prostate cancer facing first- to fourth-line chemotherapy decisions [3]. The aids were in the form of take-home printed information reviewing prognosis, the impact of treatment on outcomes, and other issues to consider such as advance directives, cardiopulmonary resuscitation, and those involving hospice care. 26 patients reviewed the aids, which improved the proportion of patients that believed advanced cancer was curable from 52 to 31 % (not statistically significant), with no impact on anxiety or hopefulness.

A randomized trial is planned or ongoing of patients with advanced colon, breast or ovarian

cancer considering supportive care with or without second-line palliative chemotherapy [31]. The planned sample size is 170 patients; the nurse will present each component of the aid (including prognosis and toxicity), and patients will select whether to review or not. Outcomes of the trial are to examine the impact of the aid on patient well-being, anxiety and depression, information preferences and satisfaction, knowledge, decision and treatment satisfaction, treatment choice, decision control, and many others.

A randomized trial is also ongoing at the Fox Chase Cancer Center (Principal Investigator Dr. N. Meropol). The study sample size is 720 patients, and patients will be randomized to one of three arms: to receive a generic computer-based survey assessing demographic data, a targeted survey and communication aid with a summary report to the physician, or the targeted survey and communication aid without a report to the physician. Primary outcomes include satisfaction, decisional conflicts, expectations of treatment benefit and risks (clinical trials.gov identifier NCT 00244868).

Finally a study of a decision aid in stage III or IV non-small cell lung cancer is being conducted through the Memorial Sloan Kettering Cancer Centre (Principal Investigator Dr. Leslie Tyson). The impact of a decision aid administered over three treatment visits in those considering lung-cancer directed therapy will be tested, examining feasibility and decision-making quality, including decreased decisional conflict compared to usual care (NCT00579215).

Decision Aids in End-of-Life Planning

Similar to palliative anticancer therapy, a number of interventions have been developed to assist end-of-life and palliative planning, again including audiotapes, letters, videos, question prompt sheets and written materials [4, 32]. DAs have also been developed to facilitate end-of-life planning decisions, directed at patients as well as caregivers.

Volandes et al. have recently published their experience in developing and testing an educational videotape aimed at helping patients understand goals in advanced cancer and clarifying preferences for resuscitation. Eighty patients reviewed the video, with more patients opting out of cardiopulmonary resuscitation or ventilation after their review (71 vs. 62 %, $p = 0.03$) [33]. This DA is currently being evaluated in a clinical trial that aims to recruit 150 patients with incurable cancer in their last year of life. Patients will be randomized to review the video about advance care planning versus a verbal description, and the primary outcome measure will be patient preferences for cardiopulmonary resuscitation (clinicaltrials.gov identifier NCT01241929). The same investigators are currently running a similar, smaller trial in advanced malignant glioma, with a sample size of 50 patients (NCT00970788, www.clinicaltrials.gov).

Korean investigators have developed a video and workbook for caregivers of terminal cancer patients, to facilitate discussion of terminal prognosis [34]. Four hundred and forty-four patients' caregivers were randomized to receive either receive the DA, entitled "Patients want to know the truth" or in the control arm, to educational information on controlling cancer pain. While the rates of discussion of terminal prognosis were similar between the groups, caregivers that received the DA had significantly less decisional conflict sustained over 6 months, and less depression at 1 month.

Current Challenges in the Use of Decision Aids in Advanced Cancer

There have been several challenges identified in the routine adoption of DAs in clinical oncology practice. Information and treatment options change over time, requiring frequent updates. Information contained in the aid may need to be personalized to the prognosis and treatment options facing a particular patient [30]. DAs available through the internet, such as Adjuvant! Online (www.adjuvantonline.com), have been more successfully used in clinical practice, and may be more amenable to an individualized approach. Also previous research has shown that patients prefer simpler interventions to more

complex versions [35]. Also the clear need for a sensitive and effective means of conveying prognostic information to terminally ill cancer patients and their families is imperative, especially with variable patient and family preferences for this information, yet a clear requirement for disclosure to allow informed consent to treatment.

But perhaps the most challenging aspect of DAs in advanced cancer is that of the timing of decision-making. Most advanced cancer DA studies have focused on the initial consultation of patients referred to specialists to discuss cancer-directed therapy. Thus, both patients and providers have an inherent bias towards anticancer therapy. Studies suggest that the majority of patients arrive at a decision during their initial consultation, yet their understanding about limited prognosis, and the modest and uncertain benefits of palliative anticancer therapy take longer than that initial meeting [30]. Furthermore, many oncologists and patients defer decisions about end-of-life and supportive care until these are the only options left for patients [2, 36]. While much of the blame for this has been attributed to physicians [2], it is likely that there is a more subtle interplay between patient, family, and the physician at work, including patient and physician collusion to defer discussion of poor prognosis and treatment outcomes for as long as possible when the treatment goal is not cure. Accelerating the transfer of knowledge about limited prognosis and treatment benefit remains a major challenge in decision-making in advanced cancer, in order to minimize false hope and unrealistic expectations, while preserving reasonable hopes of modest improvements or symptom control at the end of life.

Summary and Future Directions

Decisions in advanced cancer remain among the most complex in oncology, and misunderstanding of prognosis and treatment impact remains common among patients and physicians. DAs can be used as a reliable source of evidence-based information for advanced cancer patients, and improve patient understanding about prognosis and treatment benefits. DAs may also reduce decisional conflict, and have not been associated with an increase in patient anxiety despite greater understanding of limited prognosis.

DAs are valuable tools to promote patient involvement in decision-making, to minimize misunderstanding of key facts about metastatic cancer and therapy, and to improve the quality of decision-making in advanced cancer. Randomized trials are now being successfully conducted to evaluate the role of DAs in advanced cancer. The optimal primary outcome in these trials remains an open question. The achievement of greater patient understanding and informed consent are key goals. But improving decision quality is also a major endpoint, including decisional conflict and decision satisfaction. Treatment options selected, patient survival, symptom control and quality of life are also important, as are patient and provider satisfaction with the decision-making process, and patient and caregiver distress.

Future challenges for DAs include the ability to individualize patient information, ensuring sufficient timing for informed decision-making beyond the initial consultation about therapy, and accelerating the conversation between patient, family, and physicians about palliative goals and end-of-life planning.

References

1. Leighl NB, Butow PN, Tattersall MHN. Treatment Decision Aids in Advanced Cancer: When the Goal Is Not Cure and the Answer Is Not Clear. J Clin Oncol. 2004;22:1759–62.
2. Belanger E, Rodriguez C, Groleau D. Shared decision-making in palliative care: a systematic mixed studies review using narrative synthesis. Palliat Med. 2011;25:242–61.
3. Smith TJ, Dow LA, Virago EA, et al. A pilot trial of decision aids to give truthful prognostic and treatment information to chemotherapy patients with advanced cancer. J Support Oncol. 2011;9:79–86.
4. Gaston CM, Mitchell G. Information giving and decision-making in patients with advanced cancer: a systematic review. Soc Sci Med. 2005;61:2252–64.
5. Braddock 3rd CH, Edwards KA, Hasenberg NM, et al. Informed decision making in outpatient practice: time to get back to basics. JAMA. 1999;282:2313–20.
6. Gattellari M, Voigt K, Butow PN, et al. Are cancer patients equipped to make informed decisions? J Clin Oncol. 2002;20:503–13.
7. Audrey S, Abel J, Blazeby JM, et al. What oncologists tell patients about survival benefits of palliative chemotherapy and implications for informed consent: qualitative study. BMJ. 2008;337:a752.
8. Berland GK, Elliott MN, Morales LS, et al. Health information on the Internet: accessibility, quality and readability in English and Spanish. JAMA. 2001;285:2612–21.
9. Lawrentschuk N, Sasges D, Tasevski R, et al. Oncology health information quality on the Internet: a multilingual evaluation. Ann Surg Oncol. 2012;19:706–13.
10. MacKillop WJ, Stewart WE, Ginsberg AD, et al. Cancer patients' perceptions of their disease and its treatment. Br J Cancer. 1988;58:355–8.
11. Gattellari M, et al. Misunderstanding in cancer patients: why shoot the messenger? Ann Oncol. 1999;10:39–46.
12. Bruera E, Sweeney C, Calder K, et al. Patient preferences versus physician perceptions of treatment decisions in cancer care. J Clin Oncol. 2001;19: 2883–5.
13. Schofield P, Carey M, Love A, et al. "Would you like to talk about your future treatment options?" Discussing the transition from curative cancer treatment to palliative care. Palliat Med. 2006;20: 397–406.
14. Bruera E, Newmann CM, Mazzocato C, et al. Attitudes and belief of palliative care physicians regarding communication with terminally ill cancer patients. Palliat Med. 2000;14:287–98.
15. Lamont EB, Christakis NA. Prognostic disclosure to patients with cancer near the end of life. Ann Intern Med. 2001;34:1096–105.
16. Weeks JC, Cook EF, O'Day SJ, et al. Relationship between cancer patients' predictions of prognosis and their treatment preferences. JAMA. 1998;279: 1709–14.
17. Frankl D, Oye RK, Bellamy PE. Attitudes of hospitalized patients toward life support: a survey of 200 medical inpatients. Am J Med. 1989;86:645–8.
18. Murphy DJ, Borrows D, Santilli S, et al. The influence of the probability of survival on patients' preferences regarding cardiopulmonary resuscitation. NEJM. 1994;330:545–9.
19. O'Brien MA, Whelan TJ, Villasis-Keever M, et al. Are Cancer-Related Decision Aids Effective? A Systematic Review and Meta-analysis. J Clin Oncol. 2009;27:974–85.
20. O'Connor AM, Rostom A, Fiset V, et al. Decision aids for patients facing health treatment or screening decisions: systematic review. BMJ. 1999;319:731–4.
21. Elit LM, Levine MN, Gafni A, et al. Patients' preferences for therapy in advanced epithelial ovarian cancer: development, testing, and application of a bedside decision instrument. Gynecol Oncol. 1996;62: 329–35.

22. Fiset V, O'Connor AM, Evans W, et al. Development and evaluation of a decision aid for patients with stage IV non-small cell lung cancer. Health Exp. 2000;3:125–36.
23. Brundage MD, Feldman-Stewart D, Cosby R, et al. Phase I study of a decision aid for patients with locally advanced non-small-cell lung cancer. J Clin Oncol. 2001;19:1326–35.
24. Brundage MD, Feldman-Stewart D, Dixon P, et al. A treatment trade-off based decision aid for patients with locally advanced non-small cell lung cancer. Health Expect. 2000;3:55–68.
25. Leighl NB, Shepherd FA, Zawisza D, et al. Enhancing treatment decision-making: pilot study of a treatment decision aid in stage IV non-small cell lung cancer. Br J Cancer. 2008;98(11):1769–73.
26. Cassileth BR, Soloway MS, Vogelzang NJ, et al. Patients' choice of treatment in stage D prostate cancer. Urology. 1989;33(5 Suppl):57–62.
27. Chadwick DJ, Gillatt DA, Gingell JC. Medical or surgical orchidectomy: the patients' choice. BMJ. 1991;302:572.
28. Chiew KS, Shepherd H, Vardy J, et al. Development and evaluation of a decision aid for patients considering first-line chemotherapy for metastatic breast cancer. Health Expect. 2008;11:35–45.
29. Sepucha KR, Ozanne EM, Partridge AH, Moy B. Is there a role for decision aids in advanced breast cancer? Med Decis Making. 2009;29:475–82.
30. Leighl NB, Shepherd HL, Butow PN, et al. Supporting treatment decision making in advanced cancer: a ran-

domized trial of a decision aid for patients with advanced colorectal cancer considering chemotherapy. J Clin Oncol. 2011;29:2077–84.
31. Oostendorp LJ, Ottevanger PB, van der Graaf WT, Stalmeier PF. Assessing the information desire of patients with advanced cancer by providing information with a decision aid, which is evaluated in a randomized trial: a study protocol. BMC Med Inform Decis Mak. 2011;11:9.
32. Clayton JM, Butow PN, Tattersall MHN, et al. Randomized controlled trial of a prompt list to help advanced cancer patients and their caregivers to ask questions about prognosis and end-of-life care. J Clin Oncol. 2007;25:715–23.
33. Volandes AE, Levin TT, Slovin S, et al. Augmenting advance care planning in poor prognosis cancer with a video decision aid: a preintervention-postintervention study. Cancer. 2012;118(17):4331–8. doi:10.1002/cncr.27423.
34. Yun YH, Lee MK, Park S, et al. Use of a decision aid to help caregivers discuss terminal disease status with a family member with cancer: a randomized controlled trial. J Clin Oncol. 2011;29: 4811–9.
35. Butow PN, Brindle E, McConnell D, et al. Information booklets about cancer: factors influencing patient satisfaction and utilization. Patient Educ Couns. 1998;33:129–41.
36. Drought TS, Koenig BA. "Choice" in end-of-life decision making: researching fact or fiction? Gerontologist. 2002;43(Spec No 3):114–28.

Cancer Fatalism: Attitudes Toward Screening and Care

6

Miri Cohen

Introduction

Over the last 15 years, interest in fatalism has emerged among heath care researchers [1, 2]. This interest was generated by the search for efficient targets for intervention to increase health behaviors and screening attendance among underserved social groups [3–7]. Studies have shown that fatalistic beliefs are related to lower adherence to medical examinations and lifestyle regimens needed in the management of chronic diseases such as cardiovascular disease [8], diabetes [9] and HIV [10], and to attitudes toward health behaviors such as practicing safe sex [11, 12], smoking [13, 14] and screening for the early detection of several types of cancer [1, 3, 5–7].

Definitions of Fatalism

Although definitions vary, fatalism is usually conceptualized as a belief that events are predetermined and that human beings are unable to change their outcomes [15]. Fatalism refers to two similar but not identical beliefs: the belief that events are beyond personal control, and the

belief that a person cannot change the outcome of events. Fatalism is incompatible with free will, as individuals with a strong belief in fatalism believe that very little, or nothing, can be done to change the course of events determined by external forces [16].

Fatalism may or may not be based on belief in God. Believers tend to accept that God has control over every detail of life, while nonreligious fatalism may be expressed in the belief that things happen by chance or luck [17–21]. In a modern society, which stresses free will and self actualization, fatalism often attains a negative connotation [5], and is viewed as being related to pessimism, hopelessness and despair [3, 22].

Cancer Fatalism

Studies had defined cancer fatalism as the perception that encountering cancer is a certain death sentence and that sooner or later the individual with cancer will die [3, 23–25]. This belief is often found to be related to perceptions that screening for early detection of cancer is not necessary because if the end outcome is death, it does not matter when the cancer is detected [1, 3, 7, 26–28]. This belief may also encourage refusal or non-adherence to cancer treatment due to the same reasoning that treatments will not change the death outcome [29–32].

Less attention is given to another aspect of cancer fatalism, which is the belief that health is a matter of God's will, fate or luck and beyond an

M. Cohen Ph.D (✉)
Department of Gerontology, Faculty of Social Welfare and Health Sciences, University of Haifa, Mount Carmel 31905, Haifa, Israel
e-mail: cohenm@research.haifa.ac.il

B.I. Carr and J. Steel (eds.), *Psychological Aspects of Cancer*,
DOI 10.1007/978-1-4614-4866-2_6, © Springer Science+Business Media, LLC 2013

individual's control [15, 18, 33]. It is often accompanied by an assurance that "it will not happen to me" or by the pessimistic conviction of an individual that he or she will encounter cancer sooner or later regardless of personal actions. This perception may develop out of knowing many individuals diagnosed with cancer [7, 28], through the media [34–36] or due to being convinced that he or she carries a genetic predisposition [37, 38]. These people also believe that if occurrence or nonoccurrence of cancer is not in the individual's hands, this implies that a healthy lifestyle or screenings will not change one's personal fate [35].

Thus, cancer fatalism can act as a barrier to screening [1, 2, 18, 21, 23, 27, 33, 39–51], can be a cause for delay in seeking medical help once symptoms appear [29–32, 52, 53] or be a cause of refusing to receive all or certain treatments for cancer [54]. However, it is important to bear in mind that, similar to other health attitudes, fatalistic beliefs held by individuals vary along a continuum from extreme fatalistic beliefs to a strong belief in personal actions as determinants of one's health [17, 18, 23]. Accordingly, as a result, their effects on individuals' perceptions vary [21, 23, 39, 41, 42].

This chapter will address empirical data on cancer fatalism—its relationship to ethnicity and socioeconomic status (SES); its relationship to screening behaviors; delay in seeking help and its relation to coping with cancer once diagnosed. This will be followed by a review of the relatively new data on genetic fatalism among individuals at high risk for cancer. Finally, based on the review of existing empirical knowledge, a multidimensional conceptualization of the concept of fatalism will be suggested.

Cancer Fatalism in Diverse Population Groups

Most of the studies on cancer fatalism has been conducted in the USA, exploring the attitudes of its multicultural groups, especially Caucasians, African-Americans, and Latinas [1, 2, 27, 33, 41–49, 51, 55–58]. Several studies have also been conducted in Israel which explored fatalistic beliefs related to cancer among Jewish and Arab interviewees [21, 25, 39–41, 59, 60]. Studies assessing cancer fatalism have also been conducted in other countries such as China [61], and among indigenous people in Australia, New Zealand, and Canada [62].

In spite of the large advances in medical treatment and in cure rates, cancer fatalism is a widespread belief in Western countries [63]. In a study based on a random sample of 6,369 Americans, 27 % of the participants agreed there is "not much people can do to lower their chances of getting cancer" [35].

Several studies have been conducted by Powe, a central researcher in this study area [1, 2, 31, 47, 53, 55, 64, 65], and by other researchers [6, 24, 43, 45, 49, 51] on attitudes of African Americans to cancer. However, most of the studies assessed levels of cancer fatalism among African Americans alone, without a comparison to Caucasians or to other ethnic groups [2, 31, 43, 47, 49, 64, 65]. Few studies have focused on comparing fatalism among different groups [1, 6, 45, 51, 66]. In one of the first studies, 192 older persons, mostly African Americans, were asked to complete Powe's Fatalism Inventory (PFI). This inventory was developed to assess perceptions of cancer fatalism using 15 yes or no items that assess fear, pessimism, inevitability of death and predetermination [1, 23]. The study found higher levels of cancer fatalism in the African Americans [1]. In a study of 190 young men, significantly higher cancer fatalism was found among African Americans than Caucasians. However, the overall scores of fatalism were very low (3.0 for Caucasians and 4.5 for African Americans, on a possible scale of 0–15) [67]. In a comparison between African Americans and Hispanic men [66], moderate fatalism was reported for both groups, but it was higher for the Hispanic men as compared to the African Americans (6.6 and 4.8 respectively). However, the differences were not controlled for the higher education of the African American participants [66]. In contrast to this study, another study reported that Latina women reported higher levels of fatalism as compared to African-American women [68]. Several other studies found higher levels of fatalism in African Americans compared to Caucasians [50], but these results were not controlled for main demographic variables. In another recent study, Powe and colleagues [69] reported the results of a study on cancer knowledge and attitudes between nursing and non nursing college students, but data on comparison between African-American and Caucasian students were not provided.

In a study that focused on African Americans only, substantially higher levels of cancer fatalism were reported for older African-American women (mean score of 10.3 on a range of 0–15) [64]. However, in another study of women aged 28–78, cancer fatalism scores were closer between the younger and older participants (4.4 and 5.6 respectively) [47]. These low scores are especially interesting as 361 of the women were from primary care centers in the southeastern USA. The authors note that these centers service an underserved population, with about 66 % at or below the poverty level and 75 % uninsured or on Medicaid. In a study on breast cancer knowledge and perceptions among African Americans, only 16 % out of 179 women agreed that a "woman's chance of surviving breast cancer is very low, even if it is found early" [65]. Several other studies focused on correlates of fatalism, but did not provide details on fatalism scores [6, 19, 31, 44].

Another group of studies examined cancer fatalism in the Latina population [27, 33, 46, 48, 68, 70–72]. Several of these studies found higher levels of cancer fatalism among Latina women compared to Caucasian women [33, 68, 71, 72]. A large-scale study with a random sample, although conducted in 1989, compared Latina and Caucasian women regarding various health perceptions and beliefs [72]. It found that a higher proportion of Latinas believed that having cancer is like receiving a death sentence (46 vs. 26 %); that cancer is God's punishment (7 vs. 2 %); that there is very little one can do to prevent contracting cancer (26 vs. 18 %) and that it is uncomfortable to touch someone with cancer (13 vs. 8 %).

In another study, of 803 Latina women and 422 Caucasian women, the Latina women, especially those born outside the US, expressed more fatalistic beliefs regarding cervical cancer [33]. A study among Latina women revealed moderate levels of fatalism (mean of 2.4 on a scale of 1–5), with higher scores being obtained for less acculturated women. However, the scale was a combined fatalism and fear measure, consisting of five items, including perceived risk, fear of cancer and lack of control over developing cancer [48].

In a qualitative study of 29 rural Latina women, the majority of them believed in fate or in God as causes of breast cancer; however the report does not mention whether participants discussed the beliefs regarding the possibility of cure from cancer [70].

Several studies assessed cancer fatalism among Jewish and Arab women in Israel [39, 41, 42, 60]. Baron et al. [60] assessed cancer fatalism using two items representing fatalistic beliefs in external forces as a cause of cancer (God and fate) in a random sample of 1,550 women recruited from one of four major health care insurance companies in Israel. The sample included four culturally distinct groups: ultra-Orthodox Jewish women, Arab women, Jewish women who were secular to moderately religious, and recent Jewish immigrants. The authors found moderate fatalistic perception in the non ultra-Orthodox Jewish women (mean of 2.5, range 1–5) and higher fatalistic perceptions in ultra-Orthodox Jewish women (3.7) and Arab women (4.5). Differences were significant for the Arab group only compared to the other groups. Cohen et al. [39] conducted a qualitative study with Arab women in Israel in which the women expressed fatalistic beliefs regarding their chances of contracting cancer; they perceived that life and death were in the hands of Allah (God). Thus, cancer might be a punishment for bad deeds or it might be a test for His believers or a way of atonement. Interestingly, these beliefs were expressed by the participants together with notions regarding biomedical knowledge of causes of cancer such as genetic predisposition, lifestyle or environmental causes such as radiation. Some of the participants in the focus groups believed that cancer is a death sentence, and that medical interventions only postpone the inevitable death. This fatalistic view was strengthened by witnessing cancer patients from their own surroundings who had died from cancer.

It should be noted that some of the participants who expressed the belief that cancer is a test from God, although admitting their belief in an external force that causes cancer, believed that God places the outcome of the disease in women's hands. Thus they perceived a substantial level of control over the outcome.

In another study, a comparison was made between Palestinian women residing in Israel and the Palestinian Authority (N=697). Cancer fatalism was assessed using a two-item perceived cancer fatalism scale, which is part of the Arab culture-specific barriers scale (ASCB) [21]. The scale was developed based on focus groups' content analysis and further validated in a quantitative study using content, criterion, and divergent, convergent, and construct validity. The Israeli Arab women expressed lower cancer fatalism than the participants from the Palestinian Authority. The authors noted that although some of the differences may be explained by disparities in SES and in sociopolitical status, the results may represent differences in location along the traditional-Westernizing continuum. They also noted that while the two groups have similar cultural origins, they represent different phases of Westernization which affect their perceptions of cancer.

The existing empirical data on fatalistic beliefs among ethnic groups should be regarded with caution. Many of the studies described above reported statistical differences between ethnic groups as compared to the Caucasians or other mainstream groups. However, the review above shows that the overall levels of fatalism, when reported, were mild to moderate in most of the studies. Another misconception may arise from studies reporting on correlates of fatalism within specific ethnic groups, but not reporting the actual scores obtained for fatalism. These data may lead to a simplistic conclusion that cancer fatalism is mainly a cultural characteristic [23, 28, 73].

Moreover, several scholars argued that higher cancer fatalism in ethnic groups should be analyzed in relation to social structural factors which characterize many individuals who belong to ethnic groups [23, 28, 73]. For example, lower SES and lower education were found to be consistently related to higher cancer fatalism [18, 35, 51, 68, 74, 75]. In addition, lesser knowledge

about cancer causes and cancer treatments, lower acculturation and language barriers [28, 48, 72] were also found related to higher fatalistic perceptions of cancer. Relevant to this discussion, Pasick [76] argues that caution is needed regarding an overgeneralized look at fatalism as a cultural component, and attests that fatalism should be understood in its social and economic context. Poverty, racism, discrimination and inadequate access to health care services may be mistakenly interpreted as fatalism [28, 77]. Moreover, ethnic groups living within Western countries or even those residing in their original countries, are going through modernization processes which affect their knowledge, perceptions, beliefs about diseases and medical treatments and their health behaviors [39, 78–81]. Thus, conclusions from studies regarding health perceptions or beliefs should be reached from a deep understanding of the dynamic and changing nature of health perceptions and of the complexity of research.

Fatalism and Screening for Early Detection of Cancer

Cancer fatalism has often been reported to be related to lower performance of various health behaviors [15, 17, 35, 63]. Analysis of data from 6,369 respondents revealed that individuals with high fatalistic beliefs lead less healthy lifestyles: they perform less regular exercise, are less likely to eat fruits and vegetables and smoke more [35]. Other studies reported that higher fatalistic perceptions of cancer were related to a lower rate of attending screenings for breast cancer [43–45, 57], colorectal cancer [2, 27, 55, 56, 58] and cervical cancer [33, 48, 61]. Mixed results on the associations between fatalism and screenings were obtained in studies that controlled for possibly confounding or intervening variables in their data analysis [18, 27, 33, 41, 42, 45, 48, 50, 51]. When adjusted for demographic variables, some of the studies demonstrated significant links between fatalism and screening attendance. For example, in a study with Chinese, Malay and Indian women, adherence to mammography, clinical breast examination, breast self examination and Pap smears was predicted by fatalism (measured by the FATE [18], a seven-item scale consisting of fatalistic attitudes toward health in general, medical screen testing and individual responsibility toward well being). However, the authors did not describe the demographic variables that the regression model was adjusted for [18]. In a study of more than 1,200 Latina and Caucasian participants, adjusting for confounding variables and fatalistic beliefs predicted attendance of cervical cancer screening [33]. Similar results were obtained by Harmon et al. [48] in a study of 566 Latina women, as well as in other studies [27, 45].

In contrast, several studies found no association between fatalism and screening attendance after adjusting for demographic variables [50, 51, 82]. For example, Russel et al. [50] reported that in a multivariate logistic regression, fatalism did not predict mammography attendance in a sample of 175 African-American and Caucasian women. In Mayo et al.'s study [51] of 135 African-American women aged 70 and over, the association between fatalism and mammography attendance stopped being significant in a multivariate regression analysis when adjusted for age, education and doctors' recommendation. Also, in a study using a stratified cluster sampling to recruit 1,364 women aged 50–70 years from six ethnic groups, fatalism did not predict mammography screening in a logistic regression model [6]. However, this finding may be due to multicolinearity with several cognitive variables such as perceived risk or "cause of cancer is governed by God" entered into the regression model.

Lower attendance of mammography in Palestinian women residing in the Palestinian Authority was also found to be associated with higher cancer fatalism (measured by two items assessing belief in cancer as a fatal disease). This association remained significant after adjusting for demographic characteristics, health beliefs and situational barriers [41]. In addition, situational barriers related to the sociopolitical situation were correlated with attendance of mammography and clinical breast examinations, but did not predict their attendance in a multivariate logistic regression, while cancer fatalism remained as a significant predictor [42]. Baron et al. [60] assessed the effect of fatalistic perceptions (using two items from the PFI [1]) on mammography attendance among 1,500 women in

Israel. Similarly, adjusting for possible demographic confounders, a significant association was found between fatalistic beliefs in external forces as a cause of cancer and attendance of mammography as reported by claims records among Arab women and Jewish ultra-Orthodox women, but not among Jewish veterans or new immigrants [60].

However, comparison between results of the studies reviewed is difficult to conduct, due to principal variability in definitions and measurement tools of fatalism, size and type of samples, age ranges and methodology used. Of special concern is the divergence in defining adherence to screenings. Most of the studies relied on self-reporting [46] or face-to-face interviews [18, 41, 42, 51, 64] and only a few used claims records [60]. Most studies defined adherence to mammography, clinical breast examinations [18, 40, 41, 51, 60] or Pap smear tests [48] as ever attended or never attended, while others assessed frequency [45], being on time with screenings [83] or frequency of more than four mammograms per 10 years [6], at least one mammography in the last 5 years [49] or compliance with overall screening guidelines [44]. Flynn [19] calculated clinical breast examination adherence as the total number of clinical breast exam tests reported divided by the maximum number that a woman of her age should have if she were fully compliant with screening guidelines. This wide diversity is probably responsible to some extent for the mixed results and difficulty in coming to conclusions regarding the relationships between cancer fatalism and adherence. Also, many questions should still be investigated such as the following: do the nature and direction of these relationships differ for different screening methods, for different types of cancers screened for, or among the different ethnic groups?

Cancer Fatalism and Delay in Diagnosis

Delay in seeking medical care when, or after, symptoms are identified often leads to a later stage at diagnosis and lower survival rates [84]. Studies reported that delay in seeking help is not a rare situation. Estimated rate of delay ranges in different studies from 16 to 30 % [85]. Norsaadah [86] reported a 2-month delay of 72 % and a 6-month delay of 45 % among Malay women. Higher rates of delay were found related to lower income [85, 87], lower education [31, 53, 85, 87], lack of a regular health provider or health insurance [85, 87] and belonging to ethnic groups [85, 88–90]. Also, delay in seeking help was found to be associated with less knowledge about cancer and greater misconceptions of symptoms [85].

Only a small number of studies assessed delay in diagnosis in relation to cancer fatalism. Gullatte et al. [31, 53] studied 129 African-American women aged between 30 and 84 years who were diagnosed with breast cancer following self-detecting a breast symptom. Time elapsed from onset of symptoms to seeking medical care was 5.5 months on average. Religiosity, spirituality and fatalism did not predict length in delay or stage at diagnosis, while lower education and being unmarried were significant predictors of delay. In addition, women who talked to God only about their breast symptoms were more likely to delay seeking medical care. In contrast, women who had told a person about their breast symptom were more likely to seek medical care sooner.

Using medical records, Weinman et al. [32] reported that of 2,694 cancer patients with late and early stage breast cancer, 7 % (195 women) refused provider's advice to further examine symptoms or abnormal results. These women tended to be at a later stage of breast cancer at diagnosis, were older, and women with high parity. The most frequent reasons the women gave (as documented in the medical records) for their initial refusal were related to fatalism, avoidance or denial, fear of mammography pain or discomfort and fear of surgery.

A very small-scale study assessed 11 women with locally advanced breast cancer and 11 women with early stage cancer. The semi-structured interviews identified that late diagnosis was associated with not being aware of screening guidelines, denial, fatalism and reliance on alternative therapies. Also, the spouses of the late diagnosis women's group tended to be more

passive in their wives' medical care, and also expressed fatalistic thinking and denial [52].

Burgess and colleagues [30] conducted interviews with 46 women newly diagnosed with breast cancer. Of them, 31 had waited 12 weeks or more between noticing symptoms and approaching their physicians. The women who delayed seeking medical care differed from the non-delayers in their beliefs about the consequences of cancer treatment and in perceptions of other priorities taking precedence over personal health. In a qualitative review of 32 papers, Smith et al. [29] found that fear, either of embarrassment or of the pain, suffering or death from cancer was among the main reasons for delay, in addition to not recognizing or misconception of the symptoms.

The few studies that focused on the role of fatalism in delay in seeking help are not sufficient to draw conclusions. Gaining more knowledge on the nature of this relationship is necessary for planning future interventions among women at risk for delay in seeking medical care.

Cancer Fatalism and Cancer Patients

Although numerous studies were conducted to assess cognitive, emotional and behavioral aspects of coping with and adjustment among cancer patients, a relatively small number of studies focused on fatalistic beliefs of cancer patients and the impact of the beliefs on the process of adjustment [91–95]. Therefore, very little is actually known about perceptions of fatalism among cancer patients and their effects on psychological reactions, adherence to treatment and other relevant issues.

One of the very few studies on fatalism among cancer patients was conducted by Sheppard et al. [91]. This is a study with a small sample of 26 African-American breast cancer patients, aged 42–73 years in which the participants were at different stages of breast cancer. Cancer fatalism was assessed using the PFI [1]. The authors report that 80 % of the sample had at least one type of fatalistic belief, but the overall score of fatalism was low. Interestingly, the majority of the women believed that contracting cancer was a matter of fate, but a low rate of positive answers were given to items that referred to cancer as causing an inevitable or imminent death. For example, none of them believed that "if someone gets breast cancer, their time to die is soon" or "if someone has breast cancer, it is already too late to get treated for it."

An intriguing, but unanswered, question in this regard is whether fatalistic perceptions change in individuals once they are diagnosed with cancer [92, 93]. An indirect insight into the process of change may be gained from the contrast that exists regarding fatalistic beliefs of healthy women and those of cancer patients as depicted in qualitative studies. For example, as reported above, healthy Arab participants in focus groups reported many fatalistic beliefs regarding the causes and the fatal outcome of breast cancer [39]. In contrast, in a recent qualitative study using in-depth interviews with 40 Arab breast cancer patients who were about a year post treatment and without evident signs of disease, all the women were optimistic about the outcome of their disease and confident that they would defeat it, with God's help [94].

Another qualitative study with 16 Chinese patients with colorectal cancer revealed that most participants perceived their cancer as a predetermined destiny. This belief was followed by passive acceptance alternating with focus on positive aspects. However, the authors identified a flow in fatalistic beliefs, being strongest with early diagnosis and lowered as treatment progressed. Upon treatment completion, fatalism reemerged regarding disease recurrence [95].

Fatalism in cancer patients was also studied from a different perspective, as a coping style [96, 97]. While scholars in the area of coping usually differentiate between cognitive perceptions (such as optimism or fatalism) and coping strategies [98], Greer and colleagues [96, 97, 99] combined the cognitive perceptions and coping responses into a single construct termed coping styles (also referred to as adjustment styles) [97]. They constructed a profile of five coping responses: fighting spirit, hopelessness and helplessness, anxious preoccupation, fatalism and avoidance [96, 97, 99]. Fatalism was described as "a perception that no control can be exerted over the situation and the consequences of lack of control can and should be accepted with equanimity" [96, p13]. As a result the attitude of women with a fatalistic coping style toward cancer is one of passive acceptance, and for them the diagnosis of cancer represents a relatively minor threat [96]. Studies using this typology of coping styles reported that higher use of fatalism was associated with lower adjustment and higher emotional distress. The same was found for patients using coping styles of hopelessness/helplessness and anxious preoccupation in contrast to the use of fighting spirit [13, 100, 101]. Also, an intervention study using cognitive behavior therapy showed a significant decrease in anxiety and depression concomitant with an increase in fighting spirit and a decrease in the less adaptive coping strategies [99]. However, in a sample which included 101 women with advanced breast cancer, no association was found between emotional distress and using fatalism as a coping style [102].

In a more recent study [103], a total of 353 women treated for primary breast cancer were assessed within 1 year of diagnosis for emotional distress, anxiety and depression, adjustment and coping style. The authors combined fighting spirit with fatalism to a coping style termed "positive reappraisal." The multivariate analysis conducted suggested an association between this combined coping style and lower fatigue.

Greer and his group [96, 97, 99] conducted longitudinal studies in which cancer patients were followed for long periods in order to assess the role of coping styles in survival. They reported that patients who responded with fighting spirit or with denial were significantly more likely to be alive and free of recurrence 5, 10 and 15 years after diagnosis than patients with fatalistic or helpless responses [97, 104]. These results were obtained after controlling for demographic and disease-related variables. When the prognostic factors were examined individually, psychological response was the most important factor in predicting death from any cause, death from cancer and first recurrence.

A similar view on fatalism as a mean of coping was suggested by Sharf et al. [54]. The authors proposed that fatalism may be used by cancer patients as a mode of coping with the uncertainty imposed by cancer diagnosis. Similarly, other researchers referred to fatalism as a means of coping with self-blame [37].

The extent and nature of fatalistic views in cancer patients and their effect on psychological and physical health are still mostly unknown and understudied. The distinct ways of conceptualization of fatalism in cancer patients in the few existing studies hinder reaching conclusions, but point to the necessity of expanding the research in this area.

Genetic Fatalism and Cancer

A comparatively new aspect of fatalism—genetic fatalism—was recently presented [37]. Research in this area appeared following the identification of familial risk for specific types of cancer such as breast cancer, ovarian cancer or colorectal cancer. About 20 years ago breast cancer mutations in the BRACA1 and BRACA 2 genes were identified which increase susceptibility to breast and ovarian cancer [105]. The identification of these specific mutations has increased the sense of genetic fatalism in first degree relatives of breast or ovarian cancer sufferers [37, 106].

Previous studies concluded that people often respond in fatalistic ways when they hear about genetic causes of disease [38]. This reaction has been explained by misconceptions people often have regarding the role of genes in disease susceptibility. Walter [38] argues that once a disease is perceived to be caused solely by genes, the individuals' reaction may be one of lack of control and fatalism. One of the few similar studies is a study of parents of neonates who had received a positive screening test result informing them that their child was at-risk for having hypercholesterolaemia, an inherited predisposition to heart disease [107]. Parents who regarded this condition as a genetic problem perceived the situation as uncontrollable and, hence, more threatening.

A very small number of studies assessed fatalistic perceptions in persons with familial history of cancer or diagnosed as carriers of identified mutations of susceptibility [48, 108–110]. The existing studies were mainly conducted with women who had first-degree relatives with breast cancer and in almost all of these studies fatalism was measured indirectly or was not the primary focus of the study. For example, it was reported that women at high risk often overestimate their lifetime risk of developing breast cancer [111, 112], experiencing higher levels of anxiety and depression than matched controls [108, 113–116], although several studies did not find higher distress among high-risk individuals [117–119].

Fatalistic beliefs were examined by Ryan et al. [109] using focus groups with 29 first-degree relatives of cancer patients. The authors noted that some of the women reported fatalistic beliefs regarding their contracting breast cancer. Harmon reported that individuals who reported a family history of cancer were more likely to endorse fatalistic beliefs [48]. Cohen et al. [108] assessed cognitive perceptions, coping strategies and emotional distress in 80 adult daughters of breast cancer patients as predictors of levels of stress hormones and immune cytotoxic functions. The psychological and immune functions were examined in comparison to a control group matched by age and education. Among the cognitive perception studies, the participants were asked to grade their sense of control over contracting breast cancer. The daughters expressed a lower sense of control over contracting breast cancer than the participants in the control group. In addition, lower levels of perceived control were associated with higher psychological distress, higher levels of stress hormones and with lower natural killer activity and lower secretion of cytotoxic cytokines (interleukin- (IL-)2, IL-12, interferon-gamma). These immune functions take part in immune defense against viruses, infections and cancerous cells. Of special interest was the relationship between lower sense of control and lower interleukin-2-induced natural killer activity against breast cancer target cells [108]. It was also found that higher perceived control over contracting breast cancer predicted higher adherence to screenings for early detection of breast cancer [108].

Another study used focus groups with first-degree relatives of ovarian cancer patients. The participants in this study expressed an increased sense of vulnerability. They perceived that vulnerability to cancer was much higher than for other diseases in their family such as heart disease or other cancers. They had a fatalistic view of lack of personal control over ovarian cancer. They felt fatalistic and helpless about ovarian cancer as they believed there were no lifestyle risk factors that they could control by living a healthy lifestyle [110].

Walter [38] conducted a systematic review of qualitative studies on perceptions of familial risk of common chronic diseases. The author reported that most participants in the studies felt deeply fatalistic about familial risk of diseases. They felt especially fatalistic about cancer, particularly those cancers that have a late presentation of symptoms such as ovarian or colorectal cancer.

A view of high susceptibility and a sense of inevitability about contracting cancer among women at high risk for breast cancer may affect health behaviors in two directions: it may reinforce a sense of lack of power to affect the inevitable fate, thus health behaviors or screenings may be perceived as not needed and thus avoided. In contrast, the sense of vulnerability may encourage women to engage more in health behaviors, screening or even take prophylactic action. Informing individuals at high risk about the meaning of genetic predisposition and that cancer cannot be caused solely by genetics may reduce their sense of fatalism [38] and encourage active ways for prevention or early detection, thus increasing chances for survival.

Understanding Cancer Fatalism as a Multidimensional Construct

The mixed results on cancer fatalism and its consequences (e.g., [1, 2, 43, 44, 48, 51, 56, 57, 120]) described in this chapter point to the complexity of the structure of fatalism that requires that interrelations among cultural, structural and individual factors be considered. Moreover, it may raise a question as to whether researchers who address cancer fatalism are actually measuring the same construct, or whether it is possible that they are measuring different dimensions of the construct or even distinct constructs. The literature addresses two main dimensions of fatalism [5]. The first dimension, widely described by Powe [1, 2, 118] and by Powe and colleagues [3, 23], is defined as a belief that death is inevitable when cancer is present. The second dimension of cancer fatalism, mainly represented by Straughan and Seow [18], views cancer onset as a matter of fate, luck or God's will. Both types were often interchangeably referred to in the literature as cancer fatalism [5]. Also, when fatalism was studied in relation to culture or ethnicity, often no distinctions between the dimensions were made [28]. However, some evidence exists as to the different nature of the constructs. For example, in a study of Latina women, 54 % believed they had no control over developing cancer, while most did not express fatalistic attitudes concerning the chances of surviving breast, uterine or cervical cancer [71].

I would like to argue that each of these two dimensions of fatalism has unique origins, antecedents and unique impact on psychological reactions and on health behaviors (Fig. 6.1). The first dimension, the view that death is inevitable no matter at what the stage cancer is detected and what treatments are offered, may indeed cause unwillingness or refusal to attend screenings [23]. It is believed that if the end outcome is already known, early detection will not change the inevitable course of the disease.

Thus, individuals may logically decide that it is more worthwhile to avoid screenings [18] and thus avoid negative emotions of fear and anxiety that arise when focusing on cancer or when taking steps toward screening.

The belief that cancer is a death sentence may emerge out of different processes or conditions. According to studies that found associations between cancer fatalism and level of knowledge or education [35], lack of knowledge of options of treatment and cure or of the impact of early detection on survival, may indeed foster this type

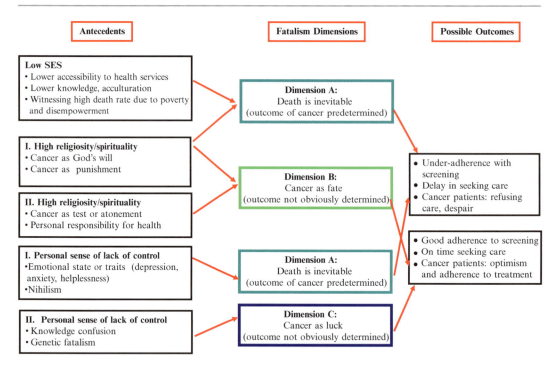

Fig. 6.1 A multidimensional model of fatalism, its consequences and possible outcomes

of fatalism [28, 48, 72]. Peek et al. [43] cites one woman as saying: "I didn't know that it was a possibility to live after you had breast cancer or had been found having breast cancer. Everybody I know who had breast cancer [has] died. I [wasn't aware] of anything different" (p. 1,851).

Higher fatalism of this kind was often found among individuals from ethnic minority groups in Western countries or ethnic groups in their original countries [1, 2, 42, 53, 55, 64, 66, 72]. Thus, fatalism was often referred to as a cultural belief. However, this specific type of fatalism may emerge as well from social structures that are characteristic of disadvantaged groups [23, 28, 73, 76], which happen to often be ethnic minorities such as African Americans [23]. Low socioeconomic circumstances may reinforce beliefs that death is inevitable when facing cancer independent of culture. Poor people have lower access to health services, they may not have health insurance or regular health providers [28], or even if they have health insurance they cannot provide themselves with the cure opportunities that people with higher incomes have. Also, studies have reported that physicians impart less

information and recommend less screening and checkups for individuals from minority groups or disadvantaged individuals [80, 121]. As a result, individuals witness around them more cases of cancer that were not cured, and this may reinforce the fatalistic belief that death is an inevitable outcome of cancer [39, 63].

The other dimension of fatalism—that cancer, as with other events in life, often occurs due to pure luck or chance, or is predetermined by fate—[18] may grow out of distinct origins other than the former fatalistic belief. Below I describe three main (but not exclusive) sources that may give rise to such beliefs: religious/spiritual beliefs [15, 31, 53, 122], the way scientific and medical knowledge is communicated to the public [34, 35, 63] and personal attitudes or characteristics [81].

The three main religions, Christianity, Judaism and Islam, share the belief that major life occurrences are in God's hands and out of personal control [15, 39, 123, 124]. However, the fate of cancer, as well as other diseases, is believed not to be a casual one, but is God's response to a person's deeds or behaviors. This may be a punishment for unfaithful or unacceptable behaviors, or it may be a test of a person's faithfulness to God, similar to Job's story. A young Arab woman said in a focus group: "God tests our patience, the same as what happened to Job. God tried him with all kinds of diseases and disasters to test how strong his belief was. God strikes those He loves, as He wishes to test them" [39, p. 37] Women in the focus groups also raised the idea that cancer may also be God's act to stimulate atonement or change in a person's attitudes and way of life [39].

Moreover, although the main religions convey the belief that everything is in God's hands, they also state that a person's body is a gift given to the individual to take care of until the time comes to give it back, thus the individual has a personal responsibility to preserve his/her own health [39, 124]. In contrast to passive acceptance and neglect of personal health often reported to be related to fatalism [1], these religious perceptions of fatalism encourage the individual to actively act to preserve or promote his or her health [39, 124]. Of course, it cannot be ruled out that religious beliefs may be used as an excuse for a passive attitude toward health [15].

This view of religious-related fatalism can provide an explanation for the unanswered paradox regarding the relationships between fatalism, religion and health: on the one hand, fatalism was reported to be more prevalent among ethnic minorities, who are often reported to be more religious [15], while on the other hand religiousness was reported to be related to a healthier lifestyle and better health indices [125, 126]. It may be that interplay exists between the first dimension of fatalism which may be influenced mainly by poverty and disempowerment and the second dimension of fatalism may be influenced by scripture writings of the main religions. Several studies revealed that the different perceptions may coexist within specific population groups [15]. For example, in focus groups and in qualitative studies with religious Arab women [39, 60] and with ultra-Orthodox Jewish women [123], women differed in the degree of their perceptions of health as a completely uncontrolled fate or as a factor within their responsibility, although governed by God.

The view of cancer as a matter of chance, not guided by higher forces, is also a spread belief. Powe and Johnson [3] connected it to a sense of nihilism common in modern Western society. Another aspect of this fatalism is genetic fatalism, which conveys the belief that genes solely determine occurrence of cancer [38, 107]. In addition, the belief of lack of control over cancer occurrence may also develop against the backdrop of bewilderment regarding cancer causes and means of prevention among the public [34, 35].

Several scholars have attributed fatalism in part to the nature of cancer research, which is difficult to communicate to the lay public [34, 35]. A mass of findings regarding causes of cancer is frequently communicated to the public by the media [36]. These findings are often conflicting and cause confusion and mistrust [34]. An example is the previously strongly disseminated knowledge that high-fiber diets have cancer-preventing properties, which scientists concede is now based on newer results of studies [63]. Therefore, as a result of conflicting mass knowledge, many people feel overwhelmed and confused. A national survey found that 47 % of the American public believed that "it seems like almost everything causes cancer" and 71 % agreed that "there are so many recommendations about preventing cancer, it's hard to know which ones to follow," [35] and therefore react with fatalistic beliefs of lack of control over cancer occurrence.

Another issue that needs consideration relates to the complex relationships between different psychological factors (such as self-efficacy, helplessness, hopelessness, sense of control, fear, anxiety, depression) and fatalism. Very little empirical knowledge exists regarding the nature of these relationships and little is known whether these factors act as antecedents to fatalism, outcome of fatalism or are perhaps coincidently related. Considerably little attention has been given in fatalism research to the role of personal perceptions, personal traits or psychological characteristics of individuals in the development of fatalism. Although most studies stress the cultural and ethnic connection of fatalism, fatalism may develop due to personal characteristics at least partially independent from the cultural perspective. Several studies found high fatalism to be related to low self-efficacy [50, 127, 128] with the underlying notion that when an individual perceives himself or herself as ineffective, he/she will believe that events in life are out of his/her control [49, 50, 127]. Also, external health locus of control was mentioned to be related to higher fatalism [129] and lower performance of good health behaviors [78, 81]. However, external locus of control may also imply higher adherence to physicians' recommendations [129] or higher belief in God which might be related to healthier lifestyle and performance of health behaviors [126].

Several other personal traits may be related but not studied yet in relation to fatalism. For example, helplessness is a personal trait that develops following early and later life experience. Due to earlier experiences of lack of control over situations, individuals may acquire a sense of inability to control their environment [130]. It provides the person with a sense of lacking in resources and power to affect life circumstances including health. Helplessness was often found to be related to lower utilization of health behaviors and worse health outcomes [131]. This personal attitude may, as a result, reinforce a fatalistic view that life happens to the individual without an option of exerting personal control over it. However, the nature of the relationships between perceived helplessness and fatalism is yet to be explored.

Emotions studied in relation to fatalism were mostly specifically cancer-related or screening-related emotions, such as fear, anxiety and embarrassment [19, 45], often referring to negative emotions as an outcome of fatalism [23, 132]. No attention has been paid to emotional states such as anxiety or depression. Examining these emotional states may provide an additional way to study fatalism from an individualized perspective. Depression is defined by categories of symptoms: emotional, cognitive and behavioral symptoms (DSM-4) [133]. Cognitive symptoms of depression consist of lack of motivation for action, perceptions of hopelessness and lack of sense of meaning. These cognitions may be translated into fatalism when a depressed individual is

asked about his beliefs. Moreover, depressed individuals engage much less in good health behaviors and screening, due to difficulty in taking decisions, planning and acting.

Based on clinical interviews [134], about 18–30 % of the adult population in the USA is reported to be distressed, and 12-month and lifetime prevalence of major depressive disorder is 5.3 and 13.2 %. Rates of depression are even higher among older adults and in individuals with low income and low-level education [135]. Thus, it may be that in studies examining fatalism among these groups, the results are confined to depression. Also, higher trait anxiety or higher cancer specific anxiety may result in higher scores of fatalism.

A lack of clear distinctions between different aspects of fatalism may explain some of the limitations of the measurement tools, which may also be responsible for the mixed and contradictory findings in fatalism literature [7]. Gaining greater understanding of the distinct dimensions of fatalism will allow the building of a multidimensional construct of fatalism. This construct may be further used to understand the fine differences between its dimensions, their specific antecedents and their unique effects on preventive behaviors, screening adherence and the adjustment of cancer patients to their illness. It will also provide tools for studying specific populations, such as individuals at high risk or individuals who delay seeking medical treatment.

A more finely tuned knowledge of different dimensions of fatalism is also essential for tailoring interventions to overcome barriers of fatalism. Since delivering preventive health care information may not be enough to increase adherence to screening, a few studies measured the effect interventions tailored to target specific fatalistic beliefs had on change in health behaviors [4, 40, 58]. For example, Azaiza and Cohen [40] used a tailored intervention to lower specific barriers of Arab women to attending mammography and clinical breast examinations. Using scripts, the interviewers reframed notions of cancer as an inevitable fate and that the notion of personal ability to control the outcomes once cancer is detected early was in their control, stressing that this notion coincides with the scripture writings of Islam and Christianity. For example, the belief that cancer is a punishment from God was reframed into the motivating notion that cancer may be a test from God. The results showed that almost 48 % of the intervention group and 12.5 % of the control group scheduled or attended a clinical examination, and 38.5 % of women in the intervention group and 21.4 % of the control group attended or scheduled a mammography post intervention. In another study with African-American women, biblical passages about the importance of staying healthy were provided and discussed in an intervention aimed at increasing attendance at colorectal cancer screenings [56]. Biblical passages selected were used to empower participants to take control of their health [56]. A total of 539 African-American men and women 50 years of age and older participated in this study. The intervention group had a significantly greater proportion of those receiving a colonoscopy within 3 months after the educational session than the control group.

Further controlled studies are needed to assess the effect of challenging the different types of fatalism among healthy participants in order to increase screening and good health behaviors, and among cancer patients to promote adaptive coping and well being.

Discussion and Conclusions

This chapter provides a review of various aspects of cancer fatalism, including its prevalence in different population groups and correlates of fatalism with socio-demographic variables. An effort has been made to critically review the role of fatalism in screening behaviors and in delay in seeking help. The effect of cancer fatalism on cancer patients' adjustment and well-being was also addressed. In addition, the relatively new concept of genetic fatalism and the few studies related to the concept were reviewed. Finally, a conceptualization of fatalism as a multidimensional construct has been suggested.

The review demonstrates the complexity of the concept of fatalism, consisting of different

dimensions that each may have a unique effect on health behaviors. Also, its various correlates and confounders call for caution in drawing conclusions from cross-sectional and correlative studies.

Most studies that assessed fatalism in ethnic groups have not addressed the dynamic nature of culture. Traditional societies are steadily going through a process of Westernization, incorporating cultural beliefs regarding health and illness with modern biomedical knowledge [79]. Thus, fatalism should be studied in this context of change.

It is suggested that further studies will examine multidimensional aspects of fatalism based on new or refined tools. In addition, attention should be given to psychological confounders of fatalism, such as depression and trait anxiety, and its interaction with coping styles such as emotional control or use of denial or avoidance. Special caution should be paid to pitfalls of overgeneralization and of too simplistic linking of fatalism to specific ethnic groups.

References

1. Powe BD. Cancer fatalism among elderly Caucasians and African Americans. Oncol Nurs Forum. 1995;22: 1355–9.
2. Powe BD. Fatalism among elderly African Americans: effects on colorectal screening. Cancer Nurs. 1995;18: 385–92.
3. Powe BD, Johnson A. Fatalism among African Americans: philosophical perspectives. J Religion Health. 1995;34(2):119–25.
4. Powe BD, Weinrich S. An intervention to decrease cancer fatalism among rural elders. Oncol Nurs Forum. 1999;26:583–8.
5. Morgan PD, Tyler ID, Fogel J. Fatalism revisited. Semin Oncol Nurs. 2008;24:237–45.
6. Magai C, Concedine N, et al. Diversity matters: unique populations of women and breast cancer screening. Cancer. 2004;100:2300–7.
7. Espinosa LMK, Gallo LC. The relevance of fatalism in the study of Latinas' cancer screening behavior: a systematic review of the literature. Int J Behav Med. 2011;18(4):310–8. doi:10.1007/s12529-010-9119-4.
8. Urizar Jr GG, Sears Jr SF. Psychological and cultural influences on cardiovascular health and quality of life among Hispanic cardiac patients in South Florida. J Behav Med. 2006;29:255–68.
9. Egede LE, Bonadonna RJ. Diabetes self-management in African Americans: an exploration of the role of fatalism. Diabetes Educ. 2003;29:105–15.

10. Sowell RL, Seals BF, Moneyham L, et al. Quality of life in HIV-infected women in the south-eastern United States. AIDS Care. 1997;9:501–12.

11. Kalichman S, Kelly J, et al. Fatalism, current life satisfaction, and risk for HIV infection among gay and bisexual men. J Consult Clin Psychol. 1997;65:542–6.

12. Varga CA. Coping with HIV/AIDS in Durban's commercial sex industry. AIDS Care. 2001;13:351–65.

13. Schnoll RA, Malstrom M, James C, et al. Correlates of tobacco use among smokers and recent quitters diagnosed with cancer. Patient Educ Couns. 2002;46:137–45.

14. Unger JB, Ritt-Olson A, et al. Cultural values and substance use in a multiethnic sample of California adolescents. Addict Res Theory. 2002;10:257–80.

15. Franklin MD, Schlundt DG, McClellan LH, et al. Religious fatalism and its association with health behaviors and outcomes. Am J Health Behav. 2007;31:563–72.

16. Taylor R. Fatalism. Philos Rev. 1962;71:56–66.

17. Davison C, Frankel S, Smith GD. The limits of lifestyle: re-accessing "fatalism" in the popular culture of illness prevention. Soc Sci Med. 1992;34:675–85.

18. Straughan PT, Seow A. Fatalism reconceptualized: a concept to predict health screening behavior. J Gend Cult Health. 1998;3:85–100.

19. Flynn PM, Betancourt HM, Ormseth SR. Culture, emotion, and cancer screening: an integrative framework for investigation health behavior. Ann Behav Med. 2011;42(1):79–90. doi:10.1007/s12160-011-9267-z.

20. Azaiza F, Cohen M. Health beliefs and rates of breast cancer screening among Arab women. J Women's Health. 2006;15:520–30.

21. Cohen M, Azaiza F. Developing and testing an instrument for identifying culture-specific barriers to breast cancer screening in Israeli Arab women. Acta Oncol. 2008;47:1570–7.

22. Scheier M, Bridges M. Person variables and health: personality predispositions and acute psychological states as shared determinants for disease. Psychosom Med. 1995;57:255–68.

23. Powe BD, Finnie R. Cancer fatalism. The state of the science. Cancer Nurs. 2003;26:454–65.

24. Phillips JM, Cohen MZ, Mozes G. Breast cancer screening and African American women: fear, fatalism, and silence. Oncol Nurs Forum. 1999;26:561–71.

25. Baron-Epel O, Friedman N, Lernau O. Fatalism and mammography in a multicultural population. Oncol Nurs Forum. 2009;36:353–61.

26. Powe BD. Cancer fatalism among African-Americans: a review of the literature. Nurs Outlook. 1996;44(1):18–21.

27. Gorin SS. Correlates of colorectal cancer screening compliance among urban Hispanics. J Behav Med. 2005;28:125–37.

28. Abraido-Lanza A, Viladrich A, Florez KR, et al. Commentary: fatalismo reconsidered: a cautionary note for health-related research and practice with Latino populations. Ethn Dis. 2007;17:153–8.

29. Smith LK, Pope C, Botha JL. Patients' help-seeking experiences and delay in cancer presentation: a qualitative synthesis. Lancet. 2005;366:825–32.

30. Burgess C, Hunter MS, Ramirez AJ. A qualitative study of delay among women reporting symptoms of breast cancer. Br J Gen Pract. 2001;51:967–71.

31. Gullatte MM, Brawley O, et al. Religiosity, spirituality, and cancer fatalism beliefs on delay in breast cancer diagnosis in African American women. J Relig Health. 2010;49:62–72.

32. Weinmann S, Taplin SH, Gilbert J, et al. Characteristics of women refusing follow-up for tests or symptoms suggestive of breast cancer. J Natl Cancer Inst Monogr. 2005;35:33–8.

33. Chavez LR, Hubbell FA, et al. The influence of fatalism on self-reported use of Papanicolaou smears. Am J Prev Med. 1997;13:418–24.

34. Jensen JD, Carcioppolo N, King AJ, et al. Including limitations in news coverage of cancer research: effects of news hedging on fatalism, medical skepticism, patient trust, and backlash. J Health Commun. 2011;16:486–503.

35. Niederdeppel J, Levy AG. Fatalistic beliefs about cancer prevention and three prevention behaviors. Cancer Epidemiol Biomarkers Prev. 2007;16:998–1003.

36. Viswanath K, Breen N, Meissner H, et al. Cancer knowledge and disparities in the information age. J Health Commun. 2006;11:1–17.

37. Keeley B, Wright L, Condit CM. Functions of health fatalism: fatalistic talk as face saving, uncertainty management, stress relief and sense making. Sociol Health Illn. 2009;31:734–47.

38. Walter FM, Emery J, et al. Lay understanding of familial risk of common chronic diseases: a systematic review and synthesis of qualitative research. Ann Fam Med. 2004;2:583–94.

39. Azaiza F, Cohen M. Between traditional and modern perceptions of breast and cervical cancer screenings: a qualitative study of Arab women in Israel. Psychooncology. 2008;17:34–41.

40. Cohen M, Azaiza F. Increasing breast examinations among Arab women using a tailored culture-based intervention. Behav Med. 2010;36:92–9.

41. Azaiza F, Cohen M, et al. Traditional-Westernizing continuum of change in screening behaviors: comparison between Arab women in Israel and the West Bank. Breast Cancer Res Treat. 2011;128(1):219–27. doi:10.1007/s10549-010-1321-1.

42. Azaiza F, Cohen M, et al. Factors associated with low screening for breast cancer in the Palestinian Authority: relations of availability, barriers fatalism. Cancer. 2010;116:4646–55.

43. Peek ME, Sayad JV, Markwardt R. Fear, fatalism and breast cancer screening in low-income African-American women: the role of clinicians and the health care system. J Gen Intern Med. 2008;23:1847–53.

44. Spurlock WR, Cullins LS. Cancer fatalism and breast cancer screening in African American women. ABNF J. 2006;17:38–43.

45. Talbert PY. The relationship of fear and fatalism with breast cancer screening among a selected target population of African American middle class women. J Soc Behav Health Sci. 2008;2:96–110.
46. Lopez-McKee G, McNeill JA, et al. Comparison of factors affecting repeat mammography screening of low-income Mexican American Women. Oncol Nurs Forum. 2008;35:941–7.
47. Powe BD, Hamilton J, Brooks P. Perceptions of cancer fatalism and cancer knowledge. J Psychosoc Oncol. 2006;24:1–13.
48. Harmon MP, Castro FG, Coe K. Acculturation and cervical cancer: knowledge, beliefs, and behaviors of Hispanic women. Women Health. 1996;24:37–57.
49. Russel KM, Champion VL, Skinner CS. Psychological factors related to repeat mammography screening over five years in African American women. Cancer Nurs. 2006;29:236–43.
50. Russel KM, Perkins SM, et al. Sociocultural context of mammography screening use. Oncol Nurs Forum. 2006;33:105–12.
51. Mayo RM, Ureda JR, Parker VG. Importance of fatalism in understanding mammography screening in rural elderly women. J Women Aging. 2001;13: 57–72.
52. Mohamed IE, Williams KS, et al. Understanding locally advanced breast cancer: what influences a woman's decision to delay treatment? Prev Med. 2005;41:399–405.
53. Gullatte MM, Hardin P, et al. Religious beliefs and delay in breast cancer diagnosis for self-detected breast changes in African-American women. J Natl Black Nurses Assoc. 2009;20:25–35.
54. Sharf BF, Stelljes LA, Gordon HS. "A little bitty spot and I'm a big man": patients' perspectives on refusing diagnosis of treatment for lung cancer. Psychooncology. 2005;14:636–46.
55. Powe BD. Promoting fecal occult blood testing in rural African American women. Cancer Pract. 2002;10:139–46.
56. Morgan PD, Fogel J, et al. Culturally targeted educational intervention to increase colorectal health awareness among African Americans. J Health Care Poor Underserved. 2010;21:132–47.
57. Fair AM, Wujcik D, Lin JMS, et al. Psychosocial determinants of mammography follow-up after receipt of abnormal mammography results in medically underserved women. J Health Care Poor Underserved. 2010;21:71–94.
58. Philip EJ, DuHamel K, Jandorf L. Evaluating the impact of an educational intervention to increase CRC screening rates in the African American community: a preliminary study. Cancer Causes Control. 2010;21:1685–91.
59. Baron-Epel O, Granot M, et al. Perceptions of breast cancer among Arab Israeli women. Women Health. 2004;40:101–16.
60. Baron-Epel O. Attitudes and beliefs associated with mammography in a multiethnic population in Israel. Health Educ Behav. 2010;37:227–42.
61. Holroyd E, Twinn S, Peymane A. Socio-cultural influences on Chinese women's attendance for cervical screening. J Adv Nurs. 2004;46:42–52.
62. Shahid S, Thompson SC. An overview of cancer and beliefs about the disease in indigenous people of Australia, Canada, New Zealand and the US. Aust N Z J Public Health. 2009;33:109–18.
63. Schmidt C. Fatalism may fuel cancer-causing behaviors. J Natl Cancer Inst. 2007;99:1222–3.
64. Powe BD. Cancer fatalism among elderly African American women: predictors of the intensity of the perceptions. J Psychosoc Oncol. 2001;19:85–96.
65. Powe BD, Daniels EC, et al. Perceptions about breast cancer among African American women: do selected educational materials challenge them? Patient Educ Couns. 2005;56:197–204.
66. Powe BD, Cooper DL, Harmond L, et al. Comparing knowledge of colorectal and prostate cancer among African American and Hispanic men. Cancer Nurs. 2009;32:412–7.
67. Powe BD, Ross L, et al. Testicular Cancer among African American college men: knowledge, perceived risk, and perceptions of cancer fatalism. Am J Mens Health. 2007;1:73–80.
68. Facione NC, Miaskowski C, et al. The self-reported likelihood of patient delay in breast cancer: new thoughts for early detection. Prev Med. 2002;34:397–407.
69. Powe BD, Underwood S, et al. Perceptions about breast cancer among college students: implications for nursing education. J Nurs Educ. 2005;44:257–65.
70. Salazar MK. Hispanic women's beliefs about breast cancer and mammography. Cancer Nurs. 1996;19: 437–46.
71. Carpenter V, Colwell B. Cancer knowledge, self-efficacy, and cancer screening behaviors among Mexican-American women. J Cancer Educ. 1995;10:217–22.
72. Pérez-Stable EJ, Sabogal R, et al. Misconceptions about cancer among Latinos and Anglos. JAMA. 1992;268:3219–23.
73. Sanders Thompson VL, Lewis T, Williams SL. Refining the use of cancer-related cultural constructs among African Americans. Health Promot Pract. 2011. doi:10.1177/1524839911399431
74. Ramirez JR, Crano WD, Quist R, et al. Effects of fatalism and family communication on HIV/AIDS awareness variations in Native American and Anglo parents and children. AIDS Educ Prev. 2002;14: 29–40.
75. Lange LJ, Piette JD. Personal models for diabetes in context and patients' health status. J Behav Med. 2006;29:239–53.
76. Pasick RJ, Burke NJ. A critical review of theory in breast cancer screening promotion across cultures. Annu Rev Public Health. 2008;29:351–68.
77. Freeman HP. Cancer in the socioeconomically disadvantaged. CA Cancer J Clin. 1989;39:266–88.
78. Azaiza F, Cohen M. Colorectal cancer screening patterns, intentions, and predictors in Jewish and Arab Israelis. Health Educ Behav. 2008;35:198–203.

79. Angel RJ, Williams K. Cultural models of health and illness. In: Cuellar I, Paniagua FA, editors. Handbook of multicultural mental health. San Diego, CA: Academic; 2000. p. 27–44.

80. Cohen M, Azaiza F. Early breast cancer detection practices, health beliefs and cancer worries in Jewish and Arab women. Prev Med. 2005;41:852–8.

81. Cohen M, Azaiza F. Health-promoting behaviors and health locus of control from a multicultural perspective. Ethn Dis. 2007;17:636–42.

82. Ramirez AG, Suarez L, et al. Hispanic women's breast and cervical cancer knowledge, attitudes, and screening behaviors. Am J Health Promot. 2000;14:292–300.

83. Terán L, Baezconde-Garbanati L, et al. On-time mammography screening with a focus on Latinas with low income: A proposed cultural model. Anticancer Res. 2007;27:4325–38.

84. Smith RA, Cokkinides V, Brooks D, et al. Cancer Screening in the United States, 2011. A review of current American Cancer Society guidelines and issues in cancer screening. CA Cancer J Clin. 2011;61:8–30.

85. Rauscher GH, Ferrans CE, Kaiser K, et al. Misconceptions about breast lumps and delayed medical presentation in urban breast cancer patients. Cancer Epidemiol Biomarkers Prev. 2010;19:640–7.

86. Norsaadah B, Rampal KG, et al. Diagnosis delay of breast cancer and its associated factors in Malaysian women. BMC Cancer. 2011;11:141.

87. Siminoff LA, Rogers HL, et al. Doctor, what's wrong with me? Factors that delay the diagnosis of colorectal cancer. Patient Educ Couns. 2011;84(3):352–8. doi:10.1016/j.pec.2011.05.002.

88. Maly RC, Leake B, Mojica CM, et al. What influences diagnostic delay in low-income women with breast cancer? J Women's Health (Larchmt). 2011;20(7):1017–23. doi:10.1089/jwh.2010.2105.

89. Bibb SC. The relationship between access and stage at diagnosis of breast cancer in African American and Caucasian women. Oncol Nurs Forum. 2001;28:711–9.

90. Fedewa SA, Edge SB, et al. Race and ethnicity are associated with delays in breast cancer treatment (2003–2006). J Health Care Poor Underserved. 2011;22:128–41.

91. Sheppard VB, Davis K. Boisvert, et al. Do recently diagnosed black breast cancer patients find questions about cancer fatalism acceptable? A Preliminary Report. J Cancer Educ. 2011;26:5–10.

92. Powe BD. Editorial: do recently diagnosed black breast cancer patients find questions about cancer fatalism acceptable? A preliminary report. J Cancer Educ. 2011;26:3–4.

93. Henderson PD, Gore SV, et al. African American women coping with breast cancer: a qualitative analysis. Oncol Nurs Forum. 2003;30:641–7.

94. Goldblatt H, Cohen M, Azaiza F, Ramon M. Being within or being between? The cultural context of Arab women's experience of coping with breast cancer in Israel. Psychooncology 2012 (Epub, ahead of print)

95. Hou WK, Lam WW, Fielding R. Adaptation process and psychosocial resources of Chinese colorectal cancer patients undergoing adjuvant treatment: a qualitative analysis. Psychooncology. 2009;18:936–44.

96. Moorey S, Greer S. Cognitive Behavior Therapy for People with Cancer. Oxford: Oxford University Press; 2002.

97. Greer S, Watson M. Mental adjustment to cancer: its measurement and prognostic importance. Cancer Surv. 1987;6:439–53.

98. Lazarus R, Folkman S. Stress, Appraisal, and Coping. New York: Springer; 1984.

99. Greer S, Moorey S, Baruch JDR, et al. Group adjuvant psychological therapy for patients with cancer: a prospective randomized trial. BMJ. 1992;304: 675–80.

100. Watson M, Greer S, Rowden L, et al. Relationships between emotional control, adjustment to cancer and depression and anxiety in breast cancer patients. Psychol Med. 1991;21:51–7.

101. Ferrero J, Barreto MP, Toledo M. Mental adjustment to cancer and quality of life in breast cancer. An exploratory study. Psychooncology. 1994;3: 223–32.

102. Classen C, Koopman C, et al. Coping styles associated with psychological adjustment to advanced breast cancer. Health Psychol. 1996;15:434–7.

103. Reuter K, Classen CC, Roscoe JA, et al. Association of coping style, pain, age and depression with fatigue in women with primary breast cancer. Psychooncology. 2006;15:772–9.

104. Pettingale KW, Morris T, Greer S. Mental attitudes to cancer: an additional prognostic factor. Lancet. 1985;30:750.

105. Miki Y, Swensen J, Shattuck-Eidens D, et al. A strong candidate for the breast and ovarian cancer susceptibility gene BRCA1. Science. 1994;266:66–71.

106. Belkic K, Cohen M, et al. Screening of high-risk groups for breast and ovarian cancer in Europe: a focus on the Jewish population. Oncol Rev. 2010;4:233–67.

107. Senior V, Marteau TM, Peters TJ. Will genetic testing for predisposition for disease result in fatalism? A qualitative study of parents' responses to neonatal screening for familial hypercholesterolaemia. Soc Sci Med. 1999;48:1857–60.

108. Cohen M, Klein E, Kuten A, et al. Increased emotional distress in daughters of breast cancer patients is associated with decreased natural cytotoxic activity, elevated level of stress hormones and decreased secretion of TH1 cytokines. Int J Cancer. 2002;100:347–54.

109. Ryan EL, Skinner SC. Risk beliefs and interest in counseling: focus-group interviews among first-degree relatives of breast cancer patients. J Cancer Educ. 1999;14:99–103.

110. Green J, Murton F, Statham H. Psychosocial issues raised by a familial ovarian cancer register. J Med Genet. 1993;30:575–9.
111. Caruso A, Vigna C, Marozzo B, et al. Subjective versus objective risk in genetic counseling for hereditary breast and/or ovarian cancers. J Exp Clin Cancer Res. 2009;28:157.
112. Lerman C, Lustbader E, Rimer B, et al. Effects of individualized breast cancer risk counseling: a randomized trial. J Natl Cancer Inst. 1995;7: 286–91.
113. Lerman C, Daly M, Sands C, et al. Mammography adherence and psychological distress among women at risk for breast cancer. J Natl Cancer Inst. 1993;85:1074–80.
114. Cohen M. First-degree relatives of breast cancer patients: cognitive perceptions, coping, and adherence to breast self-examination. Behav Med. 2002;28:15–22.
115. Cohen M. Breast cancer early detection, health beliefs, and cancer worries in randomly selected women with and without a family history of breast cancer. Psychooncology. 2006;10:873–83.
116. Kash KM, Holland JC, et al. Psychological distress and surveillance behaviors of women with a family history of breast cancer. J Natl Cancer Inst. 1992;84:24–30.
117. Gilbar O. Do attitudes toward cancer, sense of coherence and family high risk predict more psychological distress in women referred for a breast cancer examination? Women Health. 2003;38:35–46.
118. Power TE, Robinson JW, Bridge P, et al. Distress and psychosocial needs of a heterogeneous high risk familial cancer population. J Genet Couns. 2011;20:249–69.
119. Wellisch DK, Gritz ER, et al. Psychological functioning of daughters of breast cancer patients. Part I: daughters and comparison subjects. Psychosomatics. 1991;32:324–36.
120. Randolph WM, Freeman Jr DH, Freeman JL. Pap smear use in a population of older Mexican-American women. Women Health. 2002;36:21–31.
121. O'Malley MS, Earp JA, Hawley ST, et al. The association of race/ethnicity, socioeconomic status, and physician recommendation for mammography: who gets the message about breast cancer screening? Am J Public Health. 2001;91:49–54.
122. Jennings K. Getting black women to screen for cancer: incorporating health beliefs into practice. J Am Acad Nurse Pract. 1996;8:53–9.
123. Freund A, Cohen M, Azaiza F. Perceptions of barriers to screening of ultra-Orthodox Jewish women in Israel. In preparation research report (in Hebrew).
124. Rajaram SS, Rashidi A. Asian-Islamic women and breast cancer screening: a socio-cultural analysis. Women Health. 1999;28:45–58.
125. James A, Wells A. Religion and mental health: towards a cognitive-behavioral framework. Br J Health Psychol. 2003;8:359–76.
126. McCullough ME, Hoyt WT, Larson DB, et al. Religious involvement and mortality: a meta-analytic review. Health Psychol. 2000;19: 211–22.
127. Zollinger TW, Champion VL, Monahan PO, et al. Effects of personal characteristics on African-American women's beliefs about breast cancer. Am J Health Promot. 2010;24:371–7.
128. Lagos VI, Perez MA, Ricker CN, et al. Social-cognitive aspects of underserved Latinas preparing to undergo genetic cancer risk assessment for hereditary breast and ovarian cancer. Psychooncology. 2008;17:774–82.
129. Roncancio AM, Ward KK, Berenson AB. Hispanic women's health care provider control expectations: the influence of fatalism and acculturation. J Health Care Poor Underserved. 2011;22:482–90.
130. Seligman MEP. Helplessness: on depression, Development, and Death. San Francisco: W.H. Freeman; 1975.
131. Henry PC. Life stress, explanatory style, hopelessness, and occupational stress. Int J Stress Manag. 2005;12:241–56.
132. Powe BD. Cancer fatalism—spiritual perspectives. J Relig Health. 1997;36:135–7.
133. American Psychiatric Association. Diagnostic and Statistical Manual of Mental Disorders. 4th ed. Washington, DC: American Psychiatric Association; 2000.
134. Coyne JC, Thompson R, et al. Should we screen for depression? Caveats and potential pitfalls. Appl Prev Psychol. 2000;9:101–21.
135. Hasin DS, Goodwin RD, et al. The epidemiology of major depressive disorder: results from the National Epidemiologic Survey on Alcoholism and Related Conditions. Arch Gen Psychiatry. 2005;62: 1097–106.

Positive Psychology Perspectives Across the Cancer Continuum: Meaning, Spirituality, and Growth

Crystal L. Park

To live is to suffer, to survive is to find some meaning in the suffering

(attributed to both Friedrich Nietzsche and Roberta Flack)

Cancer Survivorship

Through both public health and public relations efforts, cancer survivorship has come to denote the state or process of living after a diagnosis of cancer, regardless of how long a person lives (National Cancer Institute [1]). By this definition, a person is considered to become a cancer survivor at the point of diagnosis and to remain a survivor throughout treatment and the rest of his or her life [1]. The term "survivor" was chosen with great care by the National Coalition for Cancer Survivorship to explicitly promote empowerment of those with cancer [2]. There are an estimated 12 million cancer survivors in the United States, representing approximately 4% of the US population [3], and an estimated 25 million survivors worldwide [4]. Many survivors are in longer-term survivorship; for example, approximately 14% of cancer survivors in the United States were diagnosed over 20 years ago [3].

The cancer experience from diagnosis through longer-term survivorship has been described as a continuum comprising different phases, including living with cancer, living through cancer, and living beyond cancer [5, 6].

The demands on survivors differ across these phases, leading to different emotional reactions and coping responses. Further, the roles played by each of the three positive psychology constructs considered here, meaning, spirituality, and growth, may differ across these phases (see Table 7.1).

The first phase, living with cancer, refers to the time of diagnosis and active treatment. Fear, anxiety, and pain resulting from both illness and treatment are common. While in primary treatment, cancer often becomes life's central focus not only for the cancer patient but also for his or her family and friends. Primary treatment may involve intensive and immediate coping with medical issues, decision-making, and the many chaotic emotions that ensue, including fear, hope, pain, and grief [7].

The second phase, living through cancer, refers to the time following remission or treatment completion. The transition period from primary treatment to longer-term survivorship is a critical time, setting the course of psychological adjustment for years to come. While a relief in many ways, this transition is often highly stressful in its own right [8, 9], due in part to reduced frequency of visits and access to medical providers, changes in daily routines, adjustment to treatment-related side effects, and uneasiness about being on one's own after having such close relations with medical providers [7, 10]. Psychologically, survivors are often in a state of watchful waiting, with high fears of recurrence [9, 11].

C.L. Park, Ph.D (✉)
Department of Psychology, University of Connecticut,
Storrs, CT 06269-1020, USA
e-mail: crystal.park@uconn.edu

B.I. Carr and J. Steel (eds.), *Psychological Aspects of Cancer*,
DOI 10.1007/978-1-4614-4866-2_7, © Springer Science+Business Media, LLC 2013

Table 7.1 The Roles of Meaning, Spirituality and Growth Across the Cancer Continuum

	Living with cancer	Living through cancer	Living beyond cancer
Cancer-related involvement	Diagnosis and active treatment	Transition from primary treatment and regular contact with health-care providers	Longer-term survivorship
Role of cancer in one's life	Cancer and treatment is life's central focus	Attempts to resume a "new normal" life; cancer focus reduced. Transition from patient can be jarring	Long-term implications of being a cancer survivor
Potential roles of meaning	Sources of meaning as support Violations of global meaning	Reconsideration and reconstitution of global beliefs and goals	Cancer as part of one's life narrative. Sense of life meaning often enhanced
Potential roles of spirituality	Spiritual crisis. Turning towards spirituality for strength and support	Reconsideration and reconstitution of spiritual beliefs and goals	Revised spiritual global meaning
Potential roles of growth	Possibilities of positive outcomes may provide hope Most reports illusory, function as coping	Reflection on changes experienced; identification of positive changes	Maintenance of life changes or return to pre-cancer baseline

The third phase, living beyond cancer, refers to a time when the "activity of the disease or likelihood of its return is sufficiently small that the cancer can now be considered permanently arrested" [5, p. 272]. Even after survivors enter this phase, a sense of vulnerability, fears of recurrence, and psychosocial problems related to their cancer experience are common [12]. However, longer-term survivorship affords individuals opportunities to reflect on and embellish their narratives to include their cancer experience, and to feel they have made some meaning from their cancer [13]. Being a cancer survivor often becomes an important aspect of self-identity [14].

The Meaning-Making Model

The meaning-making model addresses two levels of meaning, global and situational [15]. Global meaning refers to individuals' general orienting systems. Situational meaning comprises initial appraisals of a given situation, the processes through which global and appraised situational meanings are revised, and the outcomes of these processes. Components of the meaning-making model are illustrated in Fig. 7.1. In this section, the elements of this meaning-making model are briefly described. This model then serves as the framework to discuss the roles of meaning, spirituality, and growth in the context of cancer.

Global Meaning

Global Meaning consists of the structures through which people perceive and understand themselves and the world, encompassing beliefs, goals, and subjective feelings of purpose or meaning in life [15, 16]. Global meaning consists of cognitive, motivational, and affective components, termed, respectively, global beliefs, global goals, and a sense of meaning or purpose [17–19].

Global beliefs concerning fairness, justice, luck, control, predictability, coherence, benevolence, personal vulnerability, and identity comprise the core schemas through which people interpret their experiences of the world [20, 21]. Global goals are individuals' ideals, states, or objects towards which they work to be, obtain, accomplish, or maintain [22, 23]. Common global goals include relationships, work, health, wealth, knowledge, and achievement [24]. Subjective feelings of meaning refer to a sense of "meaningfulness" or purpose in life [19, 25]. This sense of meaningfulness comes from seeing one's life as containing those goals that one values as well as feeling one is making adequate progress towards important future goals [25, 26]. Together, global beliefs and goals, and the resultant sense of life meaning, form individuals' meaning systems, the lens through which they interpret, evaluate, and respond to their experiences.

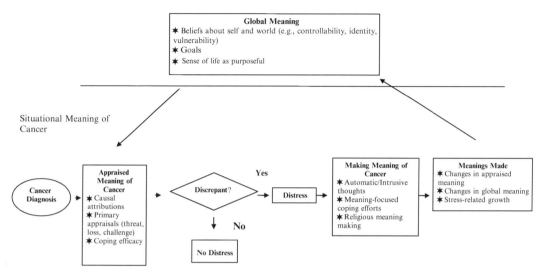

Fig. 7.1 The Meaning-making Model in the Context of Cancer

Situational Meaning: The Meaning of Potentially Stressful Encounters

Meaning is an important part of everyday life [27], informing people's ways of understanding and functioning, although such influences are typically subtle and unnoticed. However, confrontations with highly stressful experiences such as serious illness bring meaning to the fore [28, 29]. People assign meanings to, or appraise, potentially stressful situations [30]. These appraised meanings are to some extent determined by the specifics of the particular situation, but are also largely informed by individuals' global meaning.

Stress as Discrepancy Between Global and Situational Meaning

The meaning-making model is based on the notion that stress occurs when people perceive discrepancies between their global meaning (i.e., what they believe and desire) and their appraised meaning of a particular situation [17, 18]. This discrepancy-related stress motivates individuals to resolve their problems and dissipate the resultant negative emotions [31]. Confrontation with a severe stressor is thought to have the potential to

violate or even shatter global meaning systems (i.e., individuals' global beliefs about the world and themselves and their overarching goals). Such violations or discrepancies are thought to initiate individuals' cognitive and emotional processing—"meaning-making" efforts—to rebuild their meaning systems. Meaning-making involves efforts to understand and conceptualize a stressor in a way more consistent with their global meaning and to incorporate that understanding into their larger system of global meaning through assimilation and accommodation processes [15].

Resolving stressful events entails reducing discrepancies between appraised meanings and global meanings [32–34]. Discrepancies can be reduced in many ways, and, to this end, people engage in many types of coping (e.g., [13, 35]). People may engage in problem-focused coping, taking direct actions to reduce the discrepancy by changing the conditions that create or maintain the problem. When encountering stress, individuals can also engage in emotion-focused coping, much of which is targeted at directly alleviating distress, albeit temporarily, by disengaging mentally or behaviorally (e.g., focusing on some distraction). Emotion-focused coping, by definition, does not reduce discrepancies, which may be why it is generally associated with distress [36].

Stressful situations vary in the extent to which they are amenable to problem-focused coping, such as planning and actively focusing on changing the problematic situation (e.g., [37, 38]). Problem-focused coping is generally considered the most adaptive type of coping [36], but low-control situations such as trauma, loss, and serious illness are not amenable to direct repair or problem-solving. In such low-control situations, meaning-making coping is particularly relevant and potentially more adaptive [39]. Meaning-making refers to approach-oriented *intrapsychic* efforts to reduce discrepancies between appraised and global meaning. Meaning-focused coping aims to reduce discrepancy by changing either the very meaning of the stressor itself (appraised meaning) or by changing one's global beliefs and goals; either way, meaning-focused coping aims to improve the fit between the appraised meaning of the stressor and global meaning.

Following highly stressful events, individuals' meaning-making processes typically involve searching for some more favorable or consistent understanding of the event and its implications for their beliefs about themselves and their lives. Meaning-making may also entail reconsidering global beliefs and revising goals (see [40]) and questioning or revising their sense of meaning in life [25].

This rebuilding process is assumed to lead to better adjustment, particularly if adequate meaning is found or created (for reviews, see [17, 41, 42]). However, protracted attempts to assimilate or accommodate may devolve into maladaptive rumination over time if satisfactory meanings cannot be constructed [43]. That is, meaning-making is helpful to the extent that it produces a satisfactory product (i.e., *meaning made*) [17].

Meanings Made

The products that result from meaning-making, termed *meanings made*, involve changes in global or situational meaning, such as revised identity, growth, or reappraised situational or global meaning. The outcomes of the meaning-making process involve changes in global or situational meaning. As illustrated in Fig. 7.1, individuals may make many different types of meaning through their meaning-making processes. Among these are a sense of having "made sense" (e.g., [44]), a sense of acceptance (e.g., [45]), causal understanding (e.g., [20]), transformed identity that integrates the stressful experience into one's identity [46], reappraised or transformed meaning of the stressor (e.g., [35]), changed global beliefs (e.g., [47]), changed global goals (e.g., [48]), a revised or reconstituted sense of meaning in life (e.g., [20]), and perceptions of growth or positive life changes [31].

Meaning in the Context of Cancer

Both global and situational meanings influence the processes of coping with cancer across the continuum from diagnosis through treatment and longer-term survivorship. Further, these influences may vary across this continuum (see Table 7.1). A diagnosis of cancer can shatter aspects of a patient's extant global meaning. For example, most people hold views of the world as benign, predictable, and fair and their own lives as safe and controllable [33, 49]. A cancer diagnosis is typically experienced as being at extreme odds with such beliefs (e.g., [50]), setting in motion processes of distress and meaning-making that ultimately lead to changes in survivors' situational and global meaning.

Appraised Meaning of Cancer

People appraise the meaning of their cancer diagnosis based on the information they receive from their healthcare providers and other sources along with their own understanding of the disease of "cancer" (e.g., time course, severity) [51], their appraisals of their ability to manage the illness and its anticipated impact on their future [51], and their general sense of control over their life [52, 53]. Research indicates that the meanings that survivors assign to their cancer experience predict not only their coping and subsequent adjustment but also their treatment-related decisions and their well-being (e.g., [54, 55]). For example, a study of prostate cancer survivors found that those who appraised their cancer as a loss had higher levels of depression, while those who appraised their cancer as a threat had higher levels of anxiety [55]. Similarly, a study of survivors of a variety of cancers found that threat appraisals were related to higher levels of distress, although challenge appraisals were unrelated to distress [56].

Applying Lipowski's [57] taxonomy of illness appraisals in a large sample of breast cancer survivors, Degner et al. [58] found that shortly after diagnosis, most survivors appraised their cancer as a "challenge" (57.4%) or as having "value" (27.6%); few appraised their cancer as "enemy" (7.8%), "irreparable loss" (3.9%), or "punishment" (0.6%). These appraisals were mostly unchanged 3 years later, and survivors who had initially appraised their cancer as a challenge or as having value reported less anxiety at follow-up. Cross-sectionally, at follow-up, women who appraised the cancer negatively (i.e., "enemy," "loss," or "punishment") had higher levels of depression and anxiety and poorer quality of life than women who appraised their cancer in more positive ways. Similar findings were recently reported by Büssing and Fischer [59].

Control appraisals have also been linked to survivors' well-being. For example, in the above-mentioned study of survivors of various cancers [56], appraised uncontrollability of the cancer was related to higher levels of distress, although appraised self-controllability of the cancer was unrelated to distress. Similarly, a study of ovarian cancer patients found a strong negative relationship between women's appraised control over their illness and their psychological distress [60]. Some research has shown that appraisals are also related to physical health. In studies of colorectal [61] and prostate [62] cancer survivors, having a belief that nothing could cure most cancer was related to all-cause mortality 15 years later, controlling for many confounding factors. The authors speculated that these associations may be due to health protective behaviors, adherence to recommended medical protocols, or more lax monitoring of disease recurrence.

Attributions for the cancer are another type of appraisal survivors make [63]. Attributions involve assigning a cause to the cancer; such attributions may change over time through meaning-making processes. In those cases where the attribution is derived not through a fairly quick and automatic process but through cognitive processing over time, such attributions may be more accurately viewed as reattributions, a product of meaning-making [17]. Unfortunately, virtually no studies have differentiated attributions from reattributions or examined processes of timing and change. Further, most studies assessed attributions long after the initial diagnosis of cancer was made. Thus, survivors in most existing research are reporting on their reattributions rather than their initial understanding of their cancer. Therefore, the majority of research on cancer attributions is reviewed in the subsequent section on meanings made.

This section simply notes that different types of cancer may elicit different types of causal attributions, which may be evidenced in initial appraisals. For example, Costanzo and her colleagues [64] proposed that because of the lack of information on environmental or behavioral causes of gynecological cancer, women with gynecological cancers were less likely to attribute their cancer to specific causes and more likely to attribute their cancer to chance or God's will. In that study of gynecological cancer survivors, God's will was mentioned as a factor contributing to the development of cancer by 39% of the sample, ranking third only behind genetics/heredity and stress. Further, in the factors perceived to prevent a cancer recurrence, prayer was mentioned by 90% of the sample, ranking third only behind medical checkups and a positive attitude. God's will, assessed as a separate factor, was mentioned by 69% of the sample.

Cancer as Violation of Global Meaning

Receiving a diagnosis of cancer can violate important global beliefs such as the fairness, benevolence, and predictability of the world as well as one's sense of invulnerability and personal control [10, 65, 66]. Beliefs in a loving God may also be violated [67]. Further, having cancer almost invariably violates individuals' goals for their current lives and their plans for the future [68].

According to the meaning-making model, the extent to which having cancer is perceived as inconsistent with global beliefs such as those regarding identity (e.g., I live a healthy life style) and health (e.g., living a healthy lifestyle protects people from illness) and global goals (e.g., desire to live a long time with robust health and without disability) determines the extent to which the diagnosis is distressing. Different types of cancer and the specifics of an individual's illness (e.g., prognosis, treatment) likely influence the situational meaning given and the extent of discrepancy with global meaning (e.g., [69]).

Several studies of cancer survivors have examined how global meaning violations may arise from having cancer. For example, a cross-sectional study found that gastrointestinal cancer patients appraised their cancer as highly discrepant with their beliefs and goals; greater discrepancies were related to more anxiety and depression [70]. A longitudinal study of survivors of various cancers found that the extent to which the cancer was appraised as violating their beliefs in a just world was inversely related to their psychological well-being across the year of the study [13]. Similarly, a study that did not directly measure appraisals of violation but that likely reflects those found that compared to women without a diagnosis of breast cancer, women diagnosed with breast cancer reported lower levels of perceived control over their lives; findings were especially strong for breast cancer survivors who had received chemotherapy [71]. These links between discrepancy of appraised and global meaning with adjustment in cancer survivorship have seldom been directly examined, and much remains to be learned about perceptions of belief and goal violation.

Making Meaning from the Cancer Experience

Researchers have posited that meaning-making efforts are essential to adjustment to cancer by helping survivors either assimilate the cancer experience into their pre-cancer global meaning or helping them to change their global meaning to accommodate it [66]. Many researchers have proposed, therefore, that meaning-making is critical to successfully navigate these changes ([29, 66, 72, 73]. Indeed, it is hard to imagine that survivors could come through a cancer experience without some reconsideration of their lives vis-à-vis cancer [29, 72, 74, 75]. However, some researchers have suggested that survivors sometimes simply accept their cancer experience or, once it has ended, have little need to think or reflect on it [76, 77].

According to the meaning-making model, meaning-making following cancer involves survivors' attempts to integrate their understanding (appraisal) of the cancer together with their global meaning to reduce the discrepancy between them [15, 78]. Yet to assess meaning-making, many studies have employed overly simple questions, such as "How often have you found yourself searching to make sense of your illness?' and "How often have you found yourself wondering why you got cancer or asking, 'Why Me?'" (e.g., [79]).

Such assessments do not adequately measure meaning-making [17]. Survivors' meaning-making processes involve deliberate coping efforts, such as reappraising the event, reconsidering their global beliefs and goals, and searching for some understanding of the cancer and its implications for themselves and their lives (e.g., [66, 80]). In addition, meaning-making processes apparently often occur beneath the level of awareness or without conscious efforts (e.g., in the form of intrusive thoughts; [32, 66]).

In addition, although meaning-making is presumed to be adaptive [17, 66], many studies have found that survivors' searching for meaning is typically related to poorer adjustment (e.g., [79, 81, 82]). For example, a study of breast cancer survivors completing treatment found that positive reinterpretation, attempting to see the cancer in a more positive light or find benefits in it, was unrelated to adjustment, while emotional processing, attempting to understand the reasons underlying one's feelings, was actually associated with subsequently higher levels of distress [83].

A cross-sectional study of long-term breast cancer survivors found that searching for meaning was related to poorer adjustment [75], and a study of prostate cancer survivors shortly after treatment found that meaning-making efforts were related to higher levels of distress both concurrently and 3 months later [79].

Such findings are not inconsistent with the meaning-making model, however, because these studies not only failed to adequately assess meaning-making, but they also failed to comprehensively examine all of the components of the model, such as belief and goal violation. Further, many were conducted cross-sectionally, although longitudinal assessments of appraised meanings and discrepancies between situational and global meaning and examination of change in them over time are necessary to truly capture this assimilation/accommodation process.

In addition, the meaning-making model proposes that meaning-making per se is not necessarily adaptive and, in fact, may be indistinguishable from rumination, without attention to whether meaning has actually been *made*. Few studies have distinguished between adaptive meaning-making and maladaptive rumination; this lack of discrimination may account for the lack of more consistently favorable effects of meaning-making [13, 43]. According to the meaning-making model, when cancer survivors search for meaning, either through deliberate efforts or through more automatic processes, and achieve a reintegration of their cancer experience and their global meaning, they experience less distress *and* engage in less subsequent meaning-making [13]. However, when meaning-making efforts fail, the cancer experience may remain highly distressing. Unable to assimilate their cancer experience into their belief system or accommodate their previously held beliefs to account for their experience, survivors may experience a loss of personal or spiritual meaning, existential isolation, and apathy [10] and may persist in meaning-making efforts even years afterward (e.g., [75]), accounting for the positive relationship between searching for meaning and distress.

To date, few studies of cancer survivorship have assessed both the search for and the finding of meaning and tested their combined effects on adjustment in survivors. A study of breast cancer survivors in the first 18 months post diagnosis found that women who never searched for meaning and those who searched and found meaning did not differ on negative affect, but both groups had less negative affect than women who were searching but had not found meaning over time [82]. Further, the abovementioned study of younger adult survivors of various cancers assessed meaning-making (as positive reappraisal) and meanings made (growth, reduced discrepancies with global meaning). Results indicated that positive reappraisal led to increases in perceived growth and life meaning, which was related to reduced violations of a just world belief. This process was related to better psychological adjustment [13].

An intriguing but largely overlooked aspect of meaning-making in cancer survivorship is that meaning-making efforts may have different effects on well-being at different points along the survivorship continuum. For example, some researchers have proposed that during primary treatment, when patients are dealing with the impact of the diagnosis and making treatment decisions, effective coping may be more problem-focused, dealing with the immediate demands of the crisis, while meaning-making may be especially important during the transition to longer-term survivorship [10]. The transition to longer-term survivorship, as survivors return to their everyday postprimary treatment lives, may allow more time and energy for more reflective approaches to longer-term psychosocial and existential issues and may change the effects of such processing [75, 83].

Meaning Made from the Cancer Experience

People are thought to make meaning of stressful experiences primarily by changing the meaning of those experiences (i.e., their situational meaning), but sometimes violations of global meaning are too great to be assimilated, and people must turn to processes of accommodation, which produce shifts in global meaning [20]. Researchers have identified a number of products of meaning-making in cancer survivorship. The global meaning change most studied among cancer survivors is that of stress-related growth, the positive changes people report experiencing as the result of stressful encounters [31]; growth is so widely studied that it warrants its own section below. In addition, researchers have identified other psychological phenomena that may be conceptualized as outcomes or products of the search for meaning in cancer survivors. Among these are understanding regarding the cancer's occurrence (usually assessed as reattributions) and the integration of cancer and survivorship into identity [46].

Causal understanding of cancer. As noted above, many studies have focused on the attributions cancer survivors make; because these studies are usually conducted long after the diagnosis, survivors' reported attributions likely reflect considerable meaning-making. Research with cancer survivors has indicated that most survivors have ideas or explanations regarding the cause of their cancer (e.g., [63]. However, simply possessing an explanation does not necessarily reflect adequate meaning; in fact, many causal attributions are associated with *greater* distress (e.g., [64, 84]). Instead, the specific cause referred to determines an attribution's ability to establish meaning and thus its relations with adjustment. For example, one literature review on attributions made by breast cancer survivors concluded that attributions to predictable and controllable causes such as pollution, stress, or lifestyle factors such as smoking were associated with better adjustment [85]. However, feeling that one caused one's own cancer (self-blame) has consistently been shown to be negatively related to adjustment among cancer survivors (e.g., [86]).

The link between having made meaning by identifying causes of the cancer and adjustment is therefore more complicated than it might first appear. This is illustrated in the abovementioned study of women with gynecological cancers [64], in which most attributions (e.g., genetics/heredity, stress, hormones, and environmental factors) were related to elevated levels of anxiety and depression. However, survivors who attributed their cancer to potentially controllable causes

were more likely to be practicing healthy behaviors. Similarly, women citing health behaviors as important in preventing recurrence reported greater anxiety, but were also more likely to practice positive health behaviors. Further, health behavior attributions interacted with health practices in predicting distress. For example, among women who had not made positive dietary changes, appraising lifestyle as important in preventing recurrence was associated with greater distress, whereas for those who had made a positive change in diet, lifestyle attributions were associated with less distress. Thus, it appears that behaviors consistent with attributions can be effective in reducing discrepancies in meaning and therefore related to better adjustment.

Integration of cancer and survivorship into one's life narrative and identity. Another potentially important outcome of meaning-making involves the integration of the experience of cancer into survivors' ongoing life story and sense of self [87]. Surviving cancer has been described as a process of identity reconstruction through which survivors integrate the cancer experience into their self-concept, developing a sense of "living through and beyond cancer" [88, 89]. The extent to which having cancer becomes interwoven with other experiences in survivors' narratives may reflect successful making of meaning, having come to terms with the cancer. Such narrative integration is widely viewed as an important aspect of recovery (e.g., [66]). Little quantitative research has studied the cancer recovery process in terms of narrative reconstruction, although many qualitative accounts suggest that this is a promising approach (e.g., [90]).

A few studies have examined the extent to which cancer survivors embrace labels that refer to their cancer status and how that identification relates to their well-being. An early study by Deimling and his colleagues [89] examined cancer-related identities in a sample of older, long-term survivors of a variety of cancers. Asked whether they identified themselves as survivors (yes or no), 90% answered affirmatively. Other labels were endorsed less frequently: 60% identified as ex-patients, 30% as victims, and 20%

as patients. However, considering oneself a victim or a survivor was unrelated to aspects of adjustment, such as mastery, self-esteem, anxiety, depression, or hostility. It should be noted that this study was conducted prior to the mid-1990s, when the term "survivor" began to be actively promoted [2]. A more recent study of long-term survivors of colon, breast, or prostate cancer by the same group of researchers using the same measurement strategy found that 86% of the sample identified as a "cancer survivor," 13% saw themselves as a "patient," and 13% identified as "victim" [91].

Several other studies have addressed post-cancer identities. Asked which term best described them, over half of a sample of longer-term prostate cancer survivors chose "someone who has had cancer" and a quarter chose "survivor," with smaller numbers choosing "patient" or "victim" [76]. Only identifying as a survivor was related to having more positive affect, and no identity was related to negative affect. Finally, in a study of younger adult cancer survivors asked about their post-cancer identities, 83% endorsed "survivor" identity, 81% the identity of "person who has had cancer," 58% "patient," and 18% "victim" (all at least "somewhat") [14]. Endorsements of these four identities were minimally correlated with one another. Those who more strongly endorsed 'Survivor" and "Person who has had cancer" identities were more involved in many cancer-related activities, such as wearing cancer-related items and talking about prevention. Survivor identity correlated with better psychological well-being and victim identity with poorer well-being; neither identifying as a patient nor a person with cancer was related to well-being. However, the extent to which these survivors felt their cancer experience was central to their identity was inversely related to their psychological well-being [92].

Spirituality and Cancer Survivorship

The proliferating literature on spirituality in cancer survivorship provides strong evidence that spirituality typically plays myriad roles in the lives of those with cancer (for reviews, see [93–96]). Spirituality is often pervasively involved in

survivors' global and situational meaning, including their making meaning of the cancer, across the phases of survivorship [97]. Because the present chapter focuses specifically on cancer survivorship, information on how religiousness and spirituality are more generally involved in global meaning is not reviewed here; readers are referred to Park [47]. This section specifically focuses on meaning in the situational context of cancer survivorship.

Spirituality and Appraised Meaning of Cancer

At diagnosis, individuals' pre-cancer spirituality may influence the situational meaning they assign to their cancer, including its appraised meaning and the extent to which their global meaning is violated by that appraisal. Some studies have found that global religious beliefs are related to the ways that cancer patients approach their illness. For example, a study of patients in treatment for a variety of cancers found that although religious beliefs (e.g., "I believe that God will not give me a burden I cannot carry") were not directly related to psychological adjustment, those with higher religious beliefs had a higher sense of efficacy in coping with their cancer, which was related to higher levels of well-being [98]. Another study found that women diagnosed with breast cancer who viewed God as benevolent and involved in their lives appraised their cancer as more of a challenge and an opportunity to grow [67].

Religious beliefs about God's role in suffering, also known as theodicies, may also play an important role in how patients deal with their cancer. One study identified five types of theodicy beliefs: that their suffering is God's punishment for sinful behavior, that they will become a better person as a consequence of their suffering, that a reward for suffering will come in Heaven, that God has a reason for suffering that cannot be explained, and that by suffering with illness, one shares in the suffering of Christ [99]. To date, no research has examined how these different theodicies influence coping with and adjustment to cancer, but recently developed theodicy measurement tools [100] should facilitate such inquiry.

Studies assessing associations of religious causal attributions and control appraisals with well-being in cancer survivors have produced mixed results. In a sample of recently diagnosed cancer patients receiving chemotherapy, appraisals that God was in control of the cancer and that the cancer was due to chance were related to higher self-esteem and lower distress regarding the cancer, while control attributions to self, natural causes, and other people were unrelated [101], and a study focusing more specifically on different types of religious attributions in a sample of young to middle-aged adult survivors of various cancers found that attributing the cancer to an angry or punishing God was related to more anger at God and poorer psychological adjustment [102]. However, in a sample of prostate cancer survivors, causal attributions to God, regardless of their negative (God's anger) or positive (God's love) nature, were related to poorer quality of life. In addition, prostate cancer survivors who reported having a more benevolent relationship with God reported perceiving less control over their health [67]. Attributions of the cancer to God's will in the abovementioned study of gynecological cancer survivors were related to worry about recurrence, but not to anxiety or depressive symptoms [64].

Spirituality and Meaning-making from the Cancer Experience

Meaning-making often involves spiritual methods. For example, people can redefine their cancer experience as an opportunity for spiritual growth or as a punishment from God, or may reappraise whether God has control of their lives or even whether God exists [103]. Researchers typically assess religious meaning-making with subscales from the RCOPE measure [104], which includes a benevolent religious reappraisal subscale (sample item: "saw my situation as part of God's plan") as a component of a broader "positive religious coping" factor and a punishing God reappraisal subscale (sample item: "decided that God was punishing me for my sins") as a component of a broader "negative religious coping" factor.

Studies of people dealing with cancer have generally indicated that positive religious coping is weakly and inconsistently related to adjustment and well-being in cancer survivorship [93, 95]. In contrast, negative religious coping, although less frequently used, tends to be strongly and consistently associated with poorer adjustment and quality of life (e.g., [105, 106]). However, studies of coping with cancer have not separated out the religious meaning-focused coping subscales from other types of positive or negative religious coping nor examined the resultant meanings made through meaning-making.

Further, different types of spiritual and religious coping efforts may be differentially related to well-being depending on the particular phase of the continuum under study. For example, one study suggested that during the diagnostic phase, private spirituality may be particularly relevant [107]. However, few studies have examined spirituality and meaning-making across phases. One important exception, a prospective study of breast cancer patients from pre-diagnosis to 2 years post surgery, found that the use of different religious coping strategies changed over time, and that during particularly high stress points such as pre-surgery, religious coping strategies that provided comfort, such as active surrender of control to God, were highest, while religious coping processes reflecting meaning-making remained elevated or increased over time [108].

Spiritual Meanings Made from the Cancer Experience

Through the meaning-making process, survivors often make changes in how they understand their cancer (changed appraised meaning). They may also make changes in their global beliefs and goals. These changes often have a religious aspect. For example, through meaning-making, survivors may revise their initial understanding of their cancer; these reappraised meanings may be of a religious nature. Summarizing findings from a qualitative study of breast cancer survivors, Gall and Cornblat [109] noted, "When used in the creation of meaning, relationship with God allowed some women to reframe the cancer from a disruptive, crisis event to a 'blessing' and a 'gift.' These women believed that the cancer served some Divine purpose in their lives and so they were better able to accept it" (p. 531). At this point, little quantitative research on reappraised religious meanings has been conducted.

Changes in global religious or spiritual meaning in cancer survivorship are also common [110]. Cole and her colleagues have studied the myriad positive and negative religious and spiritual changes that survivors report in great detail. They have documented that cancer survivors often report that they have become more spiritual and have a stronger sense of the sacred directing their lives but survivors may also believe less strongly in their faith or feel spiritually lost because of their cancer. Interestingly, these two directions of perceived change were uncorrelated in a sample of survivors of a variety of cancers, although positive spiritual transformations were related to higher levels of emotional well-being and quality of life while negative spiritual transformations were inversely related to well-being and quality of life. Cancer survivors with a more advanced stage of cancer or with recurrence were more likely to report positive spiritual transformation, but these factors were not related to spiritual decline. That study did not report whether time since diagnosis (or place on the survivorship continuum) was related to spiritual transformations or its relations with well-being [111]. Such changes in spirituality are usually studied as part of the broader phenomenon of stress-related growth, discussed in the following section.

Stress-Related Growth and Cancer

Stress-related growth, the positive life changes that people report experiencing following stressful events, has garnered increasing research interest in recent years (see [112], for a review), particularly in the context of cancer [31, 113]. Myriad studies of survivors of many types of can-

cer have established that a majority of survivors report experiencing stress-related growth as a result of their experience with cancer [114]. Reported positive changes may occur in one's social relationships (e.g., becoming closer to family or friends), personal resources (e.g., developing patience or persistence), life philosophies (e.g., rethinking one's priorities), spirituality (e.g., feeling closer to God), coping skills (e.g., learning better ways to handle problems or manage emotions), and health behaviors or lifestyles (e.g., lessening stress and taking better care of one's self) [31].

Stress-related growth has also been referred to as "posttraumatic growth," "perceived benefits," "adversarial growth," and "benefit-finding" [113]. This growth is thought to arise as people attempt to make meaning of their cancer experience, trying to understand their cancer and its implications for their lives within the framework of their previous global meaning system or coming to grips with it by transforming their understanding of the world and themselves to enable the integration of the cancer experience into their global meaning system [13, 115].

Stress-related growth is a subjective phenomenon; that is, it reflects a survivor's *perceptions* of change rather than directly reflecting objective change. This subjective nature creates one of the controversies surrounding stress-related growth: Is it "real" or illusory [116]? Research from other areas of psychology suggests a substantial gap between perceptions of positive change and measured change [117], which has also been demonstrated in the few studies that have compared self-reported and actual growth [118, 119].

Some researchers have suggested that stress-related growth may be either an effort to cope (i.e., a form of meaning-making) or an actual outcome of coping (i.e., a form of meaning made), depending on the specifics of the person and the point at which he or she is in the cancer continuum and meaning-making process [31, 113]. For example, a cancer patient experiencing distress who is struggling to deal with difficult treatments may search for some more benign way to understand the experience, voicing how in some ways this experience is a good one because of the positive changes he or she is experiencing. Another may look back at his or her cancer experience from the vantage of posttreatment and identify ways that the experience has favorably changed him or her. The former may be more suspect as an actual meaning made while the latter may more accurately reflect meaning made from the experience. However, more research is needed to determine the conditions under which reported growth reflects meaning-making versus meaning made. One study examining growth in survivors from presurgery to 1 year later found that growth was unrelated to well-being at any point cross-sectionally, but increases in growth over time were related to higher levels of well-being [120], suggesting that "real" or adaptive growth may occur only over time.

Another controversial issue regarding stress-related growth is its relationship with indices of well-being. Although some have argued that perceptions of growth constitute a positive outcome in and of themselves (e.g., [121]), most researchers have endeavored to ascertain relations between stress-related growth and indices of well-being. Although extensive research has been conducted on this topic, results are inconclusive. Cancer survivors' reports of growth following their cancer experience are sometimes (e.g., [122]), but not always (e.g., [123, 124]), related to better psychological adjustment. Many studies on this topic fail to control for potential confounds such as optimism, positive affectivity, or neuroticism, which may account for some of the inconsistency. Also drawing skepticism regarding the relevance of stress-related growth for adjustment are the emerging findings that survivors' reports of negative changes wrought by the cancer appear to be much more potent predictors of well-being than reported positive changes [75, 125].

Positive Psychology and Interventions with Cancer Survivors

Along with the increasing recognition of the importance of meaning-making in the lives of cancer survivors has come the development of a number of meaning-based psychosocial interventions for those with cancer. Some of these interventions are existential in nature, focusing on broader issues of meaning in life (e.g., [126]; see [97], for a review). Breitbart and his colleagues (e.g., [127]) have developed a palliative care therapy for those with cancer, aiming to identify and enhance sources of meaning and patients' sense of purpose as they approach death.

Other interventions more explicitly target processes of meaning-making. For example, Virginia Lee and her colleagues have developed a brief, manualized intervention, the Meaning-Making intervention (MMi), designed to explicitly promote survivors' exploration of existential issues and their cancer experiences through the use of meaning-making coping strategies [28]. Cancer survivors receive up to four sessions in which they explore their cognitive appraisals of and emotional responses to their cancer experience within the context of their previous experiences and future goals. In several pilot studies, participants in the experimental group reported higher levels of self-esteem, optimism, and self-efficacy [28] and meaning in life [128], demonstrating preliminary effectiveness of a therapy that explicitly promotes meaning-making. Interventions specifically focusing on spirituality in survivorship have also been developed (e.g., [129]) although little empirical evaluation of such interventions is yet available.

Chan et al. [130] noted that while meaning-based interventions are proliferating, "there is a sad lack of a corresponding body of controlled outcome studies, without which we cannot answer two central questions: (1) Can meaning-making interventions facilitate or catalyze the meaning construction process? (2) How much (if any) improvement of the psychosocial well-being of patients is attributable to the catalyzed meaning construction process?" (p. 844). An important challenge for interventionists is conducting well-designed outcome studies evaluating meaning-making interventions in terms of not only their effects but also the mechanisms bringing about those effects.

Noting that some interventions focused on broader issues of stress management have demonstrated that stress-related growth is often a by-product of those interventions (e.g., [131]), some researchers have advocated for interventions that explicitly promote stress-related growth (e.g., [132]). However, given the lack of understanding of growth and controversies regarding its meaning vis-à-vis well-being, others have suggested that an explicit focus on interventions targeting stress-related growth may be premature (e.g., [65]).

Future Research in Positive Psychology and Cancer Survivorship

As this chapter makes clear, much remains to be learned about cancer survivors' meaning-making processes, spirituality, and stress-related growth. The present review is based on the meaning-making model, which provides a useful framework for examining many different phenomena relevant to survivors' psychological adjustment. To date, the literature on meaning-making does not provide strong support for meaning-making processes as requisite for psychological adjustment in cancer survivorship. However, as noted earlier, extant studies have not adequately tested the model. An adequate test of this model awaits studies that thoroughly assess the range of meaning-making efforts, both deliberate and automatic, and whether there are any meanings made (e.g., adaptive changes) resulting from efforts at meaning-making. To date, no study of cancer survivors has fully assessed the components of the meaning-making process and much remains to be learned about meaning and meaning-making in cancer survivorship. Such studies will need to attend closely to the specific characteristics of the survivors under study and the demands placed on them depending on their location within the survivorship continuum.

Research on issues of spirituality suggests that this is a very important part of survivors' adjustment across the continuum. Both existential and more traditionally religious aspects of spirituality appear to be important [133] and should be examined separately and in combination. A better understanding of spirituality and its unique place

in survivors' meaning-making and adjustment across the phases from diagnosis through survivorship is desperately needed. In addition, the phenomenon of stress-related growth, which often reflects spirituality as well as many other aspects of life, is poorly understood. The questions raised here (How do these appraisals reflect reality? Is growth helpful?) await sophisticated research approaches.

Acquiring a better understanding of the ways by which survivors create meaning through their experiences with cancer holds great promise for better appreciating the ways in which survivors differ in their adjustment and the myriad influences on this process. This knowledge should help to identify those needing more assistance in adjusting to survivorship including informing interventions for those who may need help returning to their "new normal" lives.

References

1. National Cancer Institute (2011a) Cancer survivorship research. Retrieved on February 28, 2011, from http://dccps.nci.nih.gov/ocs/definitions.html
2. Twombly R. What's in a name: who is a cancer survivor? J Natl Cancer Inst. 2004;96:1414–5.
3. National Cancer Institute (2011b) Retrieved on February 28, 2011, from http://dccps.nci.nih.gov/ocs/prevalence/prevalence.html#time
4. Stull VB, Snyder DC, Demark-Wahnefried W. Lifestyle interventions in cancer survivors: designing programs that meet the needs of this vulnerable and growing population. J Nutr. 2007;137:243S–8.
5. Mullan F. Seasons of survival: reflections of a physician with cancer. N Engl J Med. 1985;313:270–3.
6. Anderson MD (2011). http://www.mdanderson.org/patient-and-cancer-information/cancer-information/cancer-topics/survivorship/stages-of-cancer-survivorship/index.html
7. Ganz PA, Kwan L, Stanton AL, Krupnick JL, Rowland JH, Meyerowitz BE, et al. Quality of life at the end of primary treatment of breast cancer: first results from the Moving Beyond Cancer randomized trial. J Natl Cancer Inst. 2004;96:376–87.
8. Hewitt M, Greenfield S, Stovall E, editors. From cancer patient to cancer survivor: lost in transition. Washington, DC: Institute of Medicine; 2005.
9. Tross S, Holland JC. Psychological sequelae in cancer survivors. In: Holland JC, Rowland JH, editors. Handbook of psycho-oncology: psychological care for the patient with cancer. New York: Oxford University Press; 1989. p. 101–16.

10. Holland JC, Reznik I. Pathways for psychosocial care of cancer survivors. Cancer. 2005;704:2624–37.

11. Lethborg CE, Kissane D, Burns WI, Snyder R. 'Cast adrift': the experience of completing treatment among women with early stage breast cancer. J Psychosoc Oncol. 2000;18:73–90.

12. Bower JE, Meyerowitz BE, Desmond KA, Bernaards CA, Rowland JH, Ganz PA. Perceptions of positive meaning and vulnerability following breast cancer: predictors and outcomes among long-term breast cancer survivors. Ann Behav Med. 2005;29:236–45.

13. Park CL, Edmondson D, Fenster JR, Blank TO. Meaning-making and psychological adjustment following cancer: the mediating roles of growth, life meaning, and restored just world beliefs. J Consult Clin Psychol. 2008;76:863–75.

14. Park CL, Zlateva I, Blank TO. Self-Identity after cancer: "Survivor", "Victim", "Patient", and "Person with cancer". J Gen Intern Med. 2009;24(Supplement 2: special issue on survivorship):S430–5.

15. Park CL, Folkman S. Meaning in the context of stress and coping. Rev General Psychol. 1997;1:115–44.

16. Dittmann-Kohli F, Westerhof GJ. The personal meaning system in a life span perspective. In: Reker GT, Chamberlain K, editors. Exploring existential meaning: optimizing human development across the lifespan. Thousand Oaks, CA: Sage; 2000. p. 107–23.

17. Park CL. Making sense of the meaning literature: an integrative review of meaning-making and its effects on adjustment to stressful life events. Psychol Bull. 2010;136:257–301.

18. Park CL. Stress, coping, and meaning. In: Folkman S, editor. Oxford handbook of stress, health, and coping. New York: Oxford University Press; 2010. p. 227–41.

19. Reker GT, Wong PTP. Aging as an individual process: toward a theory of personal meaning. In: Birren JE, Bengston VL, editors. Emergent theories of aging. New York: Springer; 1988. p. 214–46.

20. Janoff-Bulman R, Frantz CM. The impact of trauma on meaning: from meaningless world to meaningful life. In: Power M, Brewin C, editors. The transformation of meaning in psychological therapies: integrating theory and practice. Sussex, England: Wiley & Sons; 1997.

21. Koltko-Rivera ME. The psychology of worldviews. Rev General Psychol. 2004;8:1–58.

22. Karoly P. A goal systems-self-regulatory perspective on personality, psychopathology, and change. Rev General Psychol. 1999;3:264–91.

23. Klinger E. Meaning and void: inner experience and the incentives in people's lives. Minneapolis, MN: University of Minnesota Press; 1977.

24. Emmons RA. The psychology of ultimate concerns: motivation and spirituality in personality. New York: Guilford; 1999.

25. Steger MF. Meaning in life. In: Lopez SJ, editor. Handbook of positive psychology. 2nd ed. Oxford, UK: Oxford University Press; 2009. p. 679–87.

26. Wrosch C, Scheier MF, Miller GE, Schulz R, Carver CS. Adaptive self-regulation of unattainable goals: goal disengagement, goal reengagement, and subjective well-being. Personality Soc Psychol Bull. 2003;29:1494–508.

27. Park CL, Edmondson D. Religion as a quest for meaning. In: Mikulincer M, Shaver P, editors. The psychology of meaning. Washington, DC: American Psychological Association; 2011.

28. Lee V, Cohen SR, Edgar L, Laizner AM, Gagnon AJ. Meaning-making intervention during breast or colorectal cancer treatment improves self-esteem, optimism, and self-efficacy. Soc Sci Med. 2006;62:3133–45.

29. Moadel A, Morgan C, Fatone A, Grennan J, Carter J, Laruffa G, Skummy A, Dutcher J. Seeking meaning and hope: self-reported spiritual and existential needs among an ethnically-diverse cancer patient population. Psychooncology. 1999;8:378–285.

30. Lazarus RS, Folkman S. Stress, appraisal, and coping. New York: Springer; 1984.

31. Park CL. Overview of theoretical perspectives. In: Park CL, Lechner S, Antoni MH, Stanton A, editors. Positive life change in the context of medical illness: can the experience of serious illness lead to transformation? Washington, DC: American Psychological Association; 2009. p. 11–30.

32. Greenberg MA. Cognitive processing of traumas: the role of intrusive thoughts and reappraisals. J Appl Soc Psychol. 1995;25:1262–96.

33. Janoff-Bulman R. Shattered assumptions: towards a new psychology of trauma. New York: Free Press; 1992.

34. Joseph S, Linley PA. Positive adjustment to threatening events: an organismic valuing theory of growth through adversity. Rev General Psychol. 2005;9:262–80.

35. Manne S, Ostroff J, Fox K, Grana G, Winkel G. Cognitive and social processes predicting partner psychological adaptation to early stage breast cancer. Br J Health Psychol. 2009;14:49–68.

36. Aldwin CM. Stress, coping, and development: an integrative approach. 2nd ed. New York: Guilford; 2007.

37. Moos RH, Holahan CJ. Adaptive tasks and methods of coping with illness and disability. In: Martz E, Livneh H, editors. Coping with chronic illness and disability: theoretical, empirical, and clinical aspects. New York: Springer; 2007. p. 107–26.

38. Park CL, Armeli S, Tennen H. Appraisal-coping goodness of fit: a daily Internet study. Personality and Soc Psychol Bull. 2004;30:558–69.

39. Park CL, Folkman S, Bostrom A. Appraisals of controllability and coping in caregivers and HIV+ men: testing the goodness-of-fit hypothesis. J Consult Clin Psychol. 2001;69:481–8.

40. Wrosch C. Self-regulation of unattainable goals and pathways to quality of life. In: Folkman S, editor. Oxford Handbook of Stress, Health, and Coping. New York: Oxford University Press; 2010. p. 319–33.
41. Collie KK, Long BC. Considering 'meaning' in the context of breast cancer. J Health Psychol. 2005;10:843–53.
42. Skaggs BG, Barron CR. Searching for meaning in negative events: concept analysis. J Adv Nurs. 2006;53:559–70.
43. Segerstrom SC, Stanton AL, Alden LE, Shortridge BE. A multidimensional structure for repetitive thought: what's on your mind, and how, and how much? J Pers Soc Psychol. 2003;85:909–21.
44. Davis CG, Nolen-Hoeksema S, Larson J. Making sense of loss and benefiting from the experience: two construals of meaning. J Pers Soc Psychol. 1998;75:561–74.
45. Pakenham KI. Making sense of multiple sclerosis. Rehabil Psychol. 2007;52:380–9.
46. Gillies J, Neimeyer RA. Loss, grief, and the search for significance: toward a model of meaning reconstruction in bereavement. J Constructi Psychol. 2006;19:31–65.
47. Park CL. Religion and meaning. In: Paloutzian RF, Park CL, editors. Handbook of the psychology of religion and spirituality. New York: Guilford; 2005. p. 295–314.
48. Thompson SC, Janigian AS. Life schemes: a framework for understanding the search for meaning. J Soc Clin Psychol. 1988;7:260–80.
49. Kaler ME, Frazier PA, Anders SL, Tashiro T, Tomich P, Tennen H, Park CL. Assessing the psychometric properties of the World Assumptions Scale. J Trauma Stress. 2008;21:1–7.
50. Maliski SL, Heilemann MV, McCorkle R. From "Death Sentence" to "Good Cancer": couples' transformation of a prostate cancer diagnosis. Nurs Res. 2002;51:391–7.
51. Leventhal H, Weinman J, Leventhal EA, Phillips LA. Health psychology: the search for pathways between behavior and health. Annu Rev Psychol. 2008;59:477–505.
52. Peacock EJ, Wong PTP. Anticipatory stress: the relation of locus of control, optimism, and control appraisals to coping. J Res Personality. 1996;30:204–22.
53. Weinstein SE, Quigley KS. Locus of Control predicts appraisals and cardiovascular reactivity to a novel active coping task. J Pers. 2006;74:911–32.
54. Bickell NA, Weidmann J, Fei K, Lin JJ, Leventhal H. Underuse of breast cancer adjuvant treatment: patient knowledge, beliefs, and medical mistrust. J Clin Oncol. 2009;27:5160–7.
55. Bjorck JP, Hopp D, Jones LW. Prostate cancer and emotional functioning: effects of mental adjustment, optimism, and appraisal. J Psychosoc Oncol. 1999;17:71–85.
56. Silver-Aylaian M, Cohen LH. Role of major lifetime stressors in patients' and spouses' reactions to cancer. J Trauma Stress. 2001;14:405–12.
57. Lipowski ZJ. Physical illness, the individual and the coping process. Psychiatr Med. 1970;1:91–102.
58. Degner L, Hack T, O'Neil J, Kristjanson LJ. A new approach to eliciting meaning in the context of breast cancer. Cancer Nurs. 2003;26:169–78.
59. Büssing A, Fischer J. Interpretation of illness in cancer survivors is associated with health-related variables and adaptive coping styles. BMC Womens Health. 2009;9(2).
60. Norton TR, Manne SL, Rubin S, Hernandez E, Carlson J, Bergman C, Rosenblum N. Ovarian cancer patients' psychological distress: the role of physical impairment, perceived unsupportive family and friend behaviors, perceived control, and self-esteem. Health Psychol. 2005;24:143–52.
61. Soler-Vilá H, Dubrow R, Franco VI, Saathoff AK, Kasl SV, Jones BA. Cancer-Specific beliefs and survival in nonmetastatic colorectal cancer patients. Cancer. 2009;115:4270–82.
62. Soler-Vilá H, Dubrow R, Franco VI, Kasl SV, Jones BA. The prognostic role of cancer-specific beliefs among prostate cancer survivors. Cancer Causes Control. 2010;22:251–60.
63. Ferrucci LM, Cartmel B, Turkman YE, Murphy ME, Smith T, Stein KD, McCorkle R. Causal attribution among cancer survivors of the 10 most common cancers. J Psychosoc Oncol. 2011;29:121–40.
64. Costanzo ES, Lutgendorf SK, Bradley SL, Rose SL, Anderson B. Cancer attributions, distress, and health practices among gynecologic cancer survivors. Psychosom Med. 2005;67:972–80.
65. Jim HS, Jacobsen PB. Posttraumatic stress and posttraumatic growth in cancer survivorship: a review. Cancer J. 2008;14:414–9.
66. Lepore SJ. A social-cognitive processing model of emotional adjustment to cancer. In: Baum A, Anderson B, editors. Psychosocial interventions for cancer. Washington, DC: American Psychological Association; 2001. p. 99–118.
67. Gall TL. Relationship with God and the quality of life of prostate cancer survivors. Qual Life Res. 2004;13:1357–68.
68. Carver CS. Enhancing adaptation during treatment and the role of individual differences. Cancer. 2005;104:2602–7.
69. McBride CM, Clipp E, Peterson BL, Lipkus IM, Demark-Wahnefried W. Psychological impact of diagnosis and risk reduction among cancer survivors. Psychooncology. 2000;9:418–27.
70. Nordin K, Wasteson E, Hoffman K, Glimelius B, Sjödén PO. Discrepancies between attainment and importance of life values and anxiety and depression in gastrointestinal cancer patients and their spouses. Psychooncology. 2001;10:479–89.
71. Henselmans I, Sanderman R, Baas PC, Smink A, Ranchor AV. Personal control after a breast cancer

diagnosis: stability and adaptive value. Psychooncology. 2009;18:104–8.

72. Taylor SE. Adjustment to threatening events: a theory of cognitive adaptation. Am Psychol. 1983;38: 1161–73.

73. Zebrack BJ, Ganz PA, Bernaards CA, Petersen L, Abraham L. Assessing the impact of cancer: development of a new instrument for long- term survivors. Psycho-Oncology. 2006;15:407–21.

74. Schroevers MJ, Ranchor AV, Sanderman R. The role of age at the onset of cancer in relation to survivors' long-term adjustment: a controlled comparison over an eight-year period. Psychooncology. 2004;13: 740–52.

75. Tomich PL, Helgeson VS. Five years later: a cross-sectional comparison of breast cancer survivors with healthy women. Psychooncology. 2002;11:154–69.

76. Bellizzi KM, Blank TO. Cancer-related identity and positive affect in survivors of prostate cancer. J Cancer Surviv. 2007;1:44–8.

77. Dirksen SR. Search for meaning in long-term cancer survivors. J Adv Nurs. 1995;21:628–33.

78. Horowitz MJ. Stress response syndromes: personality styles and interventions. 4th ed. Northvale, NJ: Jason Aronson; 2001.

79. Roberts KJ, Lepore SJ, Helgeson V. Social-cognitive correlates of adjustment to prostate cancer. Psychooncology. 2006;15:183–92.

80. Redd WH, DuHamel K, Johnson Vickberg SM, Ostroff JL, Smith MY, et al. Long-term adjustment in cancer survivors: integration of classical-conditioning and cognitive processing models. In: Baum A, Anderson B, editors. Psychosocial interventions for cancer. Washington, DC: American Psychological Association; 2001. p. 77–98.

81. Chan MWC, Ho SMY, Tedeschi RG, Leung CWL. The valence of attentional bias and cancer-related rumination in posttraumatic stress and posttraumatic growth among women with breast cancer. Psychooncology. 2011;20:544–52.

82. Kernan W, Lepore S. Searching for and making meaning after breast cancer: prevalence, patterns, and negative affect. Soc Sci Med. 2009;68: 1176–82.

83. Stanton AL, Danoff-Burg S, Cameron CL, Bishop M, Collins CA, Kirk SB, et al. Emotionally expressive coping predicts psychological and physical adjustment to breast cancer. J Consult Clin Psychol. 2000;68:875–82.

84. Kulik L, Kronfeld M. The contribution of resources and causal attributions regarding the illness. Soc Work Health Care. 2005;41:37–57.

85. Taylor EJ. Whys and wherefores: adult patient perspectives of the meaning of cancer. Semin Oncol Nurs. 1995;11:32–40.

86. Bennett KK, Compas BE, Beckjord E, Glinder JG. Self-blame and distress among women with newly diagnosed breast cancer. J Behav Med. 2005;28:313–23.

87. Zebrack BJ. Cancer survivor identity and quality of life. Cancer Pract. 2000;8:238–42.

88. Brennan J. Adjustment to cancer: coping or personal transition? Psychooncology. 2001;10:1–18.

89. Deimling G, Kahana B, Schumacher J. Life threatening illness: the transition from victim to survivor. J Aging Ident. 1997;2:165–86.

90. Sadler-Gerhard CJT, Reynolds CA, Britton PJ, Kruse SD. Women breast cancer survivors: stories of change and meaning. J Mental Health Counsel. 2010;32:265–82.

91. Deimling GT, Bowman KF, Wagner LJ. Cancer survivorship and identity among long-term survivors. Cancer Invest. 2007;25:758–65.

92. Park CL, Bharadwaj AK, Blank TO. Illness centrality, disclosure, and well-being in younger adult cancer survivors. Br J Health Psychol. 2011;16(4): 880–9.

93. Lavery ME, O'Hea EL. Religious/spiritual coping and adjustment in individuals with cancer: unanswered questions, important trends, and future directions. Mental Health, Religion, Culture. 2010;13: 55–65.

94. Stefanek M, McDonald PG, Hess SA. Religion, spirituality and cancer: current status and methodological challenges. Psychooncology. 2005;14:450–63.

95. Thuné-Boyle I, Stygall J, Keshtgar M, Newman S. Do religious/spiritual coping strategies affect illness adjustment in patients with cancer? A systematic review of the literature. Soc Sci Med. 2006;63: 151–64.

96. Visser A, Garssen B, Vingerhoets A. Spirituality and well-being in cancer patients: a review. Psychooncology. 2010;19:565–72.

97. Henoch I, Danielson E. Existential concerns among patients with cancer and interventions to meet them: an integrative literature review. Psychooncology. 2009;18:225–36.

98. Howsepian BA, Merluzzi TV. Religious beliefs, social support, self-efficacy and adjustment to cancer. Psychooncology. 2009;18:1069–79.

99. Moschella VD, Pressman KR, Pressman P, Weissman DE. The problem of theodicy and religious response to cancer. J Relig Health. 1997;36:17–20.

100. Hale-Smith A, Park CL, Edmondson D (in press). Measuring religious beliefs about suffering: Development of the views of suffering scale.Psychological Assessment.

101. Jenkins RA, Pargament KI. Cognitive appraisals in cancer patients. Soc Sci Med. 1988;26:625–33.

102. Exline JJ, Park CL, Smyth JM, Carey MP. Anger toward God: social-cognitive predictors, prevalence, and links with adjustment to bereavement and cancer. J Pers Soc Psychol. 2011;100:129–48.

103. Exline JJ, Rose ED. Religious and spiritual struggles. In: Paloutzian RF, Park C, editors. Handbook of the psychology of religion and spirituality. 2nd ed. New York: Guilford Press; 2010.

104. Pargament KI, Koenig HG, Perez LM. The many methods of religious coping: development and initial validation of the RCOPE. J Clin Psychol. 2000;56: 519–43.

105. Sherman AC, Plante TG, Simonton S, Latif U, Anaissie EJ. Prospective study of religious coping

among patients undergoing autologous stem cell transplantation. J Behav Med. 2009;32:118–28.

106. Zwingmann C, Wirtz M, Muller C, Korber J, Murken S. Positive and negative religious coping in German breast cancer patients. J Behav Med. 2006;29:533–47.

107. Logan J, Hackbusch-Pinto R, De Grasse CE. Women undergoing breast diagnostics: the lived experience of spirituality. Oncol Nurs Forum. 2006;33:121–6.

108. Gall TL, Guirguis-Younger M, Charbonneau C, Florack P. The trajectory of religious coping across time in response to the diagnosis of breast cancer. Psychooncology. 2009;18:1165–78.

109. Gall TL, Cornblat MW. Breast cancer survivors give voice: a qualitative analysis of spiritual factors in long-term adjustment. Psychooncology. 2002;11: 524–35.

110. Denney RM, Aten JD, Leavell K. Posttraumatic spiritual growth: a phenomenological study of cancer survivors. Mental Health, Religion Culture. 2010;14:371–91.

111. Cole BS, Hopkins CM, Tisak J, Steel JL, Carr BI. Assessing spiritual growth and spiritual decline following a diagnosis of cancer: reliability and validity of the spiritual transformation scale. Psychooncology. 2008;17:112–21.

112. Calhoun LG, Tedeschi RG. Handbook of posttraumatic growth: research and practice. Mahwah, NJ: Erlbaum; 2006.

113. Sumalla EC, Ochoa C, Blanco I. Posttraumatic growth in cancer: reality or illusion? Clin Psychol Rev. 2009;29:24–33.

114. Stanton AL, Bower JE, Low CA. Posttraumatic growth after cancer. In: Calhoun L, Tedeschi R, editors. Handbook of posttraumatic growth. Mahwah, NJ: Erlbaum; 2006. p. 138–75.

115. Rajandram RK, Jenewein J, McGrath C, Zwahlen RA. Coping processes relevant to posttraumatic growth: an evidence-based review. Support Care Cancer. 2011;19:583–9.

116. Zoellner T, Maercker A. Posttraumatic growth in clinical psychology—a critical review and introduction of a two component model. Clin Psychol Rev. 2006;26:626–53.

117. Coyne JC, Tennen H. Positive psychology in cancer care: bad science, exaggerated claims, and unproven medicine. Ann Behav Med. 2010;39:16–26.

118. Frazier P, Tennen H, Gavian M, Park CL, Tomich P, Tashiro T. Does self-reported post-traumatic growth reflect genuine positive change? Psychological Science. 2009;20:912–19.

119. Ransom S, Sheldon KM, Jacobsen PB. Actual change and inaccurate recall contribute to posttraumatic growth following radiotherapy. J Consult Clin Psychol. 2008;76:811–9.

120. Schwarzer R, Luszczynska A, Boehmer S, Taubert S, Knoll N. Changes in finding benefit after cancer surgery and the prediction of well-being one year later. Soc Sci Med. 2006;63:1614–24.

121. Aspinwall LG, Tedeschi RG. The value of positive psychology for health psychology: progress and pitfalls in examining the relation of positive phenomena to health. Ann Behav Med. 2010;39:4–15.

122. Carver CS, Antoni MH. Finding benefit in breast cancer during the year after diagnosis predicts better adjustment 5 to 8 years after diagnosis. Health Psychol. 2004;23:595–8.

123. Cordova MJ, Cunningham LLC, Carlson CR, Andrykowski MA. Posttraumatic growth following breast cancer: a controlled comparison study. Health Psychol. 2001;20:176–85.

124. Bellizzi KM, Miller MF, Arora NK, Rowland JH. Positive and negative life changes experienced by survivors of non-Hodgkin's lymphoma. Ann Behav Med. 2007;34:188–99.

125. Park CL, Blank TO. Associations of positive and negative life changes with well-being in young- and middle-aged adult cancer survivors. Psychol Health. 2012;27(4):412–29.

126. Kissane DW, Bloch S, Smith GC, Miach P, Clarke DM, Ikin JM, Love A, Ranieri N, McKenzie D. Cognitive-existential group psychotherapy for women with primary breast cancer: a randomised controlled trial. Psychooncology. 2003;12:532–46.

127. Breitbart W, Gibson C, Poppito SR, Berg A. Psychotherapeutic interventions at the end of life: a focus on meaning and spirituality. Can J Psychiatry. 2004;49:366–72.

128. Henry M, Cohen SR, Lee V, Sauthier P, Provencher D, Drouin P, Mayo N. The Meaning-Making intervention (MMi) appears to increase meaning in life in advanced ovarian cancer: a randomized controlled pilot study. Psychooncology. 2010;19:1340–7.

129. Cole B, Pargament KI. Re-creating your life: a spiritual/psychotherapeutic intervention for people diagnosed with cancer. Psychooncology. 1999;8: 395–407.

130. Chan THY, Ho RTH, Chan CLW. Developing an outcome measurement for meaning-making intervention with Chinese cancer patients. Psychooncology. 2007;16:843–50.

131. Penedo FJ, Dahn JR, Molton I, et al. Cognitive-behavioral stress management improves stress-management skills and quality of life in men recovering from treatment of prostate carcinoma. Cancer. 2004;100:192–200.

132. Tedeschi RG, Calhoun LG. The clinician as expert companion. In: Park CL, Lechner S, Antoni MH, Stanton A, editors. Positive life change in the context of medical illness: can the experience of serious illness lead to transformation? Washington, DC: American Psychological Association; 2009. p. 215–35.

133. Yanez B, Edmondson D, Stanton AL, Park CL, Kwan L, Ganz PA, Blank TO. Facets of spirituality as predictors of adjustment to cancer: relative contributions of having faith and finding meaning. J Consult Clin Psychol. 2009;77:730–41.

Stress, Coping, and Hope

8

Susan Folkman

Hope
Hope is the thing with feathers
That perches in the soul,
And sings the tune without the words,
And never stops at all,

And sweetest in the gale is heard;
And sore must be the storm
That could abash the little bird
That kept so many warm.

I've heard it in the chillest land,
And on the strangest sea;
Yet, never, in extremity,
It asked a crumb of me.

Emily Dickinson

Few would question the critical importance of hope when facing serious and prolonged threats to psychological or physical well-being, whether our own or that of a loved one (for review see [1]). The significance of hope is perhaps best understood by the consequences of its absence. Hopelessness is a dire state that gives rise to despair, depression, and ultimately loss of will to live. The assumption of the fundamental importance of hope in confronting serious threats is so embedded in our belief system that hope approaches the status of an evolutionarily adaptive mechanism wired into our genome. Indeed, that might be the case. But it is another matter to assume that hope is an automatically self-renewing resource, as suggested in the frequently quoted passage by Alexander Pope, "Hope springs eternal in the human breast." On the contrary, hope needs to be nurtured; at the very

least, it needs something from which to spring as well as something to spring towards.

In this essay, I view hope from the perspective of stress and coping theory. Hope usually appears in the stress and coping literature in the form of hopelessness, frequently as a predictor of depression or suicidal ideation (for reviews see [2, 3]). A more interesting story about hope may be the one told in terms of its dynamic and reciprocal relationship with coping in which each supports, and in turn is supported by, the other.

To provide a framework for this discussion, I begin with a very brief account of stress and coping theory. Then I shall incorporate hope, illustrating the interplay between coping and hope as stressful situations unfold over time. I have chosen the context of serious illness for this discussion, but the ideas and hypotheses I propose are likely to apply to any situation that involves prolonged psychological stress.

Reprinted with permission, John Wiley and Sons, 2010.

Based on a Keynote Address to the International Psycho-Oncology Society, May 28, 2010 Quebec City, Quebec, Canada

S. Folkman, Ph.D (✉)
Department of Medicine, University of California San Francisco, 40 West Third Ave, Apt 504, San Mateo, CA 94402, USA
e-mail: susan.folkman@ucsf.edu

Stress and Coping Theory

Stress and Coping theory [4] is a framework for studying psychological stress. The theory holds that stress is contextual, meaning that it involves a transaction between the person and the environment, and it is a process, meaning that it changes over time. Stress is defined as a situation that is appraised by the individual as personally significant and as having demands that exceed the person's resources for coping.

Appraisal

Primary appraisal is the term applied to the appraisal of the personal significance of a situation—what is happening and whether it matters and why. Primary appraisal is shaped by the person's beliefs, values, and goals. Secondary appraisal refers to the person's evaluation of options for coping. These options are determined both by the situation, such as whether there are opportunities for controlling the outcome, and by the person's physical, psychological, material, and spiritual resources for coping. The two forms of appraisal determine the extent to which the situation is appraised as a harm or loss, a threat, or a challenge, each of which is a stress appraisal. The appraisal process generates emotions. Anger or sadness, for example, is associated with loss appraisals; anxiety and fear are associated with threat appraisals; and anxiety mixed with excitement is associated with challenge appraisals. The personal quality of the appraisal process explains why a given event can have different meanings for individuals. A job interview, for example, may be considered a threat by one person and a challenge by another.

Coping

Coping refers to the thoughts and behaviors people use to manage the internal and external demands of stressful events. Stress and coping theory originally posited two kinds of coping: problem-focused coping such as planful problem to address the problem causing distress using strategies such as information gathering, and decision making, and emotion-focused coping to regulate negative emotion using strategies such as distancing, seeking emotional support, and escape-avoidance.

A third kind of coping, "meaning-focused coping," was introduced into the model based on findings that positive emotions occur alongside negative emotions throughout intensely stressful periods, including caregiving and subsequent bereavement [5–7], and in cancer patients during the months preceding their deaths [8]. As suggested by Fredrickson's [9] "Broaden and Build" theory of positive emotion, these positive emotions serve important functions in the stress process by restoring resources for coping, thereby helping to transform threat appraisals into challenge appraisals and motivating and sustaining coping efforts over the long term. Meaning-focused coping strategies are qualitatively different from emotion-focused coping strategies, such as distancing or seeking social support, that regulate negative emotions. Meaning-focused coping draws on deeply held values and beliefs in the form of strategies such as goal revision, focusing on strengths gained from life experience, and reordering priorities.

The various types of coping often work in tandem, such that the regulation of anxiety (emotion-focused coping) will allow the person to concentrate on making a decision (problem-focused coping), which in turn is informed by a review of underlying values and goals (meaning-focused coping). Ideally, there would be independence among these processes so as to permit prediction. In reality, however, we are looking at a dynamic system of processes that are highly interactive.

Hope

Hope has been defined many ways and in many literatures. (See [10] for an excellent review of definitions from diverse literatures.) In the psychology literature, for example, hope is defined as yearning for amelioration of a dreaded outcome [11], a theological virtue along with faith and charity [12], and as a positive goal-related motivational state [13]. Hope has also been characterized in the nursing literature as having a "being" dimension, something that is deep inside one's self that remains positive whatever happens; a "doing" dimension, a pragmatic, goal-setting entity in response to situations; and a "becoming" dimension, anticipating future possibilities, positive results [14]. In the medical literature, maintaining and restoring hope is seen as an important function of the physician [15].

Hope and psychological stress share many formal characteristics. Hope, like stress, is appraisal-based; it waxes and wanes, it is contextual, and, like stress, it is complex. Hope has a cognitive base that contains information and goals; it generates an energy, often described as "will," that has a motivational quality; it has both negative and positive emotional tones due to the possibility that what is hoped for might not come to pass; and for many people hope has a basis in religion or spirituality whereby it is equivalent to faith. Although I think of hope as aligned with positive emotions, I consider it to be a state of mind that has emotional tones rather than an emotion per se.

Coping and Hope: Dynamic Interdependence

A number of writers speak of hope in relationship to outcomes over which the individual believes he or she has some control. Jerome Groopman represents this point of view in his book, *The Anatomy of Hope* [16]: "To have hope, then, is to acquire a belief in your ability to have some control over your circumstances" (p. 26). However, psychological stress is at its peak in precisely those situations that offer few, if any, options for personal control [4], meaning that the situations in which hope is most needed are the ones in which hope is most likely to be at low ebb or even absent.

The revival of hope in intensely stressful situations depends at least in part on cognitive coping processes. In turn, the person's capacity to sustain coping with intensely stressful situations over time depends at least in part on having hope with respect to the desired outcome.

The interdependence of coping and hope is played out in many ways over the course of prolonged stress, as can be illustrated in the case of

serious disease. Learning that one has a serious disease changes how things are for the patient and the patient's family members and close friends, especially those who are involved directly with the patient's caregiving. The world is different. The future is suddenly filled with unknowns about what lies ahead and how it will affect the physical, psychological, and spiritual well-being of the patient and the patient's close others. The challenges to well-being may differ according to diagnosis and patient characteristics such as age, health, access to care, social support system, and psychosocial and psycho-spiritual resources. But certain adaptive tasks are common to virtually all seriously ill patients and their family members. I have chosen two of these tasks—coping with uncertainty and dealing with a changing reality—to illustrate the dynamic, interdependent relationship between hope and coping and how each would at times be difficult, if not impossible, without the other.

Coping with Uncertainty

Uncertainty travels with psychological stress. There can be uncertainty about when something will happen (temporal uncertainty), what will happen (event uncertainty), what can be done (efficacy uncertainty), and the outcome (outcome uncertainty) [4]. Although not all aspects of uncertainty are relevant in every situation, it is safe to say that every stressful situation involves some uncertainty.

The process of coping with uncertainty in the context of illness begins when the person becomes aware of a change in the *status quo*, such as when he or she receives a diagnosis or learns of the progression of an established condition. The initial response for some patients will be to minimize the significance of what they were told or to avoid thinking about it altogether. I discuss these emotion-focused strategies below. But I believe the more typical response of patients is to search for a frame of reference that allows them to appraise the seriousness of their condition. "Am I in danger? Will I be okay? How bad is this?" Answers are often in the form of odds—the odds associated with treatment options and their outcomes, the odds associated with the nature and speed of disease progression, or the odds associated with the prognosis more generally.

Odds are estimates, statements of probabilities, often conditional probabilities that are open to interpretation. Statements about odds, and the range of possibilities they imply, invite hope. Hope gains a strong toehold when the odds of a good outcome are favorable. But as noted earlier, hope is likely to be at low ebb or even absent when the odds are unfavorable. Based on the assumption that hope underlies any effort to cope with the demands posed by the illness, I suggest that when odds are unfavorable, people initiate a reappraisal process of their own personal odds that improves them. This process is significant because it gives hope its toehold within the individual's psychological milieu. I refer to this reappraisal process as "personalizing the odds." This coping strategy not only creates a toehold for hope, but it also reduces threat.

The rationales people use to personalize the odds are familiar to anyone who has been involved in conversations about diagnoses with patients and their family members. For example the person may:

1. Identify reasons why the odds do not apply in this case. For example, a person might reason that the odds do not apply to him or her because of personal attributes ("I am a strong person," "I am lucky"), attributes of the environment ("I have the best doctor, the best medical care, the best hospital in the city/state/ nation"), or because of existential beliefs ("God will protect me").
2. Search for information that contradicts the odds that were given. The Internet is a major source of such opinions. Friends and family members may also share information, advice, and beliefs that affect the patient's appraisal of his or her personal odds. Another physician may have a different assessment of the odds.
3. Read the medical literature to determine whether there are other ways of interpreting findings.

Stephen Jay Gould, the internationally renowned geologist, zoologist, paleontologist, and evolutionary biologist, illustrated the process of personalizing odds in an article he wrote about his reactions when he was diagnosed in 1982 with a rare and deadly form of cancer, an abdominal mesothelioma [17]. When he revived after surgery, he asked his doctor what the best technical literature on the cancer was. She told him that there was really nothing worth reading. His reaction was as soon as possible to go to the nearby Harvard Countway medical library. He soon realized why his doctor had tried to discourage him from looking, "The literature couldn't have been more brutally clear: mesothelioma is incurable, with a median mortality of only 8 months after discovery. I sat stunned for about 15 min … Then my mind started to work again, thank goodness." Gould, who knew about statistics, wanted to find out his chances of being in the half that survived more than 8 months, and especially its tail. "I read for a furious and nervous hour and concluded, with relief: damned good. I possessed every one of the characteristics conferring a probability of longer life: I was young; my disease had been recognized in a relatively early stage; I would receive the nation's best medical treatment; I had the world to live for; I knew how to read the data properly and not despair."

I wonder whether Dr. Gould felt any hope during the 15 min when he sat stunned. But by the end of his hour of reading and using many of the cognitive coping strategies listed above to interpret his personal odds more favorably, Dr. Gould was certainly feeling hopeful. Dr. Gould did in fact survive until 2002, when he died of an unrelated cancer.

Uncertainty and distortion of reality. Coping with uncertainty, and especially the process of personalizing odds, can involve distortion of reality, which is a red flag to those who believe that veridicality—adherence to reality—is essential for good mental and physical health. Traditionally, failure to adhere to veridicality was equated with denial. The concern was that if people engage in denial, they will fail to engage in appropriate medical treatment and also that a person engaging in denial has to expend energy on avoiding evidence to the contrary [4].

The issue about veridicality and denial actually involves two questions: Denial of what? And, what are the consequences? Breznitz [18] presents a hierarchy of denial and denial-like processes that offers options for the question: "Denial of what?" The most serious of these is the denial of information, which is probably the closest to the definition of denial of external reality, considered a psychotic defense mechanism [19]. But Breznitz goes on to list other denial-like processes in which information as such is not denied, but its implications are. Breznitz' hierarchy of denial-like processes descends from the denial of threat to the denial of personal relevance, urgency, vulnerability/responsibility, affect, and affect relevance.

Any of these denial-like processes might disturb the physician, who wants to make certain that the patient is fully informed so that the patient can make good decisions. On the other hand, the patient's need to maintain at least an approximation of equilibrium may call for regulating the flow of information into awareness, whether knowingly or unconsciously. A number of articles have been written about achieving this delicate balance [1].

It is understandable that physicians would be concerned if unrealistic hopes lead to treatment decisions that harm the patient or consume scarce resources the patient will need in the future. But the literature suggests that most people do not distort reality to this extent. In general, people's illusions tend to depart only modestly from indicators of their objective standings, show a high degree of relative accuracy, and are kept from becoming too extreme by feedback from the environment [20]. Indeed, the social psychology literature shows not only that people tend to have unrealistic optimism about their ability to manage traumatic events, but also that these illusions are associated with effective coping and psychological adjustment [20] and a sense of agency [21]. And, as Snyder and his colleagues note, people who have lofty goals often attain them [21].

The medical literature often uses the term "false hope" to refer to unrealistic hope. A more literal interpretation of false hope is suggested by Klenow [22] who refers to false hope as hope that originates from deliberate deception by the physician, as when a physician tells a patient that he or she has a less serious illness than he or she actually does. Let us assume that this form of deception is rare.

Efforts to discourage unrealistic expectations may push the patient and his or her caregivers to consider a more realistic appraisal of what the future holds. Whether this is important for the patient's health, however, depends on the reasons compelling the more realistic appraisal and the costs of not doing so. Unrealistic hope, for example, may be what the patient needs at the outset in order to have any hope at all, what I referred to earlier as giving hope a toehold, in which case the unrealistic hope may be serving an important adaptive function. Over time, as the patient and the patient's family caregivers absorb more information and its meaning, I would expect them to begin formulating more realistic expectations and to shift their focus away from hoping for unrealistic outcomes, such as a cure, to hoping for more plausible outcomes such as hope of living longer than expected, being well cared for and supported, having good pain and symptom control, and hope of getting to certain events [1].

Managing uncertainty over time. Whether uncertainty lasts just a few hours, as when a parent waits for a teenage driver to return home at night, or years, as when a cancer patient has to wait to learn whether the cancer is in remission, uncertainty is often an aversive condition that is difficult to tolerate. Uncertainty can provide a fertile milieu for doubts based on what one hears, sees, reads, or imagines. Well-intended friends can share anecdotal accounts that have the unintended effect of creating more anxiety rather than reducing it.

Theoretically, hope provides a counterbalance to both intrapersonal and interpersonal events that feed anxiety during periods of uncertainty. In this sense, hope (e.g., as faith) or hoping (e.g., actively focusing on reasons for feeling hopeful) act as emotion-focused coping strategies. The calming effects of hope can be reinforced by other kinds of emotion-focused coping strategies that are appropriate for managing anxiety in waiting situations, for example, distracting one's self by turning to other activities such as exercising, work, or gardening [23]. This example further illustrates the interplay between hope and coping, whereby each can facilitate the other.

Hope has a very special quality that is especially important in managing uncertainty over time: it allows us to hold conflicting expectations simultaneously. For example, we have reliable information that a hurricane is approaching, so we take necessary precautions—tape windows, get sandbags to ward off flooding, stock up on water, to name a few—and then relax because we also believe the hurricane will veer off its predicted path.

The concept of hope *legitimizes* holding conflicting expectations. The person who holds these conflicting expectations is not thought to be confused or delusional; the person is labeled *hopeful*. Holding both possibilities also facilitates adaptive problem-focused and emotion-focused coping. The belief that the hurricane is coming frees the person to prepare for the hurricane (problem-focused coping). The expectation that the hurricane will veer off path regulates anxiety (emotion-focused coping). By combining both expectations, the person is also likely to continue attending to information about the hurricane's path (problem-focused coping).

Dealing with a Changing Reality

When circumstances change with time, previous expectations and hopes may no longer be relevant. A cancer patient, for example, may learn that the course of chemotherapy was not effective and that a new treatment with more aversive side effects is required, or that there are no further treatments available at the moment. Perhaps the patient learns that his or her cancer has metastasized, or that there has been a recurrence following a period of remission.

The patient and the patient's family members are faced with the dual challenges of sustaining hope while coping with a changing reality. Recognizing that things are not going well means giving up hope with respect to what had been, but hope itself is not necessarily quashed. Generalized hope—hope that is based on faith, personality disposition, or developmental history—can act as a reserve that supports the efforts to revise expectations in the present situation. For example, when there is little that can be done by the patient to affect a particular outcome, religious faith can support hope by providing a sense of ultimate control through the sacred [24] or through affirming beliefs about the sacred such as "God will be by my side." Individuals who rate high on hope as a trait have the advantage of approaching situations with a hopeful bias that is protective; they show diminished stress reactivity and more effective emotional-recovery than those low in dispositional hope [25]. And a developmental history that includes experience confronting stress and coming through quite well provides the individual with confidence that the present situation can also be managed well [26, 27].

The reserve of generalized hope is important for the patient as he or she begins coping with the demands spawned by advancing illness that must be addressed to preserve physical, psychological, and spiritual health. These demands define an array of goals for the patient, ranging from proximal, concrete goals such as the ones on the weekly to-do list, to distal, abstract aspirational values, goals, beliefs, and commitments. In what might be called ideal "normal" day-to-day life, distal and proximal levels are in harmony. Proximal goals (e.g., producing an excellent report on time at work; volunteering service to a community organization) are expressions of distal values, beliefs, and commitments (e.g., valuing excellence and honoring commitments; and belief in communal responsibility) [7].

But illness has a way of perturbing the goals that organize day-to-day choices and behavior—the routine weekly to-do list. The individual needs to revise these goals [28, 29] and revisit the distal values and higher order goals that guide day-to-day choices and infuse them with meaning [7]. For example, a mother diagnosed with cancer whose top priority had been her children may now need to put attending to her own health at the top of the list in order to restore her health so that she can resume care of her children. For now, by making her own health her immediate top priority, this mother will be able to focus her time and attention on necessary tasks such as arranging for appropriate medical care; arranging finances; preparing for debilitating surgery and for side effects of a course of chemotherapy; and in some cases, even preparing for a shortened life expectancy.

Overall, the process of revising goals—letting go of goals that are no longer tenable and identifying meaningful, realistic goals that are adaptive for coping in the present circumstances—is an important form of meaning-focused coping that helps sustain a sense of control, creates a renewed sense of purpose, and, of relevance here, allows hope with respect to new goals. I call these goal-specific hopes "situational hope." The seeming simplicity of goal revision processes belies their actual complexity. As the narratives that follow illustrate, the process of goal revision may proceed in fits and starts or happen rather quickly, and the process may be intensely emotional or relatively matter-of-fact. A number of factors influence the process including beliefs, personality disposition, and previous experiences with stress as noted above; the meaning of what is now at stake; what else is going on in the person's life; interactions with close others; and the quality and sensitivity of patient–physician communications during this transition.

The following narrative from the Care Preference Study conducted by Judith Rabkin, myself, and our colleagues in New York and San Francisco [8] illustrates the outcome of a process of goal revision. Participants in this study were diagnosed with terminal illness. Note that the patient's revised goals are not trivial and reflect underlying meaning. The patient's name is Rob, and he had advanced AIDS:

> "Rob—Look at you. You're still here! You can't do all the things you used to do—you used to have all the diamonds, and gold, and all the fun you wanted—you can't do that anymore. Those days are gone. And so I try to think about, what now? What do I do now with the time I have left? In my actions—in my spiritual life—pray more, be nicer to other people, give."

Not everyone succeeds in the goal revision process. Some are unwilling to relinquish untenable goals, as illustrated by another patient with advanced AIDS from the Care Preference Study who was asked how he had spent his day. His response: "Moping, depressed, trying to get as close to the life I had before I got sick." This patient was obviously unwilling or unable to relinquish goals that are now unrealistic.

In a dialog between a patient and his wife, transcribed from a documentary about the caregivers of patients with brain tumors [30], the patient does not know what he wants, while his wife has strong feelings about what he *should* want. The exchange illustrates how interpersonal dynamics can further complicate the process of goal revision and create additional stress.

Tony was diagnosed with a glioblastoma multiforme, a brain tumor that few survive. Lisa is his wife and primary caregiver. Following Tony's surgery, Tony's doctor told him that the surgery was "a success, a complete resection."

Tony: When I asked what did that [*a success, a complete resection*] mean, will it grow back, the doctor said to me the tumor would grow back. He said he couldn't say when, but it would definitely grow back.

Lisa: I just felt contempt for that point of view. When I hear the doctor say it will definitely grow back I say, "Oh no, there is a *95 % chance* the tumor will grow back. But Tony is a 5 percenter."

Tony: And I don't want to say to her "I'm going to die," but I am going to die. Lisa wanted me to think positive. She wanted me to ally myself with anecdotal others who had beaten the odds so to speak … The trouble is, I don't know WHAT I want."

Tony's refusal to think more positively became unbearable for Lisa, and she left Tony, although she eventually returned to take care of him.

Notice that Tony cannot name a goal. He says he does not know what he wants. Tony's conundrum raises an important issue. I have been discussing goal revision as an important coping strategy for dealing with a changing reality. The underlying assumption is that goals give the person something to hope for. And in fact a body of research in psychology is based on a definition of hope offered by the late C.R. Snyder [13] that is entirely related to goals: "a positive motivational state that is based on an interactively derived sense of successful (a) agency (goal-directed energy), and (b) pathways (planning to meet goals)." (p. 287).

However, I consider the boundaries defining hope to be more porous than those defining goals. Hope's more porous boundaries open the way to exploring existential issues that clarify underlying meaning. In the case of patients whose reality is changing, for example, we need to ask questions about *what patients hope for*. Although the initial response is likely to be a response such as "a miracle cure" or "that I beat the odds and land in the tiny percentage that has a lasting remission" (see [31] for a thoughtful discussion of philosophical underpinnings of such hopes), asking patients what they hope for may also inspire them to move beyond those immediate responses and express what matters to them now in their new reality, what they value, and what they yearn for (Rachel Remen, personal communication, March, 2010). Examples might include "maintain my dignity," "be at peace with my God," or "avoid suffering." Or responses may express cosmologic hopes such as being reunited with loved ones who have died, being with their God, or entering a divine world. These aspirations give definition to underlying meaning, the foundation for hope and sustained coping. Technically, these aspirations could be termed higher order distal goals. Responses to a question about hopes may also be expressed in the form of more concrete, proximal goals such as "to find the best doctor," "to attend my grandson's graduation," or "to have a successful conversation with my insurance carrier."

Regardless of the response, the key is to allow the patient the opportunity to consider existential issues that clarify meaning, and for this purpose I believe it is important to ask about hopes in addition to goals. This meaning-clarification function may in fact be a key to the whole process of goal revision, serving to give it a jump start much as I proposed that personalizing odds can give a toe-hold for hope. With this idea in mind, consider how the following participant in our study of the caregiving partners of men with AIDS [5] might

have responded had he been asked about his hopes for himself and his partner:

Michael: As time passes we reach different plateaus. And Josh and I view this as if we are climbing down a canyon. And each time he hits a certain health problem it is another plateau that you have to kind of adjust to and face. And we know that his death is the bottom of the canyon. And then it is up to me to start my new existence.

Conclusions

I have discussed hope from the vantage of stress and coping theory and explored the dynamic and reciprocal relationship that hope has with coping. I began with the assumption that hope is essential when we need to confront stressful circumstances, but that hope is not always available. Coping plays a critical role in fostering hope when it is at low ebb, as when an individual is confronted with information that threatens well-being. Hope in turn can sustain coping, as when the individual moves forward to deal with the demands of his or her new reality. But hope is more than what is implied by this analysis.

In his *New York Times* column of March 26, 2010, David Brooks highlights the shortcomings of modern economics, most recently those of behavioral economics in which economists are interested in "those parts of emotional life that they can count and model (the activities that make them economists)." He warns "But once they're in this terrain, they'll surely find that the processes that make up the inner life are not amenable to the methodologies of social science. The moral and social yearnings of fully realized human beings are not reducible to universal laws and cannot be studied by physics."

David Brook's comment applies as well to hope. No single interpretation, perspective, or discipline has proprietary rights to hope. Hope belongs to the arts as much as it does to the sciences; its meanings range from the ordinary to the transcendent. We can study certain aspects of hope with behavioral and social science techniques, but we cannot capture all of its aspects. However, what we do learn from those aspects we are able to study can be used to help people sustain well-being through difficult times.

Acknowledgements The author declares no conflict of interest.

References

1. Clayton JM, Butow PN, Arnold RM, Tattersall MH. Fostering coping and nurturing hope when discussing the future with terminally ill cancer patients and their caregivers. Cancer. 2005;103:1965–75.
2. McMillan D, Gilbody S, Beresford E, Neilly L. Can we predict suicide and non-fatal self-harm with the Beck Hopelessness Scale? A meta-analysis. Psychol Med. 2007;37:769–78.
3. Lin HR, Bauer-Wu SM. Psycho-spiritual well-being in patients with advanced cancer: an integrative review of the literature. J Adv Nurs. 2003;44:69–80.
4. Lazarus RS, Folkman S. Stress, appraisal, and coping. New York: Springer; 1984.
5. Folkman S. Positive psychological states and coping with severe stress. Soc Sci Med. 1997;45:1207–21.
6. Moskowitz JT, Folkman S, Collette L, Vittinghoff E. Coping and mood during AIDS-related caregiving and bereavement. Ann Behav Med. 1996;18:49–57.
7. Park CL, Folkman S. Meaning in the context of stress and coping. Rev General Psychol. 1997;2:115–44.
8. Rabkin JG, McElhiney M, Moran P, Acree M, Folkman S. Depression, distress and positive mood in late-stage cancer: a longitudinal study. Psychooncology. 2009;18:79–86.
9. Fredrickson BL. What good are positive emotions? Rev General Psychol. 1998;2:300–19. Special Issue: New directions in research on emotion.
10. Eliott JA, Olver IN. The discursive properties of "hope": A qualitative analysis of cancer patients' speech. Qual Health Res. 2002;12:173–93.
11. Lazarus RS. Emotion and adaptation. New York: Oxford University Press; 1991.
12. Emmons RA. Emotion and religion. In: Park CL, editor. Handbook of the psychology of religion and spirituality. New York: Guilford; 2005. p. 235–52.
13. Snyder CR, Irving LM, Anderson JR. Hope and Health. In: Snyder CR, Forsyth DR, editors. Handbook of social and clinical psychology: The health perspective Elmsford. NY: Pergamon Press; 1991. p. 285–305.
14. Hammer K, Mogensen O, Hall EOC. The meaning of hope in nursing research: a meta-synthesis. Scand J Caring Sci. 2009;23:549–57.
15. Brooksbank MA, Cassell EJ. The place of hope in clinical medicine. In: Eliott JA, editor. Interdisciplinary perspectives on hope. New York: Nova; 2005. p. 231–9.
16. Groopman J. The anatomy of hope. New York: Random House; 2004.
17. Gould SJ (1985) The median isn't the message. Discover 1985 June:40-2.
18. Breznitz S. The seven kinds of denial. In: Breznitz S, editor. The denial of stress. New York: International Universities Press; 1983. p. 257–80.
19. Vaillant GE. Ego mechanisms of defense and personality psychopathology. J Abnorm Psychol. 1994;103:44–50.
20. Taylor SE, Armor DA. Positive illusions and coping with adversity. J Pers. 1996;64:873–98.
21. Snyder CR, Rand KL, King EA, Feldman DB, Woodward JT. "False" hope. J Clin Psychol. 2002;58:1003–22.
22. Klenow DJ. Emotion and life threatening illness: A typology of hope sources. Omega (Westport). 1991;24:49–60.
23. Folkman S, Lazarus R. S. If it changes it must be a process: Study of emotion and coping during three stages of a college examnation. J Pers Soc Psychol. 1985;48:150–70.
24. Pargament K. Religion and coping: The current state of knowledge. In: Folkman S, editor. The Oxford handbook of stress, health, and coping. New York: Oxford University Press; 2011. p. 269–88.
25. Ong AD, Edwards LM, Bergeman CS. Hope as a source of resilience in later adulthood. Personality Individ Differ. 2006;41:1263–73.
26. Aldwin CM. Stress, coping, and development. 2nd ed. New york: Guilford; 2007.
27. Aldwin CM. Stress and coping across the lifespan. In: Folkman S, editor. Stress, health, and coping. New York: Oxford University Press; 2011. p. 15–34.
28. Stein N, Folkman S, Trabasso T, Richards TA. Appraisal and goal processes as predictors of psychological well-being in bereaved caregivers. J Pers Soc Psychol. 1997;72:872–84.
29. Wrosch C, Scheier MF, Miller GE, Schulz R, Carver CS. Adaptive self-regulation of unattainable goals: goal disengagement, goal reengagement, and subjective well-being. Pers Soc Psychol Bull. 2003;29: 1494–508.
30. Wilson AA (2007) The Caregivers In. U.S: Fanlight Production Company:48 minutes
31. Eliott JA, Olver IN. Hope, life, and death: a qualitative analysis of dying cancer patients' talk about hope. Death Stud. 2009;33:609–38.

Religiousness and Spirituality in Coping with Cancer

9

Ingela C.V. Thuné-Boyle

Definitions of Religiousness and Spirituality

There has been much debate in the literature over exactly how religiousness and spirituality should be defined. Religion is often described as institutional and formal while spirituality is seen as more informal, existential and personal [1]. This may not always be the case however. Indeed, religion is a multidimensional construct that may involve spiritual experiences, meaning, values, beliefs, forgiveness, private and public religious practices, religious coping, religious support, commitments and preferences [2]. Spirituality may also be viewed as a multidimensional construct that can be divided into three main dimensions: (1) a God-orientated spirituality where thoughts and practices are premised in theologies; (2) a world-orientated spirituality stressing relationships with ecology or nature and (3) a humanistic spirituality (or people orientated) stressing human achievement or potential [3].

The use of the term "spirituality" as being apart from religion has a surprisingly short history [4, 5] and evolved mainly from a growing

I.C.V. Thuné-Boyle, B.Sc. (Hons.), M.Sc.,
Ph.D., C.Psychol. (✉)
Cancer Research UK Health Behaviour Research Centre,
Department of Epidemiology and Public Health,
University College London, 1-19 Torrington Place,
London WC1E 6BT, UK
e-mail: i.thune-boyle@ucl.ac.uk

disillusionment with religious institutions in Western society during the 1960s and 1970s. Today, it is often associated with more favourable connotations to religion [6] and appears to be the terminology favoured by health care professionals, especially within oncology and palliative care. However, viewing religiousness and spirituality as distinct and separate constructs may potentially ignore the rich and dynamic interaction between the two [7]. Studies have generally found defining religiousness and spirituality problematic and empirical studies examining people's understanding of these concepts have produced conflicting results to the notion of separate constructs. For example, Zinnbauer et al. [8] found that religiousness and spirituality were not totally independent and that as many as 74% considered themselves both religious and spiritual. A large overlap between the two concepts, with many similarities in terms of beliefs, time spent in prayer, guidance, a sense of right and wrong and a connection to God, also exists [9]. Indeed, Scott [10] found that definitions of religiousness and spirituality were evenly distributed across nine content categories: (1) experiences of connectedness or relationships; (2) processes leading to increased connectedness; (3) behavioural responses to something sacred; (4) systems of thoughts or set beliefs; (5) traditional institutional or organisational structures; (6) pleasurable states of being; (7) beliefs in the sacred or transcendent; (8) attempts at or capacities for transcendence and (9) concerns for existential questions or issues. This further demonstrates a substantial diversity in the content of people's understanding of religiousness and spirituality, and signifies a considerable overlap between the two constructs. Both may involve a search for meaning and purpose, transcendence, connectedness and values. Religious involvement can therefore be similar to spirituality. Equally, spirituality may also have communal or group expressions. When these expressions are formalised, spirituality is more like an organised religion [11].

Most studies examining definitional issues surrounding religiousness and spirituality have been conducted in the USA. Therefore, before commencing research in this area, my colleagues and I conducted a brief assessment into the definitional views of religiousness and spirituality in a UK, London, population to gain a clearer idea of how people in the UK view these concepts [12]. Although we are not in a position to generalise these findings to the UK population as a whole, in line with previous US findings, results from these interviews show that people in the UK may also have different, and often overlapping, understandings of religiousness and spirituality, although most did not view these terms in any great detail. Being religious was understood in three different ways: having a belief in God or devotion to one's faith (non-organisational), belonging to an organised religion (attending church and adhering to the doctrine of a particular religion) or it may also incorporate both of these. Equally, spirituality was viewed in different ways, as being separate from religion, where it was seen as a broader non-organisational concept with a strong dedication to one's faith. Some viewed it as providing meaning to a person's life and as being similar to religion, describing spiritual people as practicing in much the same way as a religious person might. Others found spirituality difficult to define with some tending towards a "New Age" or Eastern philosophy rather than associating it with more organised religions. Finally, some felt that spirituality was something they associated with people being "a bit phoney."

The variations in people's ideas about these concepts show that it may be more useful to concentrate on the content behind their understanding of religiousness and spirituality rather than focusing

on the label itself. Indeed, within medically ill populations, how patients use their spirituality or religiousness in the coping process has been a growing area of interest to health care researchers.

Religious/Spiritual Coping

Since 1985, 30% of coping studies in the literature have examined some aspect of coping with cancer [13]; yet despite significant interest in the coping process being evident in the last 30 years, the role of religion and spirituality in coping with illness has received relatively little attention as an area of study in its own right. For example, up until 1998, only 1% of coping studies had examined the use of faith in coping [14]. This is surprising, especially as its role in the appraisal process may lead to both cognitive (e.g. appraising an illness as part of God's plan) and behavioural (e.g. praying or attending religious services) aspects of coping. Religious/Spiritual coping can therefore be defined as "The use of cognitive and behavioural techniques, in the face of stressful life events, that arise out of one's religion or spirituality" [14]. The term "religious coping" will be used throughout this chapter simply because it is the term generally used in the literature. However, it does, of course, incorporate the coping of people who view themselves as spiritual and not religious. Other terms such as "spiritual needs" will be used as it is also the term generally used in the literature. It too includes those who regard themselves as religious and therefore have religious needs.

Nature of Religious Coping

Turning to religion during times of difficulty has been described in the literature as a form of escapism, defence, denial, avoidance, passivity or dependence [15] and the notion that religious coping is a maladaptive avoidant coping strategy was first argued by Freud [16] who believed that people who turn to religion do so from a sense of helplessness with the aim of reducing unwanted tensions and anxieties: *"Religion is a universal obsessional neurosis ... infantile helplessness ... a regression to primary narcissism"*. By 1980, attitudes had changed little; the US psychologist Albert Ellis wrote: *"Religiosity is in many respects equivalent to irrational thinking and emotional disturbance ... The elegant solution to emotional problems is to be quite unreligious ... the less religious they are, the more emotionally healthy they will be"* [17]. However, this view is simplistic and stereotypical and fails to consider the diverse roles religious/spiritual beliefs, practices and communities play in people's attempts to find some sort of significance in their lives [15]. Although religious coping can be avoidant, passive, ineffective and maladaptive, it may also be adaptive, active and problem-focused in nature [18].

Public religious/spiritual practices (e.g. attending religious services at church/synagogue/mosque/temple, Sufi meetings or bible study) and private religious/spiritual practices (e.g. prayer or meditation without the influence of other like-minded people) may be conceptualised as a form of religious coping but religious coping may also describe various religious coping cognitions. These can further be divided into positive and negative religious coping strategies. Positive religious coping is considered to be an expression of a secure relationship with a supportive God/higher power. Seeing the situation as part of God's plan, seeking God's love and care or working together with God to solve problems are examples of positive religious coping strategies. Negative religious coping (sometimes referred to in the literature as "religious struggle") is viewed as an expression of a less secure relationship with a God/higher power that is distant and punishing, or as a religious struggle in the search for significance [19]. Feeling punished or abandoned by God, reappraising God's powers or feeling let down by God are examples of negative religious coping strategies (see Table 3.4). In this chapter, the terms "negative religious coping" and "religious struggle" will be used interchangeably.

Pargament et al. [20] argue that the exploration of religious coping should be theoretically based and functionally orientated. They consider five key religious functions in coping based on various theories:

1. *Meaning.* According to theorists (e.g. Clifford Geertz, [21]), religion plays a key role in the search for meaning during suffering or during difficult life experiences. Religion offers a framework for understanding and interpretation.
2. *Control.* Theorists such as Eric Fromm [22] have stressed the role of religion in the search for control over an event that pushes an individual beyond his or her own resources.
3. *Comfort.* According to classic Freudian theory [23], religion is designed to reduce an individual's apprehensions about living in a world where disaster can strike at any moment.
4. *Intimacy.* Sociologists such as Durkheim [24] have generally emphasised the role of religion in facilitating social cohesiveness. Religion is said to be a mechanism for fostering social solidarity.
5. *Life transformation.* Religion may assist people in making major life transformations where individuals give up old objects of value to find new sources of significance [25].

Table 9.1 shows various religious coping strategies falling within Pargament et al.'s [20] five functional dimensions and examples of each are given. Researchers should not expect to find five different factors of religious coping according to these five functions as any form of religious coping may serve more than one purpose. For example, meaning in a stressful situation can be sought in many different ways: redefining the stressor as an opportunity for spiritual growth ("benevolent religious reappraisal"), or redefining the situation as a punishment from God ("punishing God reappraisal") where the former is a potentially adaptive positive religious coping strategy while the latter is a potentially maladaptive negative religious coping strategy. Empirical studies have indeed confirmed that different forms of religious coping have different implications for adjustment, at least in the short term [26, 27]. For example, collaborative religious coping has been associated with better physical and mental health [18, 28, 29] while religious coping strategies such as punish-

Table 9.1 Examples of the functions of coping and associated religious/spiritual coping strategies along Pargament et al.'s [20] five dimensions

Religious coping strategies under the five different functions	Positive/negative	Example of coping strategy
1. *To find meaning*		
Benevolent religious reappraisal	Positive	"Saw my situation as part of God's plan"
Punishing God reappraisal	Negative	"I wondered what I did for God to punish me"
Demonic reappraisal	Negative	"Believed the devil was responsible for my situation"
Reappraisal of God's powers	Negative	"Questioned the power of God"
2. *To gain control*		
Collaborative religious coping	Positive	"Tried to put my plan into action together with God"
Active religious surrender	Positive	"Did my best, then turned the situation over to God"
Passive religious deferral	Negative/Mixed	"Didn't do much, just expected God to solve my problems for me"
Pleading for direct intercession	Negative	"Pleaded with God to make things turn out okay", "Prayed for a miracle"
Self-directing religious coping	Mixed	"Tried to deal with my feelings without the help of God"
3. *To gain comfort*		
Seeking spiritual support	Positive	"Sought God's love and care"
Religious focus	Positive	"Prayed to get my mind off my problems"
Religious purification	Positive	"Confessed my sins"
Spiritual connection	Positive	"Looked for a stronger connection with God"
Spiritual discontent	Negative	"Wondered whether God had abandoned me"
Marking religious boundaries	Positive	"Avoided people who weren't of my faith"
4. *To gain intimacy with others/God*		
Seeking support from clergy or members	Positive	"Looked for spiritual support from religious leaders/ clergy"
Religious helping	Positive	"Prayed for the well-being of others"
Interpersonal religious discontent	Negative	"Disagreed with what the church wanted me to do or believe"
5. *To achieve a life transformation*		
Seeking religious direction	Positive	"Asked God to find a new purpose in life"
Religious conversion	Positive	"Tried to find a completely new life through religion"
Religious forgiving	Positive	"Sought help from God in letting go of my anger"

ing God reappraisal, demonic reappraisal, spiritual discontent, interpersonal religious discontent and pleading for direct intercession are all associated with greater levels of distress [25]. However, there is also evidence that not all forms of religious coping fall easily into negative and positive categories but may be associated with both positive and negative outcomes. For example, self-directing (i.e. dealing with a situation without relying on God), and deferring religious coping strategies (giving over control to God) have demonstrated mixed results [19], as has pleading religious coping strategies (i.e. pleading and bargaining with God or praying for a miracle) [25].

Measurement of Religious Coping

Early studies have tended to use public religious/ spiritual practices such as congregational attendance as a measure of religious coping [30, 31]. Using frequencies of religious service attendance as a coping measure is generally problematic for a number of reasons. For example, public religious/spiritual institutions/group attendance that involves meeting other like-minded people potentially expose people to social support, a variable known to predict illness adjustment which may therefore confound the results, whether the attendance is at a place of worship of an organised or non-organised religion or in someone's home (e.g. bible study). People may also follow religious/spiritual practices for social reasons, e.g. for social approval or social status often referred to as extrinsic religiousness [32]. Measuring public religious practices may therefore not necessarily inform much about *how* people use their faith in coping and how much it is involved in, for example, their cancer diagnosis or during cancer treatment. A distinction needs to be made between habitual religious/spiritual practices and those actively involved in coping with illness. Indeed, simply enquiring about service attendance does not inform about its intended purpose. It is also important to consider that people who are ill may not be well enough to take part in public religious/spiritual practices [33]. An example of a validated public religious practice scale [34] is shown in Table 9.2.

Private religious/spiritual practices such as prayer have also been used in research to represent religion/spirituality in the coping process [30, 31]. Using this approach is limited in that it only informs about the frequency of prayer and not its content, nor does it tell us about the actual cognitions used, whether they were adaptive or maladaptive. It can, however, inform researchers about the frequency of engaging in private religious practices such as frequency of prayer and whether these change as a result of being diagnosed with cancer. As with public religious practices, attention needs to be given to whether a practice is a coping or a habitual behaviour or whether it involves praying with other like-minded people whose support may contaminate the findings if not controlled for adequately in the study analyses. An example of a validated private religious practice scale [35] is shown in Table 9.2.

The importance of religious coping strategies is reflected in several commonly used coping questionnaires (e.g. the COPE by Carver et al. [36]; the Brief COPE by Carver [37]; the Ways of Coping Scale by Folkman and Lazarus [38] — Table 9.2). These questionnaire items usually involve explicit terms such as "I prayed" or "I have been trying to find comfort in my religious/spiritual beliefs". However, attempts made by "non-religious" coping scales to classify religious

coping highlight some difficulties. For example, this form of coping is often conceived as emotion focused [38], but can, as mentioned previously, also be problem focused [18]. Statements about prayer do not tell us about its content, nor does it inform about the actual coping cognitions that are used. Also, prayer is treated as a unidimensional construct when different forms of prayer may be associated with different outcomes. Some general coping measures (e.g. the Ways of Coping Scale) also ignore the possibility that religious coping might entail a unique coping dimension [37, 39–41], where religious coping items are combined within non-religious sub-scales such as "positive reappraisal" and "escape-avoidance". However, the distinct nature of religious coping in comparison to other forms of coping is evident in empirical studies. For example, the religious coping items of the COPE and Brief COPE load exclusively together onto one sub-scale [36, 37].

The specific content of potentially adaptive or maladaptive coping strategies (usually cognitive in nature but also some behavioural such as seeking religious support) can be measured using the Ways of Religious Coping Scale by Boudreaux et al. [42], the Religious Problem-Solving Scale by Pargament et al. [18], the Religious Coping Activities Scale by Pargament et al. [43] and the RCOPE by Pargament et al. [20] (Table 9.2). The Ways of Religious Coping Scale includes two sub-scales: (1) Internal/Private (e.g. "I pray", "I put my problems into God's hands") and (2) External/Social (e.g. "I get support from church/mosque/temple members", "I donate time to a religious cause or activity"). (Note that the former example is not a coping strategy, rather the possible consequence of seeking support from religious groups which, in turn, reduces the validity of this questionnaire.) Prayer is also treated as unidimensional. Although this scale has good psychometric properties (e.g. a two-factor structure and Cronbach's alpha scores of 0.93 and 0.97), it has not been extensively used.

The Religious Problem Solving Scale [18] includes three sub-scales examining various religious coping cognitions. These are labelled as follows: (1) collaborative (where the individual and God actively work together as partners, e.g. "When it comes to deciding how to solve problems, God and I work together as partners"); (2)

Table 9.2 Instruments examining religious coping strategies

Authors	Religious coping scales	Description
Idler [34]	Organisational religiousness scale	2 items examining frequency of attendance at religious services and participation in religious/spiritual activities with other people. Cronbach's alpha=0.82
Levin [35]	Private religious practices scale	4 items examining how often people pray or meditate, read religious or spiritual literature, watch or listen to religious programmes on TV or radio and say grace before meals. Cronbach's alpha=0.72
Folkman and Lazarus [38]	The ways of coping scale	2 items, 1 item as part of the "Escape-Avoidance" dimension: "Hoped a miracle would happen" and 1 item as part of the "positive reappraisal" dimension: "I prayed"
Carver et al. [36]	The COPE	4 items from the "Turning to religion" sub-scale, e.g. "I try to find comfort in my religion", "I seek God's help". Cronbach's alpha=0.92
Carver [37]	The Brief COPE	2 items from the "Religion" sub-scale, e.g. "I have been trying to find comfort in my religious beliefs", "I've been praying or meditating". Cronbach's alpha=0.82
Pargament et al. [18]	The religious problem-solving scale	22 items, 3 sub-scales labelled, (1) collaborative ("When it comes to deciding how to solve problems, God and I work together as partners". Cronbach's alpha=0.93); (2) self-directing ("When I have difficulty, I decide what it means by myself without relying on God". Cronbach's alpha=0.91); (3) deferring ("Rather than trying to come up with the right solution to a problem myself, I let God decide how to deal with it". Cronbach's alpha=0.89)
Pargament et al. [43]	The religious coping activities scale	15 items, 6 sub-scales: (1) Spiritually based (e.g. "Trusted that God would not let anything terrible happen to me"); (2) Good deeds (e.g. "Tried to be less sinful"); (3) Discontent (e.g. "Felt angry with or distant from God"); (4) Religious support (e.g. "received support from clergy"—note, not a coping strategy but its consequence); (5) plead (e.g. "Asked for a miracle") and (6) Religious avoidance (e.g. "Focused on the world to come rather than on the problems of this world"). Cronbach's alpha=0.61–0.92
Boudreaux et al. [42]	The ways of religious coping scale	25 items, 2 sub-scales: (1) Internal/Private (e.g. "I pray", "I put my problems into God's hands") and (2) External/Social (e.g. "I get support from church/mosque/temple members", "I donate time to a religious cause or activity"). Cronbach's alphas=0.93 and 0.97
Pargament et al. [20]	The RCOPE	105 items measuring positive and negative religious coping cognitions along five key religious functions in coping: (1) religious coping to give *meaning* to an event; (2) to provide a framework to achieve a sense of *control* over a difficult situation; (3) to provide *comfort* during times of difficulty; (4) to provide *intimacy* with other like-minded people and (5) to assist people in making major *life transformations*. Cronbach's alpha=0.65 or greater. Examples of items are displayed in Table 9.1
Pargament et al. [19]	The Brief RCOPE	14 items divided into two sub-scales of positive and negative religious coping strategies. Cronbach's alpha=0.87 (positive sub-scale) and 0.78 (negative sub-scale)

self-directing (where people are religious/spiritual but use coping strategies that do not involve God, e.g. "When I have difficulty, I decide what it means by myself without relying on God") and (3) deferring (where the responsibility of coping is passively deferred to God, e.g. "Rather than trying to come up with the right solution to a problem myself, I let God decide how to deal with it"). During development, the items from the scale loaded onto three separate factors and the sub-scales had Cronbach's alpha scores from 0.89 to 0.93. However, non-religious people would have trouble responding to items from the "self-directing" religious coping sub-scale as this scale assesses coping strategies of religious/spiritual people who use coping strategies without involving their faith in the coping process. The assumption is therefore that everyone has a belief in God or a higher power. It is, however, important to make sure that non-religious people can respond to religious coping items as many may indeed turn to a higher power during periods of severe illness despite not admitting to believing in a God.

The Religious Activities Scale [43] includes six sub-scales: (1) spiritually based (e.g. "Trusted that God would not let anything terrible happen to me"); (2) good deeds (e.g. "Tried to be less sinful"); (3) discontent (e.g. "Felt angry with or distant from God"); (4) religious support (e.g. "received support from clergy"—note, not a coping strategy, rather, its consequence); (5) plead (e.g. "Asked for a miracle") and (6) religious avoidance (e.g. "Focused on the world to come rather than on the problems of this world"). The items from the scale loaded onto six separate factors during development and the sub-scales had Cronbach's alpha scores from poor (0.61) to excellent (0.92).

The RCOPE [20] is the most comprehensive measure to date. It includes 21 sub-scales (see Table 9.1 for examples of items from each sub-scale and Table 9.2) and is a theoretically based measure that examines much more wide-ranging religious coping methods, including potentially harmful religious expressions. It examines the functional aspects of religious coping and attempts to answer how people make use of their religion

or spirituality to understand and deal with a stressful event which includes the five key religious functions in coping mentioned earlier (e.g. to gain meaning, control, comfort, intimacy and to achieve a life transformation). It is, however, very long (105 items) but the authors recommend that researchers can pick sub-scales of interest or pick sub-scales that are relevant to the research purpose, and can use three items (instead of five) with the highest loadings from each sub-scale (as indicated by the authors). The RCOPE was originally validated by Pargament et al. [20] using a college sample (five items per sub-scale) and a hospital sample (three items per sub-scale). The psychometric properties of the former, based on a 17-factor solution, were found to be acceptable with a Cronbach's alpha of 0.80 or greater for all but two scales: "marking religious boundaries" and "reappraisal of God's power", which had an alpha score of 0.78. The psychometric properties of the latter study, using a hospital sample, were also found to be acceptable showing alpha levels of 0.75 or greater for most factors.

Studies have found that several religious coping methods are moderately inter-correlated [19]. Therefore, specific clusters or patterns of religious coping strategies have more recently been explored using the Brief RCOPE [19]. This means that people do not make use of specific religious coping methods alone, but apply them in some combination. Items are divided into positive and negative religious coping patterns (i.e. two sub-scales) and may be useful if researchers are interested in focusing on several methods and how these relate to outcome, rather than focusing on one method in detail [19]. All of the items from this scale can be found within the sub-scales of the RCOPE. The negative sub-scale includes items measuring spiritual discontent, punishing God reappraisal, interpersonal religious discontent, demonic reappraisal and reappraisal of God's powers (see Table 9.2) and have all been empirically examined and associated with negative outcomes in the USA [25]. The positive sub-scale includes items measuring spiritual connection, seeking spiritual support, religious forgiveness, collaborative religious coping, benevolent religious reappraisal and religious purification. Again, all these sub-scales have been empirically associated with positive outcomes in the USA [25]. During development, the Brief RCOPE showed a clear two-factor structure and acceptable alpha scores of 0.87 (positive sub-scale) and 0.78 (negative sub-scale). However, considering the current lack of research outside of the USA, one potential problem with this approach is that it makes a priori assumptions about which religious coping strategies are adaptive and which are maladaptive rather than treating this as an empirical question. Also, some items may not be as relevant outside of the USA. For example, demonic religious reappraisal (e.g. "Decided that the devil made this happen") may seem alien to many people in Western Europe [44]. This combination of items may therefore not translate well to other cultures.

Most of these scales were developed on Christian populations and therefore use terms such as "church attendance" which may not be applicable to all patients with cancer. However, researchers can substitute these with more neutral terms such as "religious/spiritual service attendance" if patients from different religions or spiritual leanings are included in studies. It may also be necessary to ask patients to substitute the word God for a term they are more comfortable with (e.g. a higher power, the universe, spiritual force, etc.). Indeed, my colleagues and I have found that most patients from a variety of cultural backgrounds and religious/spiritual affiliations have no problem responding to these types of questionnaires when these minor adaptations are made.

Prevalence of Religious Coping in Cancer

Studies have reported that religious coping is one of the most commonly used coping strategies in the US cancer patients where up to 85% of women with breast cancer indicate that religion helped them cope with their illness [45]. Negative religious coping strategies on the other hand are used less often [20, 46, 47]. Fitchett et al. [47] found that only 13% of patients used "reappraisal of

God's powers" in the coping process. However, religious/spiritual beliefs and practices are very different across cultures and these findings may therefore not generalise to cancer patients outside the USA; 83% of North Americans feel God is important in their lives compared with 49% of people in Europe; 47% attend a place of worship regularly in the USA in contrast to 12% in the UK [48, 49]. In the USA, only 5% of the population are reported to be atheists [50] compared with 20% in the UK [51]. Indeed, Harcourt et al. [52] found that only 23% of the UK patients with breast cancer used religion in coping 8 weeks after diagnosis. However, this study examined religious coping in a simplistic way (e.g. by using generic questions from the Brief COPE) [37].

My colleagues and I examined various specific religious coping strategies (taken from the RCOPE) and we found a very different pattern; the use of non-religious coping strategies was, overall, more common and religious coping, despite being used by 66% of the sample, was one of the least used coping strategies when assessed using a comparable general coping measure [53]. This is probably due to a much larger proportion of non-religious/spiritual people in the UK. Indeed, 28% of patients in our study reported not having a belief in God or being unsure of God's existence. Using items from the RCOPE, we also found consistently high levels of positive religious coping strategies throughout the first year of illness. For example, "active and positive religious coping" was the most common religious coping strategy (with 73% of the sample using it to some degree at surgery), where patients attempted to find meaning, a sense of control, comfort and intimacy in their illness. This was followed by coping methods to achieve a life transformation (used by 53% of the sample), where patients used religious coping to find a new purpose in life. Indeed, the majority of patients used active non-religious coping by taking actions to try and make their situation better. It is therefore not surprising that the proportion of the sample who considered themselves religious/spiritual also used their religious/spiritual resources to achieve this. In contrast, negative religious coping strategies were, overall, relatively less common.

These findings support previous US results as well as a German study, where negative religious coping strategies were found to be overall less common than positive religious coping [20, 44, 46, 47]. However, despite being less common, negative religious coping strategies were used by as many as 53% of patients (e.g. reappraised God's powers). In addition, 37% of the sample felt, to some degree, punished and abandoned by God. This number is much higher than those reported by the US studies and may reflect the secular nature of the UK where God and religion may be viewed in more negative terms by those not practicing their faith in a more organised manner and may, as a result, have a less secure relationship with a God or may be struggling with their faith in their search for significance during periods of stress.

Change in Religious Coping Strategies Across the Illness Course

According to the "mobilisation hypothesis" [54, 55], under stressful circumstances (e.g. a health threat), people are more likely to turn to their faith for coping in response; yet there is inconsistent evidence in cancer patients that this is the case [56]. There are also inconsistencies regarding how religious coping changes during the illness course in cancer. Using a general simple measure of religious coping, Carver et al. [57] and Culver et al. [58] found that religious coping decreased over time. In contrast, Alferi et al. [59] found that levels of religious coping ("extent of turning to religion for comfort") remained stable across a 12-month period. To date, only two studies have examined the trajectory of religious coping across a range of specific religious coping strategies in cancer patients (breast cancer) [53, 60]. Gall et al. [60] found various patterns of change during the first 2 years of illness in ten specific religious coping strategies from the RCOPE. "Active religious surrender" and "spiritual support" showed an increase pre-surgery, and then a steady decline at follow-up. "Religious helping", on the other hand, increased from pre-diagnosis to 1 week pre-surgery but remained

stable from pre-surgery throughout 2 years post surgery, while "religious direction" increased pre-diagnosis to pre-surgery, followed by an increase until 6 months post surgery, where it stabilised. "Religious focus" increased from pre-diagnosis to pre-surgery and from 1 to 6 months post surgery, followed by a decrease from 6 months to 1 year. Other religious coping strategies such as "passive religious deferral", "spiritual discontent", "pleading", "benevolent religious reappraisal" and "collaborative religious coping" all remained stable. The pattern of change may therefore depend on the type of religious coping that is used.

In the second study carried out by my colleagues and me [53], we compared the use of specific religious coping strategies in the UK patients with early-stage breast cancer at the time of surgery and examined how these changed in the first year of illness. In support of previous findings by Alferi et al. [31], we found non-significant changes in four of the more specific religious coping strategies from the RCOPE; "religious coping to achieve a life transformation"; "passive religious deferral"; "reappraisal of God's powers" and "pleading for direct intercession". Gall et al [60] also found that "passive religious deferral" and "pleading" remained stable across time. However, they found significant changes in "seeking religious direction" (included in the "religious coping to achieve a life transformation" sub-scale in this study as they loaded together onto one factor) where it increased in use until 6 months post surgery when it stabilised. This demonstrates that findings from one culture may not generalise to another. We also found a significant reduction in some religious coping strategies across time; "active and positive religious coping" and "seeking support from religious leaders and members of religious group" were significantly higher at the time of surgery than at follow-up. This suggests that patients were significantly more likely to seek support from God, actively surrendering to the will of God, work together with a benevolent God to solve problems and seek support from religious/spiritual leaders and members of religious/spiritual groups in the early stages than further into the illness course. The value of emotional support in patients with breast cancer is well established and appears to have the strongest associations with illness adjustment [61, 62]. For those with a close attachment to God, asking God for support could serve as an added support resource or even a support substitute. Seeking support from God or from religious/spiritual leaders/members early in the illness course is therefore not surprising considering the potential difficulties associated with a breast diagnosis and subsequent surgery. Indeed, Gall et al. [60] also found higher levels of seeking spiritual support early in the illness course. However, in our study, religious struggles such as "feeling punished and abandoned by God" and "searching for spiritual cleansing" were both significantly higher at surgery and 12 months compared with 3 months post surgery. Gall et al. [60] found no change in spiritual discontent coping strategies across time (combined in our study with "punishing God reappraisal" as these loaded together onto one factor). Finally, the generic religious coping sub-scale from the Brief COPE only demonstrated that religious coping strategies were more common earlier in the illness course, confirming its limited usefulness as a measure of religious coping.

The above findings provide partial support for the mobilisation hypothesis. Indeed, increasing the use of religious/spiritual resources in the coping process, when faced with uncertainties about the future after a cancer diagnosis, may be the case. The majority of our participants were unaware of their prognosis at baseline assessment. Religious coping may therefore be higher as a result and may decrease as the patients become aware of the good prognosis that is associated with early-stage breast cancers. However, the mobilisation hypothesis does not explain why some religious coping strategies showed a tendency to increase at 12 months. Indeed, patterns of change may depend on the type of religious coping strategy that is used and some of these may be particularly volatile. They are also likely to be influenced by co-occurring life events. The Cognitive Phenomenological Theory of Stress and Coping by Lazarus and Folkman [63] describes coping as process-orientated that is

directed towards what an individual thinks and does within the context of a specific encounter and how these thoughts and actions change as the encounter unfolds. During the first year of cancer treatment, patients with breast cancer often undergo lengthy treatment protocols with distressing side effects and regular medical surveillance, and worries about treatment and cancer recurrence are common [64]. The postoperative period is one of recovery from the procedure but also of confrontation with, and adaptation to, loss and possible death [65]. It is likely that, as a result of searching for spiritual cleansing through religious actions earlier in the illness course, a need to repent or feelings of being punished and abandoned by God may no longer be salient a few months later. However, as a result of being under close surveillance by hospital staff, this care and attention may serve to substitute feelings of being abandoned or punished and may reduce efforts of religious purification. As this close level of attention is reduced around 12 months, negative feelings of being punished and abandoned, and a need for religious purification, may resurface as a reaction to the loss of care. There is related evidence that end-of-treatment distress may occur as a result of patients feeling vulnerable to tumour recurrence, as they are no longer monitored closely by hospital staff [66]. Indeed, patients may experience a loss of security from having treatment and loss of support relating to ongoing communication with health care providers [67–69]. What is clear from these findings is that cancer patients have different spiritual needs at different times during their illness course depending on their coping appraisals.

Cultural and Denominational Differences

It is important to note that specific religious coping strategies may vary between different ethnic groups and religious affiliations; Alferi et al. [59] found that the US Evangelical women with breast cancer reported higher levels of church attendance and religiosity across a 12-month period post surgery compared with Catholic women.

Religious denominations may also differ in the extent to which they focus on supporting and fostering the emotional well-being of their members, and in their focus on the expiation of guilt and the preparation for the hereafter [59]. There may also be differences between those who are affiliated and those who are not in how they use religious coping strategies. There is evidence that non-affiliates are less likely to express "religious consolation", i.e. seeking spiritual comfort and support. Religious affiliates, on the other hand, are more likely to be exposed to support by religious group members and rituals which may enhance the use of positive religious coping [70]. There is evidence that relying on faith during illness in the USA is also greater in some groups such as African Americans [71–73] and Hispanics [36] compared to Caucasians [58, 74]. In addition, one cannot assume that those reporting an affiliation with a particular religious denomination actually practice their faith, as they may simply be referring to their identity rather than their religious involvement, especially in countries such as the UK where regular religious service attendance is relatively low. Therefore, establishing that religious affiliation refers to the actual practice of faith is vital.

There may also be differences between those who are affiliated (e.g. Catholic, Protestant) and those who are not (e.g. those who believe in God but do not see themselves as belonging to a particular denomination) in how they use religious coping strategies. There is evidence that non-affiliates are less likely to express "religious consolation", i.e. seeking spiritual comfort and support and are less likely to be connected to religious groups and therefore less likely to use religious coping strategies, even in the light of a serious illness such as cancer. Religious affiliates, on the other hand, are more likely to be exposed to rituals which may enhance the use of religious coping [70]. In addition, in countries where a large proportion of the population do not believe in a God, it is important to include all patients in studies examining religious coping, as "non-believers" may nevertheless use religious coping during difficult and desperate times, just as those who believe may exclude their faith in the coping process [53].

Religious Coping and Adjustment in Cancer

Various religious coping strategies adopted by people and how these change during the illness course have implications for illness adjustment in cancer [44, 60, 74]. Indeed, there is increasing evidence of the importance of drawing on religious/spiritual resources in the coping process during illness. However, few studies have adequately examined these in patients with cancer, especially outside the USA [75]. A systematic review published in 2006 examining the relationship between religious coping and cancer adjustment found that many studies report mixed findings but most have various methodological shortcomings using, for example, mixed cancer groups at different stages of their illness [75]. This makes it difficult to discern the impact of the relationship between religious coping and time, as it is possible that at crucial times during the illness course, patients may rely more on their religion/spirituality as they adapt to their diagnosis, treatments and an uncertain future. Another issue is how religious coping has been conceptualised and measured. However, the potential confusion between religious coping cognitions versus behaviours such as religious service attendance is particularly important in societies with high religious service attendance, where an effect could be caused by perceived social support from the religious community rather than religious coping. Many studies have also used generic instruments (e.g. the Brief COPE [37]) that do not identify the content of prayer or the specific religious coping strategies used. Only three studies used measures developed specifically to examine religious coping [76–78], all of which produced significant results in the expected direction.

Since the review was published, further studies have been conducted examining the efficacy of religious coping on well-being in patients with cancer [44, 46, 47, 60, 74, 79–84]. These additional studies reinforce the suggestion that when better ways of measuring religious coping are used, more significant findings are evident. Particularly   noticeable   is   the   consistent relationship between negative religious coping and poorer outcomes. However, all of the above studies except Derks et al. [80], Hebert et al. [83], Sherman et al. [84] and Gall et al. [60] were cross-sectional in design and most (except Gall et al. [60]) used the Brief RCOPE to measure religious coping. Some had very large refusal rates or attrition [44, 74, 80]. Four were conducted outside the USA and found the effects of religious coping to be comparable [44, 60, 80, 82]. Although some controlled for demographic and medical variables [46] only one study [83] controlled for the potential confounding effect of perceived social support.

The Role of Non-religious Variables

Studies examining religious coping in cancer using more appropriate measures have rarely assessed the role of other important psychological variables (e.g. perceived support, non-religious coping and optimism) and how these feature in explaining the link between religious coping and adjustment. For example, Gall [79] and Sherman et al. [46] used regression analysis to assess the efficacy of religious coping in predicting adjustment. These studies controlled for demographic variables and found a significant independent effect of religious coping (Brief RCOPE) on adjustment. However, it is not known how these significant effects would appear if other variables known to affect adjustment in patients with cancer had been entered into the regression model. Indeed, researchers need to be thoughtful about which other variables should be measured alongside religious/spiritual variables and consider the order in which these are entered if regression analysis is used. Entering religious coping strategies last, after other non-religious variables, can only produce two results: an independent effect or a non-significant effect of religious coping. If a mediating effect has occurred, it would not be visible; rather a non-significant finding would be evident leading to a false conclusion.

Few studies have examined the mechanism through which religious coping affects outcome in patients with cancer. However, there is evidence

from non-cancer studies that perceived social support is correlated with various religious factors such as church attendance, church membership, subjective religiosity, religious affiliation [85] and even private religious practices such as prayer [86]. Indeed, perceived social support as well as hope and optimism were found to completely mediate the effect of positive religious coping on better adjustment in cardiac patients [87–89]. Other studies have found inconsistent results. For example, Koenig et al. [86] found that religious activity as a single construct was correlated with social support but was unrelated to depression in a sample of patients over the age of 65. In the same study, frequency of church attendance was negatively related to depression, but was surprisingly unrelated to social support. Private prayer was, however, positively related to social support but unrelated to depression. In addition, Bosworth et al. [90] found that social support was related to lower levels of negative religious coping strategies (Brief RCOPE) in a geriatric sample but negative religious coping was independently related to lower levels of depression. They also found that public religious practice was related to social support but independently related to lower levels of depression in the regression analyses once social support was controlled for.

There are cancer studies examining how religious/spiritual resources other than religious coping strategies are linked to outcome (e.g. religious involvement, strength of faith or levels of religiosity/spirituality). For example, Sherman and Simonton [91] found that optimism played a mediating role in the relationship between general religious orientation and psychological adjustment in patients but social support did not seem to play a comparable role. Sherman et al. [91] found that strength of faith was related to optimism but not to social support. However, Carver et al. [57], using a generic measure of religious coping (the Brief COPE), found that religious coping in patients with breast cancer was not related to optimism at any time point of assessment. This suggests that how religiousness/spirituality is operationalised and measured determines how and whether it is significantly related to outcome.

Various religious coping strategies are also both positively and negatively related to non-religious coping strategies such as active coping, suppressing competitive activities, planning, use of social support [57], positive reinterpretation and growth [36], positive and negative appraisal of the cancer situation, distancing coping and focusing on the positive, seeking support, behavioural avoidance, cognitive avoidance and focusing on the positive [76]. Qualitative work has also found a link between humour and spirituality [92]. Indeed, there is evidence that active coping mediates the link between religion/spirituality and functional well-being in patients with ovarian cancer [93] and between religious involvement and psychological distress in patients with HIV [94]. In addition, religious/spiritual beliefs have been shown to have a positive association with active rather than passive non-religious coping strategies in cancer patients [95, 96] and those who have strong religious/spiritual beliefs are more likely to use cognitive reframing (i.e. focusing on the positive) as a coping strategy during cancer [97].

Only two studies to date have examined the mediating role of non-religious variables between religious coping and adjustment in patients with cancer [44, 98]. Zwingman et al. [44] found a mediating effect of non-religious coping between positive and negative religious coping and psychosocial well-being. They also found that negative religious coping moderated the effect of religious commitment and anxiety. The second study was conducted by my colleagues and me. We examined the role of various specific religious coping strategies on anxious and depressed mood [98]. Previous studies have tended to find negative religious coping, as measured by the Brief RCOPE, to be related to higher levels of anxious mood in patients with cancer [44, 46, 47, 82, 84]. As mentioned earlier, this seven-item sub-scale clusters together various negative religious coping strategies. It is therefore not known which negative religious coping strategy is responsible for this effect. We were indeed able to demonstrate which negative religious coping strategy was important in predicting anxiety in patients with breast cancer living in the UK and

also how religious coping was related to this mood variable. First, it appeared that feeling punished and abandoned by God significantly explained 5% of the variance in higher levels of anxiety, but this effect was partially buffered by acceptance coping, reducing levels of distress. The effect of feeling punished and abandoned by God on anxiety was also partially mediated by denial coping, which was significantly associated with higher levels of anxiety. This suggests that a "negative" religious coping strategy can be associated with both higher and lower levels of anxious mood depending on which combination of non-religious coping strategies is used and shows that religious coping may be related to outcome in more complex ways. Referring to it as a negative religious coping strategy could therefore be misleading in some instances. These findings also reject the usefulness of clustering questionnaire items based on a priori assumptions of which coping strategies are negative and which are positive.

Previous findings have also demonstrated that negative religious coping strategies are associated with higher levels of depressed mood in patients with cancer [44, 46, 47, 84]. However, as with anxiety, most previous studies have used the Brief RCOPE to examine negative religious coping in relation to depression. It is therefore currently not known which negative religious coping strategy is responsible for this effect. In our study, "feeling punished and abandoned by God" was an independent predictor of depressed mood explaining 4% of the variance. We also found that self-blame coping was the only non-religious coping strategy to predict higher levels of depressed mood and was responsible for 5% of the variance. This demonstrates that religious coping was of equal importance to non-religious coping in predicting depressed mood in patients with breast cancer in the UK. It is important to mention, however, that these analyses were cross-sectional, so we cannot infer causality at this stage. It is, for example, possible that depressed mood may cause people to appraise their situations within a negative religious framework.

We were unable to find a significant effect of positive religious coping on adjustment in patients with breast cancer. Similar and mixed results in cancer populations are seen elsewhere [44, 46, 84]. The reason for inconsistencies is not yet clear and the presence or the absence of an effect may simply be due to difficulties in selecting the right outcome measure. Positive religious coping strategies may, for example, be more likely to be related to positive outcomes such as positive affect and life satisfaction. It is also worth mentioning that different patterns of religious coping and how these relate to various adjustment outcomes may be expected from different ethnic groups with different religious backgrounds. For example, the literal meaning of "Islam" means submission and peace which is found by accepting the will of God and accepting events that are outside of our control. For this reason, Islamic theology does not accept anger towards God as an acceptable response to suffering [99]. Currently, very little is known about how ethnic differences relate to religious coping and psychological well-being.

In our studies, perceived social support did not play an important role in explaining how religious coping is associated with adjustment variables. Indeed, previous studies have found inconsistent evidence of social support as a mediator between religious/spiritual resources and adjustment. This inconsistency raises more questions than answers. There is some evidence that church attendance and seeking support from a priest/minister are more advantageous in some denominations. For example, there is evidence that it is beneficial for Evangelical women, but detrimental for Catholics, and that obtaining emotional support from church members is related to less distress in Evangelical women only [59]. Differentiating between the sources of perceived social support may be important as these sources may serve different support functions with different types of consequences. Perhaps a support measure needs to be more explicit regarding which type of support it is measuring, i.e. specifically examine support from religious/spiritual communities. However, this is problematic in studies assessing support in a large proportion of individuals who simply do not belong to a religious community (e.g. a European sample). Future studies, especially in the USA, may never-

theless attempt to be more specific in terms of how they enquire about patients' perceived support and examine specific support from religious/spiritual communities using a measure designed specifically for this purpose [100].

Religious Coping and Growth

Until recently, research had largely focused on the negative consequences of a cancer diagnosis (e.g. negative mood) [101]. Indeed, many cancer patients experience clinical levels of distress and dysfunction including anxiety and depression and some may even suffer from post-traumatic stress disorder [102, 103]. However, there is evidence that cancer should not be viewed as a stressor with uniformly negative outcomes but rather as a transitional event which may create the potential for both positive and negative change [104, 105]. Despite the stress of coping with a cancer diagnosis and dealing with often lengthy treatment protocols, many patients are able to find meaning in their illness such as experiencing profound positive changes in themselves, in their relationships and in other life domains after cancer [106]. It is even suggested that finding meaning in a stressful event is critical for understanding illness adjustment [107].

Researchers have used a number of terms to describe individual reports of finding meaning in the face of adversity [108]. These include related concepts such as "benefit finding" [101, 109], "stress-related growth" [110], "post-traumatic growth" [111] and "gratitude" [112, 113]. Post-traumatic growth has been defined as "Positive psychological change experienced as a result of the struggle with highly challenging life circumstances" [108]. Benefit finding has been described as "the pursuit for the silver lining of adversities" [101] while gratitude has been defined as "the willingness to recognise the unearned increment of value in one's experience" [114]. Although these concepts are similar and related to a large extent, gratitude is considered a broader concept while benefit finding, stress-related and post-traumatic growth are seen as examining more specific aspects of growth and positive changes arising from a stressful event [115].

Finding meaning in the cancer experience in the form of positive benefits is a common occurrence [116]. There is also evidence that a higher level of faith/religiousness is linked to greater levels of perceived cancer-related growth and benefit finding [111, 117, 118]. However, very few studies have examined the link between religious coping and growth/benefit finding in patients with cancer although some have provided some insight using the Brief COPE. For example, studies have found that patients with breast cancer scoring high on religious coping also scored high on growth [119, 120] and religious coping pre-surgery has also been found to predict higher levels of growth 12 months later in patients with prostate cancer [121]. However, only one study to date has addressed which aspects of religious coping may facilitate growth: a prospective study carried out by my colleagues and me examining the effects of religious/spiritual coping resources on benefit finding in breast cancer along with other potentially influencing variables such as non-religious coping, optimism and social support [122]. We found that religious coping to achieve a life transformation predicted 14% of the variance but was partially mediated by strength of faith. Strength of faith at surgery on the other hand was an independent predictor of benefit finding 3 months later, predicting 6% of the variance. Seeking emotional support coping at surgery was the only non-religious variable to predict outcome, explaining 3% of the variance in higher levels of benefit finding 3 months later. Our results show that religious coping was far better than non-religious coping or indeed, other psychological variables, in predicting a positive outcome such as benefit finding. Again, this study highlights the importance of examining religious/spiritual resources in combination with other variables to fully understand their relationship to adjustment in cancer.

Addressing Cancer Patients' Spiritual Needs

Assessing the psychological needs of patients with cancer has become commonplace in clinical practice in recent years. Also, as a result of studies showing social support to be important in the adjustment process, providing support groups for those patients lacking in support is also widespread. Addressing patients' spiritual concerns is also, in relative terms, commonplace within palliative care but, as research shows, spiritual concerns can occur at any time during the cancer course. However, how and whether religious/spiritual concerns should be addressed in patients with serious illness has been much debated [123, 124]. Indeed, some academics/physicians believe that there is no place for religion/spirituality within medicine [124, 125]. Then again, critics often fail to differentiate between subjective religiousness/spirituality studies (e.g. spiritual beliefs and behaviours) and those of an objective approach examining, for example, the effect of intercessory prayer on recovery where patients in the experimental group are usually not aware they are being prayed for. Intercessory prayer studies do not examine the effect of patients' own cognitions and behaviours in relation to outcome such as psychological well-being or quality of life but attempt to test the existence of God through the power of prayer. These studies are therefore not psychological in nature; rather they belong within the theological realm. A psychological study assesses the effect of patients' own *subjective* beliefs, perceptions and behaviours on outcome. Often, these two types of studies are discussed together as if they were, in some way, comparable. It should be mentioned, however, that the effect of intercessory prayer can be important if, during a difficult time, a person is aware of others praying for him or her, as it can instil a sense of comfort from communal caring, and may reinforce a sense of belonging and personal worth in relation to significant others [126]. In addition, when critics discuss patients' subjective religious/spiritual beliefs and practices in relation to health as being problematic, the focus tends to be on the efficacy of religious/spiritual practices such as prayer in assisting with the physical recovery from disease. Prayer in this case is a form of alternative therapy, where it is used as a substitute for conventional medicine. In this instance, religion/spirituality may have severe implications for recovery [125]. If there is evidence of a conflict between religious beliefs and recommended treatments, the National Comprehensive Cancer Network's (NCCN) clinical practice guidelines in oncology—distress management, p. DIS24 [127]—describe how to deal with this issue. Indeed, Koenig [128] argues that if religious/spiritual resources serve to influence medical decision making in powerful, negative ways, these need to be understood.

It is suggested that an understanding of patients' religious/spiritual foundation can guide appropriate care [129]. If religious coping turns out to be helpful or even harmful to patients, it may be beneficial for health care professionals to acknowledge and support patients' spirituality or religious leanings [130]. For example, patients who perceive their illness as a punishment may become unable to use their faith as a coping resource. God may be seen as weak, distant or uncaring which may lead to an existential crisis. Plotnikoff [131] has provided a few specific examples of spiritual struggles and their implications: (1) Spiritual alienation ("Where is God when I need him most? Why isn't God listening?"); (2) Spiritual anxiety ("Will I ever be forgiven? Am I going to die a horrible death?"); (3) Spiritual guilt ("I deserve this. I am being punished by God. I didn't pray often enough."); (4) Spiritual anger ("I'm angry at God. I blame God for this. I hate God."); (5) Spiritual loss ("I feel empty. I don't care anymore.") and (6) Spiritual despair ("There is no way God could ever care for me."). However, deciding how to best respond to a patients' spiritual needs can raise professional and ethical issues for health care professionals about how they interact and deal with patients [123]. For example, should health professionals really discuss spiritual issues with patients and do patients want them to? If so, who is best placed to do this and what should the professional boundaries be between healthcare professionals and chaplains?

There is some evidence suggesting that addressing spiritual concerns with a physician appears to have a positive impact on perception of care and well-being in patients with cancer [132] and may enhance recovery from illness [133] and improve quality of life [134]. Further, 65% of non-cancer patients in a US pulmonary outpatient clinic said that if physicians enquired about spiritual beliefs, it would strengthen their trust in their physician [135]. Therefore, having clinical respect for patients' spirituality as an important resource for coping with illness is important. In the USA, between 58 and 77% of hospitalised patients want physicians to consider their spiritual needs [136, 137]. Further, 94% of patients want their physicians to ask about their religious/ spiritual beliefs if they become gravely ill [135], and 45% of patients who did not have religious/ spiritual beliefs still felt it appropriate that physicians should ask about them [138]. However, Koenig et al. [139] also found that up to one-third of the US patients do not want physicians to discuss spiritual issues with them. Therefore, physicians (or other health care professionals such as a nurse) may initially explore patients' general coping methods in order to discover whether their religious/spiritual beliefs play an important role in their medical decisions.

Most studies examining religious/spiritual needs in patients with medical illnesses have been conducted in the USA. There is some evidence from a German study that the majority of patients who were asked wanted their doctor to be interested in their spiritual orientation [140]. The proportion of patients in other European countries who want their spiritual needs assessed and how these issues should be addressed and by whom is unclear.

Spiritual Needs' Assessments

A spiritual assessment may contain numerous questions about religious denomination, beliefs or life philosophies, important spiritual practices or rituals, use of spirituality or religion as a source of strength, being part of a faith community of support, use of prayer or meditation, loss of faith, conflicts between spiritual or religious beliefs and cancer treatments, ways that health care providers and caregivers may help with the patient's spiritual needs, concerns about death and the afterlife and end-of-life planning [141]. There are several tools in existence that attempt to address patients' spiritual needs (see Table 9.3).

Table 9.3 Instruments providing guidelines on how to take a spiritual history, thereby addressing patients' spiritual needs

Spiritual need assessment tools		
Authors	Measures	Description
Kuhn [142]	Kuhn's Spiritual Inventory	Meaning, purpose, belief, faith, love, forgiveness, prayer, meditation and worship
Matthews and Clark [143]	Matthew's Spiritual History	Importance and influence of religious beliefs and practices and desire of physician addressing these
Puchalski and Romer [144]	FICA Spiritual Assessment Tool	FICA: F=Faith: what tradition, I=importance of faith, C=church: public religious practices, A=apply: how these apply to health and illness and A=address: how these should be addressed
Maugans [145]	Maugans's SPIRITual History	Includes six areas (SPIRIT): The spiritual belief system, personal spirituality, integration within a spiritual community, ritualised practices and restrictions, implications for medical care and terminal event planning
Anandarajah and Light [147]	HOPE Questionnaire	Source of hope, meaning and comfort, organised religion, personal spirituality and practices, the effect of these on medical care and illness and how these should be addressed
Lo et al. [148]	ACP Spiritual History	Includes four questions: The importance of faith, when and for how long, availability of someone to talk to about religious/spiritual matters and whether the patient wants to explore issues with someone
Frick et al. [140]	SPIR	A semi-structured clinical interview assessing 4 main areas: Belief/spirituality/religiosity of patient; the place of spirituality in patient's life; integration in a spiritual community; preferences of the role of health care professionals in dealing with spirituality
Büssing et al. [150]	Spiritual Needs Questionnaire (SpNQ)	19 items assessing religious needs (e.g. praying), inner peace, existential (reflection/meaning) and actively giving

These have been developed mainly by the US researchers, and provide guidelines on how to conduct a spiritual history. The earliest is the Kuhn's Spiritual Inventory [142]. This brief assessment tool enquires about religious/spiritual beliefs, how illness has influenced beliefs, how patients exercise their beliefs in their lives and how faith has influenced their behaviour during illness and regaining health. Further, Matthew and Clark [143] suggest that physicians should ask about three fundamental questions as part of the initial evaluation. Their assessment tool—the Matthew's Spiritual History—examines the importance of spirituality to the patient, how this influences the way they look at their medical problem/think about health and whether they would like the physician to address these issues. A similar tool is the FICA Spiritual Assessment

Tool [144] which, again, addresses patients' religious/spiritual traditions, the importance of faith, how it is practiced, how it is applied to health and illness and how these should be addressed. Another much more thorough instrument is the Maugans's SPIRITual History [145]. This covers six areas (SPIRIT): the *S*piritual belief system (e.g. affiliation), *P*ersonal spirituality (includes acceptability of beliefs and practices), *I*ntegration within a spiritual community, *R*itualised practices and restrictions, *I*mplications for medical care and *T*erminal events planning. This is probably the most comprehensive tool to date covering the most important areas of spiritual needs [146]. Equally, the HOPE questionnaire [147] also examines a broad range of issues considered important in medical illness and decision making: source of hope, meaning and comfort, organised religion (e.g. being a member of a religious community), personal spirituality and practices, the effect of these on medical care and illness and how they should be addressed. Finally, the ACP Spiritual History tool [148] asks patients with a serious medical illness four simple questions: the importance of faith during their illness, the importance of faith at other times of their lives, the availability of someone to talk to about religious matters and their need to explore religious matters with someone. This assessment is patient centred and brief. However, it fails to gather information in several key areas such as identifying spiritual needs, connection with religious/spiritual communities and beliefs affecting medical decision making. It was also developed for patients in a palliative care setting only.

It is important to reiterate that these tools were developed in the USA and it is therefore not currently known to what degree these questions would be perceived as acceptable in the hospital environments of other countries and cultures. Indeed, the crisis of religious institutions is more noticeable in Western Europe than in the USA [140] where Davie et al. [149] have described the phenomenon of "believing without belonging". This means that religious/spiritual beliefs become increasingly personal, detached and heterogeneous in nature and this must be taken into account when patients' religiousness/spirituality is assessed in a European context [140]. However, two European (German) assessments exist: the SPIR, a semi-structured spiritual needs interview guide [140] that examines four main areas of patients' spiritual needs: how patients would describe themselves (e.g. a believer/religious/ spiritual), the place of spirituality in their lives, whether they are integrated into a spiritual community and the role they would like to assign their health care professional in the domain of spirituality.

The second is the Spiritual Needs Questionnaire [150] which is suited to both secular and religious societies and attempts to address four aspects of cancer patients' spiritual needs: the religious (e.g. praying with others or by themselves), inner peace (e.g. a need to find peace or dwell in a quiet place), existential (e.g. reflections about a previ-

ous life or the need to talk with someone about the meaning of life) and actively giving (e.g. to give away something of yourself). As it is recent, there is currently no data to assess its general usefulness. It is also important to appreciate that, after a cancer diagnosis, a non-religious/spiritual person may, for example, interpret concepts such as finding meaning and purpose in existential or humanistic terms, while a religious/spiritual person would view the same construct as religious or spiritual in nature [150]. Non-religious cancer patients may therefore have similar needs to religious/spiritual patients but may not label these as such. This may be especially prevalent in European cancer patients.

Spiritual Distress Management

It is suggested that negative events are easier to bear when understood within a benevolent religious framework. Indeed, the current findings show that positive aspects of religious coping may be related to better adjustment. Therefore, religious counsellors, i.e. hospital chaplains, can help by reframing negative events within the will of a loving and compassionate God and help patients (who show evidence of religious struggles) to utilise more effective religious coping methods. It has been suggested that this can help individuals to maintain a theologically sound understanding of suffering and to experience better mental health outcomes in terms of their psychological adjustment in the face of stressful events [131]. The UK National Institute for Clinical Excellence (NICE) guidelines on spiritual support services in cancer care [151] state that provider organisations should adhere to the framework of best practice in meeting the religious and spiritual needs of patients and staff outlined in the National Health Service's (NHS) National Guidance directive [152]. For example, on (or before) admission to hospital, patients should be asked whether they would like to have their religious affiliation recorded. They should be informed that this data will be processed for one or more specified purposes. Patients should be asked for permission to pass this information

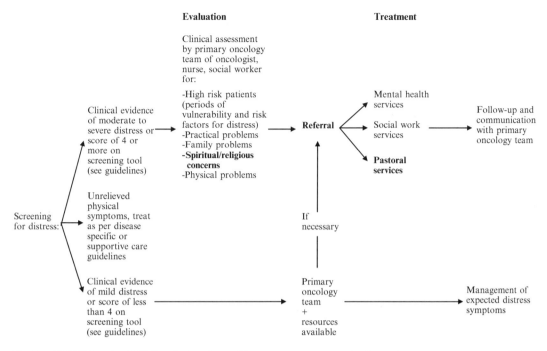

Fig. 9.1   NCCN, Practice Guidelines in Oncology—Distress management: Evaluation and treatment process, p. DIS4 [127]

on to the chaplaincy service for the purposes of spiritual care. A staff member, usually a healthcare chaplain/spiritual caregiver, should be nominated to be responsible for liaising with local faith leaders. In addition, while recognising that one individual may hold specific responsibility for ensuring the provision of spiritual care, this should also be seen as the responsibility of the whole team. Further, individual team members responsible for offering spiritual care should contribute to the team's regular review of care plans, especially for those patients with already identified spiritual needs.

In the USA, the NCCN's clinical practice guidelines in oncology—distress management [127]—also include very clear guidelines on how to manage spiritual distress. The initial evaluation process (see Fig. 9.1) describes various pathways for screening for distress: the evaluations process, through to referral, treatment and follow-up. For example, during the evaluation process, any indication of spiritual/religious concerns must be noted and appropriate referrals made to pastoral services. However, their screening tool

for measuring religious/spiritual distress asks only one very basic question, "Please indicate if any of the following has been a problem for you in the past week including today" followed by a yes/no answer for religious/spiritual concerns. Therefore, a more thorough tool (if time allows), such as those mentioned earlier in this chapter, may be implemented after the initial assessment. These assessments should also include a thorough exploration of patients' coping strategies.

The NCCN's guidelines also include very specific guidance on pastoral evaluations and treatment pathways. For example, there are guidelines designed to evaluate aspects of spiritual distress such as grief, concerns about death and the afterlife, conflicted or challenged belief systems, loss of faith, concerns with meaning/purpose of life, concerns about relationship with deity, isolation from religious community, guilt, hopelessness, conflict between religious beliefs and recommended treatments and ritual needs. They also describe how pastoral services should deal with spiritual concerns such as conflicted or challenged belief systems, loss of faith and concerns with meaning/purpose of life, how to support patients who may feel isolated from the religious community and various ways of dealing with guilt. Finally, the NCCN's guidelines illustrate pathways through which feelings of hopelessness can be adequately dealt with if these feelings are related to patients' spiritual concerns and these guidelines also demonstrate how patients' ritual needs should be met.

Evidence described in this chapter shows that cancer patients' spiritual needs may vary depending on how their situation is appraised. For example, support from their religious community may be more important early on in the illness course while religious/spiritual struggles, although more prevalent in some cancers early on, may resurface much later when healthcare professionals are no longer involved in their patients' care to the same degree. This suggests that interventions should, overall, target patients early but that healthcare professionals should also be aware of the potential resurfacing of some religious struggles later on in the illness trajectory and that these need to be re-examined and addressed at regular intervals.

Barriers to Spiritual Needs' Assessment and Management

Addressing religious/spiritual concerns is not commonplace despite the US NCCN's [127] clinical practice guidelines in oncology and the UK NICE guidelines [151] stating the importance of supporting patients' spiritual needs during the course of cancer. The UK Clinical Standards for Working in a Breast Speciality [153] further highlights the importance of understanding psychological risk factors associated with morbidity during breast cancer by understanding a variety of helpful or unhelpful coping strategies, being aware of spiritual conflicts, providing patients with appropriate emotional support and offering intervention strategies, e.g. advice regarding coping strategies or referral to other agencies. However, a recent US study found that as many as 72% of patients with advanced cancer said that their spiritual needs were either minimally met or not met at all by the medical system and 47% said

that they were supported minimally or not at all by their religious community [134]. However, health care professionals have expressed concern about lack of time, lack of skills (e.g. not knowing how to take a spiritual history) and the appropriateness of such discussions within the context of the medical encounter [137, 154, 155]. Indeed, in the USA, physicians' discomfort at addressing spiritual needs is the best predictor of whether these discussions take place or not [154]. It is also well established that religiosity/spirituality and a belief in God are much lower among physicians, healthcare professionals and academics compared with their patients or with the general population [8, 156–163]. In the UK, around 70% of people have some belief in God [49]. However, a study examining religiosity among 230 psychiatrists working in London teaching hospitals found that only 27% reported a religious affiliation and 23% reported a belief in God [164]. Another study assessing religious faith in health care professionals at a London teaching hospital found that 45% of hospital staff reported that they had a religious faith [165].

There is also a higher level of atheism among physicians. Neeleman and King [164], for example, found that 25% of doctors reported that they were atheists compared to only 9.5% of their patients. Also, Silvestri et al. [166] found that cancer patients and their caregivers ranked doctor recommendations as most important followed by faith in God second, whereas physicians placed faith in God last. These lower levels of religiosity/spirituality and higher levels of atheism may lead healthcare professionals to underestimate the importance of faith for their patients and may also explain the lack of mainstream research in the area until recently. Indeed, physicians who report addressing patients' spiritual concerns do so because of their own spirituality and because of an awareness of the scientific evidence associated with spirituality and health. Empirical findings do suggest that barriers to spiritual assessment include upbringing and culture, lack of spiritual inclination or awareness, resistance to exposing personal beliefs and the belief that spiritual discussion will not have an impact on patients and their lives [167–169].

It has also been suggested that faith may be a very personal matter for physicians due to the potential stigma associated with admitting being spiritual/religious [170]. Klitzman and Daya [170], using a qualitative methodology, examined spirituality in doctors who themselves had become seriously ill and found that they too had beliefs that ranged from being spiritual to start with; to being spiritual, but not thinking of themselves as such; to wanting, but being unable to believe. Some continued to doubt. The contents of beliefs ranged from established religious traditions to mixing beliefs, or having non-specific beliefs (e.g. concerning the power of nature). One group of doctors felt wary of organised religion, which could prove an obstacle to belief. Others felt that symptoms could be reduced through prayer. Unfortunately, there is no comparison data available for non-physicians suffering from a similar condition. However, understanding spiritual–cultural influences on health-related behaviours and illness adjustment is essential if health care professionals are to provide effective care to their patients. Overcoming barriers is therefore important as it would allow a more accepting and open discussion about patients' lives beyond the social and the psychological. Nevertheless, many physicians still practice under the biomedical model where spiritual matters may seem less relevant [133].

There are also some practical problems in meeting patients' spiritual needs. For religious/spiritual counselling to take place, someone needs to identify patients with spiritual concerns in order to refer those who struggle with their faith to a degree that it is detrimental to well-being. Current UK guidelines [152] view hospital chaplaincy as central to this role. However, chaplains may not be available in smaller hospitals or in outpatient clinics where most care is delivered, especially early in the cancer course where religious/spiritual issues may first arise [141]. In addition, patients struggling with their faith may not want to speak to hospital chaplains as they may feel alienated from religion and anyone associated with it [146]. Also, patients' spiritual concerns may not be "religious" in nature (in terms of organised beliefs and practices) but may take the form of existential and philosophical issues [171]. Therefore, having an intermediary trained to assess and deal with spiritual/existential issues may be more appropriate in the first instance. However, should more complex spiritual needs arise, or should patients wish to speak to religious/spiritual counsellors, appropriate and agreed referrals could be made. In a country such as the UK, it may be more appropriate for a senior specialist oncology nurse (e.g. a breast care nurse) to deal with spiritual needs as these health care professionals are already trained to assess and address patient's psychological and social needs. Indeed, if patients who have turned away from institutional religion would prefer to talk to a health care professional about their spiritual needs rather than a trained and certified chaplain or pastoral counsellor, there is a genuine need to provide adequate education and training to allow these professionals to competently address and uncover spiritual needs within this patient group [150].

Conclusions and Future Directions

The focus of this chapter has been on religious coping, its nature, measurement, prevalence and how it relates to adjustment in cancer. The use of religiosity and spirituality in coping is indeed common in cancer patients throughout the illness course and not just in the USA but also in European cultures where the abandonment of organised religious institutions is much more prevalent. It is also increasingly clear that it plays an important role in illness adjustment, especially the use of negative religious coping strategies. With increasing evidence of its importance, there is an argument for introducing appropriate spiritual need interventions within oncology clinics. Indeed, addressing the psychosocial needs of patients with cancer has become routine in clinical practice in recent years. However, addressing religious/spiritual concerns is not commonplace despite recommendations. Barriers to why this may be the case should be highlighted and overcome and training is needed to allow health care professionals to have confidence in their ability to assess and address cancer patients' spiritual needs within clinical practice. There is also a need to develop and test spiritual needs' interventions tailored to suit the environment in which they will be implemented. Few such interventions currently exist (but see Kristeller et al. [132]).

The relationship between religious coping and adjustment in cancer is complex [172]. Much more work is needed examining specific religious coping strategies and how these are linked to various outcomes by examining mediating/moderating relationships using longitudinal designs or by using other statistical techniques such as structural equation modelling or cluster analysis. Indeed, future studies should further examine the mechanism through which various religious coping strategies operate on outcome. Studies should investigate this by examining individual religious coping strategies rather than clusters of coping that has a priori assumptions of what is adaptive or maladaptive. Studies should also examine other psychosocial variables such as pessimism in relation to religious/spiritual variables and cancer adjustment. Optimists differ from pessimists in the manner in which they cope with situations; pessimists generally expect bad outcomes and believe that things will not go their way [36, 173]. It is therefore likely that pessimists would show a tendency to use maladaptive religious coping strategies more frequently than those with a more optimistic outlook on life. These coping strategies may, in turn, have an impact on illness adjustment. Studies should also further examine the relationships between religious coping and positive outcomes. This may provide a clearer understanding of the importance of various religious coping strategies and to which outcome they are related to.

Although there is some evidence that religious coping is more often tied to psychosocial functioning than physical functioning in patients with cancer [91], other studies have found that negative religious coping (using the Brief RCOPE), after controlling for demographic and medical variables, is associated with significantly higher levels of pain and fatigue [46]. Future studies may like to examine the link between religious coping and physical functioning further and in a more thorough manner. In addition, very little is known about differences in religious coping across cancer stages and cancer types. There are also few studies available informing us about differences in religious coping across ethnic groups and religious affiliations and how these variables impact on illness adjustment.

References

1. Stefanek M, McDonald PG, Hess SA. Religion, spirituality and cancer: current status and methodological challenges. Psychooncology. 2005;14:450–63.
2. Fetzer Institute. Multidimensional measurement of religiousness, spirituality for use in health research. A report of a National Working Group supported by the Fetzer Institute in collaboration with the National Institute on Ageing. Kalamazoo, MI: Fetzer Institute; 2003.
3. Spilka, B. Spirituality: problems and directions in operationalizing a fuzzy concept. Paper presented at the meeting of the American Psychological Association, Toronto, Ontario, 1993.
4. Sheldrake P. Spirituality and history: questions of interpretations and method. New York: Crossroads; 1992.
5. Wulff DM. Psychology of religion: classic and contemporary. 2nd ed. New York: Wiley; 1997.
6. Turner RP, Lukoff D, Barnhouse RT, Lu FG. Religious or spiritual problems: a cultural sensitive diagnostic category in the DSM-IV. J Nerv Ment Dis. 1995;183:435–44.
7. Hill PC, Pargament KI, Hood Jr RW, McCullough ME, Swyers JP, Larson DB, Zinnbauer BJ. Conceptualising religion and spirituality: points of commonality, points of departure. J Theory Soc Behav. 2000;30:51–77.
8. Zinnbauer BJ, Pargament KI, Cole BC, Rye MS, Butter EM, Belavitch TG, Hipp KM, Scott AB, Kadar JL. Religion and spirituality: unfuzzying the fuzzy. J Sci Study Relig. 1997;36:549–64.
9. Woods TE, Ironson GH. Religion and spirituality in the face of illness. How cancer, cardiac and HIV patients describe their spirituality/religiosity. J Health Psychol. 1999;4:393–412.
10. Scott AB. Categorising definitions of religion and spirituality in the psychological literature: a content analytical approach. Unpublished Manuscript. 1997.
11. Fallot R. The place of spirituality and religion in mental health services. In: Fallot R, editor. Spirituality and religion in recovery from mental illness. San Francisco: Jossey-Bass Publishers; 1998. p. 3–12.
12. Thuné-Boyle ICV, Stygall J, Newman SP. Definitions of religiousness and spirituality in a UK London population. Unpublished Manuscript. 2005

13. de Ridder DTD, Schreurs KMG. Coping en Sociale Steun van Chronisch Zieken [Coping and social support in patients with chronic diseases]. Report for the Dutch Commission for Chronic Diseases. Utrecht: Section of Clinical and heath Psychology; 1994.

14. Tix AP, Fraser PA. The use of religious coping during stressful life events: main effects, moderation, and mediation. J Consult Clin Psychol. 1998;66: 411–22.

15. Pargament KI, Park C. Merely a defence? The variety of religious means and ends. J Soc Issues. 1995;51:13–32.

16. Freud S. Obsessive actions and religious practices. In: Standard edition of the complete works of Sigmund Freud. Vol. 9. London: Hogarth; 1959, 1907/1961. p. 126–127

17. Ellis A. Psychotherapy and atheist values. J Consult Clin Psychol. 1980;48:635–9.

18. Pargament KI, Kennell J, Hathaway W, Grevengoed N, Newman J, Jones W. Religion and the problem-solving process: three styles of coping. J Sci Study Relig. 1988;27:90–104.

19. Pargament KI, Smith B, Koenig HG, Perez L. Patterns of positive and negative religious coping with major life stressors. J Sci Study Relig. 1998;37:710–24.

20. Pargament KI, Koenig HG, Perez LM. The many methods in religious coping: development and initial validation of the RCOPE. J Clin Psychol. 2000;56:519–43.

21. Geertz C. Religion as a cultural system. In: Banton M, editor. Anthropological approaches to the study of religion. London: Tavistock; 1966. p. 1–46.

22. Fromm E. Psychoanalysis and religion. New Haven: Yale University Press; 1950.

23. Freud S. The future of an illusion. New York: W. W. Norton; 1927/1961.

24. Durkheim E. The elementary forms of the religious life: a study in religious sociology. New York: Macmillan; 1915. Translated by Joseph Ward Swain.

25. Pargament KI. The psychology of religion and coping: theory, research, practice. New York: The Guildford Press; 1997.

26. Pargament KI. Religious/spiritual coping. In: The Fetzer Institute/National Institute on Ageing Working Group, editor. Multidimensional measurement of religiousness/spirituality for use in health research. Kalamazoo, MI: Fetzer Institute; 1999. p. 43–5.

27. Zinnbauer B, Pargament K. Spiritual conversion: a study of religious change among college students. J Sci Study Relig. 1998;37:161–80.

28. Hathaway WL, Pargament KI. Intrinsic religiousness, religious coping, and psychosocial competence: a covariance structure analysis. J Sci Study Relig. 1990;29:423–41.

29. McIntosh DN, Spilka B. Religion and physical health: the role of faith and control. In: Lynn ML, Moberg DC, editors. Research in the social scientific study of religion Greenwich. Greenwich, CT: JAI Press; 1990. p. 167–94.

30. Bahr HM, Harvey CD. Widowhood and perceptions of change in quality of life: evidence from the Sunshine Mine Widows. J Comp Fam Stud. 1979;10:411–28.

31. Alferi SM, Culver JL, Carver CS, Arena PL, Antoni MH. Religiosity, religious coping, and distress: A prospective study of Catholic and Evangelical Hispanic women in treatment for early-stage breast cancer. J Health Psychol 1999;4:343–56.

32. Allport GW, Ross JM. Personal religious orientation and prejudice. J Pers Soc Psychol. 1967;5:432–43.

33. Hays JC, Landerman LR, Blazer DG, Koenig HG, Carroll JW, Musick MA. Aging, health and the "electronic church". J Aging Health. 1998;10:458–82.

34. Idler E. Organisational religiousness. In: Fetzer Institute/NIA, editor. Multidimensional measurement of religiousness, spirituality for use in health research. A report of a National Working Group Supported by the Fetzer Institute in Collaboration with the National Institute on Ageing. Kalamazoo, MI: Fetzer Institute; 2003.

35. Levin JS. Private religious practices. In: Fetzer Institute/NIA, editor. Multidimensional measurement of religiousness, spirituality for use in health research. A report of a National Working Group Supported by the Fetzer Institute in Collaboration with the National Institute on Ageing. Kalamazoo, MI: Fetzer Institute; 2003.

36. Carver CS, Scheier MF, Weintraub JK. Assessing coping strategies: a theoretically-based approach. J Pers Soc Psychol. 1989;56:267–83.

37. Carver CS. You want to measure coping but your protocol is too long: consider the brief COPE. Int J Behav Med. 1997;4:92–100.

38. Folkman S, Lazarus RS. Manual for the ways of coping questionnaire. Palo Alto, CA: Consulting Psychologist Press; 1988.

39. Burker EJ, Evon DM, Loisielle MM, Finkel JB, Mill MR. Coping predict depression and disability in heart transplant candidates. J Psychosom Res. 2005;59:215–22.

40. VandeCreek L, Paget S, Horton R, Robbins L, Oettinger M, Tai K. Religious and non-religious coping methods among persons with rheumatoid arthritis. Arthritis Rheum. 2004;51:49–55.

41. Bjorck JP. Religiousness and coping: implications for clinical practice. J Psychol Christ. 1997;16: 62–7.

42. Boudreaux E, Catz S, Ryan L, Amaral-Melendez M, Brantley PJ. The ways of religious coping scale: reliability, validity and scale development. Assessment. 1995;2:233–44.

43. Pargament KI, Ensing DS, Falgout K, Olsen H, Reilly B, Van Haitsma K, Warren R. God help me: (1): Religious coping efforts as predictors of the outcomes to significant negative life events. Am J Community Psychol. 1990;18:793–824.

44. Zwingmann C, Wirtz M, Müller C, Körber J, Murken S. Positive and negative religious coping in German breast cancer patients. J Behav Med. 2006;29: 533–47.

45. Johnson SC, Spilka B. Coping with breast cancer: the roles of clergy and faith. J Relig Health. 1991;30:21–33.

46. Sherman AC, Simonton S, Latif U, Spohn R, Tricot G. Religious struggle and religious comfort in response to illness: health outcomes among stem cell transplant patients. J Behav Med. 2005;28:359–67.

47. Fitchett G, Murphy PE, Kim J, Gibbons JL, Cameron JR, Davis JA. Religious struggle: prevalence correlates and mental health risks in diabetic, congestive heart failure, and oncology patients. Int J Psychiatry Med. 2004;34:179–96.

48. Gallup International Millennium Survey. 2000. Available from: http://www.gallupinternational.com/survey15.htm. Accessed 14 Apr 2011.

49. Social Trends. Chapter 13: Lifestyles and Social Participation. 2000. Available from: http://www.statistics.gov.uk/downloads/theme_social/st30v8.pdf. Accessed 14 Apr 2011.

50. Gallup International. Voice of the people. 2005. Available from: http://www.voice-of-the-people.net/ContentFiles/files/VoP2005/Religiosity%20around%20the%20world%20VoP%2005%20press%20release.pdf. Accessed 14 Apr 2011.

51. Eurobarometer Poll. 2005. Available from: http://ec.europa.eu/public_opinion/archives/ebs/ebs_225_report_en.pdf. Accessed 16 Apr 2011.

52. Harcourt D, Rumsey N, Ambler N. Same-day diagnosis of symptomatic breast problems: psychological impact and coping strategies. Psychol Health Med. 1999;4:57–71.

53. Thuné-Boyle ICV, Stygall J, Keshtgar MRS, Davidson T, Newman SP. Religious coping strategies in patients diagnosed with breast cancer in the UK. Psychooncology. 2011;20:771–82.

54. Fitchett G, Rybarczyk BD, DeMarco GA, Nicholas JJ. The role of religion in medical rehabilitation outcomes: a longitudinal study. Rehabil Psychol. 1999;44:333–53.

55. Koenig HG, Pargament KI, Nielsen J. Religious coping and health status in medically ill hospitalized older adults. J Nerv Ment Dis. 1998;186:513–21.

56. Thuné-Boyle ICV, Stygall J, Keshtgar MRS, Davidson T, Newman SP. The impact of a breast cancer diagnosis on religious/spiritual beliefs and practices in the UK. J Relig Health. 2011;50:203–18.

57. Carver CS, Pozo C, Harris SD, Noriega V, Scheier MF, Robinson DS, Ketcham AS, Moffat Jr FL, Clark KC. How coping mediates the effect of optimism on distress: a study of women with early stage breast cancer. J Pers Soc Psychol. 1993;65:375–90.

58. Culver JL, Arena PL, Antoni MH, Carver CS. Coping and distress among women under treatment for early stage breast cancer: comparing African Americans. Hispanics and non-Hispanics whites. Psychooncology. 2002;11:495–504.

59. Alferi SM, Culver JL, Carver CS, Arena PL, Antoni MH. Religiosity, religious coping, and distress: a prospective study of Catholic and Evangelical Hispanic women in treatment for early-stage breast cancer. J Health Psychol. 1999;4:343–56.

60. Gall TL, Guirguis-Younger M, Charbonneau C, Florach P. The trajectory of religious coping across time in response to the diagnosis of breast cancer. Psychooncology. 2009;18:1165–78.

61. Nosarti C, Crayford T, Roberts JV, McKenzie K, David AS. Early psychological adjustment in breast cancer patients: a prospective study. J Psychosom Res. 2002;53:1123–30.

62. Helgeson VS, Cohen S. Social support and adjustment to cancer: reconciling descriptive, correlational and interventional research. Health Psychol. 1996;15:135–48.

63. Lazarus RS, Folkman S. Stress appraisal and coping. New York: Springer; 1984.

64. Burgess C, Cornelius V, Love S, Graham J, Richards M, Ramirez A. Depression and anxiety in women with early breast cancer: five year observational cohort study. BMJ. 2005;330:702–5.

65. Jacobsen PB, Andrykowski MA, Redd WH, Die-Trill M, Hakes TB, Kaufman RJ, Currie VE, Holland JC. Non-pharmacologic factors in the development of post-treatment nausea with adjuvant chemotherapy for breast cancer. Cancer. 1988;61:379–85.

66. Sinsheimer LM, Holland JC. Psychological issues in breast cancer. Semin Oncol. 1987;14:75–82.

67. Hart GJ, McQuellon RP, Barrett RJ. After treatment ends. Cancer Pract. 1984;2:417–20.

68. Ward SE, Viergutz G, Tormey D, de Muth J, Paulen A. Patient's reactions to completion of adjuvant breast cancer therapy. Nurs Res. 1992;41:362–6.

69. Holland JC, Rowland J, Lebovits A, Rusalem R. Reactions to cancer treatment: assessment of emotional response to adjuvant radiotherapy as a guide to planned intervention. Psychiatr Clin North Am. 1979;2:347–58.

70. Ferraro KF, Kelley-Moore J. Religious seeking among affiliates and non-affiliates: do mental and physical health problems spur religious coping? Rev Relig Res. 2001;42:229–51.

71. Bourjolly JN. Differences in religiousness among Black and White women with breast cancer. Soc Work Health Care. 1998;28:21–39.

72. Ellison CG, Taylor RJ. Turning to prayer: social and situational antecedents of religious coping among African Americans. Rev Relig Res. 1996;38:111–31.

73. Musick MA, Koenig HG, Hays JC, Cohen HJ. Religious activity and depression among community-dwelling elderly persons with cancer: the moderating effect of race. J Gerontol B Psychol Sci Soc Sci. 1998;53B:S218–27.

74. Tarakeshwar N, Vanderwerker LC, Paulk E, Pearce MJ, Kasl SV, Prigerson HG. Religious coping is associated with the quality of life of patients with advanced cancer. J Palliat Med. 2006;9:646–57.

75. Thuné-Boyle ICV, Stygall J, Keshtgar MRS, Newman SP. Do religious/spiritual coping strategies affect illness adjustment in patients with cancer?

A systematic review of the literature. Soc Sci Med. 2006;63:151–64.

76. Gall TL. Integrating religious resources within a general model of stress and coping: long-term adjustment to breast cancer. J Relig Health. 2000;39:167–82.

77. Nairn RC, Merluzzi TV. The role of religious coping in adjustment to cancer. Psychooncology. 2003;12:428–41.

78. Sherman AC, Simonton S, Plante TG, Reed Moody V, Wells P. Patterns of religious coping among multiple myeloma patients: associations with adjustment and quality of life (abstract). Psychosom Med. 2001;63:124.

79. Gall TL. The role of religious coping in adjustment to prostate cancer. Cancer Nurs. 2004;27:454–61.

80. Derks W, de Leeuw JRJ, Hordijk GJ, Winnubst JAM. Differences in coping style and locus of control between older and younger patients with head and neck cancer. Clin Otolaryngol. 2005;30:186–92.

81. Manning-Walsh J. Spiritual struggle: effect on quality of life and life satisfaction in women with breast cancer. J Holist Nurs. 2005;23:120–40.

82. Zwingmann C, Müller C, Körber J, Murken S. Religious commitment, religious coping and anxiety: a study in German patients with breast cancer. Eur J Cancer Care. 2008;17:361–70.

83. Herbert R, Zdaniuk B, Schulz R, Schemer M. Positive and negative religious coping and well-being in women with breast cancer. J Palliat Med. 2009;12:537–45.

84. Sherman AC, Plante TG, Simonton S, Latif U, Anaissie EJ. Prospective study of religious coping among patients undergoing autologous stem cell transplant. J Behav Med. 2009;32:118–28.

85. Taylor RJ, Chatters LM. Church members as a support of informal social support. Rev Relig Res. 1988;30:193–203.

86. Koenig HG, Hays JC, George LK, Blazer DG, Larson DB, Landerman LR. Modelling the cross-sectional relationships between religion, physical health, social support, and depressive symptoms. Am J Geriatr Psychiatry. 1997;5:131–44.

87. Ai AL, Peterson C, Tice TN, Bolling SF, Koenig HG. Faith-based and secular pathways to hope and optimism sub-constructs in middle-aged and older cardiac patients. J Health Psychol. 2004;9:435–50.

88. Ai AL, Park CL, Huang B, Rodgers W, Tice TN. Psychosocial mediation of religious coping styles: a study of short-term psychological distress following cardiac surgery. Pers Soc Psychol Bull. 2007;33: 867–82.

89. Hughes JW, Tomplinson A, Blumenthal JA, Davidson J, Sketch MH, Watkins LL. Social support and religiosity as coping strategies for anxiety in hospitalized cardiac patients. Ann Behav Med. 2004;28:179–85.

90. Bosworth HB, Park KS, McQuoid DR, Hays JC, Steffens DC. The impact of religious practice and religious coping on geriatric depression. Int J Geriatr Psychol. 2003;18:905–14.

91. Sherman AC, Simonton S. Religious involvement among cancer patients: associations with adjustment

and quality of life. In: Plante TG, Sherman AC, editors. Faith and health: psychological perspectives. New York: The Guildford Press; 2001. p. 167–94.

92. Johnson P. The use of humour and its influences on spirituality and coping in breast cancer survivors. Oncol Nurs Forum. 2002;29:691–5.

93. Canada AL, Parker PA, Basen-Engquist K, de Moor JS, Ramondetta LM. Active coping mediates the association between religion/spirituality and functional well-being in ovarian cancer. Gynecol Oncol. 2005;99:S125.

94. Prado G, Feaster DJ, Schwartz SJ, Pratt IA, Smith L, Szapocznik J. Religious involvement, coping, social support, and psychological distress in HIV-seropositive African American mothers. AIDS Behav. 2004;8:221–35.

95. Holland JC, Passik S, Kash KM, Russak SM, Gronert MK, Sison A, Lederberg M, Fox B, Baider L. The role of religious and spiritual beliefs in coping with malignant melanoma. Psychooncology. 1999;8:14–26.

96. Baider L, Russak SM, Perry S, Kash K, Gronert M, Fox B, Holland J, Kaplan-Denour A. The role of religious and spiritual beliefs in coping with malignant melanoma: an Israeli sample. Psychooncology. 1999;8:27–35.

97. Dunkel-Schetter C, Feinstein LG, Taylor SAE, Falke RL. Patterns of coping with cancer. Health Psychol. 1992;11:79–87.

98. Thuné-Boyle ICV, Stygall J, Keshtgar MRS, Davidson T, Newman SP. The effect of religious/spiritual coping resources on adjustment in patients newly diagnosed with breast cancer in the UK. 2012; Feb 14. doi: 10.1002/pon.3048. [Epub ahead of print].

99. Astrow AB, Mattson I, Ponet P, White M. Inter-religious perspectives on hope and limits in cancer treatment. J Clin Oncol. 2005;23:2569–73.

100. Fiala WE, Bjorck JP, Gorsuch R. The religious support scale: construction, validation, and cross validation. Am J Community Psychol. 2002;30:761–86.

101. Tomich PL, Helgeson VS. Is finding something good in the bad always good? Benefit finding among women with breast cancer. Health Psychol. 2004;23:16–23.

102. Cordova MJ, Andrykowski MA, Kenady DE, McGrath PC, Sloan DA, Redd WH. Frequency and correlates of post-traumatic stress disorder like symptoms after treatment for breast cancer. J Consult Clin Psychol. 1995;63:981–6.

103. Derogatis LR, Morrow GR, Fetting J, Penman D, Piasetsky S, Schmale A, Henrichs M, Carnicke Jr CL. The prevalence of psychiatric disorders among cancer patients. J Am Med Assoc. 1983;249:751–7.

104. Brennan J. Adjustment to cancer—coping or personal transition? Psychooncology. 2001;10:1–18.

105. Androkowski MA, Brady MJ, Hunt JW. Positive psychosocial adjustment in potential bone marrow transplant recipients: cancer as a psychosocial transition. Psychooncology. 1993;2:261–76.

106. Stanton AL, Bower JE, Low CA. Post traumatic growth after cancer. In: Calhoun LG, Tedeschi RG,

editors. Handbook of posttraumatic growth: research and practice. London: Lawrence Erlbaum Associates; 2007. p. 138–75.

107. Folkman S. Positive psychological states and coping with severe stress. Soc Sci Med. 1997;45:1207–21.

108. Tedeschi RG, Calhoun LG. Posttraumatic growth: conceptual foundations and empirical evidence. Psychol Inq. 2004;15:1–18.

109. Antoni MH, Lehman JM, Kilbourn KM, Boyers AE, Culver JL, Alferi SM, Yount SE, McGregor BA, Arena PL, Harris SD, Price AA, Carver CS. Cognitive-behavioural stress management intervention decreases the prevalence of depression and enhances benefit finding among women under treatment for early-stage breast cancer. Health Psychol. 2001;20:20–32.

110. Park CL, Cohen LH, Murch R. Assessment and prediction of stress related growth. J Pers. 1996;64:71–105.

111. Tedeschi RG, Calhoun LG. The posttraumatic growth inventory: measuring the positive legacy of trauma. J Trauma Stress. 1996;9:455–71.

112. Emmons RA, McCullough ME, Tsang J. The assessment of gratitude. In: Lopez SJ, Snyder CR, editors. Handbook of positive psychology assessment. Washington, DC: American Psychological Association; 2003. p. 327–41.

113. Emmons RA, McCullough ME. Counting blessings versus burdens: an experimental investigation of gratitude and subjective well-being in daily life. J Pers Soc Psychol. 2003;84:377–89.

114. Bertocci PA, Millard RM. Personality and the good: psychological and ethical perspectives. New York: David McKay; 1963.

115. McCullough ME, Emmons RA, Tsang J. The grateful disposition: a conceptual and empirical topography. J Pers Soc Psychol. 2002;82:112–27.

116. Collins RL, Taylor SE, Skokan LA. A better world or a shattered vision? Changes in life perspectives following victimization. Soc Cogn. 1990;8:263–85.

117. Carver CS, Antoni MH. Finding benefit in breast cancer during the year after diagnosis predicts better adjustment 5 to 8 years after diagnosis. Health Psychol. 2004;26:595–8.

118. Yanez B, Edmondson D, Stanton AL, Park CL, Kwan L, Ganz PA, Blank TO. Facets of spirituality as predictors of adjustment to cancer: relative contributions of having faith and finding meaning. J Consult Clin Psychol. 2009;77:730–41.

119. Lechner SC, Carver CS, Antoni MH, Weaver KE, Phillips KM. Curvilinear associations between benefit finding and psychosocial adjustment to breast cancer. J Consult Clin Psychol. 2006;74:828–40.

120. Urcuyo KR, Boyers AE, Carver CS, Antoni MH. Finding benefit in breast cancer: relations with personality, coping, and concurrent well-being. Psychol Health. 2005;20:175–92.

121. Thornton AA, Perez MA, Meyerowitz BE. Posttraumatic growth in prostate cancer patients and their partners. Psycooncology. 2005;15:285–95.

122. Thuné-Boyle ICV, Stygall J, Keshtgar MRS, Davidson T, Newman SP. The influence of religious/

spiritual resources on finding positive benefits from a breast cancer diagnosis. Couns Spiritual. 2011;30:107–34.

123. Post SG, Puchalski CM, Larson DB. Physicians and patients spirituality: professional boundaries, competency, and ethics. Ann Int Med. 2000;132:578–83.

124. Sloan RP, Bagiella E, Vandercreek L, Hover M, Casalone C, Jinpu Hirsch T, Hasan Y, Kreger R, Poulos P. Should physicians prescribe religious activities? N Engl J Med. 2000;432:1913–6.

125. Sloan RP, Bagiella V, Powell T. Religion, spirituality and medicine. Lancet. 1999;353:664–7.

126. Gall TL, Cornblat MW. Breast cancer survivors give voice: a qualitative analysis of spiritual factors in long-term adjustment. Psychooncology. 2002;11:524–35.

127. National Comprehensive Cancer Network (NCCN). Clinical practice guidelines in oncology: distress management. 2008. Available from: http://www.nccn.org/. Accessed 2 May 2011.

128. Koenig HG. Religion, spirituality and medicine: how are they related and what does it mean? Mayo Clin Proc. 2001;76:1189–91.

129. Woodward K. Talking to God. Newsweek. 1992;119:40.

130. Koenig HG. Meeting the spiritual needs of patient. The satisfaction monitor. July/Aug 2003. Available from: http://www.pressganey.com/research/resources/satmon/text/bin/178.shtm. Accessed 24 Apr 2011.

131. Plotnikoff GA. Should medicine reach out to the spirit? Understanding a patient's spiritual foundation can guide appropriate care. Postgrad Med. 2000;108:19–22.

132. Kristeller JL, Rhodes M, Cripe LD, Sheets V. Oncologist assisted spiritual intervention study (OASIS): patient acceptability and initial evidence of effects. Int J Psychiatry Med. 2006;35:329–47.

133. Mueller PS, Plevak DJ, Rummans TA. Religious involvement, spirituality, and medicine: implications for clinical practice. Mayo Clin Proc. 2001;76:1225–35.

134. Balboni TA, Vanderwerker LC, Block SD, Paulk ME, Lathan CS, Peteet JR, Prigerson HG. Religiousness and spiritual support among advanced cancer patients and associations with end-of-life treatment preferences and quality of life. J Clin Oncol. 2007;25:555–60.

135. Ehman JW, Ott BB, Short TH, Ciampa RC, Hansen-Flaschen J. Do patients want physicians to inquire about their spiritual or religious beliefs if they become gravely ill? Arch Intern Med. 1999;159:1803–6.

136. King DE, Bushwick B. Beliefs and attitudes of hospital inpatients about faith healing and prayer. J Fam Pract. 1994;39:349–52.

137. Ellis MR, Vinson DC, Ewigman B. Addressing spiritual concerns of patients. Family physicians' attitudes and practices. J Fam Pract. 1999;48:105–9.

138. Moadel A, Morgan C, Fatone A, Grennan J, Carter J, Laruffa G, Skummy A, Dutcher J. Seeking meaning and hope: self-reported spiritual and existential

needs among an ethnically-diverse cancer patient population. Psychooncology. 1999;8:378–85.

139. Koenig HG, Boulware LE, Cooper LA, Ratner LE, LaVeist TA, Powe NR. Race and trust in the health care system. Public Health Rep. 2003;118: 358–65.

140. Frick E, Riedner C, Fegg MJ, Hauf S, Borasio GD. A clinical interview assessing cancer patients spiritual needs and preferences. Eur J Cancer Care. 2006;15:238–43.

141. The National Cancer Institute. Available from: http://www.cancer.gov/cancertopics/pdq/supportivecare/spirituality/Patient/page3. Accessed 28 Apr 2011.

142. Kuhn CC. A spiritual inventory for the medically ill patient. Psychiatr Med. 1988;6:87–100.

143. Matthews DA, Clark C. The faith factor. New York: Viking; 1998.

144. Puchalski CM, Romer AL. Taking a spiritual history allows clinicians to understand patients more fully. J Palliat Med. 2000;3:129–37.

145. Maugans TA. The SPIRITual history. Arch Fam Med. 1996;5:11–6.

146. Koenig HG. Spirituality in patients care: why, how, when and what. Philadelphia & London: Templeton Foundation Press; 2002.

147. Anandarajah G, Hight E. Spirituality and medical practice: using the HOPE questions as a practical tool for spiritual assessment. Am Fam Physician. 2001;63:81–8.

148. Lo B, Quill T, Tulsky J. Discussing palliative care with patients. Ann Intern Med. 1999;130:744–9.

149. Davie G, Woodhead L, Heelas P. Predicting religion: Christian, secular and alternative futures. Aldershot, UK: Ashgate; 2003.

150. Büssing A, Koenig HG. Spiritual needs of patients with chronic diseases. Religions. 2010;1:18–27.

151. National Institute of Health and Clinical Excellence (NICE), Supportive and palliative care. Improving supportive and palliative care for adults with cancer. 2004. Available from: http://www.nice.org.uk/guidance/index.jsp?action=byID&o=10893. Accessed 17 Mar 2011.

152. NHS Chaplaincy. Meeting the religious and spiritual needs of patients and staff. 2003 Guidance for managers and those involved in the provision of chaplaincy spiritual care. Available from: http://www.dh.gov.uk/dr_consum_dh/groups/dh_digitalassets/@dh/@en/documents/digitalasset/dh_4062028.pdf. Accessed 12 Apr 2011.

153. Clinical Standards of Working in a Breast Speciality. RCN guidance for nursing staff. 2007. Available from: http://www.rcn.org.uk/data/assets/pdf_file/0008/78731/003110.pdf. Accessed 17 Apr 2011.

154. Chibnall JT, Brooks CA. Religion in the clinic: the role of physician beliefs. South Med J. 2001;94: 374–9.

155. Kristeller JL, Sheedy Zumbrun C, Schilling RF. I would if I could: how oncologists and oncology nurses address spiritual distress in cancer patients. Psychooncology. 1999;8:451–8.

156. Ragan C, Maloney HM, Beit-Halahmi B. Psychologist and religion: professional factors associated with personal beliefs. Rev Relig Res. 1980;21:208–17.

157. Koenig HG, Bearon LB, Hover M, Travis III JL. Religious perspectives of doctors, patients and families. J Pastoral Care. 1991;XLV:254–67.

158. Bergin AE. Values and religious issues in psychotherapy and mental health. Am Psychol. 1991;46:394–403.

159. Sheridan MJ, Bullis RK, Adcock CR, Berlin SD, Miller PC. Practitioner's personal and professional attitudes and behaviours towards religion and spirituality: issues for education and practice. J Soc Work Educ. 1992;28:190–203.

160. Shafranske EP, Malony HN. Clinical psychologists' religious and spiritual orientation and their practice of psychotherapy. Psychotherapy. 1990;27:72–8.

161. Maugans TA, Wadland WC. Religion and family medicine: a survey of physicians and patients. J Fam Pract. 1991;32:210–3.

162. Oyama O, Koenig HG. Religious beliefs and practices in family medicine. Arch Fam Med. 1998;7:431–5.

163. Frank E, Dell ML, Chopp R. Religious characteristics of US women physicians. Soc Sci Med. 1999;49:1717–22.

164. Neeleman J, King M. Psychiatrists' religious attitudes in relation to their clinical practice: a survey of 231 psychiatrists. Acta Psychiatr Scand. 1992;88:420–4.

165. King M, Speck P, Thomas A. The royal free interview for religious and spiritual beliefs: development and standardisation. Psychol Med. 1995;25:1125–34.

166. Silvestri GA, Knittig S, Zoller JS, Nietert PJ. Importance of faith on medical decisions regarding cancer care. J Clin Oncol. 2003;21:1379–82.

167. Ellis MR, Campbell JD, Detwiler-Breidenbach A. What do family physicians think about spirituality in clinical practice? J Fam Pract. 2002;51:249–54.

168. El-Nimr G, Green LL, Salib E. Spiritual care in psychiatry: professional's views. Ment Health Relig Cult. 2004;7:165–70.

169. McCauley J, Jenckes MW, Tarpley MJ, Koenig HG, Yanek LR, Becker DM. Spiritual beliefs and barriers among managed care practitioners. J Relig Health. 2005;44:137–46.

170. Klitzman RL, Daya AS. Challenges and changes in spirituality among doctors who become patients. Soc Sci Med. 2005;61:2396–406.

171. Speck P, Higginson I, Addington-Hall J. Spiritual needs in health care. BMJ. 2004;329:123–4.

172. Kristeller JL, Sheets V, Johnson T, Frank B. Understanding religious and spiritual influences on adjustment to cancer: Individual patterns and differences. J Behav Med. 2011;34:550–61.

173. Scheier MF, Weintraub JK, Carver CS. Coping with stress: divergent strategies of optimists and pessimists. J Pers Soc Psychol. 1986;51:1257–64.

Controversies in Psycho-Oncology

10

Michael Stefanek

No great advance has ever been made in science, politics, or religion, without controversy

—Lyman Beecher

No doubt science cannot admit of compromises, and can only bring out the complete truth. Hence there must be controversy, and the strife may be, and sometime must be, sharp. But must it even then be personal? Does it help science to attack the man as well as the statement? On the contrary, has not science the noble privilege of carrying on its controversies without personal quarrels?

—Rudolf Virchow

Science is saturated with controversy. Some of this "controversy" is more junk political controversy than science, such as the "debates" over climate change. Some controversy is politically or religiously driven such as the battles over evolution versus creationism or whether homosexuality is defined at birth or caused by environmental factors. If we consider issues less tainted by politics or religion, in a perfect scientific world, our knowledge would be smoothly cumulative, with each reported finding building upon prior findings until we have a pure body of knowledge ready for application in the real world. Unfortunately, this is not the case. We have varying research designs, some more rigorous than others, meta-analyses that result in attempting to summarize a series of studies that differ significantly in any number of ways (subject sample, design, measures), reviewers of articles that differ in their opinions of the value of any given submission of research

findings, and yes, even scientists who fudge data or, more benignly, are driven by their own unrecognized biases to find what they are looking for.

Behavioral science and psycho-oncology in particular is no less susceptible to controversy than any other scientific field. Certainly such controversy need not be accompanied by personal attacks or acute sensitivity to criticisms of our own scientific work. Indeed, it is our role as scientists to most aggressively attack our own theories and welcome work that challenges the assumptions behind and the results of our own findings. By supporting such challenges, we can increase the chances that our current controversies will be viewed as more settled matters of scientific fact in the future.

In this chapter, I do not assume that any of the work reported involves incompetence or an attempt to mislead the field of psycho-oncology. I hope that the criticism or questioning included in this chapter is viewed as important to the credibility and integrity of the field of behavioral science and psycho-oncology. As perhaps a scientist or clinician engaged in psycho-oncology reading this chapter, I hope you agree that we owe it to ourselves and all those involved in cancer care, including patients and family members themselves, to take the role of healthy skeptic and

M. Stefanek, Ph.D. (✉)
Office of the Vice President for Research, Carmichael Center, Indiana University, 530 E Kirkwood Avenue, Suite 202, Bloomington, IN 47408, USA

University Place Conference Center, Suite 243, Indianapolis, IN 46202-5198, USA
e-mail: mstefanek@bellsouth.net

B.I. Carr and J. Steel (eds.), *Psychological Aspects of Cancer*, DOI 10.1007/978-1-4614-4866-2_10, © Springer Science+Business Media, LLC 2013 closely examine the scientific foundations of our clinical practices and policies.

My selections in this chapter include critiques of work involving (1) psychosocial screening of cancer patients; (2) the benefit of psychosocial interventions to decrease emotional distress among cancer patients; (3) the role of positive psychology in cancer care; and (4) the role of support groups in increasing survival among cancer patients. Some of these topics are covered tangentially or directly in other chapters of this text. I encourage you to review this chapter in the context of these related contributions to arrive at your own tentative conclusions about the state of the science in these areas.

Finally, my intent in writing this chapter, given the scope of coverage across these four designated controversial areas, is not to provide an exhaustive review of each area. Rather, I attempt to summarize findings, discuss concerns that give rise to my view that this is a controversial area, provide my opinion on the state of the science, and provide solid references for readers who wish to pursue these areas in greater depth.

Screening for Emotional Distress in Cancer Patients

The argument to screen cancer patients for emotional distress seems like a straightforward one. Who could argue against the need to identify such distress among patients facing a potentially life-threatening illness? After all, depression, anxiety, and distress are common following the diagnosis of cancer [1], with overall prevalence in unselected cancer patients greater than 30 % [2, 3]. Clearly, psychosocial needs require attention due to their direct and indirect effects on health and quality of life. In addition, there is evidence that such distress is not easily recognized among oncologists [4], nurses [5], or general practitioners [6], and that errors may involve both false positives and false negatives. One meta-analysis of studies assessing clinical accuracy among general practitioners (GP) found that they had considerable difficulty accurately identifying distress and mild depression. Out of 100 consec-

utive presentations, a typical GP making a single assessment would correctly identify 19 out of 39 people with distress, missing 20, with 13 false positives [6]. Thus, it seems to make intuitive sense that in order to provide optimal care to cancer patients, using some type of screening questionnaire and initiating formal screening programs to identify cancer patients experiencing high levels of emotional distress is warranted.

Perhaps it is appropriate at this point to review briefly what we mean by screening, and the major tenets involved in "successful" screening. The most well-known are those by Wilson and Junger [7] below.

- The condition screened for should be an important health problem;
- There should be an accepted treatment for patients with the disease;
- Facilities for treatment and diagnosis should be available;
- There should be a recognizable latent or early symptomatic stage;
- There should be a suitable test or examination;
- The test should be acceptable to the population;
- The natural history of the condition should be adequately understood;
- There should be an agreed upon policy about whom to treat as patients;
- The cost should be economically balanced in relation to possible expenditure on medical care as a whole;
- Case finding should be a continuing process and not a once and for all project.

While these tenets have been set out to focus upon medical screening, they apply to screening for general emotional distress, depression, or even overall quality of life as well. For instance, issues such as which questionnaires provide solid sensitivity and specificity is key, as are other issues such as the length of questionnaires (burden to patient), whether in any given site appropriate treatment is available and cost-effective, whether such treatment is acceptable to providers, patients, etc. Thus, it is not simply the case of determining that clinical encounters by health care providers do or do not address issues of emotional distress, but also of providing evidence that formal screening of patients is superior in identifying distress relative to not screening, *and that such screening leads to superior treatment— the successful conversion of screening tests into screening programs with established benefit to patients.*

To frame the issue clearly, we know that health care providers, including oncologists, often underdiagnose and undertreat emotional distress, including depression [8]. We also know that few health care providers systematically utilize any screening instruments, even ultra-short measures, to assess emotional distress [9]. The idea of using brief, easy-to-use case finding instruments to detect such distress has wide appeal in psycho-oncology. For instance, several organizations, including the National Comprehensive Cancer Network and the Canadian Strategy for Cancer Control, have established guidelines supporting the practice of brief screening of cancer patients to attempt to detect emotional distress, endorsed by some as the "6th vital sign" for patients with cancer [10, 11]. However, despite the understandable drive to decrease emotional distress, anxiety, and depression among cancer patients, the idea of using screening as an effective way to do so has not been systematically examined. Indeed, the guidelines noted above have been based upon expert opinion rather than a systematic review of the evidence.

There are a host of studies that have assessed the accuracy of short, easily administered screening tools to identify patients with cancer who have high levels of distress. In one of the earlier analyses of "ultra-short" (less than 15 items) methods of detecting cancer-related mood disorders, Mitchell [12] identified 38 such reports involving a total of 6,414 unique patients, including 19 studies that assessed the Distress Thermometer [13], a single item measure asking patients to self-report their level of emotional distress on a 0–10 scale to the question "How distressed have you been over the last week on a scale of 0–10?" This is the main distress stress scale recommended by the National Comprehensive Cancer Network [14]. This review estimated that 12 of 20 probable cases

detected by ultra-short methods actually would have significant distress defined by an acceptable standard. Most troubling perhaps was that in the case of depression, when a patient screened positive on an ultra-short method, only 7 in every 20 "positives" were actually depressed. However, such instruments fared much better in "ruling out" depression. Of 20 patients screening negative, 19 could be correctly ruled out, with only one case of depression missed. Based upon the above, it appears that ultra-short methods are best at ruling *out* depression, anxiety, and distress, but poorer if used to confidently rule *in* depression, anxiety, and distress. Overall, findings indicated that ultra-short methods were modestly effective in screening for mood disorders, and questioned their value as a stand-alone measure to diagnose depression, anxiety, or distress in cancer patients.

There have been a number of other reports that have reviewed the use of screening instruments for emotional distress among cancer patients [15–17] since the report noted above by Mitchell [12]. These reviews focus specifically upon the ability of selected instruments to identify cancer-related distress or upon the psychometric properties of existing tools currently used for screening purposes, with the idea of encouraging screening programs to use those with strong psychometric properties. There are a number of instruments that meet such standards, although issues such as acceptability and cost-effectiveness are not addressed, and many of the cancer-specific scales require further validation with clinical interviews before they can be recommended [15, 16].

A key addition to the evidence base for screening and its impact on psychological well being is a thorough review by Bidstrup et al. [17]. This review described and discussed the findings of randomized clinical trials of screening on *psychological outcomes.* A meta-analysis was not possible, due to the heterogeneity of the designs across studies, and differences in the intervention content, site of cancer among patients in the studies reviewed, and the outcome measures applied. Only seven randomized trials were found. In this case, a randomized trial involved assignment to an intervention group that received a questionnaire to assess distress with results provided to staff or assignment to a control group that either received normal care or whose questionnaire data was not made available to staff. A distress management plan was included in four of the seven studies (e.g., contact by a social worker), while three studies provided no plan on how the staff should act on the basis of the screening results. Three of these studies showed an effect, three showed no effect and one showed an effect only for patients reporting depression at baseline. This review was the first such overview to address the issue not just of the psychometric properties of the screening instruments, acceptability, and feasibility, but also whether such screening really made a difference in the psychological outcomes of patients screened versus not screened. As noted, while many methodological differences make comparisons across studies challenging at best, the results did not provide evidence of a clear benefit for screening of cancer patients.

In addition to the valuable contribution of Bidstrup et al. [17], a recent review [18] evaluating the potential benefits of depression screening for cancer patients assessed: (1) the accuracy of depression screening tools; (2) the effectiveness of depression treatment; and (3) the effect of depression screening on depression outcomes. This review included studies that (1) compared a depression screening instrument to a valid major depression disorder criterion standard; (2) compared depression treatment with placebo or usual care in a randomized controlled trial; or (3) assessed the effect of screening interventions on depression outcomes in a randomized controlled trial. While there were 19 eligible studies on screening accuracy, there was only one depression treatment randomized control trial, and one randomized controlled trial on the effects of screening on depression outcomes. Examining the 19 trials on screening accuracy, many had small sample sizes, while the treatment trial reduced depressive symptoms moderately (effect size=0.37). Only one study assessed effects of depression screening on actual depression outcomes and found no significant improvements.

As with screening for general emotional distress, screening for depression is only useful to the degree that it leads to improved outcomes above and beyond usual care or other existing programs not including formal screening. The results reported above support the position that psychosocial screening of cancer patients does not provide benefit to patients in terms of improved psychosocial outcomes and speak to the lack of data rigorously examining this important question related to cancer patient care.

Conclusion

An Institute of Medicine report [19] and clinical guidelines from the National Comprehensive Cancer Network [10] have advocated the use of screening for emotional distress, including depression, for standard cancer care. However, none of these recommendation statements provide a systematic review of the benefits of such screening, but rather are based upon expert opinion, concern for patients suffering from emotional distress, and an emphasis on work relegated to psychometric properties of screening instruments, feasibility, and acceptability. However, despite call for the benefit of such standard screening [20], there are clearly questions as to whether such screening of patients adds value to standard care in terms of positively impacting the emotional distress cancer patients face with their cancer diagnosis and treatment. It appears that screening, while offering a seemingly simple solution for early successful treatment of emotional distress, has yet to demonstrate a clear benefit over standard approaches such as simply offering patients the chance to discuss their concerns, regardless of formal screening programs. A screening *program* is the widespread distribution of a screening test, and includes a support system post-screening across a health care system. This effort in developing and maintaining a screening program should not be underestimated and the evidence supporting such a program should be daunting. Given the brief review of the findings to date noted above, the data hardly provide a strong evidence base at this time to warrant such large scale intervention. Much work has been done examining psychometric properties of various instruments, including many "ultra-short" questionnaires. Such brief measures likely increase the chances that clinicians will find screening acceptable, and decrease the cost (time to complete, review, score) to both patients and health care providers—all necessary steps in the process to assess the cost-benefits of screening.

Where to go now? In line with the recommendations of Bidstrup et al. [17], future randomized trials need to compare the validity of different screening approaches, minimize the cost of false positives and false negatives, and most critically, evaluate the benefits of screening *linked* to standard treatments. Standardized outcome measures need to be utilized and theory-driven management/treatment plans need to be tested. Studies to date have failed to provide sufficient details on the treatment plans implemented, acceptability of the treatment plan developed, and staff training issues. At this time, without evidence from future trials, it is premature to suggest the utilization of programs to systematically screen for emotional distress among cancer patients. However, arguing for the continuation of the status quo within which patient distress can be too often ignored or addressed in an unsystematic, hit-or-miss fashion, is also unacceptable. The controversy should not involve whether to provide psychological services and support to cancer patients struggling with a disease and often treatment with significant impact on quality and quantity of life. Rather, the controversy is whether cancer patients are best served by routine screening for psychological distress or if resources may be better applied to strengthening support services for cancer patients seeking such services within and outside of the oncology setting proper.

Psychological Interventions for Emotional Distress Among Cancer Patients

Surveys going back decades present data indicating that emotional distress is common following the diagnosis of cancer and extending throughout treatment [2, 21]. The distress, anxiety, and depression accompanying the diagnosis impacts quality of life, and even satisfaction with and

adherence to treatment regimens [22, 23]. This has led not surprisingly to a call for psychosocial interventions for cancer patients, with the a priori assumption, quite reasonable, that such interventions should certainly prove no less beneficial than such interventions for individuals without cancer. However, it does behoove us to demonstrate that what we provide to patients is acceptable and of benefit to them. Without such a demonstration, the credibility of our interventions and our ability to procure resources for interventions will necessarily (and understandably) be compromised.

With the field of psychosocial oncology no longer in its infancy, it should come as no surprise that a host of psychological intervention studies have been published, and even several narrative reviews and meta-analyses completed [24, 25]. Perhaps what is surprising is that this area of psycho-oncology has made it to the list of controversial topics. Why is that the case?

One critical issue surrounding the evaluation of the scientific literature related to psychological interventions is a definitional one. That is, what do we mean by "psychological intervention" as this term relates to cancer care? In a "meta-review," Hodges et al. [26] determined how the term "psychological intervention" had been defined and used to group and compare such interventions in the context of cancer care. The authors report that they were unable to find any explicit definition of the term in over 60 narrative reviews and meta-analyses. Obviously, such a glaring problem presents a challenge in attempting to cleanly summarize research findings and utilize such findings to inform clinical practice. For the purposes of this chapter, the definition will follow the one most closely adhered to during the Society of Behavioral Medicines (Annual Meeting, 2005) "Great Debate" on this topic [27]. For this purpose, psychological intervention was defined as an interpersonal process (i.e., a relationship between a trained professional and the client or clients, if the relationship involves a group process) intended to bring about changes in behavior, feelings, cognitions, or attitudes. It includes what would be generally considered "psychological" interventions, such as cognitive-behavior therapy, psychosocial support groups, individual or group counseling, utilizing a measure or measures of emotional distress as an outcome (e.g., global distress, depression, anxiety) in adult cancer populations. To be clear, this excludes pharmacological interventions and nonpsychological interventions (e.g., medically based nurse home visits, peer support without a professional facilitator, massage, music therapy, nutritional or physical activity interventions, prayer, etc.). It also excludes interventions that focus on outcomes such as pain, increased survival, fatigue, sexual problems secondary to disease or treatment, etc.

Early meta-analyses of the effect of psychosocial interventions on measures of emotional distress or quality of life were promising [24, 25]. In the first such meta-analysis reported [24], 45 published randomized trials reporting 62 treatment–control comparisons were identified. Measures included not only emotional adjustment but also functional adjustment (e.g., socializing, return to work), treatment-and-disease-related symptoms (nausea, vomiting, pain, etc.) and medical outcomes (e.g., physician ratings of disease progression). Given our definition noted above, focusing on emotional adjustment, Meyer and Mark [24] found a small but significant benefit of psychosocial interventions (effect size $d=0.24$, 95 % CI$=0.17$–0.32). Limitations of the meta-analysis include small sample sizes that prevented examining interaction effects in many of the studies (e.g., assessing benefit by type of intervention) and over-representation of white women across studies. In addition, many types of "psychosocial" interventions were included in the meta-analysis, including music therapy, informational and educational treatments, and social support interventions by nonprofessionals. Finally, little discussion was provided by the authors of the quality of the studies reviewed, and how such quality impacted inclusion or weighing of the meta-analytic results. Of interest is the authors' conclusion that interventions benefit patients and that more studies assessing the effect of psychosocial interventions on cancer patients would be an inefficient use of resources. This is a conclusion that certainly appeared premature then, and arguably one that continues to be premature.

The second early meta-analysis assessing psychosocial interventions on quality of life [25] reported on 37 published, controlled (i.e., presence of a control group, not necessarily randomized) studies among adult cancer patients. The quality of life measures included those assessing emotional adjustment or functional adjustment and could be either global or disease specific. The measures could also include either self-report ratings or ratings by another observer (most frequently, the health care provider). Overall, the findings were generally synchronous with those of Meyer and Mark [24], supporting the hypothesis that psychosocial interventions had a positive impact on cancer patients, consistent with a small to moderate effect size. While this analysis did include patient education programs, most studies (84 %) focused upon interventions consistent with the definition we have adopted. However, again, little data was provided about the methodological quality of the studies included in the meta-analysis, and how such quality was utilized for the conclusions presented. In addition, there was little data presented on demographic variables that might be significant, although the authors did note that breast cancer patients were over-represented in the studies assessed. The authors did find that interventions of longer duration (>11 weeks) were more likely to be of benefit in decreasing emotional distress. Finally, and perhaps most critically, the selected studies varied significantly in experimental design, treatment conditions, and outcome measures.

As a result of some of the weaknesses of these early meta-analyses raised above, the Society of Behavioral Medicine convened a "Great Debate" at its annual conference in 2005 [27]. The proposition considered in the debate was that "psychological interventions for distress in cancer patients are ineffective and unaccepted by patients". This debate prompted a series of stimulating papers that served to promote differing viewpoints on the state of the science, but with some ultimate concurrence on the research needed to drive progress in this area [28–33].

The "con" position in this debate [29, 30, 32], based on the phrasing above, is that psychological interventions are indeed effective. The basic position of the "con" side noted that a plethora of studies had addressed this topic, and given the large number of such studies, single studies should not lead us to conclude that psychological interventions, in general, are not beneficial to cancer patients. Data to support the "con" position were drawn from two meta-analyses not reviewed above [34, 35], noting an overall small to medium and clinically significant effect of psychosocial interventions on emotional distress. As the debate raged, other key points of the "con" side emerged [29, 30, 32], focusing upon results from both qualitative reviews [36, 37] and the quantitative meta-analyses above [34, 35] and selected randomized controlled trials. The summary of the data reviewed indicated that while the qualitative reviews were quite tentative in supporting the benefit of psychosocial interventions, results were more definitively positive based upon the quantitative reviews. The latter found effect sizes in the small to medium range, with more benefit for outcomes specific to emotional distress and anxiety than for depression. An important point made from these meta-analyses was that more of an effect was found under conditions when (1) the studies were methodologically superior and (2) interventions were delivered to those most in need, i.e., patients reporting high levels of distress preintervention. In addition to utilizing the reviews to support the position that interventions were of benefit, a review of the highest quality randomized clinical trials published within 5 years of the debate was completed [38–42]. These trials were selected using the Consolidated Standards of Reporting Trials (CONSORT) criteria [43] in combination with evaluative criteria established for empirically based therapies by Chambless and Hollon [44]. The "con" position held that these five studies provided sufficient detail to judge the degree to which they adhered to the criteria for a rigorous empirically supported treatment. Their summary point was that four of these five interventions, focusing on cognitive-behavioral approaches, showed statistically significant beneficial effects on psychological distress outcomes when compared to a no-treatment comparison group. One study showed a beneficial effect for patients displaying higher levels of distress preintervention [38]. Two of the studies [40, 41] evidence small

effect sizes, while the Nezu et al. trial [38] reported a large effect size. Two of the studies [39, 42] did not publish effect sizes. Overall, these findings from what was considered the most rigorous investigations of psychosocial interventions led the "con" position to support the stance that cognitive-behavioral interventions for cancer patients are indeed efficacious. Moreover, data from Nezu et al. [38] are consistent with the position that such interventions are beneficial for those cancer patients presenting with high levels of baseline distress.

The "pro" position in this debate held the position that psychological interventions are not effective [28, 31, 33]. The main tenet of this position held that while dozens of studies have been conducted examining the efficacy of psychosocial interventions, and several reviews of this literature, the result of both present conflicting and inconsistent conclusions. Much of this confusion is a result of the poor quality of the studies examining intervention impact, which leaves the field in a rather murky, inconclusive scientific state. The strategy for the "pro" position was to assess a 10-year period of reviews of the psychosocial intervention literature, and focus on reviews that minimize bias by using a systematic and comprehensive search strategy while controlling for the effects of lesser quality studies on results. This was done utilizing guidelines offered by the QUORUM statement checklist [43] and the Cochrane group [45]. This process resulted in one review [46] which was clearly superior based upon the aforementioned guidelines. This review identified 129 potentially relevant trials, with only 34 trials deemed of sufficient methodological quality to fully review for efficacy, based on the Cochrane Collaboration guidelines. Across these trials, there were few statistically significant differences favoring interventions on measures of distress (anxiety, depression, global distress), with only about 25 % of tests across the various outcome measure of emotional distress reaching statistical significance. Thus, based on this high quality review of the efficacy of psychosocial intervention, results would support the "pro" position that interventions are ineffective in reducing the distress of cancer patients.

In the rebuttal to the "pro" positions findings, Manne and Andrykowksi [32] contended that finding 25 % of the analyses of individual outcome variables is not an indication of lack of benefit. Rather, they noted that no comparisons were statistically significant in the direction favoring the control group, a finding that would be expected if indeed there was no treatment effect. In addition, issue was taken with the use of the singular, albeit rigorous, review utilized by the "pro" position [46], and the argument was made that the dismissal of other meta-analyses was unreasonable. It was noted that such meta-analyses, although including flawed studies, generally supported the benefit of psychosocial interventions.

As the final rebuttal accorded the "pro" side (supporting the position that psychosocial interventions are ineffective), Coyne and Lepore [33] made the following points: (1) the "con" side relied on reviews that included nonrandomized trials to prove efficacy while the one exception [46] did not provide evidence for efficacy; and (2) four of the five intervention studies selected by the "con" side failed to provide an analysis of treatment × time interaction needed to demonstrate efficacy. That is, while the "pro" side agreed that the studies selected as the "best" by the "con" side did indeed show main treatment effects for an outcome related to emotional distress, they argued that this is potentially misleading as an indicator of efficacy. Rather, what is most critical is whether the change over time is different between groups (group × treatment interaction). Finally, they argued that the fifth trial selected by the "con" side as evidence of efficacy [38] did not provide enough evidence of efficacy as a stand-alone study to overwhelm the body of data not supporting the benefit of psychosocial intervention. Their stance remained that the data to date fail to provide even a modest case for the efficacy of psychosocial interventions to reduce distress among cancer patients.

So where does this leave us? More recent work has not served to clarify this controversy, with mixed findings of single studies [47, 48] and reviews continuing to note significant limitations in the scientific literature [49–51]. It is at best

unsettling to appreciate that after dozens of intervention studies and several systematic reviews and meta-analyses that the data linking psychosocial interventions to decreased emotional distress, anxiety, and depression remains equivocal. It does speak to our failure to systematically build a cumulative science in this important area of cancer care. In the midst of this confusion, there are some directions for research to move, clarified by the "great debate" and the thoughtful work produced by this discourse.

First, there is some data to indicate that our reviews are getting better with time [52], and it should be noted that several of the major reviews and meta-analyses referenced above were completed before the advent or major dissemination of CONSORT [53]. Thus, moving forward there is hope for more rigor in our clinical trials and more quality systematic reviews. It is hoped that the time of nonsystematic, uncritical analyses of this field (and others) is behind us, or at least moving in that direction.

Second, in terms of future trials, there is a need to clearly identify type of treatment and to consider utilizing consistent outcome measures across trials so we are not comparing "apples and oranges" when the time is ripe for a review or meta-analysis. There is indeed suggestive data that interventions, if effective, are much more likely to be effective for those cancer patients demonstrating a clear need—that is, patients reporting high levels of emotional distress, anxiety, or depression at time of entry into a psychosocial intervention. In addition, as we define our targeted populations for intervention trials, we should note that we have little information on the benefit of interventions for low-income, ethnically diverse populations, and some evidence that men are underrepresented in such trials historically.

Finally, while not specific to studies related to psychosocial interventions and cancer, increased attention to the methodology utilized in our systematic reviews and meta-analyses is needed. Such reviews and meta-analyses make life easier for researchers and clinicians alike, but come with the risk of oversimplifying complex issues. As researchers, we do need to move beyond simply linking to conclusions, and need to appraise each trial separately while looking at the consistency of the results. It is humbling to note that meta-analyses have very inconsistently predicted the results of subsequent large randomized trials [54]. Part of this involves our need to move away from interventions with small sample sizes that raise significant issues relative to confirmatory bias and other concerns relative to randomization [55, 56].

In summary, significant resources have been utilized with good intent to conduct studies to help cancer patients decrease their level of emotional distress secondary to diagnosis and treatment. As individual studies suffer from small sample size or lack of methodological rigor, subsequent meta-analyses and systematic reviews suffer in their ability to derive a solid take home message based upon these inadequately designed single studies. As a result, the quality of this work has not allowed us to derive an unqualified answer to the question of whether interventions work, what interventions, and with whom.

The Role of "Positive Psychology" in Cancer Care

A generation ago, the field of psycho-oncology was working diligently to demonstrate empirically that cancer was indeed a stressful time period, from diagnosis through survival or end of life care. It was not until the early 1980s that research began to document the prevalence of emotional distress among diagnosed cancer patients [3, 57]. Psychiatrists, psychologists, social workers, and other mental health professionals were working within a biomedical system that had yet to formally endorse the concept of "quality of life" as a research domain, and had not allocated institutional resources for such professional groups to be major players in the ongoing care of cancer patients. Thus, the evolution of psycho-oncology care necessitated a focus on demonstrating high levels of distress among cancer patients so that appropriate services could be provided and reimbursed. From a historical perspective, it is interesting to note that discussions

of patients benefitting in any way from cancer would very likely not have been embraced by the field of psycho-oncology, and such attention may have been adamantly opposed by those striving to ensure cancer patients received adequate psychosocial care.

The flip side of the above is the "tyranny of optimism" spawned by lay publications in the early-mid 1980s which essentially told cancer patients that thinking positively and having the right attitude would cure cancer [58, 59]. In the late 1980s a study by David Spiegel and colleagues supported the notion that psychosocial support groups could increase survival among women with metastatic breast cancer [60], and this study was unfortunately utilized by many in the alternative medicine community to promote the belief that cancer was a case of "mind over matter". As a practicing psychologist in a major cancer center at that time, on more than one occasion, I was clearly instructed by well-intentioned family members not to allow their relative with cancer to address the possibility of cancer progression or issues surrounding the possibility of death and dying during our counseling sessions. The fear was that such "negative" thinking would both demoralize the patient and lead to his or her physical demise. This mandate to "think positively" due to the belief that such thinking is key to survival has been appropriately labeled the "tyranny of optimism" [61], and represents a very real danger of unquestioned acceptance of "positive psychology."

It is in some ways comforting that the idea of "positive psychology," including concepts such as "posttraumatic growth" and "benefit finding" has made its way into this chapter, signaling that it is indeed undergoing empirical scrutiny. The lines of research in this area have included the conceptualization of positive psychology constructs, methodological considerations, and implications for practice. The recent attention given this exciting area in the research literature warrants its inclusion in this chapter as an ongoing psycho-oncology controversy.

A number of constructs have historically dotted the health psychology literature as "positive psychology" constructs, including "fighting spirit" [62], the related concepts of benefit finding and posttraumatic growth [63], and optimism [64]. Since "fighting spirit" has essentially been dismissed as a construct of prognostic value [65, 66], this brief review will focus upon optimism, benefit-finding, and posttraumatic growth related to coping with cancer and health outcomes.

Interest in optimism as a personality characteristic linked to psychological adjustment and health outcomes has increased over the past several decades, examining whether *dispositional* optimism (a generalized expectation that good things will happen) is linked to health. Much of this work has indeed found a protective effect for optimism when examining such outcomes as pain reports [67] or rehospitalization following coronary bypass surgery [68].

A review of this association between optimism and physical health was recently completed, with results generally supporting this optimism–health connection [64]. This review found 84 studies that met the criteria of including measures of dispositional optimism, physical health outcomes, effect size estimates (or the provision of statistics allowing transformation to an effect size), and sample size information. Overall, the mean effect size denoting the relationship between optimism and health was 0.17 (95 % CI=0.15–0.20; $p<0.001$), indicating a positive but fairly small effect for optimism. However, further analyses provided additionally interesting results. When analyzing studies utilizing subjective measures (primarily self-report measures of health) of physical health versus objective measures, the mean effect size for objective measures was significantly smaller than that for subjective measures. Although both were statistically significant overall, the mean effect size for subjective measures was nearly twice as large as the mean effect size for objective measures. Thus, these analyses indicated that the measurement mode of the health outcome assessed moderated the relationship between optimism and good health.

While this meta-analysis and other studies have linked optimism to positive health or health behaviors in a number of health domains [69, 70] there is not a wealth of data from the cancer domain.

However, one such study [71] investigated the relationship between pretreatment levels of optimism and survival in patients with non-small cell lung cancer. One hundred and seventy-nine patients ($n=179$) completed the Life Orientation Test (LOT) [72] at pretreatment, a standard questionnaire assessing dispositional optimism. There was no evidence that optimism was related to survival in this sample of patients with lung cancer, and no statistical trend in that direction. This study arguably surpasses others in this research arena, given the use of a reliable, valid measure of optimism, a reasonably large sample compared to other investigations, a single type of cancer (non-small cell lung cancer) with no evidence of metastatic disease at time of pretreatment questionnaire administration, and adjustment for a number of potential confounders in the data analysis.

A second study involving cancer patients investigated the hypothesis that head and neck cancer patients who were pessimistic had a greater probability of dying within 1 year of diagnosis than optimistic patients [73]. This prospective observational study also used the LOT [72] at baseline and tracked survival over 1 year. With a total of 96 subjects, they reported support of their hypothesis. However, the odds ratio for dying within 1 year for pessimistic patients was only 1.12 (95 % CI=1.01–1.24), raising the issue of the clinical significance of such an isolated finding. It is likely that, given the small sample size, this small difference in the odds ratio was driven by only a few study subjects.

In sum, while data is generally supportive, although less than extensive related to many health outcomes [64], studies to date in cancer have not warranted the seemingly strong belief that optimism does indeed make a difference in health outcomes related to cancer.

Dispositional optimism is of interest theoretically and clearly shows promise linking to health behaviors and health outcomes. However, defined as *dispositional* optimism, it has generally been conceptualized as more of a personality trait than a "state" measure. Thus, it is unclear how further work would lead to an intervention strategy that would change such a trait and impact survival, other than providing clinicians an awareness that differing levels of such optimism might impact intervention success.

A "positive psychology" variable with potential relevance to a psychosocial intervention is benefit finding or posttraumatic growth. These are clearly related concepts, and integral to the "positive psychology" movement. This concept refers to finding benefit or experiencing personal growth in some way as a function of stress or trauma, in this case the diagnosis and/or treatment of cancer. This benefit or growth might take the form of a greater sense of personal resilience, appreciation of one's ability to cope, enhanced relationships with family or friends, or greater appreciation of life. It may also take the form of more discrete behavior change, such as smoking cessation, eating healthier, etc. These two constructs (benefit finding and posttraumatic growth), when measured separately, have been found to be positively correlated [74], and both have been plagued by definitional challenges, measurement issues, and the lack of studies utilizing prospective designs [75, 76]. There has been recent attention focused upon determining how different concepts linked with positive psychology are related [77] and predictors of benefit finding among cancer patients [78]. However, without a clear conceptual distinction at this time between benefit finding and posttraumatic growth, the discussion below embraces both constructs examining the data linking them to positive adaptation or health outcomes.

A recent meta-analysis reviewing benefit and posttraumatic growth examined the relationship of these constructs to both psychological outcomes and physical health [63]. Results from 87 ($n=87$) cross-sectional studies found benefit finding linked to less depression and more positive well being, but no relationship of benefit finding to quality of life measures and subjective health reports. Interesting moderator analyses found that the link of benefit finding to the outcomes above were affected by how much time had elapsed since the stressor, the measure used to assess benefit finding, and racial composition. Other reviews focusing upon cancer and benefit

finding or posttraumatic growth have found inconsistent links between benefit finding and outcomes. This is true when outcomes have included both psychosocial adaptation measures and health outcomes [79], and reviews converge in noting the inconclusive data to date [80, 81]. Coyne [76] notes that such inconsistent results may be due to several factors. There may be a nonlinear relationship between benefit finding and adjustment or health outcomes, moderators unmeasured to date may be operating, or there may be something about use of this strategy that increases emotional distress in some fashion [80], an intriguing possibility given that some studies have found that benefit finding has a negative impact on psychological outcomes [79].

Given the above, we are once more in position to call for more clarity of the core concepts of "positive psychology" prior to extensive development of interventions to enhance benefit finding and promote posttraumatic growth, a position endorsed by both Tennen and Affleck [81] and Gorin [82]. If we move away for the moment from intervention studies, where might we move to promote a cumulative science in this area and determine the value of intervention development?

Aspinwall and Tedeschi [83] warn against "throwing the baby out with the bathwater" and suggest several critical directions the field might go prior to any such "tossing of the baby." First, given some supportive work linking these concepts in domains outside of cancer, it makes sense not to give up on the study of optimism or benefit finding, but rather devote more work to the pathways involved in these health domains. Second, such preintervention work should not focus solely on physical health or survival, but rather include as important outcomes those involving quality of life and psychological distress. This relationship has indeed been challenging to pin down consistently even outside of the cancer domain, and may relate to our fundamental lack of knowledge about benefit finding or the posttraumatic growth process. For example, the finding by Helgeson et al. [63] that outcomes are impacted by the amount of time since the stressor may clearly impact findings related to psychosocial outcome variables and should be considered in future work. Finally, the inclusion of positive psychology measures in a more standard fashion as we assess psychological and physical health outcomes among cancer patients would be welcome so that findings might spur additional hypotheses and directions for research.

In sum, the recommendation to return to more of a focus on theory development, measurement development and testing, and more observational prospective research designs will lead to a more solid conceptual understanding of the role of "positive psychology" variables in cancer outcomes related to physical health and psychosocial adjustment [81, 82].

Finally, it will our responsibility to temper the enthusiasm that this area of research produces among mental health clinicians and the media, and continue to be cautious as we discuss findings that link "being positive" with outcomes, particularly survival. We need only look back to the Spiegel et al. study [60] linking support group participation with increased survival to appreciate the stir such findings might create, and the challenges faced in revising beliefs when such findings are placed in a more cautious framework [84].

Support Groups and Survival in Cancer

The final area of controversy covered in this chapter has a history dating back over two decades, beginning with two studies [60, 85] with results widely interpreted as showing increased survival among cancer patients participating in group psychotherapy. This work by Spiegel et al. [60] and Fawzy et al. [85], reported that, in the case of metastatic breast cancer [60] and malignant melanoma [85], participation in a support group with other cancer patients significantly extends survival relative to a control group of patients not participating in such an intervention. These studies impacted the psychosocial and even biomedical oncology community at the time, and helped to establish the belief by some in the professional community that psychological factors could directly impact the progression of cancer and survival from the disease. These studies and much media attention helped to promote this belief in both the professional and lay communities, with a not insignificant proportion of women attending support groups noting that they did so in part to extend survival [86]. While several thorough reviews have exhaustively challenged these findings and those of others purporting to show life-extending benefits of support group interventions [84, 87], this belief in the power of support groups to extend life among cancer patients and the promotion of this belief manages to linger [88].

Given the importance of these two studies, a brief overview of each is provided. Spiegel [60] reported the effects on survival of a 1 year structured professionally led group intervention delivered to metastatic breast cancer patients ($n=50$) versus a control group ($n=36$). Very generally, this "supportive-expressive" therapy approach focused upon group members discussing coping with cancer and expressing their feelings about their experience. More specifically, content involved redefining life priorities, managing side effects of treatment and the illness, self-hypnosis for pain management, and building emotional bonds with group members. Interestingly, the study was not designed to assess survival, but was done due to the media publicity that was being accorded to the idea of "mind over matter" in disease by such alternative practitioners as Bernie Siegel, publishing books for lay consumption [58, 59]. The study found the mean time from randomization to death was approximately twice as long in the intervention group (36.6 months) compared to the no-treatment control group (18.9 months).

Fawzy et al. [85] reported on the survival of patients with malignant melanoma shortly after diagnosis and initial surgery who participated in a 6-week, 90-min structured group intervention ($n=34$) versus a control group ($n=34$). This intervention included education about melanoma and health behaviors, stress management: teaching and discussing of coping strategies, and support provided to and from other group members. Consistent with the Spiegel study [60], this intervention was also professionally led. At 6- and

10-year follow-up, risk to recurrence was significantly reduced (6-year follow-up only), as was risk of death (both 6- and 10-year follow-ups) in patients assigned to the intervention arm.

The first meta-analysis of the effects of psychosocial interventions on survival time in cancer patients [89] was completed well over a decade following the work of Spiegel [60] and Fawzy [85], and included other trials examining this same issue. This meta-analysis reviewed both randomized trials ($n=8$) and nonrandomized studies ($n=6$) of the impact of psychosocial intervention on survival among cancer patients. For inclusion in the analysis, intervention variables needed to involve some type or combination of education, social support, psychotherapy, skills training, etc. The summary of this review supported no overall treatment effect by the randomized trials or the nonrandomized trials. Indeed, the only primary study for group therapy for breast cancer which found a significant effect favoring intervention was the trial described above by Spiegel et al. [60]. Reviewing this meta-analysis, and acknowledged by the authors, this review suffered from the "apples and oranges" problem often experienced in meta-analytic attempts, i.e., significant differences across studies in cancer site, intervention, and settings, making it challenging at best to derive firm conclusions overall. This meta-analysis suffered from a small number of diverse studies, with missing data (e.g., cancer treatment) that may well have impacted individual study findings. A very conservative summation by the authors noted that conclusions about whether psychosocial interventions can increase survival were premature, driven perhaps by the finding that individual interventions (versus group) were found to be more effective.

Given the influence and lasting impact the original Spiegel study has had on the field of psycho-oncology, it is interesting to look at the replication study completed by the same investigator [90] and a replication effort by an independent investigator [91].

Goodwin [91] reported a replication of the Spiegel et al. study [60], randomly assigning 235 women with metastatic breast cancer to weekly supportive-expressive therapy or no-treatment control groups, although all participants received educational materials. Of note is that interventionists in this study received training by Spiegel to ensure integrity of the intervention content, including performance reviews and feedback. The intervention did not increase survival, with median survival in the intervention group reported as 17.9 months versus 17.6 months in the control group. Multivariate analyses incorporating a number of important variables (e.g., presence or absence of progesterone and estrogen receptors linked to differential survival, nodal stage at diagnosis, age at diagnosis, etc.) identified no significant effect of the intervention on survival and no significant interactions with treatment and study center, marital status or baseline mood disturbance.

Spiegel also designed a study [90] to replicate his earlier findings that group therapy extended survival time of women with metastatic breast cancer. With a much larger sample size than his original study, 125 ($n=125$) metastatic breast cancer patients were randomly assigned to a supportive-expressive group therapy condition ($n=64$) or a control condition ($n=61$) which received educational material. The content, length, and duration of the intervention mirrored the original investigation [60]. The earlier finding that survival was extended with supportive-expressive therapy was not replicated. Overall mortality after 14 years was 86 %, with a median survival time of 32.8 months. No statistically significant effect of support group intervention was found on survival, with median survival times for the intervention group (30.7 months) not significantly different than the 33.3 months for the control condition.

In addition to these more recent studies, interested readers are referred to an extensive recent review of the psychotherapy and survival in cancer literature [84], which includes discussions of research design, interpretation of results, and reporting of clinical trials, all issues that have not been sufficiently appreciated in this body of scientific work.

Since the extensive systematic narrative review noted above [84], Andersen et al. [92]

reported on a randomized trial of breast cancer patients with local progression who received psychosocial intervention and achieved longer recurrence-free and survival intervals over a median follow-up of 11 years compared with women randomized to no intervention. While the belief in the impact of such psychosocial intervention on the survival of cancer patients had decreased following the negative findings of the replicated works described previously [60, 85] and the extensive critical review noted above [84], this work resurrected the subdued optimism among believers in the power of such interventions. In reviewing the study and findings, this renewed optimism seems unwarranted.

Briefly, this trial randomly assigned newly diagnosed regional breast cancer patients ($n = 227$) to an intervention-with-assessment arm or assessment-only arm, measuring psychological, social, immune, and health benefits of the intervention. The intervention included professionally led groups focusing upon relaxation training, coping skills training, and strategies to improve health behaviors and adherence to treatment. Patients in the intervention arm were exposed to 39 h of psychosocial intervention (26 sessions) over 12 months. Reported results demonstrated longer recurrence-free and survival intervals over a median follow-up of 11 years compared to the women receiving no such intervention.

However, a critique of this trial [87] noted that in this trial, survival was not a primary endpoint, the observation period was not specified beforehand, and the analyses presented were post hoc, not allowing for a straightforward interpretation of the outcome. A key concern impacting validity of the findings was that there were no differences in unadjusted rates of recurrence or survival between the intervention and assessment-only groups. Overall, while the trial demonstrated that participants in the intervention were satisfied with their group experience and found the groups cohesive with some modest impact on health behaviors, mood and some selected immunological measures, it did not demonstrate decreased recurrence or improved survival.

In a follow-up study [93], the authors assessed survival among those patients who recurred, numbers that included 29 patients from the intervention group and 33 patients from the assessment-only group. Ten ($n = 10$) of the 29 patients in the intervention group survived (34 %), while 8 of the 33 in the assessment-only group survived (25 %). While the authors propose that this 59 % reduction in the risk of dying from breast cancer is statistically significant, it is challenging to appreciate the magnitude as being clinically significant when viewed in absolute terms. In addition, the results were indeed not statistically significant in simple analyses, but only in multivariate analyses in which the strategy for selection of covariates was not clear [94].

In sum, it appears that the belief that psychosocial interventions positively impacts survival among cancer patients extends beyond the data. The earlier study by Spiegel [60] was not replicated by the same investigator [90] and a second independent study [91], both replications utilizing the same diagnostic group (metastatic breast cancer patients) and intervention content (supportive-expressive group therapy). Other trials reporting positive results of psychosocial interventions on survival have significant design or analysis flaws, or do not account for outstanding confounding factors (e.g., more medical attention by those participating in the active psychosocial treatment) [84]. While critics initially seemed to make little headway on the belief that interventions were efficacious [95, 96], the evidence appears clear: No randomized trial designed with survival as a primary endpoint and in which psychotherapy was not confounded with medical care has yielded a positive effect [84].

So where do we go from here? As noted by Stefanek and McDonald [97], researchers need to appreciate the complexity and biology of the many diseases called "cancer" and work in an interdisciplinary fashion with those expert in disease and treatment issues that may impact on survival. It seems appropriate to take a step back from large clinical trials at least until we understand much more about the basic and biobehavioral science that links psychological variables to biological changes that have the potential to impact cancer progression. There are cellular and molecular studies that have identified biological processes that could potentially mediate cancer progression [98]. Chronic depression, social support, and chronic stress may influence multiple aspects of tumor growth and metastasis through neuroendocrine regulation (adrenaline, glucocorticoids, dopamine, estrogen, etc.). Work in this area may highlight how behavioral or pharmacological interventions might impact neuroendocrine effects on tumors and slow progression or increase survival [99, 100]. Exciting approaches have used results from more basic molecular and biological studies identifying signaling pathways that influence cancer growth and metastasis as a way to build our basic knowledge base. More specifically, such work explores the impact of stress on certain types of programmed cell death and considers how psychosocial factors may play a role in the avoidance of such cell death by cancer cells [101]. Such basic and translational work allows a body of knowledge to be built that may lead to more efficient, model-driven psychosocial interventions to impact cancer progression. More generally, work needs to consider the hallmarks of cancer that comprise the multistep development of human tumors [102, 103] such as the tumors ability to evade growth suppressors, resist cell death, or induce angiogenesis, and determine which of such processes are impacted by psychosocial variables prior to resorting to clinical trials uninformed by this critically important basic knowledge of tumor growth and tumor microenvironment nurturance.

Once such knowledge is gained, and if such knowledge does indeed lead to interventions that may impact tumor growth and metastasis and subsequently survival, there are other important considerations to consider in order to build a cumulative scientific base. First, too many such studies have suffered from small sample size issues. Fox [96] and Piantadosi [56] have both noted challenges with such small trials, including the fact that studies with low power are more likely to produce false positives. Second, in addition to measuring biological changes that may impact survival, it will be crucial to continue to monitor issues such as treatment adherence, changes in health behaviors, confounding by increased medical attention provided to intervention groups, etc. that may explain changes due to "psychosocial" variables. Third, careful selection

of tumor types is warranted, perhaps focusing on those that are hormonally sensitive such as breast cancer or others potentially immunogenic, such as melanoma. Targeting early stage tumors may be most productive, since the natural course of more advanced tumors, refractory to chemotherapy, or other medical treatments may dwarf the impact of psychological interventions.

If/as we move to testing psychosocial interventions based upon solid basic and translational biobehavioral work, the quality of such studies needs significant improvement. A systematic approach to the reporting of trials to ensure complete transparency in the design, conduct, analysis, and interpretation of results is sorely needed, and sorely absent from the great majority of previous work [84].

Finally, the issue of individual differences has not been extensively explored in this area of research. In this era of "personalized medicine," we do not know what key areas of such differences have physiological relevance, an area that might be informed by the more basic research noted above [99–101]. The role of each individual's genetic and experiential background may well be critical. Related to the role of individual differences, we know very little about the role of socioeconomic status, education, gender, race, and other such variables and how such variables may interact with the impact of standard psychosocial interventions. These individual variables may be important in their own right, rather than "noise" in the system in need of statistical control.

In closing this section, we should remember that there are upper limits to human longevity influenced by both nature and nurture. Quality of life and psychological distress are both worthy clinical endpoints. The role of psychological intervention to impact these important aspects of our lives is an important one, independent of the issue of increased survival.

Conclusion

This chapter has included critiques of work involving (1) psychosocial screening of cancer patients; (2) the benefit of psychosocial interventions to decrease emotional distress among cancer patients; (3) the role of positive psychology in cancer care;

and (4) the role of support groups in increasing survival among cancer patients. As noted in the introduction to this chapter, I encourage you to read other entries in this excellent text that summarize perhaps different perspectives on these areas of psycho-oncology and derive your own working hypotheses about the state of the science in each of these selected controversial areas.

My thanks are extended to the coeditors of this text for including a chapter on current controversies. There is indeed a very important role for the "healthy skeptic" in behavioral oncology [104]. Our field would be better served by more focus on post-publication critiques of our work. Relying solely on a handful of overworked volunteer reviewers, no matter how dedicated to the role, to determine the merit of work published, with no further formal comment by others most interested in a given topic, does not serve our field, or science, well. This self-evaluation, even if dominated by self-criticism, provides a more transparent and broad review, and likely would lead to superior replication attempts.

Finally, this selection of controversies was intended to focus on science, not the researchers involved in the work critiqued. I certainly did not intend to suggest incompetence or deliberate attempts on the part of any investigator to mislead the scientific field. However, I would remind us all that we should ourselves challenge our own hypotheses most strongly, and it would serve us all well and the science we engage in to be open to debate and criticism of our work. To end on a more philosophical point:

> In a controversy, the instant we feel anger we have already ceased striving for the truth and have begun striving for ourselves
>
> —Buddha

References

1. Van't Spiker A, Trijsburg RW, Duivenvoorden HJ. Psychological sequelae of cancer diagnosis: a meta-analytical review of 58 studies after 1980. Psychol Med. 1997;59:280–93.
2. Zabora J, Brintzenhofer K, Curbow B, et al. The prevalence of distress by cancer site. Psychooncology. 2001;10:19–28.
3. Stefanek ME, Derogatis LP, Shaw A. Psychological distress among oncology outpatients: prevalence and severity as measured with the brief symptom inventory. Psychosomatics. 1987;28(10):530–8.
4. Pirl WF, Muriel A, Hwang V, et al. Screening for psychological distress: a national survey of oncologists. J Support Oncol. 2007;5(10):499–504.
5. Mitchell AJ, Hussain N, Granger L, et al. Identification of patient-reported distress by clinical nurse specialists in routine oncology practice: a multicentre UK study. Psychooncology. 2011;20(10):1076–83.
6. Mitchell AJ, Rao S, Vaze A. Can general practitioners identify people with distress and mild depression? A meta-analysis of clinical accuracy. J Affect Disord. 2011;130(1–2):26–36.
7. Wilson J, Jungner G. Principles and practice of screening for disease. World Health Organization Public Health Paper 34. 1968.
8. Passik SD, Dugan W, McDonald MV, et al. Oncologists' recognition of depression in their patients with cancer. J Clin Oncol. 1998;16:1594–600.
9. Mitchell AJ, Kaar S, Coggan C, et al. Acceptability of common screening methods used to detect distress and related mood disorders: preferences of cancer specialists and non-specialists. Psychooncology. 2008;17(3):226–36.
10. Holland JC, Bultz BD. National Comprehensive Cancer Network (NCCN). The NCCN guidelines for distress management: a case for making distress the sixth vital sign. J Natl Compr Canc Netw. 2007;5:3–7.
11. MacMillan HL, Patterson CJ, Wathen CN, et al. Screening for depression in primary care: recommendation statement from the Canadian Task Force on Preventive Health Care. CMAJ. 2005;172:33–5.
12. Mitchell AJ. Pooled results from 38 analyses of the accuracy of the Distress Thermometer and other ultra-short methods of detecting cancer-related mood disorders. J Clin Oncol. 2007;25:4670–81.
13. Roth AJ, Kornblith AB, Batel-Copel L, et al. Rapid screening for psychological distress for men with prostate carcinoma: a pilot study. Cancer. 1998;82:1904–8.
14. Holland, JC, Andersen B, Breitbart WS, Compas B et al. NCCN Clinical practice guidelines in oncology: distress management. J Natl Compr Canc Netw 2010;8:448–85.
15. Vodermaier A, Linden W, Siu C. Screening for emotional distress in cancer patients: a systematic review of assessment instruments. J Natl Cancer Inst. 2009;101(21):1464–88.
16. Mitchell AJ. Short screening tools for cancer-related distress: a review and diagnostic validity meta-analysis. J Natl Compr Canc Netw. 2010;8(4):487–94.
17. Bidstrup PE, Johansen C, Mitchell AJ. Screening for cancer-related distress: summary of evidence from tools to programmes. Acta Oncol. 2011;50(2):194–204.
18. Meijer A, Roseman BA, Milette K, et al. Depression screening and patient outcomes in cancer: a systematic review. PLoS One. 2011;6(11):e27181.

19. Institute of Medicine. Cancer care for the whole patient: meeting psychosocial health needs. Washington DC: National Academy Press; 2007.

20. Bulz BD, Groff SL, Fitch M, et al. Implementing screening for distress, the 6th vital sign: a Canadian strategy for changing practice. Psychooncology. 2011;20(5):463–9.

21. Bennett GW, Stark D, Murray S, et al. Psychological distress in cancer from survivorship to end of life care: prevalence, associated factors and clinical implications. Eur J Cancer. 2010;46(11):2036–44.

22. Bui QUT, Ostir GV, Kuo YF, et al. Relationship of depression to patient satisfaction: findings from the barriers to breast cancer study. Breast Cancer Res Treat. 2005;89:23–8.

23. Kennard BD, Smith SM, Olvera R, et al. Nonadherence in adolescent oncology patients: preliminary data on psychological risk factors and relationship to outcome. J Clin Psychol Med Settings. 2004;11:30–9.

24. Meyer TJ, Mark MM. Effects of psychosocial interventions with adult cancer patients: a meta-analysis of randomized experiments. Health Psychol. 1995;14(2):101–8.

25. Rehse B, Pukrop R. Effects of psychosocial interventions on quality of life in adult cancer patients: meta-analysis of 37 published controlled outcome studies. Patient Educ Couns. 2003;50:179–86.

26. Hodges LJ, Walker J, Kleiboer AM, et al. What is a psychological intervention? A metareview and practical proposal. Psychooncology. 2011;20(5):470–8.

27. Stefanek ME, Jacobsen PB, Christensen AJ. The Society of Behavioral Medicine's "great debate": an introduction. Ann Behav Med. 2006;32(2):83–4.

28. Lepore SJ, Coyne JC. Psychological interventions for distress in cancer patients: a review of reviews. Ann Behav Med. 2006;32(2):85–92.

29. Andrykowski MA, Manne SL. Are psychological interventions effective and accepted by patients? I. Standards and levels of evidence. Ann Behav Med. 2006;32(2):93–7.

30. Manne SL, Andrykowski MA. Are psychological interventions effective and accepted by patients? II. Using empirically supported therapy guidelines to decide. Ann Behav Med. 2006;32(2):98–103.

31. Coyne JC, Lepore SJ, Palmer SC. Efficacy of psychosocial interventions in cancer care: evidence is weaker than it first looks. Ann Behav Med. 2006;32(2):104–10.

32. Manne SL, Andrykowski MA. Seeing the forest for the trees: a rebuttal. Ann Behav Med. 2006;32(2):111–4.

33. Coyne JC, Lepore SJ. Rebuttal: the black swan fallacy in evaluating psychological interventions for distress in cancer patients. Ann Behav Med. 2006;32(2):115–8.

34. Devine EC, Westlake SK. The effects of psychoeducational care provided to adults to cancer: meta-analysis of 116 studies. Oncol Nurs Forum. 1995;22:1369–81.

35. Sheard T, McGuire P. The effects of psychological interventions on anxiety and depression in cancer patients: results of two meta-analyses. Br J Cancer. 1999;80:1770–80.

36. Barsevick AM, Sweeney C, Haney E, et al. A systematic qualitative analysis of psychoeducational interventions for depression in patients with cancer. Oncol Nurs Forum. 2002;29:73–84.

37. Newell S, Sanson-Fisher RW, Savolainen NJ. Systematic review of psychological therapies for cancer patients: overview and recommendations for future research. J Natl Cancer Inst. 2002;94:558–84.

38. Nezu A, Nezu C, Felgoise S, et al. Project genesis: assessing the efficacy of problem-solving therapy for distressed adult cancer patients. J Consult Clin Psychol. 2003;71:1036–48.

39. Andersen B, Farrar W, Golden-Kreutz D, et al. Psychological, behavioral and immune changes after a psychological intervention: a clinical trial. J Clin Oncol. 2005;22:3570–80.

40. Scott J, Halford K, Ward B. United we stand? The effects of a couple-coping intervention on adjustment to early stage breast or gynecological cancer. J Consult Clin Psychol. 2004;72:112–1135.

41. Manne S, Ostroff J, Winkel G, et al. Couple-focused group intervention for women with early stage breast cancer. J Consult Clin Psychol. 2005;73:634–46.

42. Boesen E, Ross L, Frederiksen K, et al. Psychoeducational intervention for patients with cutaneous malignant melanoma: a replication study. J Clin Oncol. 2005;23:1270–7.

43. Moher D, Cook DJ, Eastwood S. Improving the quality of reports of meta-analyses of randomized controlled trials: the QUOROM statement. Quality of reporting of meta-analyses. Lancet. 1999;354:1896–900.

44. Chambless D, Hollon S. Defining empirically supported therapies. J Consult Clin Psychol. 1998;66:7–18.

45. Higgins JPT, Green S, editors. Cochrane handbook for systematic review of interventions 4.2.4. Chichester, England: Wiley; 2005.

46. Newell SA, Samson-Fisher RW, Savolainen NJ. Systematic review of psychological therapies for cancer patients: overview and recommendations for future research. J Natl Cancer Inst. 2002;94:558–84.

47. Marcus AC, Garrett KM, Cella D, et al. Can telephone counseling post-treatment improved psychosocial outcomes among early stage breast cancer survivors? Psychooncology. 2010;19(9):923–32.

48. Sherman KA, Heard G, Cavanagh KL. Psychological effects and mediators of a group multi-component program for breast cancer patients. J Behav Med. 2010;33(5):378–91.

49. Dale HL, Adair PM, Humphris GM. Systematic review of post-treatment psychosocial and behaviour change interventions for men with cancer. Psychooncology. 2010;19(3):227–37.

50. Luckett T, Britton B, Clover K, et al. Evidence for interventions to improve psychological outcomes in people with head and neck cancer: a systematic review

of the literature. Support Care Cancer. 2011;19(7): 871–81. doi:10.1007/s00520-011-1119-7.

51. Preyde M, Synnott E. Psychosocial intervention for adults with cancer: a meta-analysis. J Evid Based Soc Work. 2009;6(4):321–47.

52. Coyne JC, Thombs BD, Hagedoorn M. Ain't necessarily so: review and critique of recent meta-analyses of behavioral medicine interventions in *Health Psychology*. Health Psychol. 2010;29(2):107–16.

53. Altman DG, Schulz KF, Moher D. The revised CONSORT statement for reporting randomized trials: explanation and elaboration. Ann Intern Med. 2001;134:663–94.

54. Lelorier J, Gregoire G, Benhaddad A, et al. Discrepancies between meta-analyses and subsequent randomized controlled trials. N Eng J Med. 1997;337:536–42.

55. Kraemer HC, Gardner C, Brooks JO, et al. Advantages of excluding underpowered studies in meta-analysis: inclusionist versus exclusionist viewpoints. Psychol Methods. 1998;3:23–31.

56. Piantadosi S. Hazards of small clinical trials. J Clin Oncol. 1990;8:1–3.

57. Derogatis LR, Morrow GR, Fetting J, Penman D, Piasetsky S, Schmale AM, Henrichs M, Carnicke CL. The prevalence of psychiatric disorders among cancer patients. JAMA. 1983;249(6):751–7.

58. Siegel B. Love, medicine, and miracles. New York: Harper Collins; 1986.

59. Siegel B. Peace, love and healing. New York: Harper Collins; 1990.

60. Spiegel D, Bloom JR, Kraemer HC, et al. Effect of psychosocial treatment on survival of patients with metastatic breast cancer. Lancet. 1989;2:888–91.

61. Holland JC, Lewis S. The human side of cancer: living with hope, coping with uncertainty. New York: Harper Collins; 2000.

62. Greer S, Morris T, Pettingale KW. Psychological response to breast cancer-effect on outcome. Lancet. 1979;2(8146):785–7.

63. Helgeson V, Reynolds K, Tomich P. A meta-analytic review of benefit finding and growth. J Consult Clin Psychol. 2006;74:797–816.

64. Rasmussen HN, Scheier MF, Greenhouse JB. Optimism and physical health: a meta-analytic review. Ann Behav Med. 2009;37(3):239–56.

65. Pettigrew M, Bell R, Hunter D. Influence of psychological coping on survival and recurrence in people with cancer: systematic review. Br Med J. 2002;325(7372):1066–9.

66. Watson M, Haviland JS, Greer S, et al. Influence of psychological response on survival in breast cancer: a population-based cohort study. Lancet. 1999;354(9187):1331–6.

67. Mahler HIM, Kulik JA. Optimism, pessimism and recovery from coronary bypass surgery: prediction of affect, pain, and functional status. Psychol Health Med. 2000;5(4):347–58.

68. Scheier MF, Matthews KA, Owens JF, et al. Optimism and rehospitalization after coronary artery bypass graft surgery. Arch Intern Med. 1999; 159:829–35.

69. Taylor SE, Keneny ME, Aspinwall LG, et al. Optimism, coping, psychological distress and high risk sexual behavior among men at risk for acquired immunodeficiency syndrome (AIDS). J Pers Soc Psychol. 1992;63:460–73.

70. Gitay EJ, Gelejinse JM, Zitman FG, et al. Lifestyle and dietary correlates of dispositional optimism in men: the Zutphen Elderly Study. J Psychosom Res. 2007;63:483–90.

71. Schofield P, Ball D, Smith JG. Optimism and survival in lung carcinoma patients. Cancer. 2004;100:1276–82.

72. Scheier MF, Carver CS. Optimism, coping and health: assessment and implications of generalized outcome expectancies. Health Psychol. 1985;4:219–47.

73. Allison PJ, Guichard C, Fung K, et al. Dispositional optimism predicts survival status 1 year after diagnosis in head and neck cancer patients. J Clin Oncol. 2003;21(3):543–8.

74. Mols F, Vingerhoets AJ, Coebergh JW, et al. Wellbeing, posttraumatic growth and benefit finding in long-term breast cancer survivors. Psychol Health. 2009;24(5):583–95.

75. Sumalla EC, Ochoa C, Bianco I. Posttraumatic growth in cancer: reality or illusion? Clin Psychol Rev. 2009;29(1):24–33.

76. Coyne JC, Tennen H. Positive psychology in cancer care: bad science, exaggerated claims, and unproven medicine. Ann Behav Med. 2010;39:16–26.

77. Rinaldis M, Pakenham KI, Lynch BM. A structural model of the relationships among stress, coping, benefit-finding and quality of life in persons diagnosed with colorectal cancer. Psychol Health. 2011;4:1–19.

78. Thornton AA, Owen JE, Kernstine K, et al. Predictors of finding benefit after lung cancer diagnosis. Psychooncology. 2012;21(4):365–73. doi:10.1002/pon.1904.

79. Stanton AL, Bower JE, Low CA. Posttraumatic growth after cancer. In: Calhoun LG, Tedeschi RG, editors. Handbook of posttraumatic growth: research and practice. Mahwah: Lawrence Erlbaum Associates; 2006. p. 138–75.

80. Zoellner T, Maercker A. Posttraumatic growth in clinical psychology: a critical review and introduction of a two component model. Clin Psychol Rev. 2006;26:626–53.

81. Tennen H, Affleck G. Benefit finding and benefit-reminding. In: Snyder CR, Lopez SJ, editors. Handbook of positive psychology. New York: Oxford University Press; 2002. p. 584–97.

82. Gorin SS. Theory, measurement, and controversy in positive psychology, health psychology, and cancer: basics and next steps. Ann Behav Med. 2010;39:43–7.

83. Aspinwall LG, Tedeschi RG. Of babies and bathwater: a reply to Coyne and Tennen's views on positive psychology and health. Ann Behav Med. 2010;39:27–34.

84. Coyne JC, Stefanek M, Palmer SC. Psychotherapy and survival in cancer: the conflict between hope and evidence. Psychol Bull. 2007;133(3): 367–94.
85. Fawzy FI, Fawzy NW, Hyun CS, et al. Malignant melanoma: effects of an early structured psychiatric intervention, coping, and affective state on recurrence and survival 6 years later. Arch Gen Psychiatry. 1993;50:681–9.
86. Miller M, Boye M, Butow PN, et al. The use of unproven methods of treatment by cancer patients: frequency, expectations and cost. Support Care Cancer. 1998;6:337.
87. Stefanek ME, Palmer SC, Thombs BD, et al. Finding what is not there: unwarranted claims of an effect of psychosocial intervention on recurrence and survival. Cancer. 2009;115:5612–6.
88. Mulcahy N. In: Cancer survival, 'Mind Matters' Says Expert. Medscape Medical News February 2, 2011. http://www.medscape.com/viewarticle/736734. Accessed June 2011.
89. Smedslund G, Ringdal GI. Meta-analysis of the effects of psychosocial interventions on survival time in cancer patients. J Psychosom Res. 2004;57:123–31.
90. Spiegel D, Butler LD, Giese-Davis J, et al. Effects of supportive-expressive group therapy on survival of patients with metastatic breast cancer. Cancer. 2007;110:1130–8.
91. Goodwin PJ, Leszcz M, Ennis M, et al. The effect of group psychosocial support on survival in metastatic breast cancer. N Engl J Med. 2001;345: 1719–26.
92. Andersen BL, Yang H, Farrar W, et al. Psychologic intervention improves survival for breast cancer patients. Cancer. 2008;113:3450–8.
93. Andersen BL, Thornton LM, Shapiro CL, et al. Biobehavioral, immune and health benefits following recurrence for psychological intervention participants. Clin Cancer Res. 2010;16(12):3270–8.
94. Palmer SC, Stefanek ME, Thombs BD, et al. Psychologic intervention and survival: wishing does not make it so. Clin Cancer Res. 2010;16(21): 5364–5.
95. Stefanek ME. Psychotherapy and cancer survival: a cautionary tale. Psychosomatics. 1991;32:237–8.
96. Fox BH. A hypothesis about Spiegel et al.'s 1989 paper on psychosocial intervention and breast cancer survival. Psychooncology. 1998;7:361–70.
97. Stefanek M, McDonald P. Brain, behavior and immunity in cancer. In: Miller M, Bowen DJ, Croyle RT, Rowland JH, editors. Handbook of cancer control and behavioral science. Washington DC: APA Press; 2009. p. 499–516.
98. Antoni MH, Lutgendorf SK, Cole SW, et al. The influence of bio-behavioral factors on tumor biology: pathways and mechanisms. Nat Rev Cancer. 2006;6:240–8.
99. Thaker PH, Sood AK. Neuroendocrine influences on cancer biology. Semin Cancer Biol. 2008;18(3): 164–70.
100. Costanzo ES, Sood AK, Lutgendorf SK. Biobehavioral influences on cancer progression. Immunol Allergy Clin North Am. 2011;31(1): 109–32.
101. Sood AK, Lutgendorf SK. Stress influences on anoikis. Cancer Prev Res. 2011;4(4):481–5.
102. Hanahan D, Weinberg RA. The hallmarks of cancer. Cell. 2000;100:57–70.
103. Hanahan D, Weinberg RA. Hallmarks of cancer: the next generation. Cell. 2011;144:646–74.
104. Coyne J. The healthy scepticism project (editorial). Psychol Health. 2010;25(6):647–50.

Psychosocial Interventions for Couples Coping with Cancer: A Systematic Review

11

Hoda Badr, Cindy L. Carmack, Kathrin Milbury, and Marisol Temech

Introduction

For most individuals diagnosed with cancer, their psychological adjustment depends strongly on their interpersonal relationships. Cancer patients identify their spouses or intimate partners as their most important sources of practical and emotional support; spouses or partners are also the first persons from whom support is often sought after patients receive a cancer diagnosis [1]. However, the diagnosis and treatment of cancer can affect every aspect of both the patients' and their partners' quality of life (QOL). Patients must cope with the role changes and distress brought about by the physical side effects and increased functional disability associated with their disease and treatment. Their partners must not only confront the potential loss of a life part-

ner (the patient), but also must become adept at providing instrumental and emotional support to the patient during a time when they themselves are under extreme stress. Coping with cancer treatment can also challenge a couple's established communication patterns, roles, and responsibilities [2, 3]. Thus, it is not surprising that some couples report that the cancer experience brought them closer together, whereas other couples experience significant adjustment and communication difficulties that result in feelings of decreased intimacy and greater interpersonal conflict over time [4, 5].

Traditional approaches for addressing psychosocial adaptation after a cancer diagnosis have focused on either the patient or the patient's partner. However, a burgeoning literature involving couple-based interventions has emerged over the past two decades and there have been a number of notable reviews in this area. For example, Manne and Badr [6] conducted a thematic review of descriptive and intervention studies that focused on couples coping with cancer, although their review was not exhaustive. Both Scott and Kayser [7] and Baik and Adams [8] each conducted systematic reviews of psychosocial interventions that included randomized controlled trials (RCTs) as well as quasi-experimental studies (in which patients were not randomized or in which there was no control group). Scott and Kayser's [7] review was also narrowly focused on sexual interventions. Finally, Martire and colleagues [9] conducted a meta-analysis of interventions for couples coping with chronic illness.

This research was supported by a career development award from the National Cancer Institute K07CA124668 (Hoda Badr, Ph.D., Principal Investigator) and a pilot project grant awarded to Dr. Badr under P30 AG028741 (Albert Siu, M.D., Principal Investigator). Dr. Milbury's work was supported by American Cancer Society postdoctoral award PF-10-013-01-CPPB.

H. Badr, Ph.D. (✉) • M. Temech, B.A
Department of Oncological Sciences, Mount Sinai School of Medicine, One Gustave L. Levy Place, New York, NY, 10029, USA
e-mail: hoda.badr@mssm.edu

C.L. Carmack, Ph.D. • K. Milbury, Ph.D.
Department of Behavioral Science, The University of Texas MD Anderson Cancer Center, Houston, TX, USA

Although many of the studies focused on cancer patients and their partners, the review was broad and encompassed interventions geared toward couples with a variety of illnesses. Given the aforementioned issues, the conclusions that can be drawn from existing reviews regarding the efficacy of psychosocial interventions in couples coping with cancer are limited.

The primary goal of this chapter is to systematically review the efficacy of existing psychosocial interventions in cancer involving couples on patients' and their partners' quality of life (QOL). The secondary goal is to provide direction for future research based on identified gaps in the literature. Toward this end, we sought to identify all published reports of randomized controlled trials (RCTs) of psychosocial interventions conducted with cancer patients and their partners that were aimed at improving the patient's and/or the partner's QOL. Given that QOL is a multidimensional construct that includes physical, psychological, and social well-being [10, 11], studies that included health, psychological, or relationship outcomes were included in our review.

Systematic Review

Identification of appropriate RCTs began with electronic searches to identify English language journal articles published from January, 1980 to February, 2011 in the PubMed, Embase, PsychInfo, Web of Science, and LISTA (EBSCO) databases. The search terms, based on the interventions and outcomes of interest, were "intervention," "cancer," "couple," "dyad," "spouse," "symptom management," "behavioral," "therapy," and "psychosocial." Our strategy in selecting search terms was to balance sensitivity with specificity [12] and to verify and augment the search results by reviewing reference lists from publications retrieved, which included relevant systematic reviews and meta-analyses.

Figure 11.1 shows a flow chart depicting the process we used to identify and select journal articles that were relevant to our study. We identified 744 articles and used bibliographic software (Endnote *X*2), EPPI-Reviewer 4.0 software, and

manual review to remove duplicate publications, resulting in 275 articles. Identified articles were then screened for inclusion using the EPPI-Reviewer 4.0 software followed by manual review. The criteria for article inclusion were article was peer reviewed, study was cancer based, study participants were randomized, study was couple based, study was a psychosocial intervention, and article was available in English. Of these 275 articles, 249 did not meet these criteria and were excluded—most because they were not peer-reviewed articles (e.g., conference abstracts). We then further refined our search by manually examining the abstracts, titles, and full texts of the 26 remaining articles. An article was excluded if the article did not report original trial outcomes (i.e., it was a secondary analysis), if the article did not report on a psychological, health, or relationship outcome, or if the study reported did not include a control group. Studies that compared two interventions but did not include a control group were excluded because our goal was to examine intervention efficacy relative to either standard care (i.e., usual medical care or standard psychosocial services) or a time or attention control (i.e., standard medical education was provided). Using these criteria, seven articles were excluded; thus, 19 studies were included in our review (see Fig. 11.1). After finalizing the list of studies to be included in the review, two independent raters (HB and MT) abstracted data on intervention design, participant characteristics, theoretical basis, and key findings. Discrepancies between raters were resolved through review and discussion.

Intervention Design and Participant Characteristics

Intervention Design
As Table 11.1 shows, the vast majority of studies involved interventions conducted directly with individual couples; only one study involved a group intervention [13]. Four studies had attention control groups where educational information was provided [14–17]. The remaining studies had

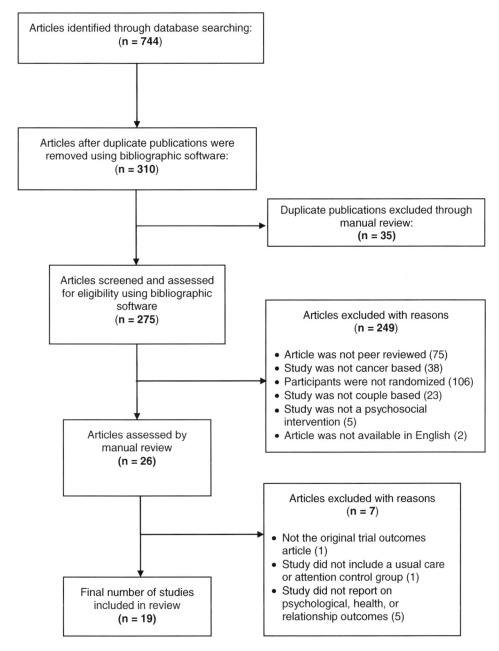

Fig. 11.1 Flow diagram depicting the systematic review process

standard care control groups where the patient received either standard psychosocial services [18, 19] or usual medical care [13, 20–31]. In two of the usual care control groups [21, 25], participants were part of a wait-list control and eventually were offered the intervention.

In terms of delivery, ten interventions involved in-person sessions (individual or group) [13, 14, 18–20, 24–27], three were exclusively over the telephone [23, 29, 32], and five involved a combination of telephone and in-person sessions [16, 17, 21, 22, 28–30, 32]. Interventions were

Table 11.1 Randomized psychosocial intervention studies of couples coping with cancer

	Sample demographics	Refusal rate, follow-up, and attrition at final follow-up	Theoretical framework, type of therapy, and who administered the intervention	Intervention and control group content
Baucom et al. [26]	*N*: 14 early-stage breast cancer patients and their spouses *Mean age*: not specified	*Refusal rate*: Not specified *Follow-up*: postintervention, 12 months *Attrition*: Not specified	*Theory*: no explicit theory; elements of communal/dyadic coping *Therapy*: cognitive behavior and behavioral marital therapy *Intervention delivery/dosage*: Six 75-min biweekly in-person sessions delivered by clinical psychology doctoral students	*Couples' intervention arm*: Couples communication training, problem-solving, and mutual-support skills, sexual functioning, and finding meaning and growth after breast cancer *Control arm*: Patients received usual medical care
Badger et al. [15]	*N*: 96 breast cancer patients and partners (63 % of partners were husbands and 14 % were significant others) *Mean age*: 53 years	*Refusal rate*: 17 % *Follow-up*: postintervention, 1 month *Attrition*: 5 % of patients and 11 % of partners	*Theory*: no explicit theory; elements of the social cognitive processing model *Therapy*: Interpersonal counseling and education *Intervention delivery/dosage*: Six weekly telephone calls for patients; three separate calls for partners. Delivered by trained nurses	*Couples' intervention arm*: Cancer education, interpersonal communication, and counseling to improve support exchanges *Second intervention arm*: Exercise protocol for patients and partners *Control arm*: Attention control; patients and partners received pamphlets and separate telephone calls for 6 weeks
Budin et al. [16]	*N*: 249 breast cancer patients and their partners (60 % spouses/significant others) *Mean age*: 52 years	*Refusal rate*: 51 % *Follow-up*: Postsurgery, adjuvant therapy, 2 weeks after completion of chemotherapy or radiation therapy or 6 months after surgery *Attrition*: 29 %	*Theory*: Individual stress and coping theory *Therapy*: Cognitive behavior Therapy *Intervention delivery/dosage*: Combination of four in-person and telephone sessions delivered to patients and partners separately. Delivered by nurses	*Couples' intervention arm*: Counseling to reduce anxiety, shape appraisals, facilitate coping strategies, improve cognitive processing, encourage behavior change, and promote functional communication *Second intervention arm*: Standardized education and telephone counseling; videotapes plus four separate sessions for patients and partners *Third intervention arm*: Standardized education; four phase-specific videotapes viewed by patients and partners separately that provided relevant evidence-based health relevant information, taught coping skills, and provided support *Control arm*: attention control where patients received education about disease management
Campbell et al. [29]	*N*: 40 prostate cancer patients (African American) and partners *Mean age*: 62 years	*Refusal rate*: 71 % *Follow-up*: postintervention *Attrition*: 25 %	*Theory*: No explicit theory *Therapy*: Education and cognitive behavioral therapy *Intervention delivery/dosage*: Six 1-h weekly sessions delivered by psychologists via telephone to patients and partners who participated together via speakerphone	*Couples' intervention arm*: Patients and partners were provided information about prostate cancer and possible long-term side effects, taught problem solving skills, and provided training in specific cognitive and behavioral coping skills (communication, relaxation, activity pacing); *Control arm*: Patients received usual medical care

Study	Sample	Follow-up data	Theory/Therapy/Intervention	Intervention and control arms
Christensen [24]	N: 20 early stage breast cancer patients (post-mastectomy) and husbands Mean age: 40 years	Refusal rate: Not specified Follow-up: Postintervention Attrition: 0 %	Theory: No explicit theory Therapy: Education and behavioral marital therapy Intervention delivery/dosage: Four in-person weekly sessions administered by a psychologist	Couples' intervention arm: Counseling focused on communication and problem-solving skills, and body image/sexuality Control arm: Patients received usual medical care
Giesler et al. [30]	N: 99 prostate cancer patients and partners Mean age: 64 years	Refusal rate: 68 % Follow-up: 4 months, 7 months, 12 months Attrition: 14 %	Theory: No explicit theory Therapy: Education and skills training Intervention delivery/dosage: Six monthly sessions (two in person and four via telephone) administered by nurses	Couples' intervention arm: Tailored couples education, support, and problem-solving Control arm: Patients received usual medical care
Kalaitzi et al. [31]	N: 40 breast cancer patients and their partners Mean age: 52 years	Refusal rate: Not specified Follow-up: Postintervention Attrition: 0 %	Framework: No explicit theory Therapy: Education and a combination of cognitive behavior couples therapy and sexual therapy Intervention delivery/dosage: Six biweekly in-person sessions administered by therapist	Couples' intervention arm: Education, communication training, and sexual counseling, including sensate focus and body imagery Control arm: Patients received usual medical care
Kayser et al. [18]	N: 63 breast cancer patients and their partners Mean age: 46 years	Refusal rate: 82 % Follow-up: 6 and 12 months after enrollment Attrition: 25 %	Theory: No explicit theory, elements of communal/dyadic coping Therapy: Cognitive behavior therapy Intervention delivery/dosage: 9 biweekly 1-h in-person sessions delivered over 5 months administered by a social worker	Couples' intervention arm: Couples coping and communication skills training, addressing impact of cancer on daily life, enhancing intimacy and sexual functioning Control arm: Patients were offered standard social work services (none of the patients in this arm requested these services)
Keefe et al. [20]	N: 78 mixed cancer patients with advanced disease and their partners Mean age: 59 years	Refusal rate: 53 % Follow-up: Postintervention Attrition: 28 %	Theory: No explicit theory Therapy: Cognitive behavioral therapy Intervention delivery/dosage: Three in-person sessions in patient's home delivered over 1–2 weeks; administered by nurses	Couples' intervention arm: Education about cancer pain and its management, pain coping strategies training, and partner taught how to help the patient acquire and maintain coping skills Control arm: Patients received usual medical care
Kuijer et al. [25]	N: 59 mixed cancer patients and partners Mean age: 50 years	Refusal rate: 3 % Follow-up: Postintervention, 3 months Attrition: 34 %	Theory: Equity theory Therapy: Cognitive behavior therapy Intervention delivery/dosage: Five 90-min biweekly in-person sessions administered by a psychologist	Couples' intervention arm: Improving the exchange of social support and restoring equity Control arm: Patients received usual medical care; wait-list control

(continued)

Table 11.1 (continued)

	Sample demographics	Refusal rate, follow-up, and attrition at final follow-up	Theoretical framework, type of therapy, and who administered the intervention	Intervention and control group content
Manne et al. [13]	N: 238 early-stage breast cancer patients and husbands Mean age: 49 years	Refusal rate: 67 % Follow-up: Postintervention, 6 months Attrition: 32 %; Note: an additional 7 % of patients randomized to the intervention completed follow-up surveys but did not attend any sessions	Theory: No explicit theory; elements of the social cognitive processing model Therapy: cognitive behavior and behavioral marital therapy Intervention delivery/dosage: Six 90-min weekly sessions delivered in a group format and administered by trained therapists	Couples' intervention arm: Couple-level stress management, problem solving as a team, respecting coping differences, enhancing support exchanges and communication skills, anticipating changes in the couple's relationship after cancer Control arm: Patients received usual medical care
Manne et al. [19]	N: 71 prostate cancer patients and their partners Mean age: 58 years	Refusal rate: 79 % Follow-up: Postintervention Attrition: 8 % of patients and 15 % of partners; Note: an additional 7 % of patients and 6 % of partners who were randomized to the intervention completed follow-up surveys but did not attend any sessions	Theory: Intimacy theory Therapy: Cognitive behavioral and behavioral marital therapy Intervention delivery/dosage: Six 90-min weekly in-person sessions delivered by trained therapists	Couples' intervention arm: Skills training in communication, improving support exchanges, enhancing emotional intimacy Control arm: Patients received standard psychosocial care (consultation with a social worker)
McCorkle et al. [22]	N: 107 men surgically treated for prostate cancer and their partners Mean age: 58 years	Refusal rate: Not specified Follow-up: 1,3, and 6 months after radical prostatectomy Attrition: 15 %	Theory: No explicit theory Therapy: Cognitive behavioral therapy Intervention delivery/dosage: Six in-person and telephone contacts delivered by nurses over 8 weeks	Couples' intervention arm: Symptom-management education, communication training, and sexual counseling Control arm: Patients received usual medical care
Mishel et al. [23]	N: 252 prostate cancer patients and partners Mean age: 64 years	Refusal rate: 33 % Follow-up: 4 months, 7 months Attrition: 5 %	Theory: No explicit theory Therapy: Cognitive behavioral therapy Intervention delivery/dosage: Eight weekly telephone sessions delivered by nurses to patients and partners separately	Couples' intervention arm: Tailored couples' education, cognitive reframing, problem solving, and patient–provider communication training Second intervention arm: Education, cognitive reframing, problem solving, and patient–provider communication training for the patient only Control arm: Patients received usual medical care
Nezu et al. [27]	N: 150 mixed cancer patients and family members (95 % spouses) Mean age: 47 years	Refusal rate: Not specified Follow-up: Postintervention, 6 months, 12 months Attrition: 12 %	Theory: No explicit theory Therapy: Cognitive behavioral therapy Intervention delivery/dosage: Ten 90-min weekly in-person sessions delivered by advanced psychology graduate students and social workers	Couples' intervention arm: Couples problem-solving training Second intervention arm: Problem-solving therapy for patients only Control arm: Patients received usual medical care, wait-list control

Study	Sample	Methods	Theory/Therapy/Intervention	Intervention arms
Northouse et al. [21]	*N*: 235 prostate cancer patients and spouses *Mean age*: 61 years	*Refusal rate*: 33 % *Follow-up*: 4 months, 8 months, 12 months *Attrition*: 17 %	*Theory*: Individual stress and coping theory *Therapy*: Cognitive behavioral and behavioral marital therapy *Intervention delivery/dosage*: Five biweekly consultations (three 90-min home visits and two 30-min telephone calls) delivered by nurses over the course of four months	*Couples' intervention arm*: Tailored education, enhancement of couples communication and support, coping effectiveness, uncertainty reduction, symptom management, family involvement, and optimism *Control arm*: Patients received usual medical care
Porter et al. [14]	*N*: 130 patients with gastrointestinal cancer and their partners *Mean age*: 59 years	*Refusal rate*: 75 % *Follow-up*: Postintervention *Attrition*: 21 %	*Theory*: No explicit theory; Elements of the Social Cognitive Processing Model *Therapy*: Cognitive behavioral therapy and behavioral marital therapy *Intervention delivery/dosage*: Four in-person sessions ranging from 45 to 75 min delivered by trained therapists (masters level social worker or psychologist)	*Couples' intervention arm*: Strategies to facilitate patient disclosure and give patients the opportunity to talk with their partners about their cancer-related concerns *Control arm*: Attention control; education, orientation to the cancer team, suggestions for communicating with providers, resources for health information, impact of cancer, financial concerns, and suggestions for maintaining quality of life
Scott et al. [17]	*N*: 94 women with early stage breast or gynecological cancer and their husbands *Mean age*: 52 years	*Refusal rate*: 6 % *Follow-up*: Postintervention, 6 months, 12 months *Attrition*: 21 % of patients and 30 % of partners	*Theory*: No explicit theory; elements of the social cognitive processing model *Therapy*: Cognitive behavior and behavioral marital therapy *Intervention delivery/dosage*: Four 120-min sessions in patients' homes and two 30-min calls delivered by psychologists	*Couples' intervention arm*: Medical information, communication skills training, social-support training, sexual counseling, discussion of existential concerns, individual coping skills training *Second intervention arm*: Medical Information, coping skills training, and supportive counseling for patients only *Control arm*: Attention Control; patients received medical information education
Ward et al. [28]	*N*: 161 mixed cancer patients and their significant others *Mean age*: 57 years	*Refusal rate*: 52 % *Follow-up*: Postintervention, 5 weeks, 9 weeks *Attrition*: 32 %	*Theory*: No explicit theory *Therapy*: Education *Intervention delivery/dosage*: One in-person session lasting 20–80 min and follow-up telephone calls administered by nurses and psychologists	*Couples' intervention arm*: Beliefs about cancer pain, barriers, pain medication misconceptions, attitudes, coping and pain management plan *Second intervention arm*: Same as couples' intervention arm except only patient received the intervention *Control arm*: Patients received usual medical care

primarily conducted in a hospital; however, a few were conducted in the patient's home [17, 20]. The interventions were administered by psychologists or therapists with masters or doctoral degrees (number [N]=11), nurses (N=7), or licensed clinical social workers (N=1) who used a variety of techniques, including cognitive behavior therapy (e.g., relaxation or cognitive restructuring), education, interpersonal counseling, and behavioral marital therapy.

One of the most frequently used treatments in the couples therapy literature is behavioral marital therapy [33]. The goal or behavioral marital therapy is to increase the ratio of positive to negative behaviors exchanged between partners [34]. Thus, behavioral exchange, improving adaptive communication, conflict resolution, and problem-solving skills are targeted [35, 36], and patients and partners are taught to be more aware of how they influence and are influenced by their interactions with one another [37].

Interventions included partners in one of two ways. The first method, used in 11 studies, treated the partner as an assistant or "coach" to facilitate learning and coping skills in the patient [14, 16, 17, 20, 23, 27–32]. In most of the interventions that used this method, the partner was present with the patient during all sessions; however, in three studies, the patient and partner each received separate instruction [15, 16, 23]. The second method, used by the remaining eight studies, treated the couple as a unit (i.e., both patient and partner were present in the room and treated together at all times during the intervention). Interventions using this method focus on improving the spousal relationship and interaction patterns by teaching skills that build teamwork, improve communication, and encourage the couple to view cancer in relational terms [6].

In terms of dosage, most interventions involved 6 weekly or biweekly sessions; however the number of sessions ranged from 1 to 16, and session-length varied from 20 to 120 min. For the most part, the number of couples who dropped out of the study before completing all of the intervention sessions was minimal. Only Manne and colleagues [13, 19] conducted questionnaire follow-ups and analyses of couples who were randomized to the intervention group but did not attend any sessions.

Participant Characteristics

As Table 11.1 shows, the mean age of participants ranged from 40 to 64 years (mean age was not specified in one study [26]), and the number enrolled varied considerably, from 14 to 252. Only eight studies had sample sizes of 100 or more [13, 14, 16, 17, 22, 23, 27, 28]. Of the 14 studies that provided descriptive data on their recruitment efforts, participation refusal rates varied widely from 3 [25] to 82 % [18]. Nine of the 14 studies had refusal rates of 50 % or more [13, 14, 16, 18–20, 28, 30], The time of follow-up ranged from postintervention to 1 year later and the number of follow-ups ranged from one to four. Regarding participant attrition at final follow-up, attrition rates for the studies that reported this information ranged from 5 [23] to 34 % [25].

Seven studies focused exclusively on couples coping with breast cancer [13, 15, 16, 18, 24, 26, 31], six studies focused exclusively on couples coping with prostate cancer [19, 21–23, 29, 30], five studies involved couples coping with different types of cancer [17, 20, 25, 27, 28], and one study focused exclusively on couples coping with gastrointestinal cancer [14]. With the exception of one study that focused exclusively on pain management at the end of life [20], all studies involved patients who had either early-stage or nonmetastatic disease. In most studies, participants were predominately white, with the exception of one study that focused exclusively on African American prostate cancer patients and their partners [29], and one study that included approximately an equal number of white and African American prostate cancer patients [23].

Even though both patients and partners participated, seven studies reported no outcomes whatsoever for partners [14, 21, 27, 28, 30, 31, 38]. However, a diverse set of patient outcomes were reported, including psychological functioning/distress, uncertainty, general QOL, relationship satisfaction, disease-specific QOL domains (e.g., pain and urinary and bowel function), sexual functioning, medication use (e.g., for erectile dysfunction), and attitudes about analgesic use.

Theoretical Bases and Description of Key Findings

Even though a variety of theoretical frameworks were used in the studies we reviewed (see Table 11.1), we classified them into three main categories based on previous reviews of the literature on couples coping with cancer [6]. First, individual stress and coping models focus on the role of stress appraisals in individual adjustment and emphasize the importance of social support provided by the partner to the patient. Second, resource theories view the marital relationship as a resource for couples to draw upon in times of stress. Third, dyadic-level theories focus on interaction patterns between patients and their partners and approaching cancer together as a team. The individual theories falling under each category are described below followed by brief descriptions and key findings of the interventions that utilized them.

Individual Stress and Coping Models

Two studies explicitly mentioned individual stress and coping models as their theoretical basis [16, 21]. These models posit that person-, social-, and illness-related factors influence how people appraise and cope with an illness, which in turn affects their QOL. They also view social support as a form of coping assistance [39]. Given this, interventions that utilize individual stress and coping models often conceptualize the healthy partner as the support provider and the patient as the support recipient [40].

Northouse and colleagues' [21] examined the efficacy of a couple-focused counseling intervention for 235 men diagnosed with prostate cancer and their spouses. The five-session intervention targeted communication skills, maintaining a positive attitude, managing stress and adopting a healthy lifestyle, obtaining information and managing uncertainty, and managing symptoms. No significant differences between the intervention arm and the control group were noted for patients' QOL, but patients enrolled in the intervention arm reported significantly less illness uncertainty and more communication with their partners about the illness than reported by patients in the

control group. Compared with spouses in the control group, spouses in the intervention group reported better QOL, more positive appraisal of care giving, less hopelessness, less illness uncertainty, more self-efficacy, better communication with the patient, fewer concerns about the patient's urinary incontinence, and less symptom distress. Some of these effects were sustained at the 8- and 12-month follow-ups.

Budin and colleagues [16] targeted both patient and partner, but intervened separately with each individual. These researchers assigned patients and partners to one of four study arms: (1) an attention control group that received education about disease management; (2) a group that watched four educational videotapes focusing on effective coping with a cancer diagnosis; recovery from surgery, adjuvant therapy, and ongoing recovery; (3) a group that received four telephone counseling sessions focusing on stress management, effective coping, and facilitating communication; or (4) a group that watched four educational videotapes and received four telephone counseling sessions. None of the patients or partners showed evidence of improvement in psychosocial functioning; however, partners in the control group reported greater distress compared with partners in the other three groups.

Resource Theories

Resource theories such as the social cognitive processing models (SCPMs) and equity theories adopt the view that the marital relationship is a resource for individuals to draw upon for assistance during difficult life events. These theories and their representative interventions are described below.

Social-Cognitive Processing Model. The SCPM posits that the social context in which recovery from cancer takes place influences emotional adjustment [41]. For many patients, cancer is experienced as a traumatic event eliciting symptoms such as intrusive thoughts and cognitive and behavioral avoidance [42, 43]. While some intrusive thoughts are an adaptive part of the cognitive processing and integration of traumatic events, these thoughts often elicit negative emotional responses. To manage emotions associated with a trauma, a person may actively avoid thinking or talking about the traumatic event. According to conditioning theories, avoidance may persist because it temporarily relieves anxiety. If avoidance continues in the long run, however, it hinders the cognitive and emotional processing of the event, causing both intrusive thoughts and psychological distress to increase [44]. Intrusive thoughts and avoidance are indicators that further cognitive processing may be needed.

According to the SCPM, a supportive spouse can serve as a resource for the patient in terms of providing assistance in cognitive processing. The spouse can also serve as a barrier to effective processing if he or she is either unavailable or unsupportive, which may be particularly problematic because of the level of importance the spouse has as both a confidante and a primary source of support [45]. Qualitative [46] and quantitative studies with cancer patients support this model [47–49]. Despite the fact that the SCPM was not explicitly mentioned as the theoretical basis for intervention, the four articles described below clearly utilized elements of this model and emphasized the role of disclosure and communication skills training as a means of reducing distress for both patients and/or their partners.

Badger and colleagues [15] conducted an RCT to examine whether telephone-delivered interventions decreased depression and anxiety in women with breast cancer and their partners. Couples participated in one of three different 6-week programs: (1) telephone interpersonal counseling, (2) self-managed physical activity, or (3) an attention control group where patients and partners received educational pamphlets and separate phone calls. Patients' and partners' symptoms of anxiety decreased over time in the telephone interpersonal counseling and exercise groups over time but not in the attention control group.

Manne and colleagues [13] conducted the only couples' group intervention study included in this review. A total of 238 women with early-stage breast cancer were randomly assigned to either a six-session couple-focused group intervention or usual care control condition. The intervention focused on support and encouragement of effective coping by facilitating communication and expression of emotions. Compared with patients receiving usual care, patients receiving the intervention reported greater reductions in symptoms of depression and these reductions persisted over the 6-month follow-up period. Subgroup analyses showed that patients who rated their partners as unsupportive benefited more from the intervention than patients with supportive partners. In addition, patients who had higher levels of physical impairment before the intervention benefited more from the intervention than did patients with lower preintervention levels of physical impairment.

Scott and colleagues [17] conducted an RCT examining the effectiveness of a six-session couple-based cognitive behavioral therapy program called Cancer Coping for Couples (CanCOPE) among 94 patients recently diagnosed with early-stage breast or gynecological cancer and their partners. Patients were randomly assigned to one of three study arms: (1) a medical information attention control group, where patients received booklets that explained their cancer and its treatment and brief telephone calls; (2) a patient-only counseling group, which involved the provision of medical information, coping education, and supportive counseling; or (3) the CanCOPE couple-based intervention group. The goal of the intervention was to enhance couples' ability to cope, reduce psychological distress, and promote better female body image and sexual adjustment. To accomplish this, CanCOPE focused largely on teaching individual coping skills and cognitive restructuring, but patients and partners were encouraged to support each other in applying these strategies. Compared with the medical information and patient-only study arms, CanCOPE produced a large increase in couples' supportive communication, a decrease in patients' psychological distress, and improvements in patients' sexual self-schema and intimacy with their partners. No differences between conditions were found with regarding couples' expression of warmth, validation, or negativity or in patients' levels of sexual responsiveness.

Porter and colleagues [14] randomly assigned 130 patients with gastrointestinal cancer and their partners to either four sessions of a partner-assisted emotional disclosure intervention or a couples' attention control group involving cancer education. The intervention was designed to systematically train patients and partners in strategies to facilitate the patients' disclosure of their cancer-related concerns and give patients the opportunity to talk with their partners about their concerns. The intervention was found to be effective for a subset of couples. Compared with couples enrolled in the attention control group, improvements in relationship quality and intimacy were found for couples in the intervention group in which the patients initially reported higher levels of holding back discussing cancer-related concerns.

Equity Theory. Some researchers have argued that for support to be beneficial, it must be reciprocal [50]. However, in the context of cancer, relationships may be affected by changes in the balance of give and take between partners [6]. Whereas support may have flowed back and forth between partners before the onset of illness, the exchange may become more one-sided with the healthy spouse's contributions to the relationship far exceeding those of the patient. According to equity theory, when the ratio of contributions to rewards for one partner differs from that of the other, the relationship is out of balance and those who are in inequitable relationships are more likely to become distressed [51], regardless of whether they are receiving more or less from their partners than what they are providing [52].

Kuijer and colleagues' [25] conducted a randomized trial with 59 couples. The intervention focused primarily on reducing feelings of inequity and restoring equity between the partners. Findings showed that the intervention significantly affected participants' perceptions of the give-and-take balance and relationship quality. However, because the perceptions of inequity between the intervention and wait-list control groups were significantly different at baseline, the authors could not conclude that the intervention was successful in reducing perceptions of inequity. Patients also reported lower levels of psychological distress after the intervention, but the intervention effects were not maintained at the 3-month follow-up.

Dyadic-Level Theories

Dyadic-level theories focus on the couple as the unit of study and examine the ongoing contributions that both partners make to preserve or improve the quality of their relationship as they strive to cope together with the cancer experience [6].

Relationship Intimacy Model. The relationship intimacy model of couples' psychosocial adaptation to cancer developed by Manne and Badr [6] posits that intimacy is a key mechanism by which relationship communication and interaction behaviors influence patient and partner adjustment. Specifically, the model proposes that relationship-enhancing and compromising behaviors can influence perceptions of relationship intimacy and that intimacy mediates the associations between these component processes and couples' psychosocial adaptation to cancer. Relationship-enhancing behaviors include the disclosure of concerns and feelings about the cancer experience, the sense that one is understood, cared for, and accepted by one's partner, and the view that cancer has implications for the relationship, whereas relationship-compromising behaviors include avoidance, criticism, and pressure-withdraw (e.g., when one partner pressures the other to discuss a cancer-related problem and the other partner withdraws).

Using this model, Manne and colleagues [19] compared a five-session intervention for men who had undergone prostatectomy and/or radiation therapy for prostate cancer and their wives to a usual care control group where patients received standard psychosocial care. The goals of the intervention were to assist couples to (1) learn ways to share their concerns about prostate cancer; (2) improve mutual understanding and support regarding one another's cancer experience; (3) engage in constructive and empathic communication regarding concerns about the loss of sexual functioning; (4) find ways to talk about feelings of shame, embarrassment, and any perceived loss of masculinity in a sensitive manner;

and (5) maintain emotional and sexual intimacy despite restrictions in sexuality. The intervention was only found to be effective for a subset of patients and partners. Specifically, patients who had higher levels of cancer concerns at pretreatment reported significant reductions in concerns posttreatment. Similarly, partners who began the intervention with higher cancer-specific distress, lower marital satisfaction, less marital intimacy, and poorer communication reported significant improvements in these outcomes after treatment.

Dyadic/Communal Coping. Broadly viewed, dyadic or communal coping recognizes mutuality and interdependence in coping responses to a specific shared stressor, indicating that couples respond to stressors as interpersonal units rather than as individuals in isolation. The construct of dyadic coping goes beyond the exchange of social support, although that is a central component in most definitions [53]. In dyadic coping, the members of the couple negotiate the emotional aspects of their shared experience [54] or engage in collaborative coping, such as joint problem solving [55], coordinating everyday demands, and relaxing together, as well as mutual calming, sharing, and expressions of solidarity. From this perspective, individual and relational well-being are believed to be affected by the couple's ability to work as a team to manage aspects of the stressor that affects both of them [56, 57]. Despite the fact that a dyadic or communal coping theory was not explicitly mentioned as the theoretical basis for intervention, three articles utilized elements of this model and are described below.

Baucom and colleagues' [26] relationship-enhancement intervention used cognitive behavioral techniques to teach couples to communicate effectively, share feelings and thoughts, and reach important decisions together as a team. The intervention also focused on both partners needs and emphasized addressing cancer-related problems as well as building positives in the couples' relationship. Results showed that both women and men in the relationship-enhancement intervention arm experienced improved psychological and relationship functioning at the postintervention and 1-year follow-ups compared to those in the control group arm where the patient received usual care. Women in the relationship-enhancement group also reported fewer medical symptoms at both follow-up time points.

Christensen [24] conducted an RCT with 20 patients with breast cancer and their partners. The therapy included educational component and a couples counseling component that was focused on communication, problem solving, and body image/sexuality. Compared with the control group who received standard care, the treatment resulted in modest decreases in emotional discomfort for both partners and patients, reduced depression in patients, and increased sexual satisfaction for both partners and patients. This study contained a number of elements common to behavioral marital therapy and dyadic-level theories; however, an explicit theoretical approach was not specified. This is likely due to the fact that this is the oldest couple-based intervention in cancer and was conducted prior to the publication of the dyadic-level theoretical models that are discussed in this chapter.

Kayser [58] examined the effects of the Partners in Coping Program (PICP) in a study of 63 patients with nonmetastatic breast cancer and their partners. The PICP consisted of nine 1-h sessions that patients and their partners attended together over the course of the first year following breast cancer diagnosis. The strategies utilized in the PICP were educational with some skills training in relaxation, communication, coping with changes in sexuality, and alternative ways of expressing intimacy. Compared to those in the control group who were offered standard social services, including the option to consult with a social worker at the hospital, patients in the PICP reported an increase in dyadic coping 6 months postbaseline, suggesting that the intervention may have facilitated a sense of *"we-ness"* in coping with the illness. However, these gains in patient-reported dyadic coping were not maintained at the 12-month follow-up. In contrast, partners in the PICP reported increases in their willingness to communicate their own stress to the patient over the 12-month period relative to those in the control group, and both patients and partners in the PICP reported improvements in psychosocial adjustment over time.

Interventions with No Explicit or Implied Theory

The seven intervention studies that did not have an explicit or implied theoretical framework are described in greater detail below. Most assessed general or cancer-specific mental health outcomes and sought to ameliorate the couple's distress. One study focused specifically on addressing attitudes about pain and analgesic use [59], and two studies included components to address cancer-specific symptoms (pain and bowel/urinary functioning) [28, 30]. Four interventions included components to address or to enhance sexual rehabilitation and body image [17, 18, 22, 31]; only two of these interventions included a component that focused explicitly on addressing changes in the couples' relationship and improving the marital relationship [22, 29].

Campbell and colleagues' [29] partner-assisted coping skills training (CST) telephone-based intervention was developed for prostate cancer survivors and their intimate partners. The goal of the six-session program was to assist couples in learning to manage symptoms by providing information about prostate cancer and possible long-term side effects, teaching problem-solving and coping skills, and improving relationship communication. Compared with the control group who received usual care, the CST intervention produced moderate to large treatment effects for disease-specific QOL, such as bowel function, and urinary, sexual, and hormonal function domains. For partners, no significant differences were found between the treatment and control groups on the general health QOL and self-efficacy scores; however partners in the intervention arm reported modest improvements in depressive symptoms and fatigue.

Giesler and colleagues [30] conducted an intervention aimed at improving QOL for prostate cancer patients and their partners. Participants in the intervention arm met once a month for 6 months with an oncology nurse who helped them identify their QOL needs using an interactive computer program. The nurse then provided education and support tailored to the individual needs of the patient. Results showed that patients in the intervention condition experienced long-term improvements in QOL outcomes related to sexual functioning and cancer worry compared with the control group who received usual care.

Keefe and colleagues [20] conducted a partner-guided pain management training intervention for patients who were facing the end of life. The three-session intervention conducted in patients' homes integrated educational information about cancer pain with systematic training of patients and partners in cognitive and behavioral pain coping skills. When compared with usual care, the intervention did not have a significant impact on patients' QOL; however, it did produce significant increases in partners' ratings of their self-efficacy for helping the patient control pain and self-efficacy for controlling other symptoms. Partners enrolled in the intervention also reported modest improvements in their levels of caregiver strain compared with partners in the control group.

McCorkle and colleagues [22] conducted an RCT to examine the effects of a standardized nursing intervention protocol designed to improve patients' and their spouses' depressive symptoms, sexual function, and marital interaction after prostate cancer. A total of 16 contacts (home visits and telephone calls) were made with patients and their spouses over 8 weeks; each intervention session had content that was specifically relevant to the patient, the spouse, and the patient and spouse as a couple. Results showed that compared to usual care, the intervention had a modest positive effect on patients' sexual function and marital interaction over time; however, patients in the intervention group reported greater distress over time. Similar outcomes were found for spouses.

Kalaitzi and colleagues [31] conducted a study on a structured combination of brief couples therapy and sex therapy for breast cancer patients and their partners. Session content included education, communication training, and sensate focus exercises and addressed body image concerns. Compared with patients in the control group who received usual medical care, patients who received the intervention experienced less depression and anxiety at follow-up; patients in the intervention arm also experienced improved body image, expressed greater satisfaction with their relationship, and reported greater orgasm frequency.

The three remaining studies that did not have an explicit or implied theoretical basis compared the efficacy of a couples' intervention condition to both a usual care control group and a patient-only intervention [23, 27, 28]. Mishel and colleagues [23] conducted an uncertainty management intervention that was delivered over the telephone to couples coping with localized prostate cancer. Patients who received the intervention—either alone (second intervention arm) or supplemented with a family member, the majority of whom were spouses (couples intervention arm)—participated in a weekly telephone call for 8 consecutive weeks with a nurse. Patients and their family members (in the couples intervention arm) received separate phone calls; nurses were matched with the patient and family member by ethnicity and gender. The nurse assessed the patient's concerns, perceived level of threat, and uncertainty related to the prostate cancer. The intervention consisted of cognitive reframing exercises, problem solving, and techniques for improving patient–provider communication. Both individual and couple interventions were effective in reducing uncertainty than was usual care; however, partners in the couples group did not fare any better than those in the individual group on the primary outcome of uncertainty.

Nezu and colleagues [27] examined the efficacy of problem-solving therapy among people diagnosed with different types of cancer. These researchers incorporated a significant other (95 % of whom were spouses) as a "coach" to assist the patient in learning coping skills. Distressed patients were randomly assigned to receive ten sessions of individual problem-solving skills training, ten sessions of problems-solving skills training with a significant other present to provide support and coaching, or a wait-list control group. Although there were no significant differences between the two problem-solving skills training groups, participants in both problem-solving skills training groups reported lower distress and better clinician ratings of functioning than did participants in the wait-list control group.

Ward and colleagues [28] attempted to overcome patient and partner attitudinal barriers to reporting cancer pain and using analgesics through education. One hundred sixty-one patients with different types of cancer were randomized to a couples intervention (patient and significant other received the intervention), solo intervention (only the patient received the intervention), or usual care. Although the intervention content was not theory-based, the authors did note that the process by which they delivered intervention materials to participants was based on a representational approach to patient education [60]. Participants received education about managing cancer pain and overcoming misconceptions and barriers. In the last session, they created a plan for changing the way they managed cancer pain. Results showed that the intervention was no more efficacious when it was presented to dyads than to patients alone. However, participants in the two intervention groups reported significant decreases in attitudinal barriers compared to those in the control group.

The conclusions that can be drawn from these three studies regarding the efficacy of couple-based interventions compared with patient-only interventions are limited because the role of the partner was primarily supportive (in terms of what he/she could do to help the patient), and the studies did not focus on addressing couples' interaction patterns or the impact of cancer on the couple's relationship. These factors would appear to be important components of a couples' intervention approach given that Scott and colleagues' [17] CanCOPE intervention had an implied theoretical basis, focused on couples' relationship and interaction patterns, and was found to be effective relative to a patient-only intervention and an attention control group. More research is thus needed to determine the circumstances under which partners should be included in interventions, the optimal degree of the partner's involvement, and whether couple-based interventions that focus on the needs of both patients and partners and their relationship interaction patterns are more effective than those targeting the patient alone.

Summary and Directions for Future Research

As our review suggests, there is a growing literature on psychological interventions for couples coping with cancer. Owing to the varied or sometimes absent theoretical basis, the varied intervention approaches used, and the diversity in outcomes reported, it is difficult to discern a clear pattern. Overall, most studies had at least some positive results. Those that were aimed at improving communication, reciprocal understanding, and intimacy appeared to be effective in reducing distress and improving relationship functioning in one or both partners. However, three studies [14, 19, 38] found that such interventions seemed to benefit only a subset of couples—particularly those who have poorer functioning relationships, greater cancer-related distress or concerns, or poor communication skills at the outset. More research is needed to determine whether there are certain profiles of at-risk couples who may benefit from such interventions.

This review highlights a number of clear limitations in the couples' intervention literature. Most studies had small sample sizes and thus were largely underpowered to examine changes in multiple outcomes over time. Several did not report on outcomes for the patient's partner; those that did often demonstrated unequal effectiveness for patients and their partners and/or a limited maintenance of improvements over time. Whereas the standard dose of cognitive behavior therapy is 8–12 sessions, the majority of interventions were comparatively brief, comprising six sessions or less. This is no doubt reflective of the difficulty of recruiting and retaining cancer patients who are often undergoing active treatment. It remains unclear how the length of treatment, number of treatments, or timing of intervention may have affected study outcomes. In addition, several studies did not include important information related to their refusal or attrition rates, suggesting that reporting standards need to improve.

Almost half of the interventions reviewed seemed to be based on theory, though several

researchers did not explicitly acknowledge a theoretical basis for their interventions. Few studies examined the mechanisms by which interventions impacted psychosocial outcomes; thus, there are limitations as to whether the theoretical basis of the intervention was as hypothesized. In the studies without a theoretical basis, intervention elements were largely dependent on cognitive behavioral techniques. Most included an educational component, and communication and symptom management training. It is interesting to note that while some interventions addressed cancer-specific issues (e.g., uncertainty, need for medical information, and problems communicating with providers or partners about cancer-related concerns), the vast majority of intervention content was similar to either couples therapy interventions developed for healthy populations or cognitive behavior interventions geared toward individuals coping with cancer. In addition, the vast majority of studies were geared toward couples where the patient was newly diagnosed and had early-stage cancer. The longest follow-up was 12-month postintervention. Given that the demands couples face change as cancer progresses [61] and long-term cancer survivors may experience different stressors than couples coping with the acute stages of the disease, it is important to assess the ongoing adaptation of couples to cancer over longer periods and to determine whether booster sessions are needed to maintain the impact of intervention.

Cognitive behavior therapy and behavioral marital therapy were the most commonly used therapeutic techniques in the studies we reviewed. It is noteworthy that none of the studies used emotion-focused therapy (which focuses on restructuring interpersonal patterns to incorporate each partner's needs for experiencing secure attachment) [62], despite it being the second most common therapeutic technique used in couples therapy [8]. Perhaps one reason for this is that the majority of studies focused on improving individual psychological outcomes; few studies examined the impact of the intervention on dyadic-level or relationship outcomes, even though most interventions included components to improve couples' interaction patterns, joint problem solving, and dyadic coping. Likewise, disease-specific QOL outcomes were rarely the primary focus of the couples' interventions.

A significant number of interventions were either offered exclusively via telephone or in combination with in-person sessions. Telephone interventions may allow therapists to reach couples who do not have local resources, who live in rural areas, or who are immobile. Additionally, couples who are not comfortable with traditional face-to-face interventions may prefer the anonymity offered through telephone counseling [63]. More research is needed to determine whether telephone interventions conducted with couples are as effective or are more effective than in-person interventions and whether telephone interventions with couples are logistically practical and cost-effective.

This review highlights a number of gaps in the literature on couples' interventions in cancer. First, there were no interventions focusing on health or lifestyle behavior changes following a cancer diagnosis. Even though the second intervention arm in the study by Badger and colleagues [15] involved an exercise component, exercise was not a component of their intervention content for couples. Second, none of the studies focused exclusively on sexual functioning issues, even though this was a component in a few studies. It is noteworthy that such studies do not examine sexual functioning from a dyadic perspective. Third, all of the studies used similar modes of intervention delivery (i.e., in-person visits or telephone calls), which might not be desirable or feasible for all couples facing cancer. We now turn our discussion to each of these issues as potential avenues for future research.

The Need for Couples' Interventions Targeting Lifestyle Behavioral Change

The social cognitive theory [64], one of the most robust models of behavior change, posits that individuals acquire behavioral routines by performing them, being reinforced for performance, and observing others. In the behavior change process, we are more likely to change when (1) we receive support from others who make us feel capable, express confidence in us, and provide specific feedback on our performance; (2) we see others modeling desired behaviors; and (3) we successfully perform the behaviors ourselves [17, 64]. Thus, interventions that include the patient's spouse, the patient's most important source of support [65], may be more powerful in promoting the cancer patient's long-term behavior change.

However, if not carefully designed and implemented, such interventions may seek to enlist the spouse to "help" the cancer patient make behavior changes but instead may leave the patient feeling controlled or overprotected. This may explain why behavior change studies enlisting spouses only as supporters have reported limited success [66]. Consideration of social support within the context of theories such as Self-Determination Theory [67] may enhance the understanding that *how* support is provided is important. Specifically, this theory emphasizes the provision of autonomous support such that the receiver of support actually feels a sense of volition, choice, and control. Exerting social control tactics (e.g., demanding, threatening, criticizing, or using guilt) can actually have a negative effect on health behavior change. For example, Helgeson and colleagues [68] found from interviews of men with prostate cancer that if their wives used social control over health-comprising behaviors like smoking, it was associated with poor health behavior. It also was associated with greater psychological distress.

Recently, it has been suggested that behavior change interventions may be most effective if they consider the interdependence of the couple—how one partner's attitude and behavior supports his/her own behavior change as well as that of the other partner. Thus, motivation for behavior change requires both members to engage in behaviors that serve the best interest of the relationship (relationship-centered) rather than the best interest of oneself (person-centered) [69]. When motivation is transformed from being self-centered to relationship-centered, it increases the couple's confidence that they can successfully cope together. For this communal coping to be effective, partners must develop a sense of confidence that together, they can plan, coordinate, and execute their strategies and that their joint behaviors will increase their mutual benefit and lessen their individual risk. Encouraging both partners to adopt and maintain healthy behaviors is particularly important since there is a strong concordance between spousal health behaviors [70] and spousal health behavior change [71].

Couple-based interventions are consistent with theories of behavior change such as Social Cognitive Theory, which emphasize the importance of social influence on the process of behavior change [64], and Self-Determination Theory [67]. The format encourages couples to model healthy behaviors for each other; observing one another's success can increase each partner's confidence. In the process, couples learn to provide one another with support and feedback regarding goal setting and to work together to solve problems and overcome barriers. They also develop skills in working together to enlist support from their environments. Finally, this process of making behavioral changes together (e.g., taking walks or preparing meals) can help couples create positive memories that make them more likely to want to continue behavior change efforts. Couples working together as they set individual and couple-focused goals will likely increase their success in changing their behaviors. Indeed, couples report that having their partner perform and model goal behaviors, join in discussions of health issues, and provide emotional support encourages their own behavior change [72].

Currently, support for such a model has shown promise for increased screening for colorectal cancer, with higher attendance rates for those invited to attend screening with their partner, compared with those who were invited to attend alone [73]. A recent review of the role of social support in smoking cessation points to the mixed results for social networks, including spouses, to enhance intervention efficacy. However, the review highlights that findings may possibly be a

function of how support was provided [74]. Thus, studies examining the efficacy of support in improving behavior change outcomes must be based on a guiding conceptual framework in which possible theoretical mediators for behavior change are studied. By using this approach, we may learn why, when, and for whom partner support promotes behavior change [9, 74].

The Need for Sexual Functioning Interventions to Take a Dyadic Perspective

Physical intimacy is vital to maintaining satisfying relationships and may reduce emotional distress [75]. Virtually all cancers and their treatments (i.e., surgery, radiation therapy, chemotherapy, and hormone therapy) either directly or indirectly affect patients' sexual function [76]. Despite this, the vast majority of studies addressing sexual problems in cancer patients have been confined to problems that directly affect the reproductive and sexual organs. This finding is surprising because cancers that do not directly involve a sexual organ (e.g., hematopoietic cancers) may also indirectly affects sexual function via treatment side effects such as fatigue, pain, nausea, decreased sexual desire, and vaginal dryness and dyspareunia in women and erectile dysfunction in men.

Although there have been no couple-based interventions meeting our search criteria that strictly target sexual concerns from a dyadic perspective, couples' interventions such as CanCOPE [17], relationship enhancement [26], and Kalaitzi's [31] sexual counseling program have included body image and sexual components and have shown to be effective. However, all of these studies were in female cancers (e.g., breast and gynecological cancer). Canada and colleagues [77] conducted a counseling intervention aimed at improving levels of sexual satisfaction for prostate cancer survivors who had been treated with radical prostatectomy or radiation therapy and their partners. Couples were randomized to attend four sessions of counseling together or to have the man attend alone. Because the study did not include a usual care control group, it did not meet our inclusion criteria and was not included in our review. Session content included education about prostate cancer, sexual function, erectile dysfunction treatment options, and sexual communication and stimulation skills. Compared with patients in the patient-only intervention arm, patients in the couples' intervention arm reported improvement in psychological distress, and patients and their partners reported improvement in sexual function at the 3-month follow-up; however, these treatment gains were not sustained at the 6-month follow-up.

Because patients and partners are likely to be of a similar age and experiencing the physical consequences of the aging process [78, 79], examining sexual concerns from a dyadic perspective is important. Indeed, it is well documented that within couples, sexual dysfunctions coexist [80, 81], and in cancer, research has shown that patient and partner sexual function is moderately to highly correlated ($r = 0.30$ to 0.74) [82]. Even in cases where the partner is not experiencing sexual problems, he or she may experience increased distress and decreased marital satisfaction as a function of the loss in sexual and nonsexual intimacy with the patient [83]. Patients and partners may avoid discussing sexual concerns because they feel that the changes in sexual and nonsexual intimacy are time limited and that they will return back to normal after treatment. However, for many, these changes are long-lasting [84], and research has shown that open discussions about sexual concerns may help to alleviate the negative impact that sexual problems have on both partners' adjustment [82]. Given this, interventions that address both partners' sexual function concerns, facilitate healthy spousal communication, and help couples to set realistic goals and manage sexual expectations after cancer treatment may prove beneficial for both partners' adjustment. Further research is needed to determine whether taking a dyadic approach is useful in both male and female cancers that affect sexual organs as well as in cancers affecting both genders that do not affect a sexual organ but still affect sexual functioning (e.g., head and neck or blood cancers).

The Need for New Intervention Modalities

While research supports the efficacy of in-person couples-based interventions for cancer patients and their partners, questions arise about generalizability, as most studies include primarily white, educated patients. Such demographics likely reflect who has access and ability to attend these programs, excluding patients residing in rural areas or areas distant from their care center, patients with limited resources and/or transportation problems, and patients with physical limitations that make travel difficult. Thus, employing interventions that can be widely disseminated is critical to advancing science and providing equal access for disparate populations. Emerging technologies—including the Internet, the telephone, and videoconferencing via the Internet or the telephone—allow for more widespread dissemination of psychosocial interventions through "remote counseling" [85].

Public Internet use continues to expand. According to the 2010 PEW Internet Report [86], Internet use was reported by 79 % of the adult population, and 66 % of adults have broadband access in their homes. The digital divide is closing in minority groups as 71 % of non-Hispanic blacks and 82 % of English-speaking Hispanics use the Internet. The multiple advantages of using the Internet for intervention delivery include reduced costs, increased convenience for users, improved access to isolated or stigmatized groups, and timeliness of access to the Internet [87]. In online support groups, participants share a high level of personal disclosure and openness, which is likely secondary to anonymity. The social equality that comes from this anonymity, the increased access to other survivors, and the potentially greater opportunity for self-expression are all features that may make the Internet a viable modality for delivering future couple-based interventions [88].

Videoconferencing is another means by which couple-based interventions could be delivered. The benefit of this modality is that communication would occur in real time with the added benefit of verbal and nonverbal cues. A counselor can moderate the discussion and ensure participants the opportunity to participate in the discussion. Such interventions could occur by Internet or telephone [85]. Internet-based videoconferencing could occur through the use of a computer with a webcam and an appropriate videoconferencing platform. Couples could access the Internet from home, work or even during travel. Another alternative is to provide the videoconferencing system through the telephone, which couples could access at a location of their choice. Existing studies with cancer patients have examined the use of videophones to deliver psychosocial interventions in an individual format [89, 90]. Studies consistently show the feasibility of using the videophone technology even with very ill patients, including terminally ill cancer patients diagnosed with adjustment disorder or major depression [89] and dying patients [90]. More research is needed to determine the intervention preferences of couples coping with cancer and whether factors such as patient advanced disease status, age, or comfort with technology affect receptivity to such interventions.

Conclusion

Cancer takes a toll on both patients and their partners, and targeting the couple in psychosocial interventions is an approach that merits further investigation. Two areas that appear to be fruitful for future intervention include expanding choice of outcomes to include health behaviors and designing sexual interventions that include both patients and their partners and that address both of their sexual functioning concerns. At the same time, efforts are needed to strengthen future studies both conceptually and methodologically. For example, few RCTs have been designed to compare couple- and patient-oriented approaches, making it difficult to evaluate the relative efficacy of a couples approach. The majority of studies reviewed did not specify how theory was used in the development of intervention materials, did not examine mediators of intervention efficacy, and did not report on outcomes for partners; thus, existing research provides an incomplete picture regarding efficacy. More research is needed to determine whether intervention modality affects intervention efficacy and whether technologically based interventions are easier to disseminate and are cost-effective. Finally, questions remain regarding at what point in the illness and treatment trajectory couples' interventions should be delivered, and how long the interventions should continue. Despite these issues, this review indicates that couples interventions appear to have beneficial effects in terms of improving psychosocial outcomes such as distress or couples functioning.

References

1. Pistrang N, Barker C. The partner relationship in psychological response to breast cancer. Soc Sci Med. 1995;40:789–97.
2. Carlson L, Bultz B, Speca M, St. Pierre M. Partners of cancer patients: part 1. Impact, adjustment, and coping across the illness trajectory. J Psychosoc Oncol. 2000;18:39–57.
3. Manne S, Badr H. Social relationships and cancer. In: Davila J, Sullivan K, editors. Support processes in intimate relationships. Oxford: Oxford Press; 2010. p. 240–64.
4. Baider L, Kaufman B, Peretz T, Manor O, Ever-Hadani P, Kaplan De-Nour A. Mutuality of fate adaptation and psychological distress in cancer patients and their partners. In: Baider L, Cooper C, Kaplan De-Nour A, editors. Cancer in the family. Chichester: Wiley; 1996. p. 173–86.
5. Ell K, Nishimoto R, Mantell J, Hamovitch M. Longitudinal analysis of psychological adaptation among family members of patients with cancer. J Psychosom Res. 1988;32:429.
6. Manne S, Badr H. Intimacy and relationship processes in couples' psychosocial adaptation to cancer. Cancer. 2008;112(11 Suppl):2541–55.
7. Scott JL, Kayser K. A review of couple-based interventions for enhancing women's sexual adjustment and body image after cancer. Cancer J. 2009;15(1):48–56.
8. Baik OM, Adams KB. Improving the well being of couples facing cancer: a review of couples based psychosocial interventions. J Marital Fam Ther. 2011;37(2):250–66.
9. Martire LM, Schulz R, Helgeson VS, Small BJ, Saghafi EM. Review and meta-analysis of couple-oriented interventions for chronic illness. Ann Behav Med. 2010;40(3):325–42.
10. Rogers SN, Ahad SA, Murphy AP. A structured review and theme analysis of papers published on 'quality of life' in head and neck cancer: 2000–2005. Oral Oncol. 2007;43(9):843–68.
11. Murphy BA, Ridner S, Wells N, Dietrich M. Quality of life research in head and neck cancer: a review of the current state of the science. Crit Rev Oncol Hematol. 2007;62(3):251–67.

12. Sutherland SE, Matthews DC. Conducting systematic reviews and creating clinical practice guidelines in dentistry: lessons learned. J Am Dent Assoc. 2004; 135(6):747.

13. Manne SL, Winkel G, Grana G, et al. Couple-focused group intervention for women with early stage breast cancer. J Consult Clin Psychol. 2005;73(4):634–46.

14. Porter LS, Keefe FJ, Baucom DH, et al. Partner assisted emotional disclosure for patients with gastro-intestinal cancer. Cancer. 2009;115(S18):4326–38.

15. Badger T, Segrin C, Dorros SM, Meek P, Lopez AM. Depression and anxiety in women with breast cancer and their partners. Nurs Res. 2007;56(1):44.

16. Budin WC, Hoskins CN, Haber J, et al. Breast cancer: education, counseling, and adjustment among patients and partners: a randomized clinical trial. Nurs Res. 2008;57(3):199.

17. Scott J, Halford W, Ward B. United we stand? The effects of a couple-coping intervention on adjustment to early stage breast or gynecological cancer. J Consult Clin Psychol. 2004;72(6):1122.

18. Kayser K, Feldman BN, Borstelmann NA, Daniels AA. Effects of a randomized couple-based intervention on quality of life of breast cancer patients and their partners. Soc Work Res. 2010;34(1):20–32.

19. Manne SL, Nelson CJ, Kissane DW, Mulhall JP, Winkel G, Zaider T. Intimacy enhancing psychological intervention for men diagnosed with prostate cancer and their partners: a pilot study. J Sex Med. 2011;8(4):1197–209.

20. Keefe FJ, Ahles TA, Sutton L, et al. Partner-guided cancer pain management at the end of life: a preliminary study. J Pain Symptom Manage. 2005;29(3):263–72.

21. Northouse L, Mood D, Schafenacker A, et al. Randomized clinical trial of a family intervention for prostate cancer patients and their spouses. Cancer. 2007;110(12):2809–18.

22. McCorkle R, Siefert M, Dowd M, Robinson J, Pickett M. Effects of advanced practice nursing on patient and spouse depressive symptoms, sexual function, and marital interaction after radical prostatectomy. Urol Nurs. 2007;27:65–77.

23. Mishel MH, Belyea M, Germino BB, et al. Helping patients with localized prostate carcinoma manage uncertainty and treatment side effects: nurse-delivered psychoeducational intervention over the telephone. Cancer. 2002;94(6):1854–66.

24. Christensen DN. Postmastectomy couple counseling: an outcome study of a structured treatment protocol. J Sex Marital Ther. 1983;9(4):266–75.

25. Kuijer RG, Buunk BP, Majella De Jong G, Ybema JF, Sanderman R. Effects of a brief intervention program for patients with cancer and their partners on feelings of inequity, relationship quality, and psychological distress. Psychooncology. 2004;13:321–34.

26. Baucom DH, Porter LS, Kirby JS, et al. A couple-based intervention for female breast cancer. Psychooncology. 2009;18(3):276–83.

27. Nezu AM, Nezu CM, Felgoise SH, McClure KS, Houts PS. Project genesis: assessing the efficacy of problem-solving therapy for distressed adult cancer patients. J Consult Clin Psychol. 2003;71(6):1036.

28. Ward SE, Serlin RC, Donovan HS, et al. A randomized trial of a representational intervention for cancer pain: does targeting the dyad make a difference? Health Psychol. 2009;28(5):588–97.

29. Campbell LC, Keefe FJ, McKee DC, et al. Prostate cancer in African Americans: relationship of patient and partner self-efficacy to quality of life. J Pain Symptom Manage. 2004;28(5):433–44.

30. Giesler RB, Given B, Given CW, et al. Improving the quality of life of patients with prostate carcinoma. Cancer. 2005;104(4):752–62.

31. Kalaitzi C, Papadopoulos VP, Michas K, Vlasis K, Skandalakis P, Filippou D. Combined brief psychosexual intervention after mastectomy: effects on sexuality, body image, and psychological well-being. J Surg Oncol. 2007;96(3):235–40.

32. Badger T, Segrin C, Meek P, Lopez AM, Bonham E. A case study of telephone interpersonal counseling for women with breast cancer and their partners. Oncol Nurs Forum. 2004;31(5):997–1003.

33. Alexander JF, Holtzworth-Munroe A, Jameson PB. The process and outcome of marital and family therapy: research review and evaluation. In: Bergin AE, Garfield SL, editors. Handbook of psychotherapy and behavior change. 4th ed. New York: Wiley; 1994. p. 595–630.

34. Jacobson NS, Margolin G. Marital therapy: strategies based on social learning and behavior exchange principles. New York: Brunner/Mazel; 1979.

35. Jacobson NS, Schmaling KB, Holtzworth-Munroe A. A component analysis of behavioral marital therapy: two-year follow-up and prediction of relapse. J Marital Fam Ther. 1987;13:187–95.

36. Gottman J, Notarius CI, Markman HJ, Banks D, Yoppi B, Rubin ME. Behavior exchange theory and marital decision making. J Pers Soc Psychol. 1976;34:14–23.

37. Christensen A. Dysfunctional interaction patterns in couples. In: Noller P, Fitzpatrick M, editors. Perspectives on marital interaction. Philadelphia: Multilingual Matters; 1988. p. 30–52.

38. Manne S, Ostroff JS, Winkel G, et al. Couple-focused group intervention for women with early stage breast cancer. J Consult Clin Psychol. 2005;73(4):634–46.

39. Thoits PA. Social support as coping assistance. J Consult Clin Psychol. 1986;54:416–23.

40. Lazarus RS, Folkman S. Stress appraisal and coping. New York: Springer; 1984.

41. Lepore SJ. A social-cognitive processing model of emotional adjustment to cancer. In: Baum A, Andersen BL, editors. Psychosocial interventions for cancer. Washington DC: American Psychological Association; 2001. p. 99–116.

42. Green BL, Epstein SA, Krupnick JL, Rowland JH. Trauma and medical illness: assessing trauma-related disorders in medical settings. In: Wilson JP, Keane TM, editors. Assessing psychological trauma and PTSD. New York: The Guilford Press; 1997. p. 160–91.

43. Redd WH, DuHamel KN, Johnson Vickberg SM, et al. Long-term adjustment in cancer survivors: integration of classical-conditioning and cognitive processing models. In: Baum A, Andersen BL, editors. Psychosocial interventions for cancer. Washington DC: American Psychological Association; 2001. p. 77–97.

44. Foa EB, Steketee G, Rothbaum BO. Behavioral/cognitive conceptualizations of post-traumatic stress disorder. Behav Ther. 1989;20:155–76.

45. Manne SL, Ostroff JS, Winkel G, Grana G, Fox K. Couple focused intervention for breast cancer patients and their spouses. Psychooncology. 2004;13(8):315.

46. Badr H, Carmack Taylor C. Social constraints and spousal communication in lung cancer. Psychooncology. 2006;15(8):673–83.

47. Cordova M, Cunningham LL, Carlson C, Andrykowski M. Posttraumatic growth following breast cancer: a controlled comparison study. Health Psychol. 2001;20:176–85.

48. Lepore SJ, Helgeson V. Social constraints, intrusive thoughts, and mental health in prostate cancer survivors. J Soc Clin Psychol. 1998;17:89–106.

49. Manne S, Alfieri T, Taylor KL, Dougherty J. Spousal negative responses to cancer patients: the role of social restriction, spouse mood, and relationship satisfaction. J Consult Clin Psychol. 1999;67(3):352–61.

50. Revenson TA, Majerovitz SD. Spouses' support provision to chronically ill patients. J Soc Pers Relat. 1990;7:575–86.

51. Walster E, Walster GW, Berscheid E. Equity: theory and research. Boston: Allyn & Bacon; 1978.

52. Buunk BP, Mutsaers W. Equity perceptions and marital satisfaction in former and current marriage: a study among the remarried. J Soc Pers Relat. 1999;16:123–32.

53. Berg CA, Upchurch R. A developmental-contextual model of couples coping with chronic illness across the adult life span. Psychol Bull. 2007;133(6):920–54.

54. Coyne JC, Smith DAF. Couples coping with a myocardial-infarction—a contextual perspective on wives distress. J Pers Soc Psychol. 1991;61(3):404–12.

55. Berg CA, Wiebe DJ, Butner J, et al. Collaborative coping and daily mood in couples dealing with prostate cancer. Psychol Aging. 2008;23(3):505–16.

56. Bodenmann G. Dyadic coping—a systemic-transactional view of stress and coping among couples: theory and empirical findings. Eur Rev Appl Psychol. 1997;47:137–40.

57. Bodenmann G. Dyadic coping and its significance for marital functioning. In: Revenson TA, Kayser K, Bodenmann G, editors. Couples coping with stress: emerging perspectives on dyadic coping. Washington DC: American Psychological Association; 2005. p. 33–50.

58. Kayser K. Enhancing dyadic coping during a time of crisis: a theory-based intervention with breast cancer patients and their partners. In: Revenson TA, Kayser K, Bodenmann G, editors. The psychology of couples

and illness. Washington DC: American Psychological Association; 2005. p. 175–91.

59. Keefe FJ, Abernethy AP, C Campbell L. Psychological approaches to understanding and treating disease-related pain. Annu Rev Psychol. 2005;56(1):601–30.

60. Donovan HS, Ward SE, Song MK, Heidrich SM, Gunnarsdottir S, Phillips CM. An update on the representational approach to patient education. J Nurs Scholarsh. 2007;39(3):259–65.

61. McLean LM, Jones JM. A review of distress and its management in couples facing end-of-life cancer. Psychooncology. 2007;16(7):603–16.

62. Johnson S, Greenberg L. The emotionally focused approach to problems in adult attachment. In: Jacobson N, Gurman A, editors. Clinical handbook of couple therapy. New York: Guilford; 1995. p. 121–41.

63. Gotay CC, Bottomley A. Providing psycho-social support by telephone: what is its potential in cancer patients? Eur J Cancer Care. 1998;7:225–31.

64. Bandura A. Social foundations of thought and action: a social-cognitive theory. Englewood Cliffs, NJ: Prentice-Hall; 1986.

65. Neuling S, Winefield H. Social support and recovery after surgery for breast cancer: frequency and correlates of supportive behaviors by family, friends, and surgeon. Soc Sci Med. 1988;27:385–92.

66. McBride CM, Baucom DH, Peterson BL, et al. Prenatal and postpartum smoking abstinence: a partner-assisted approach. Am J Prev Med. 2004;27(3):232–8.

67. Ryan RM, Deci EL. Self-determination theory and the facilitation of intrinsic motivation, social development, and well-being. Am Psychol. 2000;55(1):68–78.

68. Helgeson VS, Novak SA, Lepore SJ, Eton DT. Spouse social control efforts: relations to health behavior and well-being among men with prostate cancer. J Soc Pers Relat. 2004;21:53–68.

69. Lewis MA, McBride CM, Pollak KI, Puleo E, Butterfield RM, Emmons KM. Understanding health behavior change among couples: an interdependence and communal coping approach. Soc Sci Med. 2006;62:1369–80.

70. Meyler D, Stimpson JP, Peek MK. Health concordance within couples: a systematic review. Soc Sci Med. 2007;64:2297–310.

71. Falba TA, Sindelar JL. Spousal concordance in health behavior change. Health Serv Res. 2008;43:96–116.

72. Tucker JS, Mueller JS. Spouses' Social control of health behaviors: use and effectiveness of specific strategies. Pers Soc Psychol Bull. 2000;26:1120–30.

73. van Jaarsveld CHM, Miles A, Edwards R, Wardle J. Marriage and cancer prevention: does marital status and inviting both spouses together influence colorectal cancer screening participation? J Med Screen. 2006;13:172–6.

74. Westmaas JL, Bontemps-Jones J, Bauer JE. Social support in smoking cessation: reconciling theory and evidence. Nicotine Tob Res. 2010;12(7):695–707.

75. Hordern AJ, Currow DC. A patient-centred approach to sexuality in the face of life-limiting illness. Med J Aust. 2003;179(6):8.

76. Sadovsky R, Basson R, Krychman M, et al. Cancer and sexual problems. J Sex Med. 2010;7(1pt2):349–73.

77. Canada AL, Neese LE, Sui D, Schover LR. Pilot intervention to enhance sexual rehabilitation for couples after treatment for localized prostate carcinoma. Cancer. 2005;104(12):2689–700.

78. Revenson TA. Social support and marital coping with chronic illness. Ann Behav Med. 1994;16:122–30.

79. Hayes R, Dennerstein L. The impact of aging on sexual function and sexual dysfunction in women: a review of population-based studies. J Sex Med. 2005;2(3):317–30.

80. Fugl-Meyer A, Fugl-Meyer K. Sexual disabilities are not singularities. Int J Impot Res. 2002;14:487–93.

81. Crowe H, Costello AJ. Prostate cancer: perspectives on quality of life and impact of treatment on patients and their partners. Urol Nurs. 2003;23(4):279.

82. Badr H, Taylor CLC. Sexual dysfunction and spousal communication in couples coping with prostate cancer. Psychooncology. 2009;18(7):735–46.

83. Sanders S, Pedro LW, Bantum EO, Galbraith ME. Couples surviving prostate cancer: long-term intimacy needs and concerns following treatment. Clin J Oncol Nurs. 2006;10(4):503–8.

84. Boehmer U, Babayan RK. Facing erectile dysfunction due to prostate cancer treatment: perspectives of men and their partners. Cancer Invest. 2004;22(6):840–8.

85. Shepherd L, Goldstein D, Olver I, Parle M. Enhancing psychological care for people with cancer in rural communities: what can remote counselling offer? Aust Health Rev. 2008;32(3):423–38.

86. Pew Internet & American Life Project. http://www.pewinternet.org. Accessed 20 Oct 2010.

87. Griffiths F, Lindenmeyer A, Powell J, Lowe P, Thorogood M. Why are health care interventions delivered over the internet? A systematic review of the published literature. J Med Internet Res. 2006;8(2):e10.

88. Owen JE, Bantum EO, Golant M. Benefits and challenges experienced by professional facilitators of online support groups for cancer survivors. Psychooncology. 2009;18(2):144–55.

89. Cluver JS, Schuyler D, Frueh BC, Brescia F, Arana GW. Remote psychotherapy for terminally ill cancer patients. J Telemed Telecare. 2005;11(3):157–9.

90. Passik SD, Kirsh KL, Leibee S, et al. A feasibility study of Dignity Psychotherapy delivered via telemedicine. Palliat Support Care. 2004;2:149–55.

The Impact of Cancer and Its Therapies on Body Image and Sexuality

12

Susan V. Carr

Introduction

Sexuality is the combination of gender identity, sexual orientation, sexual attitude, knowledge, and behavior. While gender identity and sexual orientation are of biopsychosocial origin, sexual behavior is socioculturally determined, and will change over the course of a lifetime. The impact of cancer on an individual's sexuality is enormous and overwhelmingly negative in most cases.

For ease of understanding in the clinical context, sexuality can be thought of as being composed of gender identity, sexual orientation together with sexual attitudes and behavior, all of which combined are fundamental to the human sexual response [1].

Gender identity is usually described at birth with approximately half of the population being male and half female. It is biologically determined, and carries legal and societal implications. Gender identity is a fundamental determinant of future biopsychosocial development. A very small proportion of the population are transsexual or intersex; however these conditions do not become apparent until later in life, when a gender identity has already been assigned. Although most of the research and literature in

relation to sexuality focuses on women's cancers, men are 40% more likely to die of cancer than women, and prostate, testicular, and penile cancers all affect men's sexuality in particular, while all cancers have some negative effects [2].

Sexual orientation describes the likelihood of being attracted sexually to either males, females, or both.

The vast majority of the population are heterosexual, demonstrating clear sexual instincts and attraction to the opposite gender. There is, however, a proportion of men who are sexually attracted to men, and who identify as homosexual, a proportion of women who are sexually attracted to women, and around eight percent of the population who are attracted to both. Some individuals declare that they are not attracted to either sex, and are generally known as the "third gender."

There is some longstanding evidence to support a biological basis for gender identity mooted as long as 40 years ago [3]. Likewise, there are several biological factors in the origins of male homosexuality, however culture and experiences are also influential and debate still continues on this topic [4].

Cancer will not change sexual identity nor sexual orientation, but may well radically change attitudes to sex and to choices and experiences in relation to sexual behavior. All individuals are sexual beings, but vary widely in their attitudes and beliefs in relation to their own sexuality. They have an absolute right to either be sexual or nonsexual as they choose. Sadly, in some parts of the world this basic human right is not yet recognized,

S.V. Carr, M.B. Ch.B., M.Phil., MIPM., FFSRH. (✉)
Royal Womens Hospital, Locked Bag 300, Parkville, VIC, Australia
e-mail: susan.carr@thewomens.org.au

B.I. Carr and J. Steel (eds.), *Psychological Aspects of Cancer*,
DOI 10.1007/978-1-4614-4866-2_12, © Springer Science+Business Media, LLC 2013

especially in relation to women, and even in open societies most find it difficult to talk about sex, or even to accept that they have a right to a pleasurable, pain free, and autonomous sex life.

Although the majority of people have a problem free sex life, there is a recognized acceptance that a substantial proportion of the population may have a sexual problem at some time in their lives, and sadly, this is more so with cancer.

It is thus essential that clinicians are aware of sexuality in relation to cancer, the potential problems which can ensue and strategies which can be adopted, most of which are simple, in order to improve sexual well-being.

The Sexual Response

The human sexual response has been classically described as the "psychosomatic circle of sex" [5]. It depends on endocrine, vascular, and neurological integrity. The female response results from sensory input through the peripheral nerves of the autonomic and somatic nervous system, as well as the cranial nerves. Psychogenic stimulation is crucial to this process. The precise location and mechanism of transmission of afferent information within the brain and spinal cord is unknown. The temporal and frontal lobes and anterior hypothalamus also have some role in mediating the sexual response. The generalized motor responses are more obvious. The sexually aroused female has pelvic congestion and vaginal lubrication. During sexual intercourse the vagina lengthens, the labia swell, the uterus draws back and there is clitoral hood retraction. In the male the penile vessels and corpora cavernosa engorge with blood, the testes draw up and the penis becomes stiff and erect ready for intercourse.

There have been different sexual response models described over the years. Masters and Johnson [6] used a four phase model consisting of excitement, plateau, orgasm, and resolution. This was modified by Helen Singer Kaplin into a triphasic description of desire, arousal, and orgasm [7]. Desire is now thought of as the first stage of sexual arousal. These models have been used as a basis for modes of treatment, such as

sensate focus therapy, in which couples employ a series of nonsexual touching exercises to "relearn" intimate sexual contact. In appropriately selected cases improvements have been shown using this therapy.

Prevalence

Sexual problems in people with cancer are far more common than in the general population. The general prevalence of sexual problems is quoted as 30% of males and 43% of females in a US population [8], 20% in an Australian population, and 11% of both males and females in Denmark. The most common sexual problem experienced by women is that of lack of desire, followed by problems such as lack of orgasm and the presence of sexual pain [9].

Published evidence shows that at least 50% of cancer patients will have a sexual problem at some time during their cancer journey [10]. Most recognition has been paid to women with breast and gynecological cancers and men with prostate cancer as these are overtly "sexual" areas of the body; for instance, women treated for early stage breast cancer have more sexual problems than the French population in general [11]. Sexual problems, however, can affect people with all cancers, and this is an area of healthcare sadly often ignored or forgotten by the clinical team.

Sexual problems with cancer need not be permanent, and can improve over time [12] or, conversely, can be more ongoing over a long period [13]. Which will be dependent not only on physical treatments but also on the emotional and relationship status of the patient.

Gynecological cancer survivors have a greater incidence of fecal incontinence than controls, and also experience less sexual desire and less ability to orgasm [14]. However after 3 years women who had radiotherapy for gynecological cancers showed improved sexual function over baseline [15], possibly helped by feelings of being "cancer free."

Severe sexual dysfunctions are common for long-term survivors of hematopoetic stem cell transplantation, and women seem to suffer more than the men [16]. This may be because of altered hormonal levels, but may also be due to the emotional impact of the severity of the disease and its treatment. A single study of patients with hepatocellular carcinoma showed a higher prevalence of sexual problems than comparison groups, some of which was related to drug therapy [17]. Reduced libido and sexual enjoyment is described in patients with total or partial laryngectomy [18]. With major head and neck cancers, sexual and intimacy problems were not linked to site of the lesion [19].

Site of cancer, stage of cancer, and treatment of each cancer all significantly impact sexuality and no one cancer is without this effect. Interventions commenced de novo from the cancer diagnosis have the potential to reverse this often devastating impact on well-being and should be an important part of the overall multidisciplinary approach to patient care.

What Are Sexual Problems?

Physical changes as a result of cancer and its treatments can be many and varied, leading to a wide variety of sexual problems. Women with cancer can experience disruption to sexual arousal, lubrication, orgasm, and develop pain on intercourse particularly if they have experienced menopause as a result of chemotherapy or surgery. This functional disruption leads to lack of pleasure in sex and can result in total loss of libido, or sexual interest, as a subconscious way of avoiding something which has become an unpleasant or painful experience.

It is useful to be aware of some of the commonest sexual problems that may be seen in practice, and the treatment options available.

Female Sexual Problems

Anorgasmia

This is the clinical term for inability to reach a sexual climax. It is common and affects up to 20% of woman globally. Some women complain of inability to reach sexual climax, and report that they have never experienced, or are unsure whether or not they have experienced, the intense feelings leading up to and culminating in orgasm. Others may experience orgasm only when masturbating, but not with a partner during penetrative coitus. Usually education around sexual anatomy, and simple masturbation exercises will help, as can the use of vibrators.

If anorgasmia is the result of antidepressant use such as selective serotonin reuptake inhibitors (SSRIs) then sildenafil treatment may be effective in highly selected cases [20]. Otherwise educational, behavioral, and emotional therapy is of benefit.

Primary Vaginismus

Vaginismus is described as the involuntary contraction of the vaginal muscles, and may be psychogenic in origin. Primary vaginismus is a condition where nothing is able to enter the vagina. This woman will never have used a tampon for menstruation, or have had any sort of penetrative sex. In this situation there is no organic disease, the woman has a healthy vagina and vulva, and treatment should focus on the emotional blocks to having sex.

Secondary Vaginismus and Dyspareunia

Secondary vaginismus, however, is a far more likely diagnosis when a woman complains of inability to have penetrative intercourse after cancer. A woman with cancer may have been able to have penetrative sex prior to diagnosis and treatment, but at some point on her cancer journey, she finds herself unable to have sex as it was before. This can be due to pain after surgery or radiotherapy, or discomfort due to vaginal dryness following sudden menopause as a result of ovarian surgery or chemotherapy.

Dyspareunia is pain on sexual intercourse. It may or may not have an organic origin, such as cancer or dermatological problems including atrophic vaginitis and moniliasis. The pain may also derive from surgical scarring or alteration in vaginal length and/or caliber.

Dyspareunia and secondary vaginismus are often linked by cause and effect. Thus diagnosis may be confused leading to inappropriate treatment [21]. If there is pain due to organic problems, the woman will expect pain on intercourse, will subconsciously contract her vaginal muscles, and any attempts at penetration will be met by a strong wall of contracted muscle… "a brick wall", The erect penis tries to penetrate and further pain is caused thus distressing both partners. These conditions should be looked at as a possible continuum.

It is essential for the patient to have a thorough physical check to ensure no organic lesion is left untreated.

A cause of painful sexual intercourse can be one of the many vulvar pain syndromes, which can occur in women with or without cancer. It is generally recognized that the ideal approach to all of these conditions is multidisciplinary, paying as much attention, if not more, to the emotional as well as the physical aspects.

Male Sexual Problems

Erectile Failure described as failure to achieve and sustain penile erections for long enough to have satisfying sexual intercourse can be a devastating situation for any man. It can be a common side effect of some cancers, especially cancer of the prostate but is also a common accompaniment to medical conditions including obesity, diabetes, and vascular disease.

This is a condition which becomes commoner with age, with around 25% of men in their 50s and 40% in their 60s having some degree of failure.

As over 60% of erectile dysfunction is organic in origin, the mainstay of treatment is medication such as phosphodiesterase type 5 cyclic GMP inhibitors, which are facilitators not initiators of erections. If a man is not attracted to his partner, the medication is unlikely to work. Locally acting injectables, such as prostaglandin E can be injected into the base of the penis, or used as an intra-urethral pellet. The efficacy rates are high.

Vacuum devices together with penile constriction rings can produce an erection, but are cumbersome to use, and consequently not very popular.

It is important to recognize that 25% of erectile dysfunction is partially psychogenic and 15% purely pschogenic in origin, and even men with wholly organic disease will sustain an emotional impact if having erectile difficulties.

Psychosexual medicine is the mainstay of treatment for the emotional aspects of the dysfunction. The partner can be included if the patient wishes, and complex underlying emotional issues can be explored.

Premature Ejaculation

The commonest male sexual problem worldwide is premature ejaculation. The latency period, i.e., the time between achieving an erection and ejaculation is too short for satisfying sexual intercourse to take place. This condition can be very frustrating for both partners, and can cause a loss of self-esteem for the man, and feelings of dissatisfaction for his partner.

Treatment is mainly the use of SSRIs, which can lengthen the latency period. These have high efficacy rates, and it is easy to take the medication [22]. Behavioral therapy has only short-term benefits which disappear when therapy is concluded. Other techniques such as squeezing firmly at the base of the penis at the point of orgasm are widely recommended, but there is no good published evidence to support their use, and in clinical practice the technique appears to be fairly useless.

Delayed Ejaculation

This condition has a completely different presentation from that of the premature ejaculator. The condition has often been longstanding, and except for a few instances, when it can be a side effect of medication, tends to be due to issues of control.

The man has a strong subconscious block to ejaculation, which is often situational. If he can ejaculate through masturbation but not inside his partner, then the problem is clearly psychogenic, and should be treated with psychosexual or counseling therapy.

Loss of Libido: Male and Female

This is loss of sexual interest or desire, a clinical condition for which there are no physiological markers. It is sometimes called "sexual desire disorder." It can affect both males and females, regardless of gender, age sexual orientation, or ethnicity. It tends to occur more commonly in people with cancer or chronic disease and can be either caused by cancer and its treatments or brought to the surface by underlying emotional issues being highlighted by the cancer.

The only evidence-based drug treatment is for loss of libido following sudden menopause, often as a result of cancer therapy. In these cases, if appropriate, then hormone replacement, with the addition of testosterone can restore libido. Males with low testosterone levels can benefit from hormone replacement also, but there is no direct measurable link between hormone levels and libido. If a couple have had longstanding relationship problems, some hormones given after menopause will not make these problems disappear!

Emotional issues require appropriate therapies, and psychosexual interventions can help the patient gain insight.

Treatments

There are a variety of treatments which are used for sexual problems. It is essential to treat any organic disease or dysfunction before embarking on therapy for the sexual problem. All cancer symptoms and manifestations have to be assessed and treated before embarking on sexual therapy.

Treatments depend on the etiology of the problem and can be medical, surgical, psychological, analytical, behavioral, or a combination of some of these.

Vaginal dilators are commonly used for women following radiation therapy. It is thought they help to stretch the vagina and prevent adhesions. Many women, however, don't like using them and the evidence for their use is flimsy [23]. When dilators are used in women who have no vaginal pathology, as in the women with primary vaginismus, they are known as vaginal "trainers," because they are being used to teach the woman that she can in fact allow something to enter into the vagina, and that she herself can be in control. There is often concern about vaginal length in relation to penetrative intercourse, but current literature does not show any association between postsurgical vaginal length and sexual satisfaction [24].

A neurotoxic protein such as Botulinum toxin A, injected intravaginally has been show to help in vaginismus which is a result of vulvar vestibulitis [25].

Cognitive behavioral therapy (CBT) is useful in female sexual dysfunction, but procedures differ depending on the nature of the problem. Only a few CBT treatments have been empirically investigated, and as a result it is not known which components of the treatment are most effective [26]. Broader approaches can be taken which focus on the construct of flexibility in behavioral and coping strategies [27]. The current trends amongst health psychologists to use psychoeducational interventions using combinations of cognitive and behavioral therapy, and mindfulness training seem to be effective [28].

Psychosocial interventions can improve sexual outcomes, even if medication is being used. When group therapy was given to men using sildenafil for erectile dysfunction following prostatic cancer, the sexual outcomes were improved [29]; however, greater focus on the psychosocial aspects of this disease has not been adequately researched [30], despite erectile dysfunction having such a major negative impact on these men lives [31]. A Supportive–expressive group therapy intervention offered to lesbians with primary breast cancer showed reduced emotional distress and improved coping, but had no effect on sexual issues [32]. A peer counseling intervention for African American breast cancer survivors showed improved sexual functioning after

6 months, but not after a year. Peer counseling in this group showed no advantage over telephone counseling [33].

The consensus on therapy for sexual problems, however, is that, as sexuality is complex and multifaceted, whatever therapeutic modality is used, then a multidisciplinary approach to treatment must be taken [34].

Body Image

Body image and sexual self-confidence are intrinsically linked. Cancer and its therapies can cause major alterations in body image which in turn can have negative impact on sexuality and sexual satisfaction [35]. About 50% of young women with breast cancer, all of whom had stable partners, experienced body image problems within 7 months of diagnosis, regardless of stage of cancer [36]. Over half of these women also experienced problems with sex. Postmastectomy patients can experience of loss of sexual desire, and require support to restore their positive body image and sense of femininity [37].

The obvious physical changes associated with cancer can be either transient or permanent. They include baldness following chemotherapy, weight fluctuations, body shape changes such as loss of breast, stoma onto the skin, lymphoedema, or some disfiguring features following head and neck cancer. One study in Italy showed that the degree of disfigurement in head and neck cancer lead to greater problems with sex, self-image and relationship with partner compared to those with less obvious outward changes [38]; however, another study showed that age rather than degree of disfigurement was more significant in relation to sexual dissatisfaction , with men under 65 having poorer sexual functioning and satisfaction [39]. Interestingly only 58% of the sample were satisfied with their current sexual partner, the reasons for which were not explained!

In areas such as Africa where presentation of cancer can be late and incurable, sexual problems, and body image disturbance, "I don't look like myself", were ranked as of prime importance to the patients [40]. It is so easy to dismiss these concerns in the face of the life-threatening potential of the disease, but patients should be given the opportunity to discuss what is important to them, even in the palliative phase of care.

Changes in body self-perception, however, need not necessarily stem from outward change, and for a lot of young women, loss of fertility can greatly lower their feelings of femininity [41]. The impact on body image following cancer is multifactorial, and issues such as age, physical, and psychosocial factors are all relevant [42]. In adolescent and young adult survivors of testicular cancer, sexual function was closely bound to fertility issues and masculinity resulting in body image problems in this particular group [43]. What is encouraging is that many survivors of various childhood cancers successfully go on to produce healthy children [44]. It is therefore crucially important that individuals in this group have access to expert and accurate information about their fertility options, which may well alleviate many of their concerns, and avert negative sexual impact. Young people with cancer have particularly difficult issues in relation to body image as it is so integral to romantic attractions and establishing relationships [45], and where fertility issues are yet to become relevant.

Body image can stem from the patient's own feelings or can be a reflection of real or supposed feelings of a partner. If there is a regular partner, however, couple-based interventions are known to be the better therapeutic option [46], especially if they educate both partners about the cancer and its treatments and support mutual coping.

Can Different Cancer Treatments Alter Body Image and Increase Sexual Difficulties?

Different treatments can cause differing body image and sexual outcomes, for instance patients treated for rectal cancer have a high rate of sexual problems. These problems both in males and females seem to be exacerbated by nerve damage and are associated with preoperative radiotherapy [47]. Preoperative radiotherapy causes higher levels of poor body image and poorer sexual function in males being treated for rectal cancer, than in those having surgery alone [48], and all patients suffered more sexual problems than the non-cancer population. Many cancer patients have a stoma, but it has been shown that not everyone in this situation experiences negative body image and sexual problems [49].

Sexual function posttreatment in men with prostate cancer is an enormously important issue, yet there are still unmet needs for appropriate and accurate information in making treatment choices [50]. Men with nonseminomatous testicular cancer had fluctuations in sexual functioning, but not desire in the first year after diagnosis. In this case the type of treatment did not matter [51].

Women with early stage breast cancer in a US study showed less problems with sexual attractiveness over time than women without cancer; however those with mastectomies had a higher incidence of sexual problems [12]. In Turkey, 41% of women undergoing treatment for breast cancer had a deterioration of sexual functioning; however those undergoing mastectomy had a greater loss of libido than those undergoing breast conserving treatment. There was no significant change in body image, however, between the two groups [52].

Sexual abuse in childhood can have significant effect on self-esteem and body image. It has been suggested that women opting for breast reconstruction may have a higher likelihood of abuse than those who choose mastectomy alone [53]. This is a very sensitive area which needs more exploration.

Women with breast cancer did not experience a worsening of sexual feelings after surgery, but did progressively after chemotherapy and hormonal treatment [54]. Interestingly no body image deterioration was noted, but there were many physical changes in contrast to other studies.

A study undertaken in Italy comparing radical hysterectomy by either laparoscopy or laparotomy, concluded not surprisingly that radical hysterectomy lessens sexual function, regardless of type of surgical approach [55]. In another study comparing the treatment of women with early stage cervical cancer with either radical trachelectomy or radical hysterectomy, the measurements of mood, sexual function, and quality of life did not differ by treatment [56]. Women treated with neoadjuvant chemotherapy and type c2/type 111 radical hysterectomy for locally advanced cervical cancer showed no difference in sexual enjoyment to benign gynecological disease patients [57].

Regardless of type of treatment, across all cancers the most commonly discussed symptoms in relation to sexual problems were fatigue, hair loss, weight gain, and scarring [58]. Other symptoms which are out of the patients control, such as fecal and urinary incontinence are major inhibitors to sexual contact, as the sufferer is highly anxious of causing embarrassment to themselves or their partner. This alone can cause avoidance of all sexual contact. Although much of human sexual activity is an intimate and "messy" activity involving body fluids, when faced with additional excreta many people find sex unacceptable.

Symptoms such as shortness of breath due to lung involvement or severe pain are also major physical inhibitors to sex. None of this fails to have an emotional impact on the patient and their partner, and should always be recognized when treating anyone with these problems.

Emotional Aspects of Sex

Many clinicians are well versed in treating sexual problems which seem to have an obvious physical cause. Examples of this include the use of local estrogen for vaginal application following menopause or systemic estrogen and/or progestagens for hormone replacement.

What clinicians find more difficult, however, is dealing with the emotional aspects, either causative or as a consequence of sexual disturbances.

Whether or not a sexual problem has a physical cause, it will have an emotional impact. A man who has suffered erectile dysfunction after prostate cancer will not only have to deal with the potential life-threatening disease, unpleasant treatment and anxiety for the future, he will find his sexual life is altered, which impacts on his sense of self and his masculinity. Likewise a woman who finds sex too painful following radiotherapy to the genital area, will feel she is "letting herself and her partner down."

Cancer produces a list of losses which the patient may experience throughout their cancer journey. There is the loss of health, loss of freedom if having to undergo treatment, potentially loss of life expectancy and loss of plans for the future. Added to this can be the loss of self-esteem, lowering of self-worth, and feelings of being subsumed by the cancer. One of the most common sexual problems, loss of sexual interest, or loss of libido can follow major life losses, and is commonly seen in cancer patients.

There are no physiological markers for this condition [5]. In most case it is psychogenic, and will respond to appropriate psychosexual, psychological or counseling therapy.

Even when all physical symptoms have been appropriately diagnosed and treated, the sexual problem may remain. Sexual morbidity in gynecological cancer is associated with poorer psychological adjustment amongst survivors [59]. Cancer often acts as a trigger for deeply buried emotional issues to come to the fore. Previous losses may often come to light as the client undergoes counseling. These may be past loss of pregnancy, either termination of pregnancy or miscarriage, loss of job or unresolved bereavement issues around a family member. Many patients throughout therapy confront loss of a carefree childhood, with physical and verbal abuse, alcoholism in the family or a traumatic parental divorce which may be underlying factors in their current sexual condition. These are just a few examples but underline the important issue that sexual problems in cancer patients may take a broader approach than may be currently available in many centers.

Many sexual problems are of primary psychogenic origin, but with the cancer disease process in the background, there is an anxiety in making this diagnosis in case some organic disease is "missed." There is also a prevailing attitude in some cancer units that sexual problems are being treated, when in fact the depth of the emotional impact has not been recognized. It consequently may take a long time before the patient is able to access appropriate treatment for a psychosexual problem increased awareness and training, however, should eventually improve access.

Partners

When an individual has cancer, not only are they affected, but in most cases there is a substantial impact on their family, friends, and social and work contacts. In relation to sexuality, if there is a partner then the partner will almost invariably be affected. The impact of cancer on a sexual partner is enormous. Seventy-six percent of partners with nonreproductive site cancers, and 84% of partners with reproductive site cancers had sexual problems [60] is the presence or absence of a partner may be a major issue for the patient, either before, during, or after their cancer treatment.

A Danish population study showed that the male partners of women with breast cancer had an increased risk of severe depression, which was even higher in those whose partners had died [61]. The high rate of sexual problems associated with prostate cancer leads to couples spousal communication levels dropping significantly [62], as it is easier to avoid the topic than cover emotionally painful ground. The partners of cancer sufferers who had hemopoetic stem cell transplantation suffered more depression and sexual problems than controls [63].

Infertility can be an outcome of cancer or its therapy. This adds another major loss to a couple who are already dealing with loss of health and a possibly altered vision of their future together. In many, parenthood is a natural and primeval drive, and the desire to found and care for a family is profound. When faced with the inability to bear children with ones partner directly or indirectly because of malignancy, the couple are more likely to suffer anxiety, stress, and sexual problems, especially the woman [64]. Service providers should be sensitive to the fact sexual and reproductive concerns may be present, and should give the couple an opportunity to speak of their difficulties.

Treatment for sexual problems in relation to cancer should always offer the option of involving the partner. Not everyone wishes this, especially in the early stages of discussion where individuals are anxious as to the form of the consultation. In a psychosexual clinic it is a common fear of the patient that they may be made to have sex in the clinic setting. Alternatives to penetrative intercourse can be suggested, but some couples find they cannot contemplate such a radical change [65]. Simple suggestions like the use of books and modern media for ideas and information can be helpful and fun, but all of these suggestions need partner compliance. The deeper emotional issues will not be addressed in this way, but can provide some positive input into very disrupted sexual lives.

When couples are willingly involved, however, treatment outcomes can be very good. Post breast cancer it is the quality of the woman's partnered relationship which predicts sexual outcomes [66].

Sexual Minority Groups

As the majority of the population are heterosexual, when talking about sexual and relationship issues it is sometimes forgotten that the groups with minority sexual orientation, gay men, lesbians, and bisexuals are equally, or maybe more likely to be the victims of cancer There are no clear data on whether gay, lesbian, and bisexuals are more susceptible to cancer than the general population ,due to a paucity of good and routinely collected statistics, but it has been suggested that appropriate information could be acquired by using cancer registry data [67]. This is important, because lesbian and bisexual women may perceive their cancer risk to be lower than reality [68], particularly bisexual women, who are having sex with both men and women and are at high risk of HPV infection. They also feel that they are excluded from dominant sexual scripts that inform the negotiation of safer sex practice [69]. In another study, only the women who had had abnormal smear test results saw themselves at possible risk of cancer [70].

For some years now lesbian and bisexual women have been shown to be a greater risk of diseases linked to smoking and obesity, both of which have associations with cancer [71]; however despite awareness this may continue to be the case. Tobacco and alcohol misuse has clearly been associated with a variety of cancers. Lesbian and bisexual orientation and sexual abuse before the age of 11 were shown to be associated with an increased risk of tobacco and alcohol use during adolescence, greater than heterosexual women [72].

A comparison of lesbian and heterosexual women's response to newly diagnosed breast cancer showed no differences in mood, sexual activity, or relationship issues [73]. The women who openly identified themselves as lesbian or bisexual had better coping mechanisms and lower distress than women who identified themselves as actually heterosexual but also have sex with women [74].

There have been differences demonstrated in sexual minority women, and their sexual functioning after cancer. These women may experience less sexual disruption such as lubrication and orgasmic problems, and less problems with body image than heterosexual women. Their partners are often more supportive and understanding [75]. It is not unknown for both women in a same sex relationship to suffer the same cancers at the same time, and have to cope with a complex, patient, partner, and carer role. There can be robust community support for a lesbian woman with cancer, but there have been reports of isolation linked to fear of cancer and homophobia in the greater community [76]. Additional anxiety can be provoked by fear of disclosing their sexual orientation to healthcare providers, and there is often unconscious heterosexual bias in healthcare settings, as physicians do not ask or make assumptions [77] which can make the patient feel uncomfortable in facing the unknown.

Men who have sex with men are at high risk of anal cancer, especially if HIV infected. In general anal cancer screening was not associated with greater psychological stress in HIV-infected men; however it was an issue amongst younger men and those whose HIV symptomatology was greater [78]. Although men are traditionally reluctant to come forward for screening, when invited in a healthcare setting it is feasible without undue psychological stress.

Generally overt homophobia is not experienced by gay and lesbian people with cancer [79], but there can still be an unintended insensitivity to sexual minorities amongst the caring professions which only appropriate education and training can address.

Communication About Sex

Many cancer patients wish to communicate about sex to their clinician, but find it very difficult to do so. It is also difficult communicating about sex in a routine cancer consultation. There are often family members, or close friends present to support the patient, but this can clearly inhibit discussion about sex which is about the most intimate level of interaction between the patient and their partner.

It is often thought that poor communication levels can stop the patient from getting the help they need. Doctors and nurse know that they should communicate about sexual problems with their cancer patients, but they fail to do so. This can be due to personal feelings of discomfort about sex, or an embarrassment at talking about sex to others. Age disparity makes it hard to talk about sex; a young doctor is unlikely to ask an octogenarian if she is having a sexual problem, and the octogenarian lady is unlikely to bring up the subject with a doctor or nurse in their twenties. Older men with prostate cancer said they were rarely invited to talk about sex, and it became a more important issue over time, with the patients saying, "I wish I had told them" [80]. Men find it particularly difficult to talk about intimate issues due to "the barrier of masculinity" [81]. It is therefore incumbent on the professional to make sure they are adequately trained in this field, and are able to bring up the subject in a timely and positive way. When students have formal communication training, the outcomes for the patient are better.

Information from the care provider about sex varies depending on the cancer site. In one study 79% of prostate cancer sufferers were given appropriate sexual information, yet only 23% of lung cancer patients received the same help [82]. Asking routinely if patients have a partner, if they are sexually active and if they have any problems is a certain way to give the Patient permission to discuss the topic. They may not wish to at that particular point, but they know it is a "permitted" topic, and may choose to bring it up later.

In certain situations it becomes even more difficult to discuss sex. One of the great taboos in cancer care is still talk of sex during the palliative phase. Some patients who are dying do wish to talk about sex [83]. It is to them a reaffirmation of life, and a powerful bond with the person they love. In some enlightened cancer units a double bed is provided to give comfort and sexual dignity to the dying.

A major problem is the attitude of health professionals who tend to 'medicalise' sex [84]. As anyone engaged in psychodynamic work will understand, this is an easy way for the clinician to escape the emotional aspects of the problem, and to retreat into nonthreatening areas of clinical discussion. Clinicians are very skilled at "running away" from emotional issues by focusing on physical and physiological signs and symptoms. The standard clinician led question and answer session in a consultation does not allow the patient any opportunity to express any sensitive or deeper sexual or emotional issues. Allowing silence and space in questioning allows the patient better opportunity to disclose sexual issues.

Problems in communication about sex can only be addressed by formal and compulsory training for the whole clinical team, within a fully evaluated framework such as medical or nursing school, or in postgraduate training. One cannot opt in or out of training in specific diseases, nor be permitted to ignore physical symptoms. Likewise sexual problems should be regarded in the same light and should be a compulsory and integral part of education particularly in the oncological setting.

Conclusion

Sexual problems are now, finally being acknowledged by both patients and their clinicians as an intrinsic part of the life of a cancer survivor, and deserve as much, if not more attention than some of the other issues being faced. On sheer statistics alone, if around half of all cancer sufferers with a problem of a sexual nature, it is imperative that these issues are addressed.

The evidence is clear and prolific in documenting the burden of sexual distress in patients with cancer. These effects can be improved by taking a multidisciplinary approach, not only by clear diagnosis and treatment of the physical aspects of the disease, but by approaching the patient as an autonomous individual, and accepting the emotional impact on them of sexual problems within their own social, economic, and cultural setting.

Despite this ongoing knowledge, in general the provision of professional training and service provision in this field is woefully inadequate. Much help, however, can be given by the individual clinician to their patient by utilizing their core professional skills. By encouraging disclosure of sexual concerns, listening empathetically, and treating each one as an individual much ongoing suffering can be alleviated.

References

1. Carr SV. Psychosexual medicine. In: Shaw R, Luesley D, Monga, editors. Gynaecology. 4th ed. 2010. Oxford: UK, Churchill Livingstone (Elsevier).
2. Peate I. Men and cancer: the gender dimension. Br J Nurs. 2011;20(6):340–3.
3. Green R. Robert stoller's sex and gender: 40 years on. Arch Sex Behave. 2010;39(60):1457–65.
4. Jannini EA, Blanchard R, Camperio-Ciani A, Bancroft J. Male homosexuality: nature or culture? J Sex Med. 2010;7(10):3245–53.
5. Bancroft J. Human sexuality. Edinburgh: Churchill Livingstone; 1989.
6. Masters WH, Johnson VE. Human sexual inadequacy. Toronto, New York: Bantam Books; 1970.
7. Kaplan HS. The new sex therapy. New York: Brunner-Routledge; 1974.
8. Laumann EO, Paik A, Rosen RC. Sexual dysfunction in the United States: prevalence and predictors. JAMA. 1999;281:537–44.
9. Hayes RD, Bennett CM, Fairley CK, Dennerstein L. What can prevalence studies tell us about female sexual difficulty and dysfunction? J Sex Med. 2006;3(4):589–95.
10. Huyghe E, Sui D, Odensky E, Schover R. Needs assessment to justify establishing a reproductive health clinic at a comprehensive cancer centre. J Sex Med. 2009;6(1):149–63.
11. Bredart A, Dolbeault S, Savignoni A, Besancenet C, This P, Giami A, Michaels S, Flahault C, Falcou MC, Asselain B, Copel L. Prevalence and associated factors of sexual problems after early-stage breast cancer treatment: results of a French exploratory survey. Psychooncology. 2011;20(8):841–50.
12. Perez M, Liu Y, Schootman M, Aft RL, Schechtman KB, Gillanders WE, Jeffe DB. Changes in sexual problems over time in women with and without early-stage breast cancer. Menopause. 2010;17(5):924–37.
13. Harrington CB, Hansen JA, Moskowitz M, Todd BL, Feuerstein BL. Its not over when its over: long term symptoms in cancer survivors – a systematic review. Int J Psychiatry Med. 2010;40(2):163–81.
14. Rutledge TL, Heckman SR, Qualis C, Muller CY, Rogers RG. Pelvic floor disorders and sexual function in gynecologic cancer survivors: a cohort study. Am J Obstet Gynecol. 2010;203(5):514e1–7.
15. Vaz AF, Pinto-Neto AM, Conde DM, Costa-Paiva L, Morais SS, Pedro AO, Esteves SB. Quality of life and menopausal and sexual symptoms in gynaecologic cancer survivors: a cohort study. Menopause. 2011;18(6):662–9.
16. Yi JC, Syrjala KL. Sexuality after hematopoetic stem cell transplantation. Cancer J. 2009;15(1):57–64.
17. Steel J, Hess SA, Tunke L, Chopra K, Carr BI. Sexual functioning in patients with hepatocellular carcinoma. Cancer. 2005;104(10):2234–43.
18. Singer S, Danker H, Dietz A, Kienast U, Pabst F, Meister EF, Oeken J, Thiele A, Schwartz R. Sexual problems after total or partial laryngectomy. Laryngoscope. 2008;118(12):2218–24.
19. Low C, Fullarton M, Parkinson E, O'Brien K, Jackson SR, Lowe D, Rogers SN. Issues of intimacy and sexual dysfunction following major head and neck cancer treatment. Oral Oncol. 2009;45(10):898–903.
20. Nurnberg HG, Hensley PL, Heiman JR, Croft HA, Debattista C, Paine S. Sildenafil treatment of women with antidepressant-associated sexual dysfunction: a randomised controlled trial. JAMA. 2008;300(4):395–404.
21. Hope ME, Farmer L, Mc Allister KF, Cumming GP. Vaginismus in peri-and post menopausal women: a pragmatic approach for general practitioners and gynaecologists. Menopause Int. 2010;16(2):68–73.
22. Linton KD, Wylie KR. Recent advances in the treatment of premature ejaculation. Drug Des Devel Ther. 2010;4:1–6.
23. Miles T, Johnson N (2010) Vaginal dilator therapy for women receiving pelvic radiotherapy. Cochrane Database Syst Rev. 2000; Issue 9.
24. Tunuguntla HS, Gousse AE. Female sexual dysfunction following vaginal surgery: a review. J Urol. 2006;175(2):439–46.
25. Bertolasi L, Frasson E, Cappelletti JY, Vicentini S, Bordignon M, Grazziotin A. Botulinum neurotoxin type A injections for vaginismus secondary to vulvar vestibulitis syndrome. Obstet Gynecol. 2009;114(5):1008–16.

26. ter Kuile MM, Both S, van Lankveld JJ. Cognitive behavioural therapy for sexual dysfunctions in women. Psychiatr Clin North Am. 2010;33(3):595–610.

27. Reese JB, Keefe FJ, Somers TJ, Abernethy AP. Coping with sexual concerns after cancer: the use of flexible coping. Support Care Cancer. 2010;18(7): 785–800.

28. Ratner ES, Foran KA, Schwartz PE, Minkin MJ. Sexuality and intimacy after gynaecological cancer. Maturitas. 2010;66(1):23–6.

29. Melnik T, Soares BG, Nasselo AG. Psychosocial interventions for erectile dysfunction. Cochrane Database Syst Rev. 2007; (3):cd004825.

30. Wittman D, Northouse L, Foley S, Gilbert S, Wood Jr DP, Balon R, Montie JE. The psychosocial aspects of sexual recovery after prostate cancer treatment. Int J Impot Res. 2009;21(2):99–106.

31. Bokhour BG, Clark JA, et al. Sexuality after treatment for early prostate cancer: exploring the meanings of "erectile dysfunction". J Gen Intern Med. 2001;16(10):649–55.

32. Fobair P, Koopman C, DiMiceli S, O'Hanlan K, Butler LD, Classen C, Drooker N, Davids HR, Loulan J, Wallsten D, Spiegel D. Psychosocial intervention for lesbians with primary breast cancer. Psychooncology. 2002;11(5):427–38.

33. Schover LR, Rhodes MM, Baum G, Adams JH, Jenkins R, Lewis P, Jackson KO. Sisters peer counseling in reproduction issues after treatment (SPIRIT): a peer counseling programme to improve reproductive health amongst African American breast cancer survivors. Cancer. 2011;117(21):4983–92.

34. Sadovsky R, Basson R, Krychman M, Morales AM, Schover L, Wang R, Incrocci L. Cancer and sexual problems. J Sex Med. 2010;7(2):349–73.

35. Cleary V, Hegarty J, McCarthy G. Sexuality in Irish women with gynaecologic cancer. Oncol Nurs Forum. 2011;38(2):E87–96.

36. Fobair P, Stewart SL, Chang S, D'Onofrio C, Banks PJ, Bloom JR. Body image and sexual problems in young women with breast cancer. Psychooncology. 2006;15(7):579–94.

37. Karabulut N, Erici B. Sexual desire and satisfaction in sexual life affecting factors in breast cancer survivors after mastectomy. J Psychosoc Oncol. 2009;27(3):332–43.

38. Gamba A, Romano M, Grosso IM, Tamburini M, Cantu G, Molinari R, Ventafridda V. Psychosocial adjustments of patients surgically treated for head and neck cancer. Head Neck. 1992;14(3):218–23.

39. Monga U, Tan G, Ostermann HJ, Monga TN. Sexuality in head and neck cancer patients. Arch Phys Med Rehabil. 1997;78(3):298–304.

40. Harding R, Selman L, Agupio G, Dinat N, Downing J, Gwyther L, Mashao T, Mmoledi K, Sebuyira LM, Ikin B, Higginson IJ. The prevalence and burden of symptoms amongst cancer patients attending palliative care in two African countries. Eur J Cancer. 2011;47(1):51–6.

41. Schover LR. Sexuality and body image in young women with cancer. J Natl Cancer Inst Monogr. 1994;16:177–82.

42. Li CC, Rew L. A feminist perspective on sexuality and body image in females with colorectal cancer: an integrative review. J Wound Ostomy Continence Nurs. 2010;37950:519–25.

43. Carpentier MY, Fortenberry JD. Romantic and sexual relationships, body image, and fertility in the adolescent and young adult testicular cancer survivors: a review of the literature. J Adolesc Health. 2010;47(2):115–25.

44. Green DM, Sklar CA, Boice Jr JD, Mulvihill JJ, Whitton JA, Stovall M, Yasui Y. Ovarian failure and reproductive outcomes after childhood cancer treatment: results from the Childhood Cancer Survivor Study. J Clin Oncol. 2009;27(14):2374–81.

45. Tindle D, Denver K, Lilley F. Identity, image and sexuality in young adults with cancer. Semin Oncol. 2009;36(3):281–8.

46. Scott JL, Kayser K. A review of couple-based interventions for enhancing womans sexual adjustment and body image after cancer. Cancer J. 2009;15(1): 48–56.

47. Lange MM, Marijnen CA, Maas CP, Putter H, Rutten HJ, Stiggelbout AM, Meershoek-Klein Kranenbarg E, van de Velde CJ. Cooperative clinical investigators of the Dutch. Eur J Cancer. 2009;45(9):1578–88.

48. Thong MS, Mois F, Lemmens VE, Rutten HJ, Roukema JA, Martijn H, van de Poll-Franse LV. Impact of pre-operative radiotherapy on general and disease specific health status of rectal cancer survivors: a population based study. Int J Radiat Oncol Biol Phys. 2011;81(3):e49–58.

49. Ramirez M, McMullen C, Grant M, Altschuler A, Hornbrook MC, Krouse RS. Figuring out sex in a reconfigured body: experiences of female colorectal survivors with ostomies. Womens Health. 2009; 49(8):6008–24.

50. Knight SJ, Latini DM. Sexual side effects and prostate cancer treatment decisions; patient information needs and preferences. Cancer J. 2009;15(1):41–4.

51. Tuinman MA, Hoekstra HJ, Vidrine DJ, Gritz ER, Sleijf DT, Fleer J, Hoekstra-Weebers JE. Sexual function, depressive symptoms and marital status in non-seminoma testicular cancer patients: a longitudinal study. Psychooncology. 2010;19(3):238–47.

52. Alicikus ZA, Gorken IB, Sen RC, Kentli S, Kinay M, Alanyali H, Harmancioglu O. Psychosexual and body image aspects of quality of life in Turkish breast cancer patients: a comparison of breast conserving treatment and mastectomy. Tumori. 2009;95(2):212–8.

53. Clark L, Holcome C, Fisher JJ, Seward J, Salmon P. Sexual abuse in childhood and postoperative depression in women with breast cancer who opt for immediate reconstruction after mastectomy. Ann R Coll Surg Engl. 2011;93(2):106–10.

54. Biglia N, Moggio G, Peano E, Sgandurra P, Ponzone R, Nappi RE, Sismondi P. Effects of surgical and adjuvant therapies for breast cancer on sexuality, cognitive functions, and body weight. J Sex Med. 2010;7(5):1891–900.

55. Serati M, Salvatore S, Ucella S, Laterza RM, Cromi A, Ghezzi F, Bolis P. Sexual function after radical hysterectomy for early stage cervical cancer: is there

a difference between laparoscopy and laparotomy? J Sex Med. 2009;6(9):2516–22.

56. Carter J, Sonoda Y, Baser RE, Raviv L, Chi DS, Barakat RR, Iasonos A, Brown CL, Abu-Rustum CL. A 2 tear prospective study assessing the emotional, sexual and quality of life concerns of women undergoing radical trachelectomy versus radical hysterectomy for treatment of early stage cervical cancer. Gynaecol Oncol. 2010;119(2):358–65.

57. Plotti F, Sansone M, Di Donato V, Antonelli E, Altavilla T, Angioli R, Panici PB. Quality of life and sexual function after Type c2/Type 111 radical hysterectomy for locally advanced cervical cancer: a prospective study. J Sex Med. 2011;8(3):894–904.

58. Flynn KE, Jeffrey DD, Keele FJ, Porter LS, Shelby RA, Fawzy MR, Gosselin TK, Reeve BB, Weinfurt KP. Sexual functioning along the cancer continuum: focus group results from the cancer Patient-Reported Outcomes Measurement Information System (PROMIS). Psychooncology. 2011;20(4):378–86.

59. Levin AO, Carpenter KM, Fowler JM, Brothers BM, Andersen BL, Maxwell GL. Sexual morbidity associated with poorer psychological adjustment among gynaecological cancer survivors. Int J Gynecol Cancer. 2010;20(3):461–70.

60. Hawkins Y, Ussher J, Gilbert E, Perz J, Sandoval M, Sundquist K. Changes in sexuality and intimacy after the diagnosis of and treatment of cancer: the experience of partners in a sexual relationship with a person with cancer. Cancer Nurs. 2009;32(4):271–80.

61. Nakaya N, Saito-Nakaya K, Bidstrup PE, Dalton SO, Frederiksen K, Steding-Jessen M, Uchitomi Y, Johansen C. Increased risk of severe depression in male partners of women with breast cancer. Cancer. 2010;116(23):5527–34.

62. Badr H, Taylor CL. Sexual dysfunction and spousal communication in couples coping with prostate cancer. Psychooncology. 2009;18(7):735–46.

63. Bishop MM, Beaumont JL, Hahn EA, Cella D, Andrykowski MA, Brady MJ, Horowitz MM, Sobocinski KA, Rizzo JD, Wingard JR. Late effects of cancer and hemopoetic stem-cell transplantation on spouses or partners compared with survivors and survivor-matched controls. J Clin Oncol. 2007;25(11):1403–11.

64. Nelson C, Shindel A, McNaughton C, Ohelshalom M, Mulhall J. Prevalence and predictors of sexual problems, relationship stress and depression in female partners of infertile couples. J Sex Med. 2008;5(8):1904–19.

65. Gilbert E, Ussher JH, Perz J. Renegotiating sexuality and intimacy in the context of cancer: the experience of carers. Arch Sex Behav. 2010;39(4):998–1009.

66. Emilee G, Ussher JM, Perz J. Sexuality after breast cancer: a review. Maturitas. 2010;66(4):397–407.

67. Boehmer U, Clark M, Glickman M, Timm A, Sullivan M, Bradfoed J, Bowen DJ. Using cancer registry data for recruitment of sexual minority women: successes and limitations. J Womens Health. 2010;19(7):1289–97.

68. McNair R, Power J, Carr S. Comparing knowledge and perceived risk related to the human papilloma virus among Australian women of diverse sexual orientations. Aust N Z J Public Health. 2009;33(1):87–93.

69. Power J, McNair R, Carr S. Absent sexual scripts:lesbian and bisexual womens knowledge, attitudes and action regarding safer sex and sexual health information. Cult Health Sex. 2009;11(1):67–81.

70. Eaton L, Kalichman S, Cain D, Cherry C, Pope H, Fuhrel A, Kaufman M. J Womens Health. 2008;17(1):75–83.

71. Cochran SD, Mays VM, Bowen D, Gage S, Bybee D, Roberts SJ, Goldstein RS, Robison A, Rankow EJ, White J. Cancer related risk-indicators and preventive screening behaviours among lesbians and bisexual women. Am J Public Health. 2001;91(4):591–7.

72. Jun HJ, Austin SB, Wylie SA, Corliss HJ, Jackson B, Spiegelman B, Pazaris MJ, Wright RJ. The mediating effect of childhood abuse in sexual orientation disparities in tobacco and alcohol use during adolescence: results from the Nurses Health study 11. Cancer Causes Control. 2010;21(11):1817–28.

73. Fobair P, O'Hanlan K, Koopman C, Classen C, Dimiceli S, Drooker N, Warner D, Davids H, Loulan J, Wallsten D, Goffinet D, Morrow G, Spiegel D. Comparison of lesbian and heterosexual womens response to newly diagnosed breast cancer. Psychooncology. 2001;10(1):40–51.

74. Boehmer U, Linde R, Freund KM. Sexual minority womens coping and physiological adjustment after a diagnosis of breast câncer. J Womens Health. 2005;14(3):214–24.

75. Boehmer U, Potter J, Bowen DJ. Sexual functioning after cancer in sexual minority women. Cancer J. 2009;15(1):65–9.

76. Sinding C, Grassau P, Barnoff L. Community support, community values: the experiences of lesbians diagnosed with cancer. Womens Health. 2006;44(2): 59–79.

77. Boehmer U. Physicians don't ask, sometimes patients tell: disclosure of sexual orientation amongst women with breast carcinoma. Cancer. 2004;101(8):1882–9.

78. Tinmouth J, Raboud J, Ali M, Malloch L, Su D, Sano M, Lytwyn A, Rourke SB, Rabeneck L, Salit I. The psychological impact of being screened for anal cancer in HIV infected men who have sex with men. Dis Colon Rectum. 2011;54(3):352–9.

79. Katz A. Gay and lesbian patients with cancer. Oncol Nurs Forum. 2009;36(2):203–7.

80. O'Brien R, Rose P, Campbell C, Weller D, Neal RD, Wilkinson C, McIntosh H, Watson E, on behalf of Prostate Cancer Follow Up Group. 'I wish I'd told them' A qualitative study examining the unmet psychosexual needs of prostate cancer patients during follow up after treatment. Patient Educ Couns. 2011;84(2):200–7.

81. Nobis R, Sand I, Stoffson K. Masculinity and urogenital cancer: sensitive issues in healthcare. Contemp Nurse. 2007;24(1):79–88.

82. Flynn KE, Reese JB, Jeffrey DD, et al. Patient experiences with communication about sex during and after treatment for cancer. Psychooncology. 2012;21(6): 594–601.

83. Mercadante S, Vitrano V, Catania V. Sexual issues in early and late stage cancer: a review. Support Care Cancer. 2010;18(6):659–65.

84. Hordern AJ, Street AF. Communicating about patient sexuality and intimacy after cancer: mismatched expections and unmet needs. Med J Aust. 2007; 186(5):224–7.

85. Yang H, Toy E, Baker B. Sexual dysfunction in the elderly patient. 1y care update for OG/GYN. 2000; 7;(6):269–74.

Youngmee Kim

An illness affects the quality of life (QOL) of not only individuals with the disease but also their family members and close friends who care for the patients. Approximately 3.7 % of the US population has personally experienced cancer, which consists of over 11 million in the United States alone [1]. Thus, cancer-related concerns are a substantial problem not only to this large population of cancer survivors but also to their families.

Cancer Caregivership

Cancer caregivership encompasses a broad spectrum of concerns and diverse groups of people who are involved in dealing with cancer, mainly the family caregivers and cancer survivors themselves who take care of themselves without help from external resources. The caregiver role incorporates diverse aspects involved in dealing with issues brought up by the cancer. This role includes providing the patient with cognitive/informational, emotional, financial/legal, daily activity, medical, and spiritual support, as well as facilitating communication with medical professionals and other family members and assisting in the maintenance of social relationships [2].

Y. Kim, Ph.D. (✉)
Department of Psychology, University of Miami,
5665 Ponce de Leon Boulevard, Coral Gables,
FL 33124-0751, USA
e-mail: ykim@miami.edu

All of these aspects of caregiving can contribute to caregivers' stress when they perceive it difficult to mobilize their personal and social resources to carry out each of the caregiving-related tasks. Although most research in this area has focused on the negative experiences of providing care, a number of studies have also reported on the benefits of taking care of family members who are ill. Family members have reported benefit finding in providing care, post-traumatic growth, an improved sense of self-worth, and increased personal satisfaction [3, 4].

The degree to which family caregivers have negative and positive experiences in caregiving may affect their ability to care for the survivor. Being able to care for the survivor also relates to the caregivers' own QOL, which is multidimensional [2, 5] with psychological, mental, social, physical, spiritual, and behavioral components. These diverse aspects of caregivers' QOL can vary across different phases of the illness trajectory. Thorough examination of cancer caregivership throughout the illness trajectory is the first step to enhancing the efficacy of caregiving and to optimizing the QOL of survivors and their caregivers [2, 6].

Demographic Correlates of Cancer Caregivership

The degree to which family caregivers have negative and positive experiences in caregiving may depend on the gaps between the resources available for caregiving and the caregiving demands. Unmet needs in caregiving can also affect caregivers' ability to care for the patient, which also relates to their own QOL. For example, basic demographic and caregiving factors were found to be a set of compact yet powerful predictors of the QOL of caregivers about 2 years post diagnosis [7].

For example, caregivers' age was a strong predictor of their QOL [7]. Although older individuals report better mental health or psychological adjustment in general [8] and in the cancer caregiving context in particular, caregiving stress has a disproportionately burdensome impact on their physical health. The findings with respect to the effect of caregivers' age may be particularly important when coupled with the noticeable social trend of the aging of the US population. Future studies are needed to investigate the extent to which the acute but intensive nature of cancer caregiving [9] or chronic psychological concerns about the relative's cancer recurring years after the initial diagnosis could deteriorate the caregivers' physical health by impairing their immune function or causing premature aging.

Another significant predictor of diverse aspects of caregivers' QOL was household income: relatively poor caregivers reported poorer QOL at 2 years post diagnosis. A few studies have documented family caregivers' losses of employment benefits and health insurance due to their involvement with cancer care (with exception, [10]), but this information is limited to the early phase of the survivorship. Future studies are warranted to examine the economic ramifications of cancer for the family after the completion of treatment. Issues include managing the survivor's late effects, financial burden from out-of-pocket costs, and lost income related to the disability of the survivor, and even the need of the caregiver to limit employment in order to care for the survivor.

Caregivers who have been providing care for a longer period, or those who were actively providing care approximately 2 years post diagnosis, were more likely to report higher levels of psychological distress. Factors that may heighten emotional stress among cancer caregivers include the perceived unpredictability of the course of cancer; its life-threatening nature; the risk of recurrence or treatment-related second cancers, which may occur even when the patient is apparently doing well; or the cancer survivor requiring extended help after treatment ends [2, 11]. Such findings suggest that programs to help mitigate caregivers' psychological distress should be continued for family members actively engaged in cancer care beyond the early phase of survivorship.

Beyond caregiving duration and current caregiving status, other caregiving characteristics, such as providing instrumental care to the survivor and providing care to family members other than the survivor, were also significant predictors of caregivers' QOL 2 years after the initial diagnosis of the relative. Frequent provision of information about the survivor's cancer and related concerns was associated with better mental and psychological well-being, whereas providing care to multiple family members related to poorer physical health [7].

Evidence of the differential impact of the caregiving experience on various components of QOL suggests that it is important to identify the demographic and caregiving-related factors that are related to adverse versus optimal caregivership outcomes as an initial step in the development of programs to reduce caregivers' stress and enhance their QOL. A systematic understanding of the role of caregivers' demographic characteristics in caregivership outcomes will suggest certain subgroups of caregivers who might be more vulnerable to negative caregivership experience.

Cancer Caregivership Across the Illness Trajectory

The cancer caregivership experience varies depending on the illness trajectory of the survivor [12–14]. For example, in the early phase of caregivership, caregivers' stress experience is often associated with providing informational and medical support to the patients. During the remission of cancer, dealing with uncertainty about the future, fear that the disease may come back, the financial burden of extended treatment needs of the patients, and changes in social relationships are major sources of caregivers' stress. These differences in caregivership along the illness trajectory vary by caregivers' demographic characteristics. For instance, younger caregivers reported greater stress in providing psychosocial, medical, financial, and daily activity support during the early phase of the illness trajectory. During the remission years after the illness onset, however, younger caregivers reported greater stress only in daily activity.

Gender of caregivers has been also an important factor during long-term cancer survivorship but less so during the early phase of survivorship. At about 5 years after the initial diagnosis, female caregivers reported greater stress from dealing with psychosocial concerns of the patients, other family members, and themselves.

Other demographic factors, however, appear to have stable influence on caregivers' QOL. Across different trajectory of the illness, ethnic minorities tend to report lower levels of psychological stress but greater levels of physical stress from caregiving. Older caregivers reported better psychosocial adjustment but poorer physical adjustment than younger caregivers. These findings suggest that factors associated with ethnicity and chronological age might have stronger impact on persons' QOL than differences wherein the family members stand in their caregiving status or the illness trajectory as years pass by. Future studies should elucidate the nuanced relation between ethnicity, age, and cancer caregiving.

The status of being a spouse was another consistent predictor of caregivers' QOL, but only among those who were actively providing care to cancer survivors around 5 years after the initial diagnosis. The majority of the existing cancer caregiving literature includes only spousal caregivers, thus precluding the possibility of examining effects of different familial relationships with the cancer care recipient. Our findings thus add an important point to the literature: spousal caregivers (who were approximately two-thirds of our study sample) are especially vulnerable to poorer QOL, particularly when involved in long-term cancer care, compared to caregivers who are

adult offspring (about one-fifth of the sample), parents, or siblings (each about one-twentieth of the sample). Further investigation is needed to elucidate the medical and social circumstances of spousal caregivers who are involved in long-term cancer care.

Another important aspect of caregivership is the caregiver's own unmet needs—things that are not directly related to caring for the patient but represent important personal needs to the caregivers. That is, in addition to caring for the individual with an illness, family caregivers likely have responsibilities for self-care and care for other family members that may have to be set aside or ignored in order to carry out the caregiver role.

Among caregiving-related factors, the extent to which the caregivers perceived providing cancer care to be overwhelming, namely, caregiving stress, has been a strong predictor of diverse aspects of QOL, after taking into consideration the variations in caregiving stress related to demographic characteristics [12, 13]. This was particularly true among caregivers whose care recipients are alive during the long-term survivorship. In contrast to the consistent adverse impact of caregiving stress, the boost associated with feeling good about oneself as a caregiver related only to better spiritual adjustment, and only when the care recipient was alive. In general, caregivers who reported higher levels of psychosocial stress from caregiving have shown poorer mental health consistently and strongly across different phases of the illness trajectory. Caregivers' poorer mental health has also been related to higher levels of stress from meeting the medical needs of the patients during the early phase of illness, whereas during remission, poorer mental health has been related to financial stress from caregiving.

Cancer caregiving is portrayed as an intense yet acute type of stressor [9]. These findings suggest, however, that this stressor can have a long-term impact on the caregivers' QOL even after they cease their caregiver role. Investigating the ways in which perceived caregiving stress predicts various aspects of QOL years later, including attention to potential biobehavioral mechanisms influencing physical health, may be a fruitful area for future studies.

With regard to the self-reported physical health of the caregivers, caregivers' perceived stress has been a fairly weak contributor [12, 13]. However, the physical burden of caregiving, documented in objective measures, is considerable. For example, compared with matched non-caregivers, caregivers for a spouse with dementia report more infectious illness episodes, have poorer immune responses to influenza virus and pneumococcal pneumonia vaccines, show slower healing for small standardized wounds, have greater depressive symptoms, and are at greater risk for coronary heart disease [15]. A meta-analysis [15] concluded that compared with demographically similar non-caregivers, caregivers of dementia patients had a 9 % greater risk of health problems, a 23 % higher level of stress hormones, and a 15 % poorer antibody production. Moreover, caregivers' relative risk for all-cause mortality was 63 % higher than non-caregiver controls. The impact of caregiving stress can be manifested both while caregivers are actively involved in care and years after concluding the caregiver role. Prospective longitudinal studies examining different phases of caregivership will be particularly useful in teasing out the effect of caregiving stress from normative aging in caregivers' physical health outcomes.

Another aspect of cancer caregivership that has received limited attention to date is spiritual adjustment. A small number of existing studies have found that spousal caregivers reported similar levels of existential experience from their partner's illness as the patient did, and also had personal growth experiences years after their partner's illness diagnosis [3, 4, 16]. Furthermore, various domains of the experience of benefit finding among caregivers were uniquely associated with life satisfaction and depression. For example, coming to accept what happened and appreciating new relationships with others related to greater adaptation. Becoming more empathic toward others and reprioritizing values related to greater symptoms of depression [3]. These associations were significant above and beyond the variance in adjustment that was explained by

stressor, demographic, religious coping, or social support variables. These findings suggest that accepting new possibilities of emotional and spiritual growth, appreciation for new relationships with others, and maintaining core priorities in life are key elements in caregivers' thriving when faced with the challenges of cancer in their family.

On the other hand, the findings that empathy and reprioritizing are linked to greater depressive symptoms suggest that some caregivers may develop a heightened sense of vulnerability as a result of their experience with a relative with cancer. Becoming aware of the vulnerability of the self and others, or having fewer positive illusions, appears to relate to greater depressive symptoms [3]. In addition, changing one's long-standing core priorities in life, although possibly resulting in improvement in one's QOL, may come with the cost of some degree of life disruption and psychological distress. These findings provide a more nuanced picture of how psychological adjustment relates to positive or negative experiences from providing care. These findings suggest that different domains of benefit finding may function differently, through an evolving process of adaptation.

Potential Biobehavioral Pathways of Cancer Caregivership

Studies, although mainly from caregivers of persons with dementia, have suggested that the link between negative caregiving experience and poor physical health is mediated by immune dysregulation. For example, chronically stressed dementia caregivers have numerous immune deficits compared to demographically matched non-caregivers, including lower T cell proliferation, higher production of immune regulatory cytokines (interleukin-2 [IL-2], C-reactive protein [CRP], tumor necrosis factor-alpha [TNF-α], IL-10, IL-6, D-dimer), decreased antibody and virus-specific T-cell responses to influenza virus vaccination, and a shift from a Th1 to Th2 cytokine response (i.e., an increase in the percentage and total number of IL10+/CD4+ and IL10+/CD8+ cells)

[16, 17]. A 6-year longitudinal community study [18] documented that caregivers' average rate of increase in IL-6 was about four times as large as that of non-caregivers. The mean change in IL-6 among former caregivers did not differ from that of current caregivers, even several years after the death of the spouse. There were no systematic group differences in chronic health problems, medications, or health-relevant behaviors that might otherwise account for changes in caregivers' IL-6 levels during the 6 years of the study period [18].

Another mechanism linking caregiving stress to poor physical health is lifestyle behaviors. Family members with chronic strain from caring for dementia patients increase health-risk behaviors, such as smoking and alcohol consumption [19]. They also get inadequate rest, inadequate exercise, and forget to take prescription drugs to manage their own health conditions, resulting in poorer physical health [20, 21]. Although the immunological and behavioral pathways from caregiving stress to poor physical health are convincing, the generalizability of such findings that are primarily derived from dementia caregivers to cancer caregivers is uncertain.

Caregivership Goes Beyond Survivorship

At the start of the end-of-life (palliative) care period, which begins after a poor prognosis is given, caregivers report heightened levels of caregiving burden, which continue during the entire palliative care period [22]. Overall, caregiving burden is the strongest predictor of caregiver *psychological* distress during this phase of caregivership, even more than the patient's physical and emotional status [22, 23]. However, one study found that the effectiveness of the use of certain coping strategies on caregivers' QOL depended on the level of patient's symptom distress: use of avoidant coping strategies related to poorer mental health of caregivers when the patient had low levels of symptom distress [24].

Although survivorship ends at the death of the person with the disease, the caregivership

continues. The death of a close family member is one of the most stressful of life events [25]. Not surprisingly, then, bereavement in general has been widely studied for several decades [26, 27]. Existing findings [2, 28], although inconsistent, suggest that poor psychological adjustment to bereavement (i.e., depression, anxiety, and complicated grief) relates to numerous demographic and psychosocial factors. These include older age, female gender, being a spouse, youth of the lost family member, past grief experience, close bonds to the deceased, lack of self-efficacy in coping with bereavement, lower religiousness, lack of social support, greater number of other adverse life events, shorter time between diagnosis and death, greater severity of the patient's illness, perceived caregiving burden, and being unprepared for the relative's death.

After the death of the patients, the challenges that caregivers face include spiritual concerns and psychological and physical recovery efforts from caregiving strain. Among cancer caregivers, however, once again, studies of outcomes other than psychological distress at the bereavement phase are sparse. One study with recently bereaved older persons showed that health *behaviors*, such as consistent exercise, monitoring caloric intake, and proper amount of sleep at 6 and 11 months post loss, were related to better QOL at 19 months post loss [29]. Among recently bereaved adults (on average, 6 months post loss), greater use of religious/spiritual coping was associated with more functional disabilities and fewer outpatient physical health care visits at baseline, which was not related to the health status at 4-month follow-up [30].

Efforts have been made to identify particularly vulnerable family caregivers before the relative's death, based on the presence of a dysfunctional family system [31, 32] and the demographic characteristics previously mentioned. These efforts have helped in creating interventions to protect these caregivers from severe levels of grief and bereavement symptoms at 4 months [33], 6 months [34], and 12 months after the loss [35]. In addition, an intervention designed to provide psychosocial support and information to assist in the bereavement process for family members and friends of recently deceased cancer patients has demonstrated its efficacy in improving their QOL at 3 months after completion of the eight-session psychoeducational group [36].

Methodological Concerns in Cancer Caregivership Research

Concern is increasing about the well-being of long-term cancer survivors (5 years or more), as reflected in the National Cancer Institute's Request for Applications (RFA) on long-term survivors in 2003. This call encouraged researchers to pay more attention to this population. As a result, evidence has begun to accumulate on the QOL of long-term cancer survivors [5, 6, 37]. Similar issues arise about long-term well-being among cancer caregivers, but a similar research initiative has not addressed the well-being of this group. The existing body of work on family caregivers of cancer survivors focuses primarily on the caregiver's adjustment during the early survivorship phase. Most of the existing research has one or more problems. These include small sample sizes (with some exceptions: [3, 38]), cross-sectional study designs (with some exceptions: [39–41]), and examining only survivors' or caregivers' QOL, rather than both (with certain exceptions: [41, 42]).

Issues about small sample sizes often involve convenient rather than representative sampling methods and descriptive rather than theory-testing research. These limit the validity and generalizability of findings. The family caregiver's role usually changes as the disease trajectory proceeds, and cross-sectional information necessarily prevents a full understanding of the impact of cancer on the family across the trajectory of the illness. For example, recruiting caregivers during treatment often results in an assessment of caregiving in the earlier phase of survivorship, but because of the cross-sectional nature of the studies, their QOL is rarely assessed beyond the acute treatment phase [41, 43]. Similarly, recruiting caregivers at palliative care units usually results in assessment of end-of-life caregiving [35], but with caregivers terminating the study at the death of the patient

[23]. For those studies that followed up after the care recipient's death, the follow-up period typically extended no more than a year after the death of the patient [33, 35], with the exception of one study that followed bereaved caregivers for 25 months after the patient's death [44].

Bereavement researchers in general rarely examine the extent to which providing care prior to the end-of-life phase affects bereavement outcomes. Even when they do, only relatively short-term outcomes are examined. Similar pitfalls apply to caregivership research. Although researchers have documented the psychological and physical health effects of caregiving [45, 46], they rarely follow the caregivers long enough to assess the effects of the care recipient's death on the caregiver.

Three studies, however, have demonstrated the adverse impact of caregiving strain on bereavement adjustment with dementia, a disability, or mixed illnesses [47]. Studies have also shown the efficacy of a caregiving skills intervention in reducing caregiving burden and in helping the caregiver recover from a depressed mood after the death of the care recipient [48]. The extent to which these findings would be replicated with cancer caregivers, however, remains unknown.

Issues about examining survivors' and their caregivers' QOL separately involve the conceptual pitfall of ignoring mutuality in QOL between care recipients and care providers, as well as statistical violation of the assumption of independence in unit of analysis (with some exceptions: [42]). Testing theory-driven research questions and employing proper analytic strategies (e.g., Actor Partner Interdependence Model: [49]; Multilevel Modeling: [50]) will help advance our understanding of the impact of cancer on the family and complete the picture of cancer caregivership.

Conclusion

Accumulating evidence supports the view that cancer affects not only the patients/survivors but also their family members. The cancer caregivership is a multidimensional construct that varies in nature across the illness trajectory. Several approaches can be fruitful for systematic understanding of the QOL of family caregivers. First, it can be useful identifying certain caregivers by their demographic characteristics as a vulnerable subgroup to greater caregiving stress. Second, determining significant psychosocial factors that are related to various aspects of caregivership across different phases of the illness trajectory will help in designing tailored interventions effective in facilitating optimal cancer caregivership experiences among family members of cancer patients and survivors. Third, employing proper analytic strategies addressing the nature of patient–caregiver data that are interdependent to each other will help advance our understanding of the impact of illness on the family. Fourth, although it is the general consensus that major illness affects not only the individual but also family and friends, it remains unknown whether such an impact is equally significant across different ethnic groups. Fifth, theoretically and methodologically rigorous research on various aspects of the family's QOL, including physical, spiritual, and behavioral adjustment to illness in the family, remains sparse. Family-based interventions across trajectory of the illness are also needed.

References

1. American Cancer Society. Cancer facts and figures, 2011. Atlanta, GA: American Cancer Society; 2011.
2. Kim Y, Given BA. Quality of life of family caregivers of cancer survivors across the trajectory of the illness. Cancer. 2008;112(11 suppl):2556–68.
3. Kim Y, Schulz R, Carver CS. Benefit finding in the cancer caregiving experience. Psychosom Med. 2007;69:283–91.
4. McCausland J, Pakenham KI. Investigation of the benefits of HIV/AIDS caregiving and relations among caregiving adjustment, benefit finding, and stress and coping variables. AIDS Care. 2003;15:853–69.
5. Ferrell BR, Dow KH, Grant M. Measurement of the quality of life in cancer survivors. Qual Life Res. 1995;4:523–31.
6. Bloom JR. Surviving and thriving? Psychooncology. 2002;11:89–92.
7. Kim Y, Spillers RL. Quality of life of family caregivers at 2 years after a relative's cancer diagnosis. Psychooncology. 2010;19:431–40.
8. Baltes MM, Carstensen LL. The process of successful aging: selection, optimization and compensation. In: Staudinger UM, Lindenberger U, editors. Understanding human development: dialogues with lifespan psychology. Dordrecht, Netherlands: Kluwer Academic Publishers; 2003.
9. Kim Y, Schulz R. Family caregivers' strains: comparative analysis of cancer caregiving with dementia, diabetes, and frail elderly caregiving. J Aging Health. 2008;20:483–503.
10. Yabroff KR, Kim Y. Time costs associated with informal caregiving for cancer patients. Cancer. 2009;115(18 suppl):4362–73.
11. Wolfson C, Wolfson DB, Asgharian M, et al. A reevaluation of the duration of survival after the onset of dementia. N Engl J Med. 2001;344:1111–6.
12. Kim Y, Kashy DA, Spillers RL, Evans TV. Needs assessment of family caregivers of cancer survivors: three cohorts comparison. Psychooncology. 2010;19:573–82.
13. Pinquart M, Sörensen S. Associations of stressors and uplifts of caregiving with caregiver burden and depressive mood: a meta-analysis. J Gerontol B Psychol Sci Soc Sci. 2003;58(2):112–28.
14. Pinquart M, Sörensen S. Ethnic differences in stressors, resources, and psychological outcomes of family caregiving: a meta-analysis. Gerontologist. 2005;45:90–106.
15. Vitaliano PP, Zhang J, Scanlan JM. Is caregiving hazardous to one's physical health? A meta-analysis. Psychol Bull. 2003;129:946–72.
16. Manne SL, Ostroff J, Winkel G, Goldstein L, Fox K, Grana G. Posttraumatic growth after breast cancer: patient, partner, and couple perspectives. Psychosom Med. 2004;66:442–54.
17. Segerstrom SC, Miller GE. Psychological stress and the human immune system: a meta-analytic study of 30 years of inquiry. Psychol Bull. 2004;130:601–30.
18. Kicolt-Glaser JK, Preacher KJ, MacCallum RC, Atkinson C, Malarkey WB, Glaser R. Chronic stress and age-related increases in the proinflammatory cytokine IL-6. Proc Nat Acad Sci U S A. 2003;100:9090–5.
19. Carter PA. Caregivers' descriptions of sleep changes and depressive symptoms. Oncol Nurs Forum. 2002;29:1277–83.
20. Beach SR, Schulz R, Yee JL, Jackson S. Negative and positive health effects of caring for a disabled spouse: longitudinal findings from the caregiver health effects study. Psychol Aging. 2000;15:259–71.
21. Burton LC, Newsom JT, Schulz R, Hirsch CH, German PS. Preventive health behaviors among spousal caregivers. Prev Med. 1997;26:162–9.
22. Grunfeld E, Coyle D, Whelan T, Clinch J, Reyno L, Earle CC, et al. Family caregiver burden: results of a longitudinal study of breast cancer patients and their principal caregivers. Can Med Assoc J. 2004;170:1795–801.
23. Raveis VH, Karus DG, Siegel K. Correlates of depressive symptomatology among adult daughter caregivers of a parent with cancer. Cancer. 1998;83:1652–63.

24. Kershaw T, Northouse L, Kritpracha C, Schafenacker A, Mood D. Coping strategies and quality of life in women with advanced breast cancer and their family caregivers. Psychol Health. 2004;19:139–55.
25. Holmes TH, Rahe RH. The social readjustment rating scale. J Psychosom Res. 1967;11:213–8.
26. Parkes CM. Bereavement in adult life. BMJ. 1998;316:856–9.
27. Stroebe W, Stroebe WS. Determinants of adjustment to bereavement in younger widows and widowers. In: Stroebe MD, Stroebe W, Hansson RO, editors. Handbook of bereavement: theory, research and intervention. New York: Cambridge University Press; 1993. p. 208–26.
28. Hebert RS, Prigerson HG, Schulz R, Arnold RM. Preparing caregivers for the death of a loved one: a theoretical framework and suggestions for future research. J Palliat Med. 2006;9:1164–71.
29. Chen JH, Gill TM, Prigerson HG. Health behaviors associated with better quality of life for older bereaved persons. J Palliat Med. 2005;8:96–106.
30. Pearce MJ, Chen J, Silverman GK, Kasl SV, Rosenheck R, Prigerson HG. Religious coping, health, and health service use among bereaved adults. Int J Psychiatry Med. 2002;32:179–99.
31. Chan EK, O'Neill I, McKenzie M, Love A, Kissane DW. What works for therapists conducting family meetings: treatment integrity in family-focused grief therapy during palliative care and bereavement. J Pain Symptom Manage. 2004;27:502–12.
32. Kissane DW, Bloch S, McKenzie M, McDowall AC, Nitzan R. Family grief therapy: a preliminary account of a new model to promote healthy family functioning during palliative care and bereavement. Psychooncology. 1998;7:14–25.
33. Kelly B, Edwards P, Synott R, Neil C, Baillie R, Battistutta D. Predictors of bereavement outcome for family carers of cancer patients. Psychooncology. 1999;8:237–49.
34. Maciejewski PK, Zhang B, Block SD, Prigerson HG. An empirical examination of the stage theory of grief. JAMA. 2007;297:716–23.
35. Rossi FS, Zotti AM, Massara G, Nuvolone G. A comparative assessment of psychological and psychosocial characteristics of cancer patients and their caregivers. Psychooncology. 2003;12:1–7.
36. Goldstein J, Alter CL, Axelrod R. A psychoeducational bereavement-support group for families provided in an outpatient cancer center. J Cancer Educ. 1996;11:233–7.
37. Carver CS, Smith RG, Petronis VM, Antoni MH. Quality of life among long-term survivors of breast cancer: different types of antecedents predict different classes of outcomes. Psychooncology. 2006;15:749–58.
38. Mellon S, Northouse LL, Weiss LK. A population-based study of the quality of life of cancer survivors and their family caregivers. Cancer Nurs. 2006;29:120–31.
39. Baider L, Bengel J. Cancer and the spouse: gender-related differences in dealing with health care and illness. Crit Rev Oncol Hematol. 2001;40:115–23.
40. Hagedoorn M, Buunk BP, Kuijer RG, Wobbes T, Sanderman R. Couples dealing with cancer: role and gender differences regarding psychological distress and quality of life. Psychooncology. 2000;9:232–42.
41. Northouse LL, Mood D, Templin T, Mellon S, George T. Couples' patterns of adjustment to colon cancer. Soc Sci Med. 2000;50:271–84.
42. Kim Y, Kashy DA, Wellisch DK, Spillers RL, Kaw C, Smith T. Quality of life of couples dealing with cancer: dyadic and individual adjustment among breast and prostate cancer survivors and their spousal caregivers. Ann Behav Med. 2008;35:230–8.
43. Weitzner MA, McMillan SC, Jacobsen PB. Family caregiver quality of life: differences between curative and palliative cancer treatment settings. J Pain Symptom Manage. 1999;17:418–28.
44. McCorkle R, Robinson L, Nuamah I, Lev E, Benoliel JQ. The effects of home nursing care for patients during terminal illness on the bereaved's psychological distress. Nurs Res. 1998;47:2–10.
45. Given BA, Given CW, Kozachik S. Family support in advanced cancer. CA Cancer J Clin. 2001;51:213–31.
46. Schulz R, Beach SR. Caregiving as a risk factor for mortality: the Caregiver Health Effects Study. JAMA. 1999;282:2215–9.
47. Schulz R, Mendelsohn AB, Haley WE, Mahoney D, Allen RS, Zhang S, et al. End-of-life care and the effects of bereavement on family caregivers of persons with dementia. N Engl J Med. 2003;349:1936–42.
48. Czaja SJ, Schulz R, Lee CC, Belle SH. A methodology for describing and decomposing complex psychosocial and behavioral interventions. Psychol Aging. 2003;18:385–95.
49. Kenny DA, Kashy DA, Cook WL. Dyadic data analysis. New York, NY: Guilford Press; 2006.
50. Bryk AS, Raudenbush SW. Hierarchical linear models for social and behavioral research: applications and data analysis methods. 1st ed. Newbury Park: Sage Publications; 1992.

Psychosocial Interventions in Cancer

14

Catherine Benedict and Frank J. Penedo

Introduction

Cancer survivors are faced with significant disease- and treatment-related symptoms that challenge the quality of life and often lead to psychosocial distress or dysfunction. At all points in the cancer experience, from diagnosis and active treatment to long-term survivorship, there are a number of stressors that may affect psychological well-being. This refers to unpleasant emotional experiences as a result of physical, psychological, social, and existential or spiritual difficulties that interfere with the ability to cope effectively with a cancer diagnosis, treatment sequelae, and transition into survivorship. A significant number of cancer survivors report psychological responses that range from normal feelings of vulnerability, sadness, and fear to problems that can become disabling, such as clinical levels of depression, anxiety and panic disorder/attacks, interpersonal

dysfunction, sexual dysfunction, social isolation, and existential or spiritual crisis. Distress may be experienced as a reaction to the disease and its treatment as well as to the disruptions in quality of life. Importantly, not all psychological reactions are negative and many cancer survivors report finding some benefit in their cancer experience, such as a new appreciation of life and improved self-esteem and sense of mastery [1].

Psychosocial distress associated with cancer exists on a continuum ranging from normal adjustment issues to clinically significant symptoms that meet the full diagnostic criteria for a mental disorder. At one end of the spectrum, individuals express "normal" adjustment reactions and experience transient feelings of distress such as fear and sadness. Although there may be some impairment in functional domains, ongoing emotional reactions are not severe enough to significantly impair functioning. At the other end of the spectrum, individuals experience symptoms that are severe and frequent enough to meet diagnostic criteria for a debilitating mental health disorder such as major depressive disorder or anxiety disorder. Between both ends of the continuum lay adjustment disorders and subclinical symptoms of more severe mental health conditions. Research has indicated that up to 47% of cancer survivors indicate clinically significant psychiatric disorders and 90% of observable psychiatric syndromes were determined to be in response to cancer diagnosis and treatment [2]. Over one-third of cancer survivors meet diagnostic

C. Benedict, M.S.
Department of Psychology, College of Arts
& Sciences, University of Miami,
5665 Ponce de Leon Boulevard, Coral Gables,
FL 33146, USA

F.J. Penedo, Ph.D. (✉)
Department of Medical Social Sciences,
Northwestern University, 710 N Lakeshore Drive,
IL 60211, Chicago
e-mail: fpenedo@northwestern.edu

B.I. Carr and J. Steel (eds.), *Psychological Aspects of Cancer*,
DOI 10.1007/978-1-4614-4866-2_14, © Springer Science+Business Media, LLC 2013

criteria for adjustment disorder with depressed or anxious mood and about 70% of those diagnosed with any mental disorder have a diagnosis of adjustment disorder [2, 3]. Additionally, estimates indicate that up to 25% of individuals with cancer report depression and 7% meet diagnostic criteria for current major depressive disorder (NCI 2011), while up to 48% report clinically relevant symptoms of anxiety and 18% meet the criteria for an anxiety disorder [4]. Other syndromes experienced include dysthymia and subsyndromal depression (also called minor depression or subclinical depression). Mental health disorders are often accompanied by distressing symptoms such as dyspnea, fatigue, nausea, and pain [1, 5, 6]. The psychological and emotional reactions to cancer are considered briefly below.

The impact of cancer on psychological and emotional well-being is highly variable and often depends on a number of factors. Cancer site and stage as well as treatment course and prognostic medical factors account for many of the challenges individuals will face following their diagnosis and are often among the strongest predictors of emotional reactions. For example, depression is more likely to occur in younger survivors and in those with poorly controlled pain, physical impairment or discomfort, limited social support, and more advanced stage disease [3]. Among individuals receiving palliative care, estimates suggest that approximately 20% [7] meet diagnostic criteria for depression. Those with a premorbid history of depression or anxiety or who present with current and ongoing symptoms at the time of cancer diagnosis are also at increased risk for experiencing adjustment difficulties and more severe emotional reactions [3, 8]. Similarly, current life stressors may exacerbate cancer-related stress and lead to feelings of being overwhelmed and more clinically significant symptoms of distress and dysfunction.

Despite this, the majority of cancer survivors adjust relatively well. Though the initial reaction to a cancer diagnosis may be that of alarm and distress and coping with treatment-related side effects may be difficult, most never meet full diagnostic criteria for a mental health disorder.

However, the fact that most survivors do not experience symptoms that are severe enough to be clinically diagnosed should not undermine the severity of their emotional responses. Even mild symptoms of distress can lead to impairment in several areas of functioning. For example, avoidant behaviors may affect cancer treatment (e.g., missed medical visits, non-adherence to treatment) as well as interpersonal functioning (e.g., social avoidance and isolation, loss of social support), both of which may impact disease course and prognosis [3]. It is important to highlight the continuum within which emotional well-being and psychological distress occur and to approach clinical care with this variability in mind. Psychosocial interventions may be best utilized by targeting the specific needs and stressors of individuals at different levels of psychological functioning at each phase of the cancer experience.

A number of common psychosocial factors have been shown to predict adjustment and well-being. Styles of coping and the availability of inter- and intrapersonal resources have been shown to greatly influence the degree to which individuals are able to adjust to disease- and treatment-related changes and transition to long-term survivorship following the end of treatment. Greater optimism and active coping styles have been associated with positive adjustment at various stages of disease and treatment [9, 10]. Similarly, higher levels of social support from partners, family members, and loved ones have been associated with better general and disease-specific quality of life. Conversely, social constraints (e.g., avoidance of cancer-related discussions) have been associated with worse emotional well-being and quality of life [11]. At each phase of the cancer experience, psychosocial interventions may play a critical role in addressing the various factors related to psychological adjustment to promote adaptive coping and enhanced quality of life.

Psychosocial interventions for cancer survivors generally aim to reduce emotional distress, enhance coping skills, and improve quality of life. Many different types of interventions have been conducted among individuals, couples, and families, including supportive-expressive group therapy, psychoeducational interventions, and multimodal intervention approaches. Therapy components typically involve an emotionally supportive context to address fears and anxieties, information about the disease and treatment, cognitive and behavioral coping strategies, and relaxation training. Reviews of the literature have suggested that interventions promote improvements in a range of physical and psychosocial outcomes, including emotional adjustment (e.g., distress, depression, anxiety, fear, denial, or repression), functional adjustment (e.g., resumption of social and professional activities), disease- and treatment-related symptoms (e.g., fatigue, nausea, pain), and immunologic outcomes, and limited evidence suggests positive effects on recurrence and survival time [3, 11–13]. Participants have reported reduced stress, improved cognitive reframing and problem-solving skills, less uncertainty, better communication with spouses, and improved self-efficacy. Cancer survivors who have participated in support groups have also reported having a more positive outlook, a better understanding of their illness, and feeling more involved in their treatment [3, 11, 14, 15]. Although psychosocial interventions have been shown to improve adjustment and well-being at all stages of diagnosis and treatment, findings have been mixed with reports of nonsignificant intervention effects as well [16, 17]. This may be due to the variability among survivors in sociodemographic and health-related characteristics and in their baseline (pre-intervention) levels of adjustment and well-being. As individuals' needs change at different stages of the cancer experience, different intervention components may be needed at different stages of the cancer experience and for different "types" of survivors (e.g., those experiencing high versus low levels of stress). Although this chapter reviews some identified moderators of intervention effects, further research is needed to better inform targeted intervention components and enhance treatment efficacy at all phases of the cancer experience. The term survivor is used to refer to any individual with a history of a cancer diagnosis [18].

Psychosocial Responses in Cancer Survivors

Diagnosis

The initial diagnosis of cancer is often a traumatic and distressing experience. Emotional reactions include feelings of disbelief, denial, and despair. The spectrum of emotional reactions ranges from depressive symptoms, such as normal sadness, to clinically significant symptoms of adjustment disorder or major depressive disorder. Individuals must adjust to the idea of being diagnosed with a devastating illness that may be life threatening and often struggle with feelings of uncertainty and fear for the future. This time period may be more difficult for those who are unpartnered, are in an emotionally unsupportive relationship, or lack an adequate social support network; social isolation is associated with poorer physical and mental health outcomes. Conversely, survivors may feel additional distress due to worrying or anxious thoughts in anticipation of how disease- and treatment-related changes will impact their partner and/or family members. For example, older individuals may need to depend on the care and support of their children and this change in roles may be distressing, particularly if they perceive that their loved ones will experience financial strain or be burdened by the additional responsibilities. These challenges often extend beyond the initial diagnosis period and may exacerbate treatment-related difficulties or pose significant challenges in the transition to survivorship phases of the cancer continuum.

Although distressing, the initial emotional response to a diagnosis of cancer is often brief, extending over several days to weeks [11]. Nevertheless, individuals may still benefit from interventions designed to enhance adjustment and coping skills and prepare them for the challenges and stressors that they will likely face, such as sharing the news with loved ones and work colleagues/employers and deciding on a course of treatment. A recent review of the literature indicated that relaxation techniques, alone or in combination with education and skills training, is effective in preventing and relieving anxiety and depression in newly diagnosed survivors [19]. Psychoeducational interventions designed to prepare individuals for cancer treatment have also been shown to be effective in reducing anxiety and depression and improving satisfaction with cancer care [19, 20]. Evidence suggests that even brief interventions (e.g., one session, 15–20 min long) may be beneficial [11, 19, 21–23].

Treatment Decision and Pretreatment Preparation

The beginning phases of the cancer continuum require individuals to make decisions regarding treatment options and to plan for their upcoming medical care. It is common to experience significant stress related to treatment decision-making due to a lack of information or confusing guidelines, particularly for those with inadequate medical care or poor communication with their oncology specialists or medical team. Survivors may be further confused or misled by unsubstantiated Internet sources or anecdotal information from other cancer survivors. Likewise, different treatment options may be relatively equivalent and the treatment decision, therefore, may depend on individual preferences in relation to expected posttreatment side effects. Research has shown that survivors often do not have sufficient information or an adequate understanding of potential treatment-related side effects and often underestimate the impact side effects will have on their emotional well-being and quality of life. Individuals often make uninformed decisions that put them at increased risk for posttreatment distress and/or feeling unprepared to cope with side effects, changes to their physical and functional ability, and quality of life. For example, the majority of prostate cancer survivors who undergo radiation therapy or radical prostatectomy will experience some sexual dysfunction that often lasts for years after treatment [21–23]. Prior to treatment, however, men often do not have a clear understanding of potential sexual side effects and many expect to be able to treat erectile dysfunction with assistive aids (e.g., Viagra)

[24, 25]. Research shows that most men are unsatisfied with improvements from assistive aids and discontinue use within a year, suggesting that they must learn to adjust to permanent changes in their sexual functioning [24–26]. Those who are unprepared or ill equipped to adjust to sexual dysfunction and changes in their intimate relationship may experience significant decrements in emotional well-being. Similarly, women diagnosed with breast cancer who undergo surgery to remove the cancerous tissue often do not anticipate how difficult it will be to adjust to the physical changes to their bodies. They are often unprepared for the magnitude of their emotional reactions related to the impact treatment has had on their body image and self-esteem as well as to their sexuality and functioning within their intimate relationships [27–29].

Although this time period poses significant challenges, there are a limited number of interventions designed to target the diagnosis and treatment-decision phases of the cancer continuum. The majority of psychosocial interventions for cancer survivors have been administered after the termination of primary treatment. Of those that have been conducted prior to treatment, most have attempted to improve preparedness for treatment (e.g., stress management and relaxation techniques prior to surgery) and have not considered the treatment-decision making phase as a point of intervention. As decisions regarding the course of treatment have significant implications for disease-specific and general well-being, this may be an important area for future interventions.

Psychosocial interventions delivered prior to the start of treatment have mostly been conducted among breast and prostate cancer survivors and typically involve relaxation training (e.g., progressive muscle relaxation techniques, guided imagery) and stress management to prepare survivors for their treatment(s). Reviews of the literature have suggested positive effects on disease-specific and general quality of life outcomes, including reduced posttreatment side effects such as nausea and vomiting and less psychological distress [3, 11]. This is reviewed in later sections of this chapter.

Active Treatment

The active treatment phase often involves additional stressors that impact psychosocial well-being and quality of life. Depending on the site and stage of cancer as well as on the specific treatments and medical regimen, survivors are almost inevitably faced with some degree of treatment-related side effects, such as pain, nausea and vomiting, insomnia, fatigue, bodily disfigurement, urinary incontinence, and sexual dysfunction. Not surprisingly, the sequelae of side effects vary between early- and more advanced stage disease. Advances in screening and early detection have led to increases in the proportion of individuals diagnosed with early-stage disease and treatment typically involves a less complicated medical regimen. Though still challenging, side effects are often less burdensome than for those diagnosed with more advanced stage disease and those who require multimodal treatments or a combination of therapeutic agents. Survivors living with advanced disease face additional physical (e.g., pain, functional limitations) and emotional (e.g., fear of dying, end-of-life issues) consequences that often lead to further decrements in emotional well-being and quality of life. Despite this, adjustment disorders and concerns related to physical and functional disability, uncertainty, loss of control, and social disruption are common across all cancer types, stages, and treatments.

Along with the physical challenges associated with side effects, additional stressors include negotiating changes in occupational and family roles, managing household and childcare responsibilities, and interference with future life plans. Comorbid conditions (e.g., arthritis, diabetes, cardiovascular disease) may be exacerbated by treatment and lead to greater decrements in physical and emotional well-being. However, even for those survivors who do not experience chronic or debilitating side effects, physical disability in specific areas of functioning may still be distressing. For example, localized prostate cancer survivors often experience chronic sexual side effects following treatment. Despite reporting posttreatment levels of vitality, physical well-being, and levels of general quality of life that are comparable to or above age-matched normative levels, men often indicate distress related to sexual dysfunction [24, 25]. Treatment-related changes may affect specific domains of quality of life, even if more general domains remain fairly intact.

Some of the most common psychosocial concerns reported by cancer survivors are related to feelings of uncertainty and a diminished sense of control and predictability. Again, the specific nature of these concerns often depends on cancer site and stage and other medical factors. Individuals may experience feelings of uncertainty related to treatment efficacy or anticipated side effects and, particularly among those diagnosed with more advanced stage disease or with poor prognostic indicators, worry about the effects of complicated treatment regimens on their quality of life and fears related to end of life and dying may be present. These feelings are inherently connected to feeling a loss of control over one's body and/or one's future. Individuals often feel a sense of reduced autonomy and self-efficacy related to their physical condition and health outcomes, particularly if they feel uninvolved in the decision-making process of treatment planning and medical care.

Finally, social disruption may result from a number of factors related to cancer and its treatment. Due to disease- and treatment-related effects on physical and emotional well-being, cancer survivors often experience a loss of daily routines and work life. This may further contribute to negative emotional reactions related to cancer and changed roles, particularly for those who place a great deal of self-worth and esteem on work-related activities and/or bringing income into the household (e.g., feeling like a burden to others). Cancer survivors are often also limited in their social activities, which may lead to distancing of relationships and/or social isolation. Furthermore, high levels of cancer-related distress have been associated with interpersonal dysfunction, including reduced support-seeking behaviors and lowered perceptions of support. For example, treatment for head and neck cancer often results in facial disfigurement and functional limitations (e.g., problems with speech, breathing, and/or eating) that have been associated with significant psychological distress, a loss of independence, and social isolation as individuals often limit their social activities due to lowered self-esteem, concerns about body image, and functional disability related to chewing and eating in public [30, 31]. Research has shown that head and neck cancer survivors often perceive inadequate levels of social support during treatment and that this may continue to decline posttreatment (i.e., perceptions of support following treatment are often below pretreatment levels) [30, 32]. As social support is consistently related to disease-specific and general quality of life and has been shown to facilitate posttreatment adjustment and influence physiologic mechanisms of recovery, this is an important area to be aware of and address through targeted psychosocial interventions.

Psychosocial interventions in cancer survivors undergoing treatment have shown positive effects on physical and emotional well-being. Evidence suggests that relaxation training, psychoeducation, supportive or supportive-expressive therapy, and cognitive behavioral therapy have all been found to be effective in preventing or relieving anxiety and depression; evidence is strongest for relaxation training in reducing anxiety [19]. This is reviewed in more detail in later sections of this chapter.

Advanced-Stage Disease

As suggested, individuals experiencing progressing or advanced cancer with poorer treatment outcomes report the greatest levels of psychological distress and decrements in quality of life. Aside from the emotional difficulty of coping with end-of-life concerns, advanced cancer survivors often experience more significant physical side effects, such as pain, nausea and vomiting, urinary incontinence, fatigue and difficulties breathing, eating, and/or swallowing, and declining functional abilities. As individuals continue to feel debilitated and are unable to manage their self-care and the caregiver burden becomes too great, discussions regarding care and assistance with daily activities may need to take place and cause additional distress. For those who are in the

hospital, additional concerns include bed sores, difficulty sleeping due to an uncomfortable, disruptive, or unfamiliar environment (e.g., nurses checking in periodically through the night), as well as the added stress of spending time with and interacting with family members and loved ones outside the comfort of one's home or familiar environment. Furthermore, couples dealing with advanced disease face stressors of having to negotiate difficult choices regarding end-of-life treatments and care, coping with anticipatory grief as well as the emotional reactions of children and other family members, and discussions surrounding the patient's legacy in both psychological and practical terms.

Those coping with progressive disease and death also face a number of existential fears and/ or threats to their spiritual beliefs that challenge psychological well-being and interpersonal functioning at the end of life. Aspects of existential/ spiritual concerns refer to survivors' sense of peace, purpose, and connection to others as well as their beliefs about the meaning of life. Progressive disease and invasive medical procedures and treatments often result in survivors feeling like they have lost control over their sense of self and body and may struggle to maintain their self-identity, dignity, and self-esteem. Other elements include a loss of autonomy, control over the future, and life satisfaction. Particularly with end-stage disease in which care is often transferred to an inpatient medical setting, survivors may experience a loss of relationships, both with friends and family, as well as spiritual relationships that may lead to a perceived loss of support and social isolation [33, 34]. Those who experience significant threats to their existential and spiritual well-being are at increased risk for feelings of despair and hopelessness, feeling like a burden to others, loss of their sense of dignity and will to live, and desire for death [34, 35]. They may feel overwhelmed by suffering and unable to cope with the situation. Research has suggested that "feeling like a burden to others" is associated with depression, hopelessness, level of fatigue, and current quality of life [35]. Alternatively, those who are able to find a sense of meaning and peace of mind in their cancer experience may be better equipped for handling end-of-life concerns and maintaining their quality of life. The degree to which survivors are able to cope with existential and spiritual concerns has been related to cancer-related adjustment, total health and well-being, and quality of life.

Posttreatment Survivorship

Although the medical and psychosocial effects of cancer and its treatment have been long recognized, it is only recently that "posttreatment survivorship" has been identified as a distinct phase of the cancer experience. There is a substantial increase in the number of cancer survivors due to early detection and improvements in treatment. It is now recognized that management of the unique medical and psychosocial needs of survivors should be viewed within a long-term care approach. Posttreatment cancer survivorship is now characterized as a chronic condition requiring specific and targeted efforts to address the long-term issues and late effects survivors experience [36]. This is a departure from how cancer care has been conceptualized in the past, as an acute and time-limited course of treatment that is managed by oncology specialists. Factors unique to cancer care, such as the variety of diseases and treatment options depending on cancer type and stage, individualized patient profiles, long-term and late effects, and need for ongoing surveillance, suggest that survivors face a number of distinct psychosocial challenges that persist well past the acute phase of disease and treatment.

For survivors who enter the posttreatment survivorship phase, psychological distress often results from a number of cancer-specific concerns that persist well past the acute phases of illness and treatment. Negotiating the transition back to "normal" life is often the primary challenge. This involves resuming daily activities and relationships, including intimate and sexual relationships, discussing changes in life plans, implementing health behavior changes, coping with long-standing or permanent disease- and treatment-related effects, and managing fears and concerns related

to disease recurrence. It also involves coming to an understanding of how cancer has affected personal and interpersonal life narratives (e.g., finding meaning in the cancer experience and closure; negotiating any changes in existential beliefs). Many survivors need to actively integrate this new aspect of their identity as a "cancer survivor" into their self-concept while acknowledging and accepting the changes they may have encountered or endured throughout their cancer experience (e.g., cognitive declines, new outlook on life). Cancer survivors report that fear of recurrence is one of the universal psychosocial challenges at this time and have identified it as a root cause of posttreatment psychological distress [37]. This may negatively impact transition back to normal routines as well as long-term health outcomes. At high levels of distress, survivors may avoid medical care or resist long-term surveillance and may be unmotivated to participate in health risk-reduction behaviors (e.g., physical activity, smoking cessation).

Sexual health, in particular, is often cited as a particularly challenging domain of survivorship. Factors related to sexual functioning and renewal of sexually intimate relationships include decreased sexual interest and activity, openness, responsiveness, and emotional involvement. Functional impairment and body image concerns all contribute to sexual impairment. Furthermore, for younger survivors, treatment-related infertility may pose additional distress and has the potential of creating emotional distress in partners as well as marital discord related to family planning and hopes for the future.

There is a clear rationale for continued psychosocial support after the active treatment. Psychological distress should be assessed, monitored, and treated promptly at all stages of cancer, including the survivorship phases.

Distress management in the survivorship phase of cancer care
- Need for routine screening to assess psychological distress and psychosocial needs.
- Screening should identify the level and nature of the distress.
- Referrals for psychosocial interventions should be specific to the survivorship needs.

Importantly, many cancer survivors report beneficial effects of cancer. It is a common finding that survivors feel stronger and more able to handle future life challenges. Positive psychological consequences reported in the literature include better interpersonal relationships, including quality of marital relationships, changes in values and priorities, greater appreciation of life, and improved quality of life [38, 39]. Of note, cancer survivors may indicate both positive and negative effects across different domains of physical and emotional well-being and quality of life [38, 39], suggesting that psychological assessment and intervention may be required even among those who indicate some benefit of cancer.

Critical Transition Period

The transition from active treatment to the posttreatment phase of the cancer continuum is often a time of change and uncertainty for many cancer survivors. The first few months may be filled with mixed emotions. Survivors feel relieved to be finished with the demands of treatment and welcome the resolution of side effects while at the same time may feel unease and worry regarding the reduction in medical care. Many survivors may experience an increase in fear of recurrence after active treatment is withdrawn and it is common that survivors have feelings of hesitation in celebrating being cancer-free. As individuals move from frequent to more infrequent medical visits, they may feel a loss of accessibility to their oncologists and medical team and the reassurance that those relationships provide and may, as a result, feel an increased sense of vulnerability. Likewise, many individuals have feelings of uncertainty regarding posttreatment health behavior and medical regimen recommendations (e.g., "Now what do I do?") and how to resume their "normal" lives. For many, this may be impossible. Due to permanent physical changes (e.g., disfigurement, limb amputation) and long-term and late effects of treatment as well as psychological changes (e.g., new outlook on life; changed priorities), survivors often need to settle into a new normal. This can be challenging and stressful for some, particularly regarding interpersonal relationships. Couples

are often incongruent in their adjustment to cancer-related changes and that incongruence is associated with increased distress in survivors and their partners as well as interpersonal dysfunction. For example, unrealistic expectations regarding physical recovery may exacerbate adjustment-related difficulties and lead to decrements in emotional well-being. Internal or external pressures to resume pre-cancer activities such as full-time employment or resumption of household or childcare responsibilities may increase distress (discussed in more detail below in reference to long-term and late effects of treatment). Friends and family members may expect that survivors will be able to resume all of their activities at pre-cancer levels of functioning once treatment is over. Survivors may also expect this from themselves and may be surprised by physical and emotional limitations following treatment.

Rationale for posttreatment psychosocial assessment and referral
- Provides opportunity for education and early intervention
- Extends continuum for cancer care
- Facilitates reentry transition
- Facilitates referral for specialized survivorship services

Thus, the critical transition from active treatment to posttreatment survivorship is a unique time period characterized by paradoxical feelings of both positive and negative emotional reactions. Clinical trials that have targeted survivors immediately following the end of primary treatment have suggested that relatively simple interventions (e.g., videotape on issues related to reentry transitions, individual sessions with a cancer educator) may help to reduce common adjustment difficulties [11, 19]. As survivors may feel reluctant or lack the opportunity to discuss posttreatment psychosocial concerns with their cancer care providers, psychosocial interventions may fill an important void.

Short-Term Survivorship (<1 Year Post Treatment)

As suggested, the transition to survivorship has a number of unique psychosocial challenges that may persist beyond the first few months following the end of active treatment and prove to be chronic sources of stress. Many survivors feel "lost in transition." Although they continue to cope with cancer-related difficulties (e.g., feelings of uncertainty and fear of recurrence, continued physical effects of treatment), there is often a marked reduction in medical care and social support as time goes on. The transition from "sick role" to "well role" is frequently more difficult than survivors expect and navigating the practical issues related to reentry into social and professional networks can be distressing. Many of the physical and emotional difficulties noted above may persist and/or become more apparent as survivors take on more and more of their pre-cancer activities and responsibilities. For example, cognitive changes (e.g., attention or memory problems; "chemo brain") may become more distressing if they interfere with work-related activities and job performance.

Although many studies have described the quality of life of cancer survivors in the first year following primary treatment, this research has largely focused on a few cancers (i.e., breast and prostate) and generalizations to other cancer types that involve different treatment regimens are limited. As treatments are constantly evolving, becoming more complex and, at times, more toxic, caution should also be taken regarding interpretation and applicability of older reports. Nevertheless, there have been many psychosocial interventions targeting this stage of the cancer continuum. Interventions typically aim to increase physical and emotional well-being and quality of life by providing psychoeducational information related to long-term side effects, improving effective coping and stress management, and increasing social support. These are reviewed in more detail in later sections of this chapter.

Aftereffects of Cancer

Aftereffects refer to any long-term or late effects of cancer and its treatment and may range from very mild to serious in terms of their impact on physical and emotional well-being and quality of life (see Table 14.1) [36]. The occurrence of

Table 14.1 Institute of Medicine Defining long-term and late effects of cancer treatment [36]

- *Long-term effects* refer to any side effects or complications of treatment that begin during treatment and continue beyond the end of treatment; also known as persistent effects
- *Late effects* refer specifically to unrecognized toxicities that are absent or subclinical at the end of treatment and become manifest later because of any of the following factors: developmental processes, failure of compensatory mechanisms with the passage of time, or organ senescence. Late effects may appear months to years after the completion of treatment

aftereffects and how long they last are often difficult to predict and vary across disease and treatment types as well as relevant individual characteristics. Long-term and late effects impact a range of physical and emotional domains and may have practical implications for survivors related to accomplishing day-to-day life activities, employment and job performance, and obtaining or maintaining health insurance [36]. Common long-term and late effects are listed in Table 14.2.

Long-term effects develop during treatment and are persistent or chronic side effects that continue for months or even years past the end of treatment. Common long-term effects are listed below and include physical (e.g., anemia, fatigue, and neuropathy) and emotional (e.g., depressive symptoms) domains of well-being. Many long-term effects improve or resolve with time, whereas others are permanent such as limb loss, muscular weakness, or nerve damage. The prevalence of long-term effects is associated with cancer and treatment type and is influenced by the health and well-being of the individual (e.g., pre-morbid physical and psychological condition).

Late effects refer to any disease- or treatment-related difficulties that are absent or subclinical at the end of treatment but manifest anywhere from months to years later. The increasing complexity of treatment regimens has led to increased prevalence of late effects, which are often dose and modality specific [36]. The increased risk of a second cancer is the most life-threatening late effect, but other disabling conditions occur and

Table 14.2 Aftereffects of Cancer Treatment

Aftereffects of surgery include:

- Scarring at the incision site and internally
- Lymphedema or swelling of the arms or legs
- Problems with movement or activity
- Nutritional problems if part of the bowel is removed
- Cognitive problems such as memory loss and difficulty concentration
- Changes in sexual function and fertility
- Pain that may be acute (sudden), long-term, or chronic
- Emotional effects that may be related to feeling self-conscious about physical changes

Aftereffects of chemotherapy include:

- Fatigue
- Sexual problems
- Early or premature menopause
- Infertility
- Reduced lung capacity with difficulty breathing
- Kidney and urinary problems
- Neuropathy or numbness, tingling, and other sensations in certain areas of the body, especially the hands and feet
- Muscle weakness
- Cognitive problems such as memory loss or inability to concentrate
- Osteoporosis
- Changes in texture and appearance of hair and nails
- Secondary cancers

Aftereffects of radiation include:

- Cataracts, if treated near the eyes, cranial-spinal, or if given Total Body Irradiation (TBI)
- Permanent hair loss if the scalp is radiated over certain dose levels
- Dental decay, tooth loss, receding gums if radiated near the mouth
- Loss of tears and the ability to produce saliva if lacrimal or salivary glands in the face are radiated or there has been TBI
- Problems with thyroid and adrenal glands if the neck is radiated
- Slowed or halted bone growth in children if bone is radiated
- Effects on the pituitary gland and multiple hormonal effects if the hypothalamic-pituitary region is radiated
- Decreased range of motion in the treated area
- Skin sensitivity to sun exposure in area of skin that is radiated
- Problems with the bowel system if the abdomen is radiated
- Secondary cancers in the areas radiated
- Infertility, if ovaries, testes, cranial-spinal area, or TBI is directly radiated

(continued)

Table 14.2 (continued)

Emotional aftereffects following cancer treatment may include:

- Anger
- Sadness, depression, or loneliness
- Anxiety
- Post-traumatic stress
- Health worries and fear of recurrence
- Sense of loss for what might have been
- Uncertainty and vulnerability (e.g., "my body let me down")
- Uncertainty about the future; feeling unable to plan for the future
- Concerns about pain, fatigue, or physical side effects
- Concerns about body image
- Concerns about the future or having a new orientation to time and future
- Existential or spiritual concerns (e.g., "Why me?"; "Why now?")
- Concerns about death and dying
- Search for meaning and purpose; appreciation of life

Social aftereffects may include:

- Loss of support; isolation
- Alienation or stigma
- Altered social relationships, including intimate relationships and those with family members, friends, and peers
- Comparisons with peers or other cancer survivors

Practical aftereffects may include:

- Job performance; difficulty working due to physical or emotional aftereffects
- Problems getting health or life insurance coverage
- Challenges communicating concerns to your health care team
- Financial stressors
- Employment discrimination

need to be monitored for and addressed through medical and psychosocial interventions. Other common late effects include chronic fatigue and neuropathy, cognitive dysfunction, and declines in cardiovascular health [40, 41]. Female cancer survivors may experience premature menopause and both male and female survivors may experience infertility as a result of treatment [41]. The risk of late effects depends on the tissue exposed as well as the age and health condition of the patient at the time of treatment [40]. Many older survivors have comorbid medical conditions that may exacerbate treatment-related effects or complicate recovery of pre-morbid functioning. Tissues at risk for late toxicity include bone/soft tissues, cardiovascular, dental, endocrine, gastrointestinal, hepatic, hematological, immune system, neurocognitive, and nervous system tissue [36, 40, 41]. As cancer survivors are at increased risk for future health decrements, there is an ongoing need to monitor for and prevent late effects and promote healthy lifestyles.

There are relatively few longitudinal cohort studies evaluating the prevalence rates of long-term and late effects by disease and treatment type. The relationships between specific treatment regimens, patient characteristics, and physical and psychological aftereffects are not well understood. Some aftereffects may be expected given the nature of disease and treatment; brain and spine tumors, for example, increase the risk of neurologic deficits [42]; survivors of head and neck cancer are at increased risk for impaired eating, communication, and musculoskeletal functions of the neck and shoulder [31]; and individuals with bone cancers are more likely to experience mobility problems due to amputations or limb-sparing procedures [43]. Beyond general predictions like this, the degree of risk of long-term and late effects is difficult to calculate. Many of the aftereffects mentioned in this section extend well into long-term survivorship phases (>5 years post treatment) [36] and require continued monitoring.

Aftereffects of cancer treatment have the capacity to impact all domains of life, including physical and medical, psychological, social, existential, and spiritual domains. Some aftereffects may be easily identified because they are visible or have direct effects on function and well-being. Other effects, however, can be subtle and not readily apparent to the untrained observer (e.g., postural changes due to osteoporosis) or are not directly observable and only detectable through diagnostic testing (e.g., infertility, hypothyroidism). Likewise, emotional difficulties are often difficult to pinpoint and may go unrecognized or be misunderstood by survivors or by family members and loved ones. Important con-

siderations in dealing with long-term and late effects of cancer treatment, particularly with respect to emotional and psychological effects, include pre-morbid mental health functioning, personal and interpersonal resources, and coping strategies.

The role of psychosocial interventions in the first year following the end of treatment typically is to address concerns related to survivorship transition and coping with residual side effects of treatment. Research suggests that participation is associated with a number of benefits to physical and emotional well-being; this is reviewed in more detail in later sections of this chapter.

Long-Term Survivorship (>5 Years Post Treatment)

While many of the physical and psychosocial challenges of long-term survivorship are similar to those of earlier phases of the cancer experience, others may develop over time. Both the extended time period of which survivors have been coping with disease-related difficulties and the experience of new challenges (e.g., late effects) may cause distress and dysfunction even years after the end of treatment [44]. For example, infertility following cancer treatment may cause an increase in distress among younger survivors as they approach the age of reproduction and family planning [45]. Without adequate coping skills, survivors may experience increasing distress associated with social and functional difficulties as time goes on.

Additionally, long-term cancer survivors are at increased risk for poor overall health and health-related complications and may have to cope with exacerbated physical difficulties (e.g., comorbid medical conditions) and practical issues (e.g., ability to work and job performance; problems with health insurance). Furthermore, as cancer becomes more of a distance memory, survivors may be less likely to engage in healthy behaviors that are beneficial to their long-term health and well-being. As cancer survivors are at increased risk for experiencing negative health consequences, this is a vulnerable population. Evidence

Table 14.3 Physical and psychosocial challenges of long-term survivorship

- Adjustment to physical compromise, health worries, sense of loss for what might have been
- Body image concerns
- Long-term and late effects of treatment such as fatigue and cognitive difficulties
- Increased risk of poor overall health and health-related complications of treatment
- Alterations in social support and perceived loss of support from loved ones as well as cancer care medical team
- Interpersonal disruption and social isolation
- Sexuality and fertility issues and related effects on intimate relationship functioning
- Stigma of cancers associated with risk behaviors such as smoking and alcohol consumption
- Fear of recurrence and concerns about future and death
- Uncertainty and heightened sense of vulnerability
- Existential and spiritual issues
- Employment and insurance problems

suggests that despite making healthy behavior changes after diagnosis and at the end of active treatment, many longer term survivors do not maintain these changes and often resume the unhealthy lifestyle behaviors (e.g., smoking, being sedentary, being overweight or obese) they participated in prior to cancer. Common long-term survivorship difficulties are listed in Table 14.3.

While many survivors may be able to adjust to aftereffects and manage lingering fears and concerns with time, others may find that they are "stuck" and that their cope strategies are proving ineffective. This requires ongoing monitoring and interventions designed to target the specific fears and concerns of survivors coping with long-term and late effects of cancer including both physical and psychosocial areas of functioning. Many of the interventions that have been conducted among long-term survivors have been lifestyle interventions that promote healthy behavior changes. Results suggest that dietary and exercise interventions are effective [46, 47], though dissemination of interventions is often difficult as survivors become more and more removed from their cancer care [48]. Home-based interventions may be one way to overcome

barriers and promote adaptive changes in this population. These are discussed in more detail in later sections of this chapter.

Psychosocial Interventions in Cancer

Targets of Interventions

As a cancer diagnosis and its treatment pose significant short- and long-term challenges for survivors, their family members, and loved ones, psychosocial interventions that attempt to minimize the negative impact of cancer and promote positive adjustment and well-being have become increasingly common. Interventions typically aim to improve adjustment and well-being by:
- Promoting adaptive coping strategies
- Improving support-seeking behaviors and reducing social isolation
- Addressing maladaptive cognitions related to disease- or treatment-related outcomes
- Improving engagement with services and/or promotion of healthy lifestyle behaviors

The model in Fig. 14.1 proposes that cancer survivors may benefit from psychosocial interventions that target multiple components. For example, teaching anxiety reduction skills can provide a way to reduce anxiety, tension, and other forms of stress responses and thus help the survivor achieve a sense of mastery over disease-related and general stressors. The use of cognitive restructuring techniques can help survivors identify links between thoughts, emotions, and behaviors, and increase their ability to identify commonly used distorted thoughts that can interfere with effective management of their disease. Participants can benefit from increased awareness of the use of maladaptive coping strategies to deal with stress and disease-related challenges. Attention is given to replacing inefficient and indirect ways of dealing with stressors and promoting both emotion- and problem-focused strategies while also increasing survivors' ability to adaptively express both positive and negative emotions. Additionally, these intervention models promote the identification and utilization of beneficial social support resources, as well as providing

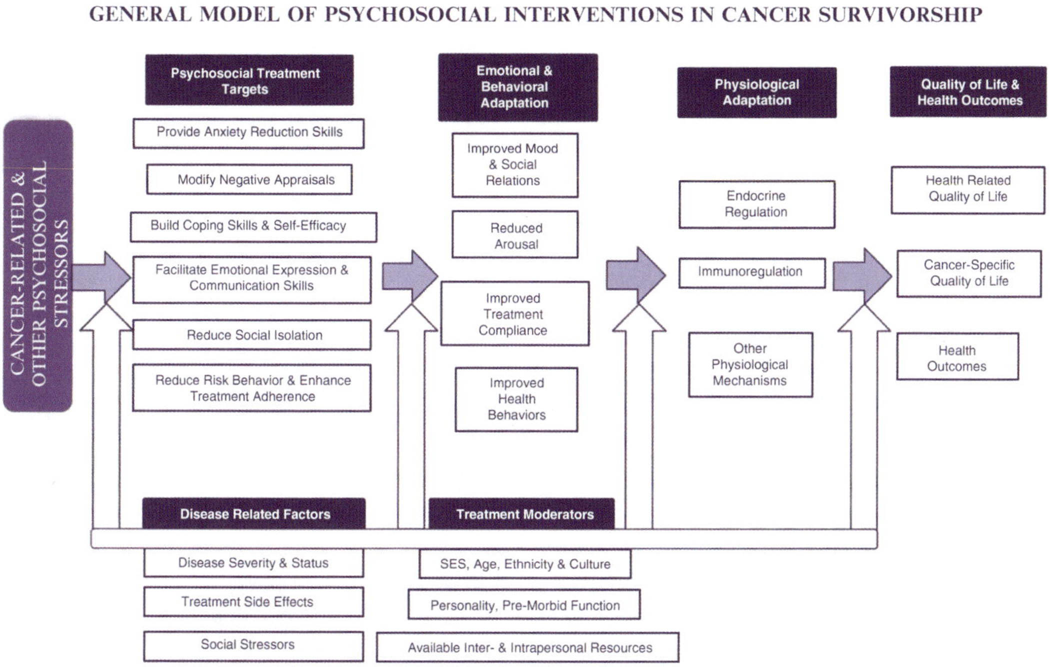

GENERAL MODEL OF PSYCHOSOCIAL INTERVENTIONS IN CANCER SURVIVORSHIP

Fig. 14.1   Conceptual model of psychosocial treatment interventions

self-management skills to engage in positive lifestyle changes and behaviors. Communication skills are also targeted, particularly those specific to interacting with health care professionals and communicating concerns about functional limitations and treatment-related side effects with the spouse/partner, family, and friends.

Psychosocial interventions typically aim to improve adjustment and well-being through the provision of disease- and treatment-related information and acquisition of intra- and interpersonal coping skills. Outcome measures often include a range of physical and emotional health indices as well as disease-specific and general quality of life. Another important target of psychosocial interventions following a cancer diagnosis is the promotion of healthy lifestyle behavior changes. Research indicates that the majority of cancer survivors continue to engage in unhealthy lifestyles (e.g., poor diet, inactivity) after the end of treatment, despite indicating a desire to make healthy changes during active treatment. Among head and neck cancer survivors, in particular, rates of alcohol and substance use are higher than normative rates and evidence suggests that many

survivors continue to smoke and drink hazardously after their diagnosis [49, 50].

Importance of health promotion following cancer treatment [48, 51]

- Engaging in health-promoting behaviors may improve health outcomes and decrease morbidity and mortality (e.g., tobacco and alcohol cessation, nutrition and diet, exercise, sun protection, cancer screening and prevention, medical surveillance).
- Engaging in health-promoting behaviors can empower active partnership with health care providers and may enhance perceived control over health outcomes.

Interventions that target existential and spiritual concerns related to disease- and treatment-related changes in quality of life as well as end-of-life fears and concerns typically focus on issues related to control, sense of meaning and peace of mind, identity, dignity, relationships, and hope or meaninglessness [34]. The goals of these interventions are largely the same as those of other psychosocial interventions and aim to improve adjustment, physical and emotional well-being, and quality of life, though some evidence suggests that physical outcomes are less of a focus than in other psychosocial interventions [52, 53]. Outcome measures have also included assessment of self-esteem, purpose in life, optimism, and hope for the future [53]. A recent review of the literature of existential and spiritual interventions indicated that the majority of the outcome measures assessed either improved or remained stable in intervention groups and declined in control groups [35]. It appears that psychosocial interventions that target existential and spiritual concerns may have positive effects on emotional well-being and quality of life [35, 53] and limited evidence suggested their utility in improving physical outcomes [35, 52].

Finally, given the interpersonal nature of cancer, couple-based interventions have also been conducted and aim to assist couples in adjusting to and coping with cancer-related changes in order to avoid or minimize individual distress and relationship dysfunction. Interventions may either be at the individual or couple level. Individual-level interventions that include both members of the couple typically target individual adjustment and well-being based on the logic that a couple will adjust to cancer most effectively if each partner adjusts well [54]. Alternatively, couple-level interventions identify relationship functioning as the primary therapeutic focus and target couple-level issues and skills, such as problem solving, promoting effective communication, and addressing concerns related to sexual interactions and intimacy. Intervention material typically addresses cancer-related problems as well as positive relationship functioning in general. The ways in which couples engage in relationship maintenance strategies (e.g., positivity, openness, assurance) after a diagnosis of cancer have been shown to impact their psychological and relational adjustment over time [54–57].

Types of Interventions

Many different types of interventions have been conducted among cancer survivors but therapy components typically involve an emotionally supportive context to address fears and anxieties, provision of information about the disease and its treatment, and promotion of cognitive and behavioral coping strategies, including stress management and relaxation training. The benefits of psychosocial interventions have been achieved through a number of therapeutic techniques that are based on theoretical models of stress and coping, psychological well-being, and health behavior change [11, 14, 58]. Supportive interventions primarily aim to provide survivors with the opportunity to acknowledge their experiences and express their emotions and concerns to other cancer survivors. Therapeutic processes by which participants benefit from an intervention and adjust to their cancer experience include sharing experiences, giving and receiving information, and reducing social isolation [3]. Psycho-educational interventions build on this but tend to be more structured in nature, often focusing on cognitive and behavioral techniques to facilitate adjustment and coping with which participants gain a greater sense of control over their illness experience [11, 58]. Participants are typically provided with information pertinent to their disease and its treatment and engage in lessons that teach and promote adaptive coping skills to help participants accept and effectively manage cancer-related changes. Cognitive behavioral approaches emphasize skill acquisition and behavioral change through goal setting, self-monitoring, coping skills, and social skills training [11, 59]. The majority of studies that have assessed the efficacy of cognitive behavioral techniques or psychoeducational methods that include or are based on cognitive behavioral techniques have found significant positive effects on a range of physical and emotional well-being outcomes (e.g., fatigue, pain, anxiety, depression, and general cancer distress) [5, 20, 60, 61]. Some evidence suggests that cancer survivors may benefit more from structured interventions than purely supportive ones [62]. This may be due to the acquisition of new skills with which survivors can more effectively cope with stress and the cancer experience after the intervention has ended (e.g., stress management, relaxation techniques) [59].

Cognitive behavioral approaches have also been combined with relaxation training and stress management techniques. For example, a manualized cognitive behavioral stress management (CBSM) group intervention developed and tailored to meet the specific needs of several medical populations, including breast cancer [63] and localized prostate cancer [64, 65], has shown a number of positive effects. The intervention consists of 10 weekly group meetings that include a 90-min didactic portion and 30 min of relaxation training. During the didactic portion of each session, participants were taught a variety of cognitive behavioral stress-management techniques, including identification of distorted thoughts, rational thought replacement, effective coping, anger management, assertiveness training, and development of social support. Information specific to disease physiology, diagnosis, treatment, and side effects was also provided. During the relaxation portion, participants learned and practiced a variety of relaxation techniques, including progressive muscle relaxation (PMR), guided imagery, meditation, and diaphragmatic breathing, and were encouraged to practice the techniques on a daily basis. The concepts and techniques introduced in each session built upon information covered in prior sessions and were reinforced through group discussions, exercises (e.g., role-plays), and weekly homework assignments. Discussions were tailored to address the specific needs and concerns of survivors given their phase along the cancer continuum. For example, among men with prostate cancer, the intervention aimed to provide an opportunity to help men accept post-treatment sexual dysfunction, normalize feelings of anxiety or depression surrounding a perceived loss of male identity, reframe intrusive or distorted thoughts of disappointment or inadequacy, and learn adaptive coping strategies to effectively communicate with sexual partners and adjust to altered sexual patterns [38, 64–67].

Individual Support and Self-Administered Interventions

Individual interventions include any form of therapy, counseling, or support that is delivered on a one-to-one basis. This may involve therapy or counseling with a qualified professional or volunteer-based support from a fellow cancer survivor

(i.e., peer-based programs) or other type of volunteer. Individual psychotherapy offers an opportunity to provide survivors with more attention and support than group therapy often allows and therapeutic efforts may be targeted to the specific needs of the individual. This may be particularly relevant among survivors who indicate clinically significant levels of distress or meet diagnostic criteria for a mental health disorder. Likewise, individuals for whom a group context provokes symptoms of distress or those unwilling to disclose information related to their feelings and experiences to group participants may benefit from individual therapy as an alternative. The disadvantages include the added time and resources that individual therapy requires. Peer-based interventions may offer an alternative. It has been reported that peer support helps to increase knowledge about the cancer experience and possible coping strategies, decrease patient's sense of isolation, and provides a sense of hope to cancer survivors [68]. Preliminary evidence suggests that regardless of whether volunteers are cancer survivors or not, one-to-one volunteer-based support interventions are well received and provide some benefit, including reduced distress and improved well-being. With regard to peer-based programs specifically, participants have indicated positive feelings towards having an opportunity to speak with someone who has shared similar experiences and seeing someone who has survived cancer [68]. However, there is limited empirical evidence supporting the effectiveness of volunteer-based support programs as very few well-designed randomized-controlled trials have been conducted. Although this may offer a cost-effective alternative to individual psychotherapy, disadvantages of peer-based programs include the lack of formal training of the volunteer support providers; the success of peer-based interventions may depend on their training and supervision.

Peer-based interventions represent an effort to increase the availability of psychosocial interventions by reducing costs and required resources. This may also be achieved through self-administered interventions. Self-administered interventions provide survivors with information to increase their knowledge and develop skills on their own to facilitate their adjustment and well-being. For example, the effect of a patient self-administered stress management intervention (SSMT) was compared to a professionally administered stress management intervention (PSMT) and a usual care control (UC) condition among cancer survivors undergoing chemotherapy [69]. The PSMT condition consisted of a single 60-min session conducted by a mental health professional in which discussion included psychoeducation regarding stress and stress management (e.g., common sources and manifestations of stress; stress management techniques to improve mental and physical well-being), guided relaxation exercises (e.g., paced abdominal breathing, abbreviated progressive muscle relaxation, relaxing mental imagery), and a brief instruction in the use of "coping self-statements" [69]. In the SSMT condition, survivors were given a package of instructional resources by a mental health professional during a 10-min session in which a booklet and prerecorded audiotapes that covered the same material and training exercises reviewed in the PSMT were provided [69]. Results indicated that participation in the SSMT condition was associated with positive effects on a range of quality of life (i.e., better physical functioning, greater vitality, fewer role limitations because of emotional problems, and better mental health) compared to the UC condition [69]. Differences between the SSMT and PSMT conditions were not directly compared, though results indicated that the SSMT intervention led to improvements in quality of life similar to previously reported PSMT intervention effects but at a much more favorable cost [69]. Although this is a relatively new area of intervention research, promising findings support the benefit and favorable cost of self-administered stress management interventions. This is may prove to be a viable alternative for survivors with reduced access to psychosocial interventions due to disease- or treatment-related disability or other limitations (e.g., lack of transportation or childcare). The efficacy and cost advantages of patient self-administered interventions warrant further investigation of techniques that require limited professional time or experience to deliver.

Group Interventions

Group-based psychosocial interventions provide an opportunity for survivors to express feelings and concerns related to disease and treatment in an emotionally supportive and safe context. As avoidant coping and emotional suppression are associated with poorer mood and adjustment outcomes [3, 70], interventions may facilitate adaptive coping strategies in which survivors may express both positive and negative emotions related to their cancer experience. Cancer survivors often struggle with feelings of uncertainty and loss of control. These feelings, albeit normal in reaction to cancer diagnosis and treatment, can be overwhelming. Furthermore, negative emotional reactions may be exacerbated without a strong social support network or amidst feelings of social isolation. While interventions delivered in both an individual and group format provide the opportunity for survivors to share their feelings and concerns while also acquiring disease-specific information and specific coping skills with which to improve their adjustment and well-being; group interventions provide a distinct advantage in several key domains. First, groups provide a setting where survivors may express their feelings to others who share similar experiences and understanding, which serves to normalize these feelings and reduce the degree of distress and interference they may cause [3]. Intervention participants can find others who are going through the same or similar experiences with regard to specific treatment regimens and side effects, disruptions to daily routines and functional limitations, and feelings of uncertainty and future-planning concerns. This may buffer the social isolation that frequently occurs after a cancer diagnosis and provide valuable support during difficult times. Cancer survivors often report feeling a loss of connection to their natural support networks either due to their own diminished energy and/or mobility to keep up old routines and social engagements or others' withdrawal out of fear or awkwardness. Social support is needed for successful coping and group interventions may provide a new and very important social connection and sense of community.

Moreover, many survivors take great pleasure in providing support to fellow group members.

This has been termed the "helper-therapy principle" and suggests that survivors benefit from being in a position to share their experiences and help others undergoing similar difficulties [3]. As such, group interventions provide an opportunity for members to learn from one another's experiences while also gaining a sense of accomplishment and self-esteem by helping others in similar and reciprocal ways.

Finally, group composition appears to be an important determinant of intervention efficacy. Differential effects of interventions that include homogeneous (e.g., all distressed) versus hetero- geneous (e.g., both distressed and non-distressed) participants have been evaluated but recommen- dations regarding the optimal conditions under which to conduct group interventions are incon- clusive. Based on theories of social comparison, some studies have shown a greater benefit for participants who report high psychosocial dis- tress at baseline and little or no benefit for those who report low distress (i.e., distressed patients benefit from the presence of non-distressed patients) [71]. The effects of social comparison have been found to be dependent on a number of different factors (e.g., need for comparison, direc- tion of the comparison [upward or downward], whether the individual identifies or contrasts with the comparison individual, the degree to which the individual feels change with regard to the comparison is possible) [71, 72]. Interpretations of these findings are limited, however, as research- based group interventions are typically homoge- neous with regard to cancer type and often distinguish between early- and advanced-stage diseases.

Couples Interventions

Undoubtedly, the impact of cancer is not limited to the individual patient. Instead, the entire fam- ily is often affected and each family member must adjust to cancer-related changes in roles and responsibilities and overall family functioning and well-being. Partners, in particular, must cope with challenges related to worry and fear about the potential loss of their partner and their ability to provide emotional and practical support. Family members routinely provide personal care and are often the primary sources of support for

the cancer survivor. Taking on these responsibili- ties may be stressful and distressing for caregiv- ers and affected family members. Additionally, financial concerns related to family income, insurance status, and employment may also arise, adding to the stress and burden of a cancer diag- nosis and its treatment. Although spouses/part- ners and family members are often negatively affected, they typically fail to receive the respite and support they need.

Psychosocial challenges associated with cancer- related changes may be different at different stages of the cancer continuum. Through and transition to survivorship, partners may take a more active caretaker role. After the end of treat- ment, however, as survivors regain their strength and resume pre-cancer activities and responsi- bilities, couples must navigate the transition in roles and relationship functioning. All phases of the cancer experience are characterized by significant challenges that can be distressing to survivors and partners on an individual level as well as to the relationship as a whole. Stressors include changes in role functions, communica- tion difficulties (e.g., avoidance of discussions of cancer-related concerns and fears), and sexual dysfunction [54, 55, 57, 73]. At times, relation- ship distress may continue even after individual distress is alleviated [54]. Importantly, couples have reported beneficial effects of cancer such as increased intimacy and marital satisfaction [74]. Nevertheless, despite some indication of overall benefit, many couples will experience some difficulty adjusting to cancer-related changes in their relationship, particularly those who face more advanced stage disease, greater treatment- related side effects, or poor prognostic factors.

Couple-based psychosocial interventions have reported a number of beneficial outcomes, includ- ing improvements in individual psychological and relationship functioning. Specifically, inter- ventions have shown positive effects on commu- nication and marital functioning, distress, appraisal of illness, appraisal of caregiving, feel- ings of uncertainty and hopelessness, and general and disease-specific quality of life [54, 75–78]. Although these results are promising, the major- ity of couple-based interventions have included couples coping with breast and prostate cancers and interpretations may not generalize to other cancers. Depending on the cancer site and stage as well as treatment and prognostic factors, couples face a wide range of challenges. Localized prostate cancer, for example, has a high survival rate and couples are more likely to focus on treatment-related side effects and long-term adjustment issues, whereas couples coping with lung or pancreatic cancer will most likely have to face end-of-life concerns and open communication about grief and loss. Couples' concerns and demands on the relationship will differ depending on disease and treatment factors. Individual and relationship moderators of psychosocial interventions are discussed in more detail below, though little research has evaluated factors associated with couple-based intervention efficacy.

Modes of Delivery

An important consideration regarding the delivery of psychosocial interventions to cancer populations concerns their availability and accessibility. Traditionally, interventions have been conducted in-person by a mental health professional. However, there are several barriers that often prevent cancer survivors from attending in-person intervention sessions such as debilitating side effects, geographic distance, and access to transportation as well as work- and family-related responsibilities (e.g., need for childcare) [69, 79–84]. Distance represents a significant barrier particularly for older cancer survivors, while younger survivors are more likely to experience competing demands on their time such as work commitments and care of young children. Widespread availability of psychosocial interventions is unlikely due to these barriers as well as to the limited number of qualified mental health professionals working in oncology settings and the costs of conducting interventions facilitated by mental health professionals. Volunteer-based interventions, discussed earlier, address some of these barriers. Home-based interventions that utilize telephone- or computer-based approaches or rely on mailed

materials may be another alternative and help to increase the accessibility to those that would otherwise be unable to participate.

There are several advantages to home-based versus in-person interventions. The modality of delivery is relatively flexible. For example, psychoeducational material may be delivered synchronously (e.g., real-time telephone calls or chat rooms) or asynchronously (e.g., materials that are mailed home or "newsgroups"). There is also a greater variety of facilitation options, including increased scheduling convenience, which may translate to increased access for individuals with poor health status, competing demands, and/or lack of transportation. Home-based interventions typically require fewer resources and costs than in-person interventions [81, 82].

Evidence suggests that the use of telephone- and Web-based interventions is efficacious across a range of outcomes Breast cancer survivors have demonstrated significant improvements in depression, cancer-related trauma, and perceived stress following a Web-based psycheducational support group (12-week intervention) [83], as well as significant improvements in exercise behaviors and weight gain following a telephone-based physical activity intervention even during adjuvant treatment phases that included chemotherapy and/or radiation [85]. Similarly, a telephone-based cognitive behavioral intervention that was combined with pharmacologic treatment for nicotine use and depression as needed, conducted in head and neck cancer survivors diagnosed with stage III/IV disease, demonstrated significant effects on smoking cessation; nonsignificant effects were reported for alcohol use and depression [49]. Findings suggest that Web- and telephone-based interventions may be effective in improving disease-specific and general quality of life among survivors undergoing adjuvant treatment and among those with advanced-stage disease. However, the majority of studies have been conducted among breast cancer survivors and more research is needed to determine the acceptability and efficacy of home-based interventions in other cancer populations. Similarly, most home-based interventions have targeted cancer survivors within the first year post diagnosis. Such interventions are well designed to improve adjustment and well-being related to cancer diagnosis and active treatment. Limited work has demonstrated that home-based interventions are feasible among long-term cancer survivors (>5 years post diagnosis). More work is needed in other cancer populations and among those who are in the later phases of the cancer continuum.

It is important to note that there are some disadvantages and limitations to consider with telephone- and Web-based interventions. The most obvious is that individuals must have access to and knowledge of the technology that is required to participate in the intervention. This is particularly relevant to older populations who may not be as familiar with or comfortable using more advanced technology (e.g., "Webcams"). Technological mishaps may be frustrating for intervention participants and disruptive to group processes and cohesion. Facilitators should be aware of potential difficulties and prepared to adjust to whatever problems may arise during the course of the session. Finally, the use of the telephone and Internet to deliver an intervention adds additional concerns regarding confidentiality. For example, group-based interventions via telephone conference calls carry the inherent risk that non-group members may overhear group discussions. Likewise, despite using passwords to protect intervention Web sites, group members may allow non-group members to view the Webpage and read postings or see photographs of other members. Participants should be reminded of the limitations of confidentiality and that their postings should be treated as potentially public documents. Despite these limitations and given the barriers to dissemination of in-person interventions, there is a distinct need for home-based interventions. Preliminary evidence indicates that home-based interventions are feasible, affordable, and acceptable to survivors, with promising effects on disease-specific and general quality of life outcomes. Home-based interventions provide an efficient means of reaching survivors who may otherwise be physically and/or socially isolated or lack the self-efficacy to report problems and seek support.

Interventions Across the Cancer Continuum

Pretreatment Interventions

As suggested, the number of interventions that have targeted survivors in the pretreatment phase of their cancer experience is limited. This may be a stressful time period, however, in which survivors are still adjusting to their cancer diagnosis, deciding on their course of treatment, and coping with the idea of anticipated treatment side effects. A few psychosocial interventions have been used to prepare survivors for the likely sequelae of physical and functional side effects and emotional reactions following treatment and shown positive results. A review of pretreatment interventions suggests that several different types (e.g., psychoeducation, behavioral, coping skills training, relaxation, and guided imagery) administered prior to the start of chemotherapy demonstrated positive effects on treatment side effects (e.g., nausea, vomiting), emotional distress and depression, functional limitations due to disease and/or treatment, and better overall QOL [69].

Psychoeducation interventions, specifically, have been shown to reduce fear and uncertainty; reviews suggest that psychoeducation intervention efforts that focus on what to expect post treatment and ways to cope with disease- and treatment-related stress are beneficial. For example, a 90-min "coping preparation" intervention for survivors about to start chemotherapy included a tour of the oncology clinic, provision of videotaped and written materials about coping with the effects of treatment, and a discussion session with a therapist and was combined with a relaxation training intervention. Compared to relaxation training alone and a standard treatment control condition, the combined coping preparation plus relaxation training intervention resulted in less anticipatory nausea, less depression, and less interference in daily life from effects [86]. Similarly, a psychoeducation intervention consisting of only a brief (15–20 min) meeting with a counselor delivered at the time of the initial treatment consultation with the medical oncologist, designed to orient the survivors with the facility and prepare them for their treatment (i.e., included a tour of the oncology clinic, description of clinic procedures, provision of contact information for clinic services and local and national support services, and a question and answer session), demonstrated positive effects on anxiety and depressive symptoms and satisfaction with medical care compared to usual care alone [87].

Behavioral interventions that consist of relaxation training (e.g., progressive muscle relaxation and guided imagery techniques) prior to the start of chemotherapy result in fewer side effects (e.g., nausea, vomiting), less psychological distress, and better overall quality of life compared to standard treatment control conditions [19, 88]. Likewise, relaxation and stress management interventions administered prior to surgery have been shown to improve postoperative mood and quality of life and some evidence suggests that benefits may extend beyond the perioperative period. For example, a preoperative interview with either a 30-min psychotherapeutic intervention or chat with a consultant surgeon trained in listening and counseling skills was effective in improving adaptive coping strategies and reducing body image distress, depression, and anxiety compared to standard care alone among breast cancer survivors at 3 months post surgery (some effects continued up to 12 months post surgery) [89]. The intervention was superior to the chat with a surgeon condition only among participants who reported severe stressful life events, highlighting the increased need for intervention in at-risk survivors depending on pretreatment psychosocial factors [89].

Interventions administered prior to the start of treatment that attempt to prepare survivors in their coping with treatment-related challenges and posttreatment side effects may have a beneficial impact on physical and psychosocial outcomes. Findings support the utility of cognitive behavioral and relaxation techniques, specifically, to enhance stress management and adaptive coping, and suggest that interventions do not necessarily have to be extensive in nature (i.e., one to two sessions). However, interventions have primarily been conducted among breast and prostate cancer survivors and it is largely unknown how pretreatment interventions may be efficacious in improving response to treatment and posttreatment well-being in other cancers. Further investigation is also warranted to determine the specific timing of optimal intervention design (e.g., time-limited prior to treatment versus ongoing throughout treatment course) and to identify those survivors most likely to benefit from different treatment components (e.g., relaxation training versus cognitive stress management techniques). Finally, although pretreatment interventions are limited, similar interventions in other medical populations further support their utility. For example, the provision of stress management techniques prior to surgery in various non-cancer patient populations has been associated with less pain and use of analgesic medication, lowered blood pressure, less distress, and better quality of life following surgery [90].

Interventions Conducted During and Immediately Following Treatment

The vast majority of psychosocial interventions in cancer survivors has been conducted either during active treatment or in the first year following the termination of primary treatment. Reviews of the literature suggest positive effects on a range of outcomes, including psychosocial and behavioral well-being, and general and disease-specific quality of life [91]. These are reviewed below.

Emotional and Physical Well-Being and Quality of Life

Emotional well-being outcomes have included distress, anxiety and depression, anger, self-esteem, optimism, and self-efficacy. Interventions have been shown to promote better understanding of illness, feeling involved in treatment, self-efficacy, having a more positive outlook, benefit finding, and hope for the future. Important physical outcomes include pain, sleep disruption or insomnia, vigor, and fatigue. Group-based cognitive behavioral interventions appear to be efficacious in improving emotional well-being and quality of life in cancer survivors in the posttreatment period. Some evidence suggests that improvements in physical functioning may be less prominent [92]. Cognitive behavioral interventions, specifically, have been related to short-term effects on anxiety and depression and both short- and long-term effects on depression and quality of life [19]. Group interventions that utilize cognitive behavioral approaches have considerable potential to be incorporated as a routine part of clinical care offered to survivors finishing treatment to promote positive adjustment to cancer survivorship. Similarly, stress management training is an effective and feasible intervention improve emotional well-being and quality of life among survivors undergoing active treatment and in the transition to posttreatment survivorship. Despite promising findings, there is a need for more well-controlled clinical trials based on the history and patterns of common problems experienced by cancer survivors. The majority of psychosocial interventions focus on dimensions of psychological distress and health-related quality of life; greater attention should be paid to mechanisms of action (i.e., psychological and physiological processes that promote positive outcomes) [93]. Although cognitive behavioral and stress management approaches are suggested as viable and effective interventions, further research is needed to improve long-term benefit.

Immune Function

For some time now it has been recognized that psychosocial factors are associated with immune functioning. Depressive symptoms, anger suppression, negative personality traits (e.g., lack of sociability), and greater illness-related disruptions in marital or partner relationships have been associated with lower immune functioning; optimism has been related to better immune functioning [3, 58, 94]. Furthermore, some research indicates that psychosocial interventions have immunological benefits, though results are variable and reliable relationships cannot be determined [58, 94, 95]. Although the impact of psychosocial interventions on immune function appears to be modest at best in the existing literature, more research and further clarification of important conceptual and methodological issues are needed before drawing definitive conclusions.

Survival

Very few psychosocial or behavioral intervention studies conducted in cancer survivors have examined survival as an outcome and conclusions regarding improvement in survival time following participation in an intervention are preliminary. Although some studies have reported beneficial effects on survival (e.g., supportive-expressive group therapy [13, 96–98]; psychosocial behavioral intervention [99, 100]; psychoeducational intervention [101]; intervention to improve medication compliance [102]), other studies have not found significant benefit of participation [97, 103, 104]. Efficacious studies have been conducted in several cancer populations, including breast and malignant melanoma, with follow-up times of up to 10 years post intervention. Common factors among those interventions that demonstrated significant effects on survival have been identified [105] and include (1) group compositions that were homogeneous with respect to cancer type and stage and (2) interventions that included an educational component, stress management, and coping skills training [105]. However, in a meta-analysis of the effect of psychosocial interventions on survival time in cancer, neither randomized nor nonrandomized studies indicated a significant effect [105]. Notably, the authors highlight several methodological limitations in making comparisons across studies due to significant variability with respect to cancer types and stage, intervention components, and follow-up times [105].

Several psychosocial factors have been linked to the development and progression of cancer and have been shown to be important considerations in cancer care (e.g., helplessness/hopelessness coping style, social isolation). It is plausible that interventions that alter modifiable risk factors may significantly impact prognosis and survival. For example, high levels of perceived stress have been shown to have suppressive effects on immune function and this relationship may be modulated by social support [106]. Therefore, interventions that aim to reduce perceptions of stress, improve physical and emotional well-being, and achieve optimal immune function may very well influence relevant disease-related factors related to survival. Although conclusions regarding the benefit of psychosocial interventions on survival should be interpreted with caution, theory and empirical evidence provide rationale for further investigation.

Mixed Findings

While there have been many reviews that have strongly supported the benefit of psychosocial interventions on emotional and physical well-being, adjustment to disease- and treatment-related side effects, and quality of life, others have offered only tentative recommendations or have cited insufficient evidence with which to make recommendations for or against their use. Meta-analyses have cited several problems in how results are reported in the literature such as low quality of methodology and inconsistent findings regarding intervention efficacy [16, 17, 107]. One reason for inconsistent findings is the inclusion of survivors who are not in need of psychosocial support and reviewers have recommended that large-scale studies should screen participants for distress prior to enrollment [104]. Additionally, few interventions have reported mechanisms of change associated with positive outcomes.

Taken together, evidence suggests that psychosocial interventions need to be employed with greater awareness of moderating factors related to emotional distress and intervention efficacy as well as mechanisms of change associated with active versus inactive intervention components. To this end, intervention components may be developed with greater specificity to target cancer populations and subpopulations characterized by different sociodemographic and health-related factors and psychosocial needs. Sources of emotional distress and the intervention components needed to address them may vary considerably across different cancer types and stages and treatment status. A greater understanding of factors that are associated with increased risk of poor adjustment and active therapeutic mechanisms will result in refinements to interventions that enhance efficacy and inform underlying theory.

What Works for Whom?
Sociodemographic Factors
Age. Younger survivors are more likely to experience emotional distress (e.g., depression and anxiety) in response to cancer and its treatment than older survivors, particularly among women [11]. This may be due to younger survivors feeling more unprepared to cope with a serious threat to their health and mortality, particularly if other responsibilities (e.g., parenting of younger children) are a concern. Conversely, older survivors (>65 years) may already be coping with age-related declines in physical health or may have peers that have faced similar (or worse) health challenges and therefore are better equipped to negotiate cancer-related changes. For example, despite experiencing significant treatment-related disruptions to physical well-being, localized prostate cancer survivors often report above average levels of emotional well-being compared to age-matched normative populations [108].

Socioeconomic Status. Recent evidence suggests that disparities in quality of life among cancer survivors are explained, in part, by differences in socioeconomic status (SES); high-income survivors are not only more likely to survive cancer but also report higher levels of quality of life than low-income survivors [36]. Cancer diagnosis and treatment may exacerbate prior socioeconomic difficulties or socioeconomic concerns may arise from cancer treatment such as financial stress related to costs of care, access to health insurance, and the ability to continue or return to work or school. Thus, individuals characterized by lower SES may be in more need of psychosocial interventions designed to address stress management and active coping skills. Some evidence suggests that survivors who report lower SES may benefit more from interventions than those who report higher SES [109].

Ethnicity and Cultural Backgrounds. Ethnic minorities are more likely to experience more difficulty adjusting to cancer and its treatment and greater decrements in quality of life, including worse mental health and physical functioning, as well as worse health outcomes, including more frequent recurrence, shorter disease-free survival, and higher mortality rates [110–112]. Despite this, few interventions have been tailored to meet the specific needs of ethnic minorities characterized by different cultural backgrounds and limited evidence has evaluated the extent to which ethnic and cultural differences are associated with intervention efficacy. Although many studies have evaluated differences in intervention effects across racial/ethnicity groups, few have tailored intervention efforts to meet the specific ethnic and cultural needs among different groups. Furthermore, strategies to achieve cultural appropriateness within psychosocial interventions for ethnic minorities have largely focused on recruitment and retention efforts and have not focused enough on ensuring that sociocultural concepts are incorporated into the content of the intervention [113, 114]. This remains a critical gap in the literature and warrants further investigation.

Medical Factors

As noted previously, more advanced disease is associated with greater likelihood of psychological distress and worse physical functioning and overall quality of life. As such, there is an increased need for effective psychosocial interventions in this patient population. A recent review of the literature suggested that support-expressive therapies and cognitive behavioral therapy are effective in preventing or relieving depression and anxiety among survivors with metastatic disease; relaxation techniques, alone or in combination with education/skills training, may be more effective in preventing or relieving depression and anxiety among survivors in the terminal phase of their disease [19].

Physical and Emotional Well-Being

Cancer survivors who report significant distress and/or disability throughout the cancer continuum are likely to be in need of psychosocial interventions and limited evidence suggests that intervention efficacy may vary depending on baseline levels of physical and emotional well-being. For example, the effects of a coping and communication-enhancing intervention (CCI)

with supportive counseling among women with gynecologic cancer and supportive counseling alone demonstrated significant improvements in depression symptoms (nonsignificant effects on cancer-specific distress); however, women who experienced decreases in functional ability over time reported greater improvements following supportive counseling [77]. The researchers hypothesized that the less structured nature of the supportive counseling may have given women more of an opportunity to discuss worries related to their increasing disability, whereas the more structured nature of the CCI may have limited those opportunities in the other condition [77]. Results suggest that under conditions in which intervention components fail to match the specific needs of participants, interventions that allow greater flexibility and freedom to address specific concerns may be more beneficial. Furthermore, interventions designed for cancer survivors experiencing heightened levels of psychological distress have demonstrated immediate and sustained benefit [8, 19]. Finally, as cancer diagnosis and its treatment often exacerbate prior psychiatric symptoms or mental health disorders, identifying those who may be at increased risk for clinically significant symptoms based on their mental health history may also be important.

Perceived Stress

The degree to which cancer survivors appraise their situation as being unpredictable, uncontrollable, or overwhelming has significant implications for their emotional well-being [100, 115, 116]. Perceived stress has been shown to be a significant moderator of intervention effects on emotional well-being; such that those with higher levels of perceived stress at baseline report greater improvements in emotional well-being following participation than those with lower levels of perceived stress at baseline [117]. Similarly, greater severity of lifetime stressful events has been associated with greater benefit from interventions including improvements in adaptive coping skills and emotional well-being (e.g., depression, anxiety, body image distress) [89]. As perceptions of stress and stress management skills are related to lowered emotional well-being, physical functioning, and lowered quality of life, findings suggest an increased need for interventions that target survivors who report higher levels of perceived stress and/or lack the skills to manage that stress.

Social Support

Cancer survivors with fewer inter- and intrapersonal resources with which to cope with cancer-related stressors are at increased risk for experiencing emotional difficulties and decrements in quality of life and are more likely to benefit from psychosocial interventions. For example, social isolation, living alone, and being unmarried or unpartnered were shown to negatively affect psychosocial outcomes and mortality [118]. Among breast cancer survivors, lack of personal resources (i.e., low self-esteem, low body image, low perceived control, and high illness uncertainty), low partner-specific emotional support, and lack of physician informational support were related to intervention efficacy, independent of SES and disease stage [119]. Similar findings have been reported among male cancer survivors suggesting that single men, compared to single women and married or partnered men and women, may be highly vulnerable to psychosocial and health-related morbidity due to low levels of social support [30, 118]. Although gender differences in social support needs often indicate that men are more likely to report a desire for informational support over emotional support, men are also more likely to have emotional support deficits. It remains unclear whether men would also benefit from emotional support interventions despite reluctance to admit as much. Nevertheless, evidence suggests the importance of considering social support as a moderator of intervention effects.

Personality Traits

Limited work has evaluated the influence of different personality traits on adjustment and well-being in cancer survivors. A recent study evaluated the predictive relationships between psychosocial traits and health-related quality of life among localized prostate cancer survivors post treatment and reported that personality traits

characterized by inhibition or avoidance, dependency, depression, passive-aggressiveness, or low self-regard (self-denigration) were significantly associated with worse emotional and social domains of health-related quality of life (i.e., nonsignificant effects on physical domains); men who indicated a tendency to have psychological difficulties with invasive medical procedures and to overutilize healthcare services also reported lower levels of health-related quality of life [120]. Among colorectal cancer survivors, personality traits defined as "sense of coherence" and "denial defense" were positively associated with multiple domains of health-related quality of life and hostility; "repression defense" was negatively associated with physical HRQOL, independent of psychological distress and disease severity [121]. These results are similar to analyses conducted in non-cancer populations in which personality traits related to neuroticism (e.g., pessimistic, depressive, and anxious traits) were found to be associated with an increased risk of all-cause mortality even when measured early in life [122, 123]. Screening for personality traits that are associated with an increased risk of experiencing disease- and treatment-related distress and lowered quality of life may be an important consideration for clinicians and targets of intervention efforts to facilitate adjustment and well-being.

Neuroticism. Consistent with above, higher neuroticism has been shown to predict poorer quality of life up to 2 years post surgery in breast cancer survivors [124]; and a population-based cohort study reported a positive association between neuroticism and cancer-related death, particularly among women [125]. Neuroticism has also been associated with somatic complaints, physical and emotional well-being (e.g., reduced functional ability, peripheral neuropathy, sexual problems, self-esteem concerns), and several indicators of unhealthy lifestyle (e.g., hazardous alcohol use, daily use of medication, use of sedatives and hypnotics) among testicular cancer survivors [126].

Interpersonal Sensitivity and Social Inhibition. Limited work has considered the effects of interpersonal sensitivity and social inhibition on adjustment and well-being in cancer. Among localized prostate cancer survivors post treatment, men who were characterized by higher levels of interpersonal sensitivity (i.e., were more sensitive to their interpersonal environment) were more likely to perceive their sexual side effects as a threat to core masculinity and experienced greater difficulty adjusting to treatment-related changes in sexual functioning [22]. Similarly, among the same sample of localized prostate cancer survivors, social inhibition was a significant moderator of CBSM intervention effects on sexual functioning such that those who were high in social inhibition demonstrated significantly larger pre- to post-intervention treatment gains in sexual functioning [23].

Unmitigated Agency. Recent work has evaluated the role of unmitigated agency and its association with poorer adjustment and well-being in cancer populations (e.g., higher levels of depressive symptoms and substance use) [127, 128]. Unmitigated agency is a gender-linked personality trait characterized by a tendency to focus on oneself to the point of exclusion of other people and is associated with stereotypical concepts of masculinity and the male gender role. It includes traits such as greed, hostility, and arrogance that represent underlying personalities characterized by self-absorption (e.g., egotistical) and a negative orientation towards others (e.g., cynicism) [127, 128]. Unmitigated agency has been shown to interact with social support among male cancer survivors; men who endorse a high degree of unmitigated agency are negatively affected by increases in perceived social support, whereas those with low unmitigated agency benefit from increases in support [129–131]. By definition, those characterized by high unmitigated agency are more likely to prefer interpersonal disengagement and less likely to accept or seek support. Increases in social support may be characterized by expectations to express difficult emotions or to be receptive to and grateful for the support [130]. As such, offers of assistance and emotional support may be negatively received. Likewise, group-based interventions that promote adjust-

ment and well-being, in part, through social support may also be negatively received and have unintended consequences. Findings suggest that differences in personality traits may moderate the impact of intervention-related increases in social support and indicate a need to match individual preferences and needs for support when considering the effects of interventions on adjustment and well-being.

Coping Styles

Different coping styles are differentially related to various indicators of adjustment and well-being. Approach, problem-focused, and emotion-focused coping strategies (e.g., seeking social support) are generally associated with better physical and emotional well-being, whereas avoidant coping (e.g., disengagement, cognitive avoidance) is associated with worse outcomes [9, 39, 70, 132]. For example, approach coping was related to better self-esteem, positive affect, depression, and anxiety compared to avoidance coping, which was related to worse psychological adjustment and physical functioning [132]. Among a mixed sample of male cancer survivors, avoidant coping was associated with greater severity of sleep disruption and more interference with daily functioning; increased depression was identified as a significant mediator of the relationship between avoidant coping and sleep disruption [133]. Women with gynecologic cancer undergoing extensive chemotherapy who reported greater use of avoidant coping were also more likely to report poorer physical and emotional well-being and greater anxiety, depression, fatigue, and total mood disturbance; those using active coping reported less distress, better social well-being, and closer relationships with their doctors [134]. Evidence also suggests that negative effects associated with avoidant coping may be more pronounced among survivors with advanced-stage disease and/or extensive treatment regimens [135]. A recent review of the literature suggested that emotion-focused coping may be more effective among survivors with advanced cancer than problem-focused coping [70]. Findings are mixed regarding the effects of religious or spiritual coping, though evidence suggests that this type of coping may be particularly relevant in advanced-stage disease and during end-of-life care [33, 34]. Of note, some studies have indicated that cancer survivors who decline to participate in psychosocial interventions are more likely to use coping styles characterized by avoidance and denial (e.g., expressed wish to avoid discussing feelings related to cancer, denial of having feelings related to cancer) [11]. Alternatively, it has been shown that avoidance and denial coping may be beneficial to some individuals, particularly those who may not have adequate intra- or interpersonal resources with which to acknowledge and accept the full extent of disease- and treatment-related changes [70]. The effectiveness of these coping strategies among subgroups characterized by different psychosocial needs requires further evaluation.

Stepped Care Approach

Psychosocial interventions among cancer survivors have shown promise in improving emotional well-being, and both general and disease-specific

quality of life. Most approaches involved group therapy interventions following cognitive behavioral, stress and coping, stress management, and supportive group environment theories and models. Some work has also included psychoeducational components, engaged spouses/partners, or provided phone-based and Web-based delivery of the interventions. Regardless of the intervention approach, it is important to consider the distress continuum among cancer survivors to determine the most optimal level of care based on their needs (see Fig. 14.2).

Psychosocial intervention is not necessary for all survivors and a stepped care model of intervention delivery is recommended. This involves a collaborative care approach to intervention efforts in which survivors are involved in treatment planning and therapeutic resources are utilized based on systematic assessment and monitoring of survivors' psychosocial well-being. Stepped care approaches require that treatments of different intensity are provided depending on the need of the individual. Treatments are initially implemented that are of minimal intensity but still likely to provide benefit

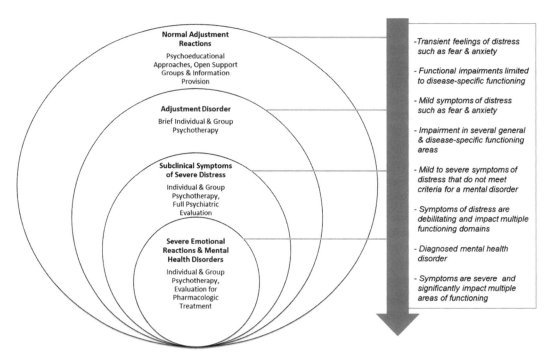

Fig. 14.2 Psychological intervention stepped approaches as a function of emotional reactions across the cancer distress continuum

and progress to more intensive interventions only if survivors do not demonstrate improvement from simpler approaches or for those who are not likely to benefit. An important feature of the stepped care model is that progress and decisions regarding intervention efforts are systematically monitored and assessed. More comprehensive intervention components are only initiated when there are no significant gains observed in the targeted outcomes. Stepped care may involve increasing intensity of a single intervention component, transition to a different intervention component, or using several intervention components additively. Likewise, different interventions may be applied to address different aspects of a patient's problem. Psychosocial needs also change as survivors move from through their cancer experience and either transition to survivorship or face advanced disease and end-of-life concerns. Utilizing a stepped care approach to promote adjustment and well-being at all phases of the cancer continuum may enhance intervention efficacy through more rigorous assessment methods and appropriateness of intervention techniques while also using the least amount of resources.

The model in Fig. 14.2 proposes that treatment planning and intervention efforts must consider the distress continuum among cancer survivors to determine the most optimal level of care based on their needs. Most cancer survivors adjust relatively well to cancer diagnosis and its treatment. The majority of individuals experience some transient levels of distress characterized by mild symptoms of anxiety and depression, fear, and interpersonal disruption specific to disease-related functioning (e.g., sexual dysfunction). Because their emotional reactions are transient and significantly below clinical levels, these survivors are likely to benefit from information provision or psychoeducational approaches that offer information on what to expect from treatment and the recovery process, available options for coping with treatment-related side effects (e.g., sexual aids), and communication skills to effectively navigate the medical system or voice concerns with a spouse/partner and family and friends.

A minority but yet significant number of cancer survivors may experience emotional reactions that warrant a more structured approach at psychological care. Those lacking in social resources, presenting with high levels of perceived stress, and enduring long-standing interpersonal dysfunction—likely driven by deficits in interpersonal skills and personality traits—are more likely to benefit from such interventions. Similarly, individuals with pre-morbid psychopathology and physical limitations, greater treatment-related functional limitations, and recurrent disease are more likely to experience greater levels of distress and benefit the most from interventions. Those who meet the criteria for a mental health disorder are likely to be experiencing an adjustment disorder characterized by clinically significant symptoms of distress. In such cases, brief individual and group psychotherapeutic approaches can be useful in ameliorating persistent symptoms of distress that. If untreated, these symptoms can interfere with multiple domains of health-related quality of life. Cancer survivors who experience subclinical manifestations of mental health disorders such as anxiety, depression, and PTSD (i.e., experience severe symptomatology but not meeting diagnostic criteria) may benefit from a full psychiatric evaluation to determine the most appropriate level of care. For these survivors, individual and group psychotherapeutic approaches can positively impact mental health and health-related quality of life outcomes. Among the small number of survivors who experience severe emotional reactions and are diagnosed with a mental health disorder, evaluation for pharmacologic treatment, in addition to individual and group psychotherapeutic approaches, is warranted.

Summary and Future Directions

Psychosocial intervention approaches have ranged from open support groups and psychoeducational programs that are based on information provision to supportive group therapy approaches and individual treatments that are structured to provide a nurturing environment to express concerns over the multiple challenges associated with cancer survivorship. Both individual- and group-based interventions based on cognitive behavioral intervention models that blend a variety of therapeutic techniques (e.g., cognitive restructuring, relaxation training) have shown success in improving health-related quality of life across multiple cancer populations. Other intervention approaches include mindfulness-based stress reduction, emotional expression, symptom management, health behavior change, and motivational interviewing. A significant amount of research has shown that effective therapy components in multimodal intervention efforts include techniques such as relaxation training to lower arousal, disease information and management, an emotionally supportive environment where participants can address fears and anxieties, behavioral and cognitive coping strategies, and social support skills training. Therapeutic processes by which participants benefit from intervention include giving and receiving information, sharing experiences, reducing social isolation, and providing survivors with coping skills that facilitate self-efficacy and sense of control over their cancer experience. Some evidence suggests that cancer survivors may benefit more from structured interventions than purely supportive ones; this may be due to learning skills with which they can more effectively cope with cancer-related changes after the intervention has ended (e.g., stress management). Interventions may also be couple or family based, depending on the goals of therapy and targeted outcomes, and may be administered at all phases of the cancer continuum, from post-diagnosis and treatment decision making to end-of-life or long-term survivorship time periods. Such interventions can be delivered via several modalities including face-to-face and technology-based individual- and group-based formats.

There is a large literature documenting the effectiveness of psychosocial intervention with cancer survivors. Interventions have demonstrated positive effects across a range of psychosocial and physical outcomes, including symptoms of depression and anxiety, and cancer-related fear, social functioning, and disease- and treatment-related symptoms (e.g., fatigue, nausea, pain). Although findings have been mixed with reports of nonsignificant effects as well,

reviews of the literature have concluded that the majority of interventions among cancer survivors demonstrate some improvement in psychosocial adjustment. Notably, sociodemographic factors (e.g., age, education, and socioeconomic status), pre-morbid psychological and physical functioning, social support, coping styles, and certain personality traits (e.g., neuroticism, interpersonal sensitivity, and social inhibition) have been associated with increased risk of adjustment difficulties following cancer diagnosis and its treatment, suggesting that there may also be considerable variability in baseline functioning and response to intervention efforts.

There are also notable gaps in the literature regarding benefits of psychosocial interventions for survivors with certain demographic, disease, and treatment characteristics. This is particularly true for ethnic and racial minorities and there is a critical gap in our understanding of how interventions may be tailored for ethnic and racial minority groups. A significant amount of the work has also focused on more common cancers and less is known about intervention techniques and efficacy among cancer survivors diagnosed with less common cancers, which are typically associated with greater treatment-related compromises, greater distress, and poorer survival rates.

References

1. Andrykowski M. The role of anxiety in the development of anticipatory nausea in cancer chemotherapy: a review and synthesis. Psychosom Med. 1990; 52(4):458–75.
2. Derogatis LR, Morrow GR, Fetting J, et al. The prevalence of psychiatric disorders among cancer patients. JAMA. 1983;249(6):751–7.
3. Spiegel D, Diamond S. Psychosocial interventions in cancer. In: Baum A, Anderson AL, editors. Psychosocial interventions for cancer. Washington, DC: American Psychological Association; 2001. p. 215–33.
4. Stark D, Kiely M, Smith A, Velikova G, House A, Selby P. Anxiety disorders in cancer patients: their nature, associations, and relation to quality of life. J Clin Oncol. 2002;20(14):3137–48.
5. Kangas M, Bovbjerg DH, Montgomery GH. Cancer-related fatigue: a systematic and meta-analytic review of non-pharmacological therapies for cancer patients. Psychol Bull. 2008;134(5):700–41.

6. Bruera E, Schmitz B, Pither J, Neumann CM, Hanson J. The frequency and correlates of dyspnea in patients with advanced cancer. J Pain Symptom Manage. 2000;19(5):357–62.

7. Chochinov HM, Wilson KG, Enns M, et al. Desire for death in the terminally ill. Am J Psychiatry. 1995; 152(8):1185–91.

8. Greer JA, Park ER, Prigerson HG, Safren SA. Tailoring cognitive-behavioral therapy to treat anxiety comorbid with advanced cancer. J Cogn Psychother. 2010;24(4):294–313.

9. Classen C, Koopman C, Angell K, Spiegel D. Coping styles associated with psychological adjustment to advanced breast cancer. Health Psychol. 1996;15(6): 434–7.

10. Hack TF, Degner LF. Coping responses following breast cancer diagnosis predict psychological adjustment three years later. Psychooncology. 2004; 13(4):235–47.

11. Andrykowski M. The role of anxiety in the development of anticipatory nausea in cancer chemotherapy: a review and synthesis. Psychosom Med. 1990;52(4): 458–75.

12. Spiegel D. Psychosocial interventions with cancer patients. J Psychosoc Oncol. 1996;4:83–95.

13. Spiegel D, Butler LD, Giese-Davis J, et al. Effects of supportive-expressive group therapy on survival of patients with metastatic breast cancer. Cancer. 2007;110(5):1130–8.

14. Anderson BL. Psychological interventions for cancer patients to enhance quality of life. J Consult Clin Psychol. 1992;60(4):552–68.

15. Rehse B, Pukrop R. Effects of psychosocial interventions on quality of life in adult cancer patients: meta analysis of 37 published controlled outcome studies. Patient Educ Couns. 2003;50(2):179–86.

16. Coyne J, Lepore S, Palmer S. Efficacy of psychosocial interventions in cancer care: evidence is weaker than it first looks. Ann Behav Med. 2006;32(2):104–10.

17. Lepore S, Coyne J. Psychological interventions for distress in cancer patients: a review of reviews. Ann Behav Med. 2006;32(2):85–92.

18. National cancer institute SEER cancer statistics review 1975–2006. http://seer.cancer.gov. Accessed June 2011.

19. Jacobsen PB, Jim HS. Psychosocial interventions for anxiety and depression in adult cancer patients: achievements and challenges. CA Cancer J Clin. 2008;58(4):214–30.

20. Dowrick C, Dunn G, Ayuso-Mateos JL, et al. Problem solving treatment and group psychoeducation for depression: multicentre randomised controlled trial. BMJ. 2000;321(7274):1450. doi:10.1136/bmj.321.7274.1450.

21. Badr H, Taylor CL. Sexual dysfunction and spousal communication in couples coping with prostate cancer. Psychooncology. 2009;18(7):735–46.

22. Molton IR, Siegel SD, Penedo FJ, et al. Promoting recovery of sexual functioning after radical prostatectomy with group-based stress management: the role of interpersonal sensitivity. J Psychosom Res. 2008;64(5):527–36.

23. Siegel SS, Molton I, Penedo FJ, et al. Interpersonal sensitivity, partner support, patient–physician communication, and sexual functioning in men recovering from prostate carcinoma. J Pers Assess. 2007;89(3):303.

24. Nelson CJ, Mulhall JP, Roth AJ. The association between erectile dysfunction and depressive symptoms in men treated for prostate cancer. J Sex Med. 2011;8(2):560–6.

25. Nelson CJ, Choi JM, Mulhall JP, Roth AJ. Determinants of sexual satisfaction in men with prostate cancer. J Sex Med. 2007;4(5):1422–7.

26. Boehmer U, Babayan RK. Facing erectile dysfunction due to prostate cancer treatment: perspectives of men and their partners. Cancer Invest. 2004;22(6): 840–8.

27. Schover LR, Yetman RJ, Tuason LJ, et al. Partial mastectomy and breast reconstruction. A comparison of their effects on psychosocial adjustment, body image, and sexuality. Cancer. 1995;75(1):54–64.

28. Schover LR. The impact of breast cancer on sexuality, body image, and intimate relationships. CA Cancer J Clin. 1991;41(2):112–20.

29. Fobair P, Stewart SL, Chang S, D'Onofrio C, Banks PJ, Bloom JR. Body image and sexual problems in young women with breast cancer. Psychooncology. 2006;15(7):579–94.

30. Katz MR, Irish JC, Devins GM, Rodin GM, Gullane PJ. Psychosocial adjustment in head and neck cancer: the impact of disfigurement, gender and social support. Head Neck. 2003;25(2):103–12.

31. Fingeret MC, Yuan Y, Urbauer D, Weston J, Nipomnick S, Weber R. The nature and extent of body image concerns among surgically treated patients with head and neck cancer. Psychooncology. 2011;21(8):836–44.

32. Penedo FJ, Traeger L, Benedict C, et al. Perceived social support as a predictor of disease-specific quality of life in head-and-neck cancer patients. J Support Oncol. 2012;10(3):119–23.

33. Phelps AC, Maciejewski PK, Nilsson M, et al. Religious coping and use of intensive life-prolonging care near death in patients with advanced cancer. JAMA. 2009;301(11):1140–7.

34. Thuné-Boyle IC, Stygall JA, Keshtgar MR, Newman SP. Do religious/spiritual coping strategies affect illness adjustment in patients with cancer? A systematic review of the literature. Soc Sci Med. 2006;63(1):151–64.

35. Henoch I, Danielson E. Existential concerns among patients with cancer and interventions to meet them: an integrative literature review. Psychooncology. 2009;18(3):225–36.

36. From cancer patient to cancer survivor: lost in transition of the institute of medicine (IOM). Institute of Medicine Website. http://www.iom.edu/Reports/2005/From-Cancer-Patient-to-Cancer-Survivor-Lost-in-Transition.aspx. Accessed June 2011.

37. Lee-Jones C, Humphris G, Dixon R, Hatcher MB. Fear of cancer recurrence? A literature review and proposed cognitive formulation to explain exacerbation of recurrence fears. Psychooncology. 1997;6(2): 95–105.

38. Carver CS, Antoni MH. Finding benefit in breast cancer during the year after diagnosis predicts better adjustment 5 to 8 years after diagnosis. Health Psychol. 2004;23(6):595–8.

39. Sears SR, Stanton AL, Danoff-Burg S. The yellow brick road and the emerald city: benefit finding, positive reappraisal coping and posttraumatic growth in women with early-stage breast cancer. Health Psychol. 2003;22(5):487–97.

40. Ganz PA. Late effects of cancer and its treatment. Semin Oncol Nurs. 2001;17(4):241–8.

41. Stein KD, Syrjala KL, Andrykowski MA. Physical and psychological long-term and late effects of cancer. Cancer. 2008;112(S11):2577–92.

42. Johannesen TB, Rasmussen K, Winther FØ, Halvorsen U, Lote K. Late radiation effects on hearing, vestibular function, and taste in brain tumor patients. Int J Radiat Oncol Biol Phys. 2002;53(1):86–90.

43. Felder-Puig R, Formann AK, Mildner A, et al. Quality of life and psychosocial adjustment of young patients after treatment of bone cancer. Cancer. 1998;83(1):69–75.

44. Tomich PL, Helgeson VS. Five years later: a cross-sectional comparison of breast cancer survivors with healthy women. Psychooncology. 2002;11(2): 154–69.

45. Partridge AH, Gelber S, Peppercorn J, et al. Web-based survey of fertility issues in young women with breast cancer. J Clin Oncol. 2004;22(20):4174–83.

46. Jones LW, Demark-Wahnefried W. Diet, exercise, and complementary therapies after primary treatment for cancer. Lancet Oncol. 2006;7(12): 1017–26.

47. Courneya KS. Exercise interventions during cancer treatment: biopsychosocial outcomes. Exerc Sport Sci Rev. 2001;29(2):60–4.

48. Demark-Wahnefried W, Aziz NM, Rowland JH, Pinto BM. Riding the crest of the teachable moment: promoting long-term health after the diagnosis of cancer. J Clin Oncol. 2005;23(24):5814–30.

49. Duffy SA, Ronis DL, Valenstein M, et al. A tailored smoking, alcohol, and depression intervention for head and neck cancer patients. Cancer Epidemiol Biomarkers Prev. 2006;15(11):2203–8.

50. Gritz ER, Carr CR, Rapkin D, et al. Predictors of long-term smoking cessation in head and neck cancer patients. Cancer Epidemiol Biomarkers Prev. 1993;2(3):261–70.

51. Stull VB, Snyder DC, Demark-Wahnefried W. Lifestyle interventions in cancer survivors: designing programs that meet the needs of this vulnerable and growing population. J Nutr. 2007;137(1): 243S–8.

52. Tarakeshwar N, Vanderwerker LC, Paulk E, Pearce MJ, Kasl SV, Prigerson HG. Religious coping is associated with the quality of life of patients with advanced cancer. J Palliat Med. 2006;9(3):646–57.

53. Weaver AJ, Flannelly KJ. The role of religion/spirituality for cancer patients and their caregivers. South Med J. 2004;97(12):1210–4.

54. Manne S, Badr H. Intimacy and relationship processes in couples' psychosocial adaptation to cancer. Cancer. 2008;112(S11):2541–55.

55. Manne S, Badr H, Zaider T, Nelson C, Kissane D. Cancer-related communication, relationship intimacy, and psychological distress among couples coping with localized prostate cancer. J Cancer Surviv. 2010;4(1):74–85.

56. Fang CY, Manne SL, Pape SJ. Functional impairment, marital quality, and patient psychological distress as predictors of psychological distress among cancer patients' spouses. Health Psychol. 2001; 20(6):452–7.

57. Badr H, Taylor CLC. Effects of relationship maintenance on psychological distress and dyadic adjustment among couples coping with lung cancer. Health Psychol. 2008;27(5):616–27.

58. Fawzy FI, Fawzy NW, Arndt LA, Pasnau RO. Critical review of psychosocial interventions in cancer care. Arch Gen Psychiatry. 1995;52(2):100–13.

59. Bottomley A. Where are we now? Evaluating two decades of group interventions with adult cancer patients. J Psychiatr Ment Health Nurs. 1997;4(4): 251–65.

60. Stanton AL. Psychosocial concerns and interventions for cancer survivors. J Clin Oncol. 2006; 24(32):5132–7.

61. Dalton JA, Keefe FJ, Carlson J, Youngblood R. Tailoring cognitive-behavioral treatment for cancer pain. Pain Manag Nurs. 2004;5(1):3–18.

62. Bottomly, A. Where are we now? Evaluating two decades of group interventions with adult cancer patients. J of Psychiatry and Mental Health Nurs.1997;4:251–65.

63. Antoni MH, Lehman JM, Klibourn KM, et al. Cognitive-behavioral stress management intervention decreases the prevalence of depression and enhances benefit finding among women under treatment for early-stage breast cancer. Health Psychol. 2001;20(1):20–32.

64. Penedo FJ, Antoni MH, Schneiderman N. Cognitive-behavioral stress management for prostate cancer recovery. New York, NY: Oxford University Press, Inc.; 2008.

65. Penedo FJ, Molton I, Dahn JR, et al. A randomized clinical trial of group-based cognitive-behavioral stress management in localized prostate cancer: development of stress management skills improves quality of life and benefit finding. Ann Behav Med. 2006;31(3):261–70.

66. Penedo F, Traeger L, Dahn J, et al. Cognitive behavioral stress management intervention improves quality of life in spanish monolingual hispanic men treated for localized prostate cancer: results of a randomized controlled trial. Int J Behav Med. 2007;14(3):164–72.

67. Penedo FJ, Dahn JR, Molton I, et al. Cognitive-behavioral stress management improves stress-management skills and quality of life in men recovering from treatment of prostate carcinoma. Cancer. 2004;100(1):192–200.
68. Macvean ML, White VM, Sanson-Fisher R. One-to-one volunteer support programs for people with cancer: a review of the literature. Patient Educ Couns. 2008;70(1):10–24.
69. Jacobsen PB, Meade CD, Stein KD, Chirikos TN, Small BJ, Ruckdeschel JC. Efficacy and costs of two forms of stress management training for cancer patients undergoing chemotherapy. J Clin Oncol. 2002;20(12):2851–62.
70. Thomsen TG, Rydahl-Hansen S, Wagner L. A review of potential factors relevant to coping in patients with advanced cancer. J Clin Nurs. 2010;19(23–24): 3410–26.
71. Taylor SE, Lobel M. Social comparison activity under threat: downward evaluation and upward contacts. Psychol Rev. 1989;96(4):569–75.
72. Buunk AP, Gibbons FX. Social comparison: the end of a theory and the emergence of a field. Organ Behav Hum Decis Process. 2007;102(1):3–21.
73. Giese-Davis J, Hermanson K, Koopman C, Weibel D, Spiegel D. Quality of couples' relationship and adjustment to metastatic breast cancer. J Fam Psychol. 2000;14(2):251–66.
74. Dorval M, Guay S, Mondor M, et al. Couples who get closer after breast cancer: frequency and predictors in a prospective investigation. J Clin Oncol. 2005;23(15):3588–96.
75. Badr H, Acitelli L, Taylor C. Does talking about their relationship affect couples' marital and psychological adjustment to lung cancer? J Cancer Surviv. 2008;2(1):53–64.
76. Baucom DH, Porter LS, Kirby JS, et al. A couple-based intervention for female breast cancer. Psychooncology. 2009;18(3):276–83.
77. Manne SL, Rubin S, Edelson M, et al. Coping and communication-enhancing intervention versus supportive counseling for women diagnosed with gynecological cancers. J Consult Clin Psychol. 2007; 75(4):615–28.
78. McLean LM, Walton T, Rodin G, Esplen MJ, Jones JM. A couple-based intervention for patients and caregivers facing end-stage cancer: outcomes of a randomized controlled trial. Psychooncology. 2011.
79. Campbell M, Tessaro I, Gellin M, et al. Adult cancer survivorship care: experiences from the LIVESTRONG centers of excellence network. J Cancer Surviv. 2011;5(3):271–82.
80. Christensen H, Griffiths KM, Jorm AF. Delivering interventions for depression by using the internet: randomised controlled trial. BMJ. 2004;328(7434):265. doi:10.1136/bmj.37945.566632.EE.
81. Ganz PA, Casillas J, Hahn EE. Ensuring quality care for cancer survivors: implementing the survivorship care plan. Semin Oncol Nurs. 2008;24(3):208–17.
82. Ganz PA. Quality of care and cancer survivorship: the challenge of implementing the institute of medicine recommendations. J Oncol Pract. 2009;5(3): 101–5.
83. Winzelberg AJ, Classen C, Alpers GW, et al. Evaluation of an internet support group for women with primary breast cancer. Cancer. 2003;97(5): 1164–73.
84. Livestrong foundation. http://www.livestrong.org. Accessed June 2011.
85. Ligibel JA, Partridge A, Giobbie-Hurder A, et al. Physical and psychological outcomes among women in a telephone-based exercise intervention during adjuvant therapy for early stage breast cancer. J Womens Health. 2010;19(8):1553–9.
86. Burish TG, Snyder SL, Jenkins RA. Preparing patients for cancer chemotherapy: Effect of coping preparation and relaxation interventions. J Consult Clin Psychol. 1991;59:518–25.
87. McQuellon RP, Wells M, Hoffman S, et al. Reducing distress in cancer patients with an orientation program. Psychooncology. 1998;7(3):207–17.
88. Jacobsen PB, Donovan KA, Vadaparampil ST, Small BJ. Systematic review and meta-analysis of psychological and activity-based interventions for cancer-related fatigue. Health Psychol. 2007;26(6):660–7.
89. Burton MV, Parker RW, Farrell A, et al. A randomized controlled trial of preoperative psychological preparation for mastectomy. Psychooncology. 1995;4(1):1–19.
90. Parker PA, Pettaway CA, Babaian RJ, et al. The effects of a presurgical stress management intervention for men with prostate cancer undergoing radical prostatectomy. J Clin Oncol. 2009;27(19):3169–76.
91. Stanton AL, Ganz PA, Kwan L, et al. Outcomes from the moving beyond cancer psychoeducational, randomized, controlled trial with breast cancer patients. J Clin Oncol. 2005;23(25):6009–18.
92. Osborn RL, Demoncada AC, Feuerstein M. Psychosocial interventions for depression, anxiety, and quality of life in cancer survivors: meta-analyses. Int J Psychiatry Med. 2006;36(1):13–34.
93. Owen JE, Klapow JC, Hicken B, Tucker DC. Psychosocial interventions for cancer: review and analysis using a three-tiered outcomes model. Psychooncology. 2001;10(3):218–30.
94. Miller GE, Cohen S. Psychological interventions and the immune system: a meta-analytic review and critique. Health Psychol. 2001;20(1):47–63.
95. Andersen BL, Farrar WB, Golden-Kreutz DM, et al. Psychological, behavioral, and immune changes after a psychological intervention: a clinical trial. J Clin Oncol. 2004;22(17):3570–80.
96. Spiegel D, Kraemer HC, Bloom JR, Gottheil E. Effects of psychosocial treatment on survival of patients with metastatic breast cancer. Lancet. 1989;334(8668):888–91.
97. Goodwin PJ, Leszcz M, Ennis M, et al. The effect of group psychosocial support on survival in metastatic

breast cancer. N Engl J Med. 2001;345(24): 1719–26.

98. Kogon MM, Biswas A, Pearl D, Carlson RW, Spiegel D. Effects of medical and psychotherapeutic treatment on the survival of women with metastatic breast carcinoma. Cancer. 1997;80(2):225–30.

99. Andersen BL, Thornton LM, Shapiro CL, et al. Biobehavioral, immune, and health benefits following recurrence for psychological intervention participants. Clin Cancer Res. 2010;16(12):3270–8.

100. Andersen BL, Farrar WB, Golden-Kreutz D, et al. Distress reduction from a psychological intervention contributes to improved health for cancer patients. Brain Behav Immun. 2007;21(7):953–61.

101. Fawzy FI, Canada AL, Fawzy NW. Malignant melanoma: effects of a brief, structured psychiatric intervention on survival and recurrence at 10-year follow-up. Arch Gen Psychiatry. 2003;60(1):100–3.

102. Richardson JL, Shelton DR, Krailo M, Levine AM. The effect of compliance with treatment on survival among patients with hematologic malignancies. J Clin Oncol. 1990;8(2):356–64.

103. Cunningham AJ, Edmonds CVI, Jenkins GP, Pollack H, Lockwood GA, Warr D. A randomized controlled trial of the effects of group psychological therapy on survival in women with metastatic breast cancer. Psychooncology. 1998;7(6):508–17.

104. Ross L, Boesen EH, Dalton SO, Johansen C. Mind and cancer: does psychosocial intervention improve survival and psychological well-being? Eur J Cancer. 2002;38(11):1447–57.

105. Smedslund G, Ringdal GI. Meta-analysis of the effects of psychosocial interventions on survival time in cancer patients. J Psychosom Res. 2004; 57(2):123–31.

106. Spiegel D, Stroud P, Fyfe A. Complimentary medicine. West J Med. 1998;168(4):241–7.

107. Raingruber B. The effectiveness of psychosocial interventions with cancer patients: an integrative review of the literature (2006–2011). ISRN Nurs. 2011;2011:638218.

108. Korfage IJ, Essink-Bot M, Borsboom GJJM, et al. Five-year follow-up of health-related quality of life after primary treatment of localized prostate cancer. Int J Cancer. 2005;116(2):291–6.

109. Scheier MF, Helgeson VS, Schulz R, et al. Moderators of interventions designed to enhance physical and psychological functioning among younger women with early-stage breast cancer. J Clin Oncol. 2007;25(36):5710–4.

110. Blackman DJ, Masi CM. Racial and ethnic disparities in breast cancer mortality: are we doing enough to address the root causes? J Clin Oncol. 2006;24(14):2170–8.

111. Shavers VL, Brown ML. Racial and ethnic disparities in the receipt of cancer treatment. J Natl Cancer Inst. 2002;94(5):334–57.

112. Ward E, Jemal A, Cokkinides V, et al. Cancer disparities by race/ethnicity and socioeconomic status. CA Cancer J Clin. 2004;54(2):78–93.

113. Barrera Jr M, Castro FG, Strycker LA, Toobert DJ. Cultural adaptations of behavioral health interventions: a progress report. J Consult Clin Psychol. 2012.

114. Hamilton JB, Agarwal M, Song L, Moore AD, Best N. Are psychosocial interventions targeting older african american cancer survivors culturally appropriate?: a review of the literature. Cancer Nurs. 2011;35(2):E12–23.

115. Kangas M, Henry JL, Bryant RA. Posttraumatic stress disorder following cancer: a conceptual and empirical review. Clin Psychol Rev. 2002;22(4):499–524.

116. Golden-Kreutz DM, Andersen BL. Depressive symptoms after breast cancer surgery: relationships with global, cancer-related, and life event stress. Psychooncology. 2004;13(3):211–20.

117. Traeger L. Effects of a psychosocial intervention on implicit models of illness and emotional well being in men recently treated for prostate cancer. Master's thesis. Coral Gables, FL: University of Miami; 2006.

118. Dale HL, Adair PM, Humphris GM. Systematic review of post-treatment psychosocial and behaviour change interventions for men with cancer. Psychooncology. 2010;19(3):227–37.

119. Helgeson VS, Cohen S, Schulz R, Yasko J. Group support interventions for women with breast cancer: who benefits from what? Health Psychol. 2000; 19(2):107–14.

120. Creuss D, Benedict C, Lattie EG. Millon Behavioral Medicine Diagnostic (MBMD) predicts health-related quality of life (HrQoL) over time among men treated for localized prostate cancer. J of Personality Assessment. 2012;DOI: 10.1080/00223891.2012. 681819.

121. Paika V, Almyroudi A, Tomenson B, et al. Personality variables are associated with colorectal cancer patients' quality of life independent of psychological distress and disease severity. Psychooncology. 2010;19(3):273–82.

122. Grossardt BR, Bower JH, Geda YE, Colligan RC, Rocca WA. Pessimistic, anxious, and depressive personality traits predict all-cause mortality: the mayo clinic cohort study of personality and aging. Psychosom Med. 2009;71(5):491–500.

123. Roberts BW, Kuncel NR, Shiner R, Caspi A, Goldberg LR. The power of personality: the comparative validity of personality traits, socioeconomic status, and cognitive ability for predicting important life outcomes. Perspect Psychol Sci. 2007;2(4):313–45.

124. Härtl K, Engel J, Herschbach P, Reinecker H, Sommer H, Friese K. Personality traits and psychosocial stress: quality of life over 2 years following breast cancer diagnosis and psychological impact factors. Psychooncology. 2010;19(2):160–9.

125. Nakaya N, Hansen PE, Schapiro IR, et al. Personality traits and cancer survival: a Danish cohort study. Br J Cancer. 2006;95(2):146–52.

126. Grov EK, Fosså SD, Bremnes RM, et al. The personality trait of neuroticism is strongly associated with long-term morbidity in testicular cancer survivors. Acta Oncol. 2009;48(6):842–9.

127. Helgeson VS, Fritz HL. Unmitigated agency and unmitigated communion: distinctions from agency and communion. J Res Pers. 1999;33(2):131–58.

128. Bruch MA. The relevance of mitigated and unmitigated agency and communion for depression vulnerabilities and dysphoria. J Couns Psychol. 2002; 49(4):449–59.

129. Hoyt MA, Stanton AL. Unmitigated agency, social support, and psychological adjustment in men with cancer. J Pers. 2011;79(2):259–76.

130. Helgeson VS, Lepore SJ. Quality of life following prostate cancer: the role of agency and unmitigated agency. J Appl Soc Psychol. 2004;34(12):2559–85.

131. Helgeson VS, Lepore SJ. Men's adjustment to prostate cancer: the role of agency and unmitigated agency. Sex Roles. 1997;37(3):251–67.

132. Roesch SC, Adams L, Hines A, et al. Coping with prostate cancer: a meta-analytic review. J Behav Med. 2005;28(3):281–93.

133. Hoyt MA, Thomas KS, Epstein DR, Dirksen SR. Coping style and sleep quality in men with cancer. Ann Behav Med. 2009;37(1):88–93.

134. Lutgendorf SK, Anderson B, Rothrock N, Buller RE, Sood AK, Sorosky JI. Quality of life and mood in women receiving extensive chemotherapy for gynecologic cancer. Cancer. 2000;89(6): 1402–11.

135. Costanzo ES, Lutgendorf SK, Rothrock NE, Anderson B. Coping and quality of life among women extensively treated for gynecologic cancer. Psychooncology. 2006;15(2):132–42.

Quality of Life

15

John M. Salsman, Timothy Pearman,
and David Cella

Introduction

Over the past 30 years quality of life has emerged as an important outcome for evaluating the impact of cancer across the continuum of cancer care. With improvements in early detection and advances in

J.M. Salsman, Ph.D. (✉)
Department of Medical Social Sciences,
Robert H. Lurie Comprehensive Cancer Center,
Northwestern University Feinberg School of Medicine,
625 North Michigan Avenue, Suite 2700,
Chicago, IL 60611-3110, USA
e-mail: j-salsman@northwestern.edu

T. Pearman, Ph.D.
Department of Medical Social Sciences,
Robert H. Lurie Comprehensive Cancer Center,
Northwestern University Feinberg School of Medicine,
625 North Michigan Avenue, Suite 2700,
Chicago, IL 60611-3110, USA

Department of Psychiatry and Behavioral Sciences,
Northwestern University Feinberg School of Medicine,
Chicago, IL, USA

D. Cella, Ph.D.
Department of Medical Social Sciences,
Robert H. Lurie Comprehensive Cancer Center,
Northwestern University Feinberg School of Medicine,
625 North Michigan Avenue, Suite 2700,
Chicago, IL 60611-3110, USA

Department of Psychiatry and Behavioral Sciences,
Institute for Healthcare Studies, Chicago, IL, USA

Division of Health and Biomedical Informatics,
Department of Preventive Medicine, Northwestern
University Feinberg School of Medicine,
Chicago, IL, USA

diagnosis and treatment, more and more people are surviving cancer and living longer. The National Cancer Institute estimates that approximately 11.9 million Americans with a history of cancer were alive in January 2009 [1], and the current 5-year survival rate is 68%, up from 50% in the 1970s [2]. Whereas survival time or *quantity* of life was an early and important objective indicator of treatment success, *quality* of life has proven to be a recent and meaningful subjective complement to survival benefits derived from treatments. In fact, weighing survival vs. quality of life benefits is a critical part of medical decision-making for cancer patients [3], and measuring quality of life has thus taken on added significance. Accordingly, in 2009 the Food and Drug Administration (FDA) coined the term "patient-reported outcomes" (PROs) as "measurement of any aspect of a patient's health status that comes directly from the patient" (e.g., quality of life) and proposed criteria for selecting PRO measures when effectiveness criteria for approval of medical product labeling claims are based on PROs [4].

Of course given the subjective nature of quality of life, efforts to operationalize the construct have led to multiple, overlapping definitions. The World Health Organization defined quality of life as an "individual's perception of their position in life in the context of the culture and value systems in which they live and in relation to their goals, expectations, standards and concerns. It is a broad-ranging concept affected in a complex way by the persons' physical health, psychological state, level of independence, social relationships, and their relationship to salient features of their environment." [5]. Others have noted the importance to quality of life of the subjective comparison between an individual's current level of functioning or well-being and his or her expected level of functioning or well-being [6]. For the purposes of this chapter, we are primarily concerned with health-related quality of life (HRQOL), succinctly defined as the extent to which one's usual or expected physical, emotional, and social well-being are affected by a medical condition or its treatment [7, 8]. Collectively, these definitions highlight two critical aspects of HRQOL: (1) the individual's subjective judgment of his/her well-being, and (2) the multiple components of HRQOL.

Dimensions of HRQOL

Many different dimensions have been proposed within the quality of life literature. An earlier review found over 30 different names for HRQOL dimensions [9]. This same review suggested that seven HRQOL dimensions were independent contributors to overall HRQOL: physical concerns (symptoms, pain, etc.), functional ability (activity), family well-being, emotional well-being, treatment satisfaction, sexuality (including body image), and social functioning. Also, many HRQOL instruments include a global evaluation of HRQOL (a single question rating the patient's overall perception of HRQOL) and a total score (summary of domain scores).

More recently, three or four dimensions of HRQOL have been proposed as adequate to fully describe HRQOL: physical, emotional, social, and, in some cases, spiritual [10]. The physical domain refers to perceived physical function, including pain, nausea and fatigue. The emotional domain refers to positive and negative mood and other emotional symptoms. The social domain measures relationships with friends and family, continued enjoyment of social activities and sexuality. The spiritual domain refers to the degree to which an individual finds comfort in his/her spiritual beliefs when coping with illness.

When selecting a measure of HRQOL to use, researchers and clinicians should consider the reliability, validity, and responsiveness of the measure. Reliability is primarily concerned with the stability and reproducibility of a measure over time. Two common forms of test reliability are the degree to which repeated administrations of a measure yield comparable scores (test-retest) and the degree to which items from the same measure are homogenous or "hang together" (internal consistency). Reliability is a necessary but not sufficient condition for the validity of a measure. Validity refers to an instrument's ability to accurately measure what it claims to measure. Several types of validity can be considered when evaluating the relative strengths of a measure with content, criterion, and construct validity among the most common. Content validity is the degree to which items accurately capture the range of attributes for a given concept. Measures whose items have a superficial appearance of content validity are said to have face validity. Criterion validity refers to how well an instrument's scores correlate with an external standard and can be subdivided into concurrent (criterion data collected simultaneously with instrument data) and predictive (criterion data collected some time after instrument data) validity. Construct validity is the degree to which test items reflect the underlying or latent variable in question and can be established in part through convergent and discriminant associations with measures of similar and dissimilar constructs, respectively. Finally, the responsiveness or sensitivity of a measure is the ability of the measure to differentiate between groups of patients expected to provide different HRQOL scores as a result of disease or treatment characteristics.

Levels of Measurement

The measurement of HRQOL can be organized conceptually under broad domains of generic and cancer-specific concepts (Fig. 15.1). Generic concepts include global evaluations of HRQOL as well as the commonly used dimensions of physical (symptoms and function), mental (affect,

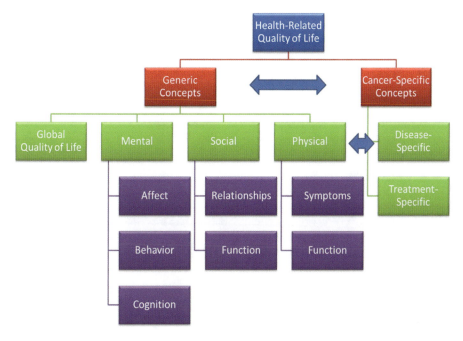

Fig. 15.1 Conceptual representation of HRQOL

behavior, cognition), and social (relationships and function) HRQOL. Cancer-specific concepts include both disease- and treatment-specific measures of HRQOL. While this framework provides a useful model for conceptualizing the hierarchical relationships among various dimensions of HRQOL, it does not readily capture the number and type of HRQOL questionnaires available for use with cancer patients and survivors. These questionnaires can be appropriately grouped within generic and cancer-specific domains, but within each of these domains there is much overlap of the physical, mental, and social dimensions, and thus they resist simple categorizations. In the subsequent sections, we summarize and highlight several frequently used measures of HRQOL as well as several promising new measures of HRQOL from the patient's perspective.

Generic

Medical Outcomes Study 36-Item (SF-36) and 12-Item (SF-12) Short-Form Health Surveys [11–13]. The SF-36 is a widely used self-report instrument for assessing generic quality of life.

It contains 36 items drawn from a larger pool of items used by RAND in the Medical Outcomes Study (MOS) [14]. The SF-36 yields summary scores for physical (PCS) and mental (MCS) components of HRQOL as well as eight subscale scores for physical functioning, role limitations due to physical problems, bodily pain, general health perceptions, vitality, social functioning, role limitations due to emotional problems, and general mental health. The SF-12 is a 12-item short-form health survey derived from the longer SF-36 instrument and encompassing the same eight dimensions [12]. Convergent validity and reliability characteristics of the SF-36 have been well established (Cronbach's alpha = .78 to .93). The SF-36 has previously been used with cancer patients, including breast [15], lung [16], and prostate cancer [17], as well as a mixed group of cancer survivors [18].

Nottingham Health Profile (NHP) [19]. The NHP is a 38-item self-report questionnaire that measures lay perceptions of health status across six domains: energy level, emotional reactions, physical mobility, pain, social isolation, and sleep. Responses are based on yes/no statements about one's subjective health. Research with various medical conditions has yielded good reliability evidence (Cronbach's alpha=.68 to .74 [20]; .63 to .80 [21]) and research with breast [22], colorectal [23], and lung cancer patients [24] has helped establish criterion-related validity.

Psychological Adjustment to Illness Scale — Self Report (PAIS-SR) [25]. The PAIS-SR is a 46-item self-report scale that measures psychosocial adjustment across seven domains: domestic environment, extended family environment, health orientation, psychological distress, sexual relationship, social environment and vocational environment. Respondents are instructed to indicate whether they have no problems or multiple problems using a four-point rating scale (0–3). Internal consistency for PAIS-SR scores was adequate to good (Cronbach's alpha range=.68 to .93) in a sample of lung and mixed cancer patients [25]. Construct validity was also reported for the PAIS-SR, which has been used in a variety of studies with cancer patients and survivors [26–33].

Sickness Impact Profile (SIP) [34]. The SIP is a 136-item instrument that provides information about how one's illness impacts activities and behaviors across 12 categories of function over three dimensions—physical (ambulation, mobility, body care and movement), psychosocial (communication, social interaction, alertness behavior, and emotional behavior), and independent (sleep and rest, eating, work, home management, recreation and pastimes). The SIP yields a total, two dimension (physical and psychosocial) and 12 category scores. Like the MOS, there are normative data using the SIP for a wide range of types and severities of illness. The SIP has good to excellent reliability (Cronbach's alpha=.60 to .90 for the categories, .91 for the dimensions, and .94 for the overall score) and construct validity [35], and recent recommendations for scoring the measure have helped minimize concerns about inconsistent and illogical scores [36]. The SIP has been used in adults with COPD [37] and muscular dystrophy [38] as well as with mixed groups of cancer patients and survivors [39–42].

Spitzer Quality of Life Index (QL-I) [43]. The QL-I is a 5-item quality of life index originally developed for use by clinicians. It differs from standard performance status measures in that it measures additional aspects of quality of life such as support and outlook and can be rated by both clinicians and patients using a three-point scale (0–2). Good correlations have been found between assessments made by clinicians and self-assessments [43]. The QL-I has shown discriminant validity as well as adequate internal consistency reliability (Cronbach's alpha=.78) [43] and been used primarily in palliative care settings and with advanced cancer patients [44–46].

Cancer-Specific

Cancer Rehabilitation Evaluation System (CARES) [47, 48]. The CARES is a self-administered rehabilitation and HRQOL instrument which has 139- and 59-item versions. Both versions are highly correlated (Pearson's r=.98), composed of a list of statements reflecting problems experienced by cancer patients, and yield a total HRQOL score and five summary scores across physical, psychosocial, medical interaction, marital, and sexual dimensions [48]. Adequate test-retest reliability, internal consistency (Cronbach's alpha=.88) and concurrent validity have been reported [47–49]. Schag et al. [48] described the sensitivity of the CARES to HRQOL improvements in breast cancer patients 1, 7, and 13 months after surgery. Moreover, the CARES discriminates between extent of disease in colon and prostate cancer survivors [50]. The CARES has also been used in patients with cervical cancer [51] and with leukemia and lymphoma [52] but is primarily used with breast cancer patients and survivors [53–56].

European Organization for Research and Treatment of Cancer Quality of Life Questionnaire-CORE 30 (EORTC QLQ-C30) [57]. The EORTC QLQ-C30 was developed to measure aspects of HRQOL relevant to patients with a wide variety of cancers who are participating in clinical trials. This 30-item questionnaire measures physical, emotional, cognitive, role, and social functioning, along with disease-specific symptoms, financial impact, and global HRQOL. Aaronson et al. [57] reported acceptable to good reliability coefficients for individual scales (Cronbach's alpha = .65 to .92) and seven scales predicted differences in patient clinical status [57, 58]. It is one of the most widely used measures of cancer-specific HRQOL, and a number of disease-specific modules have been developed and validated including: brain cancer (QLQ-BN20) [59], breast cancer (QLQ-BR23) [60], cervical cancer (QLQ-CX24) [61], colorectal cancer (QLQ-CR38) [62], endometrial cancer (QLQ-EN24) [63], head and neck cancer (QLQ-H&N35) [64], lung cancer (QLQ-LC13) [65], multiple myeloma (QLQ-MY24) [66], oesophago-gastric cancers (QLQ-OG25) [67], ovarian cancer (QLQ-OV28) [68], pancreatic cancer (QLQ-PAN26) [69], and prostate cancer (QLQ-PR25) [70]. Modules related to treatment approach or a specific HRQOL domain may also be administered.

Functional Assessment of Cancer Therapy-General, Version 4 (FACT-G) [71]. Also one of the most widely used measures of cancer-specific HRQOL, the FACT-G is a 27-item self-report measure of general questions divided into four primary HRQOL domains: Physical Well-Being, Functional Well-Being, Emotional Well-Being, and Social/Family Well-Being. The core measure has been validated in cancer and other chronic diseases and has thereby allowed for the evolution of multiple disease, treatment, condition, and non-cancer-specific subscales (over 86 different FACIT scales, including disease-specific symptom indices), which are considered to be part of a larger measurement system called the Functional Assessment of Chronic Illness Therapy (FACIT). Each is intended to be as specific as necessary to capture the clinically relevant problems associated with a given condition or symptom, yet general enough to allow for comparison across diseases, and, as appropriate, extension to other chronic medical conditions. The FACT-G and FACIT scales and indices have demonstrated adequate internal consistency (Cronbach's alpha = .56 to .89) and test-retest reliability (Pearson's r = .92), as well as evidence of validity (criterion, concurrent, known groups, and discriminant) and responsiveness [72–80]. Several disease specific modules have been developed and include the following: breast cancer (FACT-B) [81], bladder cancer (FACT-Bl), brain cancer (FACT-Br) [82], colorectal cancer (FACT-C) [83], cancer of the central nervous system (FACT-CNS), cervical cancer (FACT-Cx), esophageal cancer (FACT-E) [84], endometrial cancer (FACT-En), gastric cancer (FACT-Ga), head and neck cancer (FACT-H&N) [85], hepatobiliary cancer (FACT-Hep) [86], lung cancer (FACT-L) [87], leukemia (FACT-Leu) [88], lymphoma (FACT-Lym) [89], melanoma (FACT-M) [90], multiple myeloma (FACT-MM), nasopharyngeal cancer (FACT-NP) [91], ovarian cancer (FACT-O) [92], prostate cancer (FACT-P) [76], and vulvar cancer (FACT-V) [93].

Functional Living Index-Cancer (FLIC) [94]. Also known as the Manitoba Functional Living Cancer Questionnaire, the FLIC is a 22-item measure developed to assess cancer-related symptoms and the extent to which they disrupt one's life. Participants use a 7-point Likert response option on a linear analogue scale, and responses yield a total score as well as five subscale scores (physical well-being, psychological well-being, hardship due to cancer, social well-being, and nausea). The FLIC has demonstrated satisfactory psychometric properties, including adequate internal consistency reliability (Cronbach's alpha = .78 to .83), validity (criterion and convergent) and sensitivity to change [94–98]. It has been used widely with cancer patients and survivors, including breast [28, 99], prostate [100], lung [101], and gynecologic cancers [102].

McGill Quality of Life Questionnaire-Revised (MQOL) [103, 104]. The MQOL is a 17-item self-report scale specifically developed to measure HRQOL of patients at all stages of a life-threatening illness, from diagnosis to cure or death. The MQOL assesses general HRQOL dimensions applicable to all patients, includes both positive and negative influences on HRQOL, balances physical and nonphysical dimensions of HRQOL, and incorporates the existential dimension. Each question uses a 0–10 scale with anchors at each end. The MQOL yields four subscale scores (physical symptoms, psychological symptoms, existential well-being, and support), a single-item global HRQOL item, and an overall index score. Adequate to good test-retest reliability and internal consistency have been reported. Cronbach's alpha is > .70 for the total measure and all subscales but physical symptoms (Cronbach's alpha = .62) [105]. The physical symptoms subscale asks about the three most troublesome symptoms. Since these symptoms may be unrelated, the lower internal consistency is not surprising. Construct validity and responsiveness to change have been adequately described [104, 105]. The MQOL has been used in a number of palliative care and end-of-life studies with cancer patients [106–109].

Quality of Life Index-Cancer Version III (QLI-CV III) [110]. The QLI-CV III is a 66-item self-report scale that measures satisfaction with and importance of different aspects of one's HRQOL. The QLI-CV III yields a total score and four subscale scores (health and functioning, psychological/spiritual, social/economic and family), and respondents rate each item on a 6-point scale from 1 (very dissatisfied/very unimportant) to 6 (very satisfied/very important) [110–112]. The QLI-III-CV has demonstrated good internal consistency (Cronbach's alpha) for the total score (.95) and subscale scores: health and functioning (.90), psychological/spiritual (.84), social/economic (.93) and family (.66) [111]. Content and construct validity have also been reported, as well as sensitivity to change [110, 112, 113]. The QLI-III-CV has been used in studies of breast [114, 115], colorectal [113], and mixed groups of cancer patients [116].

As the number of cancer survivors continues to increase, there is a growing need to understand the long-term physical and psychological sequelae of the cancer experience (see Stein et al. [117]). In addition, there is concern that neither of the two most widely used measures of cancer-specific HRQOL (FACT-G, EORTC) assess important concerns of post-treatment survivors such as fear of recurrence, sexual functioning, changes in body image and genetic risk to family members [118]. In response to this need, a number of relatively new measures have been developed to measure these important concerns of cancer survivors:

Cancer Problems in Living Scale (CPILS) [119]. The CPILS is a 29-item self-report scale used to assess common physical, psychological,

and reintegration problems experienced by cancer survivors post-treatment. Using a Likert scale format, respondents indicate how much of a problem various concerns have been for them in the past 12 months (0 = not a problem to 2 = severe problem). Items can be summed for a total problem burden score or individual items can be examined as part of a needs assessment tool. Exploratory factor analysis identified four factors from the CPILS: physical distress, emotional distress, employment/financial problems, and fear of recurrence. These factors have good internal consistency (Cronbach's alpha = .78 to .87) as well as convergent and divergent validity [120]. The CPILS has been used in studies with mixed groups of cancer survivors, including breast, colorectal, lung, and prostate cancer [121, 122].

Impact of Cancer version 2 (IOCv2) [123, 124]. The IOCv2 is a 47-item self-report scale that measures the influence of cancer on HRQOL. The IOCv2 consists of a Positive Impact Summary scale with four subscales (Altruism and Empathy, Health Awareness, Meaning of Cancer, and Positive Self-Evaluation), a Negative Impact Summary scale with four subscales (Appearance Concerns, Body Change Concerns, Life Interferences, and Worry), and subscales for Employment and Relationship Concerns. High internal consistency (Cronbach's alpha = .76 to .89) has been reported across all subscales and content, criterion, and construct validity have also been established [124]. The IOCv2 has been used with mixed groups of cancer survivors as well as with long-term breast cancer survivors and non-Hodgkin lymphoma survivors [124–126]. More recently, a module for adult survivors of childhood cancers (IOC-CS) has been developed and validated [127, 128].

Long Term Quality of Life Scale (LTQL) [129–131]. The LTQL is a 34-item self-report measure designed to assess long term quality of life for female cancer survivors. The LTQL contains four subscales (somatic concerns, spiritual/philosophical views of life, fitness, and social support), and items are rated on a five-point Likert scale (0 = not at all to 4 = very much). Good reliability evidence has been reported (Cronbach's alpha = .86 to .92) and content, construct, and concurrent validity have also been established [131].

Quality of Life in Adult Cancer Survivors (QLACS) [132]. The QLACS is a 47-item self-report measure that assesses quality of life domains relevant to long-term cancer survivors. There are seven generic domains (negative feelings, positive feelings, cognitive problems, sexual problems, physical pain, fatigue, and social avoidance) and five cancer-specific domains (financial problems, benefits of cancer, distress about family, distress about recurrence, and appearance concerns). Scores are rated on a seven-point Likert scale from 1=never to 7=always. The QLACS has demonstrated good internal consistency (Cronbach's alpha≥.72 for each domain) as well as construct validity, convergent validity, and responsiveness [132, 133]. The QLACS was developed with a heterogeneous sample of male and female long-term cancer survivors (>5 years post-diagnosis) with a range of ages and cancer types represented (i.e., breast, bladder, colorectal, head and neck, gynecologic, and prostate).

Quality of Life—Cancer Survivors (QOL-CS) [134, 135]. The QOL-CS is a 41-item self-report measure designed to assess physical, psychological, social, and spiritual well-being among cancer survivors. Response options are based on an 11-point scale ranging from 0=worst outcome to 10=best outcome for each item and a total score and subscale scores can be produced. The QOL-CS has demonstrated excellent test-retest reliability (r=.81 to .90 across subscales), internal consistency (Crobach's alpha=.71 to .89 across subscales) as well as content, criterion, and construct validity [134, 135]. The QOL-CS has been used in a number of survivorship studies, including survivors of bone marrow transplants [136], childhood cancer [137], breast cancer [75], and lung cancer [16].

Disease-Specific

The impact cancer may have on one's HRQOL can often vary as a function of the specific type of cancer and the resulting physical and emotional sequelae. In order to more effectively assess these concerns, a number of disease or site-specific measures have been developed. The EORTC and the FACT-G each have several validated disease-specific modules (see above for examples) and are among the most widely used measures for evaluating HRQOL outcomes in cancer clinical trials. Other disease-specific measures of note are the UCLA Prostate Cancer Index (UCLA PCI) [138], the HNQoL (Head and Neck Quality of Life Instrument) [139], the Lung Cancer Symptom Scale (LCSS) [140], Quality of Life-Breast Cancer (QOL-BC) [75, 135], and a Colorectal Cancer-Specific Scale [141].

Symptom and Treatment Specific

While too numerous to describe as part of an exhaustive review, symptom- and treatment-specific categories of HRQOL measurement also merit discussion. These measures are more narrowly focused in their scope, but they provide important information about patient experiences which can be used to further complement general and cancer-specific levels of HRQOL assessment. More specifically, symptom-specific measures provide targeted assessment of physical and psychological sequealae secondary to the cancer experience and can include broad-based symptom indices such as the McCorkle and Young Symptom Distress Scale (SDS) [142, 143], M.D. Anderson Symptom Inventory (MDASI) [144], Edmonton Symptom Assessment Scale (ESAS) [145], Memorial Symptom Assessment Scale (MSAS) [146], Rotterdam Symptom Checklist [147], Symptom Checklist 90 (SCL-90) [148], and the Brief Symptom Inventory (BSI) [149, 150]. Similarly, broad-based assessment of psychological symptoms is frequently conducted with the use of measures such as the Profile of Mood States-Short Form (POMS-SF) [151], Mental Health Inventory (MHI) [152], Affect Balance Scale [153, 154], as well as with targeted assessments of specific clusters of mood symptoms such as depression or anxiety (Center for Epidemiological Studies-Depression Scale (CES-D) [155], Hospital Anxiety and Depression Scale

(HADS) [156], State-Trait Anxiety Inventory (STAI)) [157], including PTSD-symptomatology (Impact of Event Scale (IES) [158], Posttraumatic Stress Disorder Checklist-Civilian (PCL-C)) [159]. Pain and fatigue are common physical symptoms for cancer patients and survivors and, as a result, measures of these symptoms are often included in clinical trials with the Brief Fatigue Inventory (BFI) [160] and the Brief Pain Inventory (BPI) [161] among the more frequently selected measures.

Treatment-specific measures focus on the impact of various cancer treatments and can include measures addressing the effect of radiation, chemotherapy, and hormonal treatments on cancer patients. Much like the extensive number of cancer-specific measures provided by the EORTC and the FACT measurement systems, there are a several validated treatment-specific modules within these larger measurement frameworks.

Pediatric Measures

Lastly, measures of HRQOL for adults require adaptation and additional data collection in order to determine the psychometric utility and appropriateness of these measures for children and adolescents. A growing literature is focusing on the special needs and challenges of managing cancer for pediatric patients and survivors. Among the more common cancer-related measures of HRQOL for children are the Miami Pediatric Quality of Life Questionnaire (MPQOLQ) [162], the Minneapolis–Manchester Quality of Life Form (MMQL) [163, 164], the PedsQL Cancer Module [165–168], and the Pediatric Oncology Quality of Life Scale (POQOLS) [169, 170]. For a detailed review of these and other measures available for HRQOL for children with cancer, see Klassen et al. [171].

Selecting Measures

Since there is no gold standard when it comes to measuring HRQOL, selecting an appropriate measure can be a challenge because the clinician or researcher has a considerable number of available options. For example, there has been some debate as to whether dimensional assessment (i.e., separate scores for each dimension, evaluated independently) or aggregated assessment (i.e., evaluation of only the total HRQOL score incorporating all four dimensions) is most clinically relevant. While dimensional assessment gives a richer and more detailed picture of HRQOL, and is often preferred by clinicians, aggregated scores may be more meaningful in areas such as clinical trials research in order to enable decisions to be made adjusting survival time for its quality [172].

Dimension scores provide more data than an aggregated score, but also have differential sensitivity to various cancer symptoms. For instance, compared with physical scales (e.g., physical functioning, functional ability, sexuality, etc.), psychosocial scales such as emotional well-being and social functioning are less sensitive to changes in performance status or other primarily physical ratings. Psychosocial dimension scales are also less sensitive to disease-related characteristics, such as stage of disease [173]. Several studies have found that the EORTC is unable to detect change in performance status rating or extent of disease [174, 175]. Similar findings have emerged for the FACT measurement system [71, 87].

These findings make logical sense in the context of findings suggesting that emotional well-being may be no different in individuals diagnosed with cancer and those without cancer [176, 177]. It should be noted, however, that this finding has not always been replicated in all disease types and stages of illness (e.g., Lee et al. [178]). When the physical components of well-being are evaluated alongside measures of mental well-being, the relationship between the two is modest [10]. The fact that earlier and less refined measures of HRQOL may not adequately measure psychological distress is precisely due to the fact that these measures are composed largely of physical symptoms such as nausea, appetite, and sleep.

In summary, if focusing on aggregate HRQOL scores only, the significant impact of cancer on dimension of HRQOL may be obscured. Including more targeted disease or treatment-specific measures along with general measures of HRQOL will permit comparisons across diseases while allowing for a level of sensitivity to particular issues or symptoms arising from a given disease or treatment. In addition, including multiple measures enhances the breadth of content coverage which may maximize one's ability to identify the efficacy of a particular treatment or intervention on HRQOL outcomes. A useful strategy is to select the measure which is most closely aligned with study objectives, confirm the relevant psychometric properties, and augment the selected measure(s) with a few additional questions targeted to the condition, disease, or treatment under study.

Emerging Issues

Item Response Theory and Computerized Adaptive Testing

Advances in measurement using item response theory (IRT) and advances in computer technology make it possible to enhance measurement of HRQOL at a global level as well as at dimensional levels. IRT is an alternative to classical test theory and models the likelihood that a person at a specific latent trait or symptom level will respond to an item in a particular way [179–182]. Based upon one's overall pattern of responses to measure items, IRT modeling can produce a more precise estimate of a particular symptom or domain of HRQOL. This information can then be used to evaluate the quality of individual items, to calibrate test scoring, and to develop item banks for HRQOL domains. An item bank is composed of carefully calibrated questions that can be used for item comparison and selection. Calibrated item banks permit the application of computerized adaptive testing (CAT) tools, thus enabling tailored individual assessment while maintaining measurement precision and content validity. In short, item banks offer the potential for efficient, flexible, and precise measurement of commonly studied measures of HRQOL. They are efficient because they minimize the number of items administered without compromising reliability,

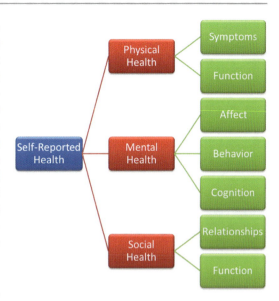

Fig. 15.2 PROMIS domain framework

flexible because they allow the use of interchangeable items, and precise because they minimize the standard error of estimate [183]. Consequently, application of IRT and CAT tools may allow for briefer assessments, more efficient assessments, and assessment of more symptoms and HRQOL domains of interest than has been typical in traditional assessments. Valid, generalizable item banks and CAT tools can stimulate and standardize clinical research across academic cancer centers and community-based practices utilizing PROs. They also may assist individual clinical practitioners and other cancer care providers to assess patient response to interventions and modify treatment plans accordingly.

PROMIS

The Patient-Reported Outcomes Measurement Information System (PROMIS) is an NIH Roadmap initiative designed to improve PROs using state-of-the-art psychometric methods (see http://www.nihpromis.org). The PROMIS domain framework is informed by the World Health Organization's tripartite model of physical, mental, and social health, but is further divided into a variety of symptom, affective, and interpersonal banks (see Fig. 15.2). In addition to a ten-item measure of global health which yields physical and mental health summary scores, PROMIS has thus far developed and calibrated 21 different items banks, including banks for emotional distress (anger, anxiety, depression), psychosocial illness impact (positive, negative), physical function, fatigue, pain (behavior, interference), sleep function (sleep disturbance, sleep-related impairment), and social function (ability to participate in social roles and activities, satisfaction with participation in social roles and activities) [183–185]. The National Cancer Institute (NCI) provided supplemental PROMIS funding to ensure that the PROs developed were valid for cancer patients and survivors. PROMIS is the most ambitious attempt to date to apply IRT models to HRQOL assessment. The PROMIS approach involves iterative steps of comprehensive literature searches, the development of conceptual frameworks, item pooling, qualitative assessment of items using focus groups and cognitive interviewing, and quantitative evaluation of items using techniques from both classical test theory and IRT [186–188]. Valid, generalizable item banks and CAT tools can stimulate and standardize clinical research across academic cancer centers and community-based practices. They also may assist individual clinical practitioners to assess patient response to interventions and modify treatment plans accordingly.

Symptom Monitoring

A measurement tool such as PROMIS can also be particularly beneficial for real-time symptom monitoring. One of the challenges of supportive care services can be responding to acute or emergent issues when a patient is not in-clinic. Due to the infrequency of medical visits and time constraints during these visits, it is difficult for clinicians to comprehensively assess and manage symptoms from the oncology clinic alone. These limitations can be moderated with a patient-oriented, technology-based, symptom-monitoring system that provides precise-yet-brief assessment in "real-time," is easily accessed by patients, and provides relevant reports to clinicians. Moreover,

such a system can facilitate identifying patient symptom burden more promptly, encourage communication between patients and their clinicians, and promote patient self-management, all key components of enhancing patient HRQOL.

Barriers to effective symptom management exist at both the health care provider and patient levels. Health care provider barriers include limitations on time available during a typical patient encounter [189], staff ability and willingness to elicit relevant information from patients [190–192], and infrequent use of systematic symptom assessment [193, 194]. Even when treatments are implemented for symptoms, instructions provided to patients in the clinic are often not tailored to the patient's specific symptom experience, are forgotten, or are ineffective in promoting continued self-management outside of the clinic [195]. Patients also experience a number of barriers to effective symptom management. For example, patients may not spontaneously report symptoms to physicians due to forgetfulness [196], desire to be a "good patient" [190, 197–199], concern over distracting the physician from treating the disease [197, 200], and concern about the side effects of or fear of becoming addicted to the prescription medications for symptom management [190, 196–198, 200–202]. Patients may also maintain fatalistic or stoic beliefs about their symptoms, believing the symptom is an inevitable consequence of having cancer, or that a symptom must be endured because nothing can be done to relieve it [196, 198].

The National Comprehensive Cancer Network, Institute of Medicine, and the Joint Commission for the Accreditation of Hospital Organizations, have recommended routine monitoring of symptoms to ensure overall good quality of patient care. Unfortunately, despite the potential benefits of active, systematic assessment with PROs [194, 203], and the feasibility and acceptability of HRQOL assessments in oncology settings, [204–210] this is seldom conducted in clinical practice settings [190, 211, 212]. While this is likely influenced by patient and provider barriers described above, patients consider HRQOL issues important and worthy of discussion with physicians [213–215]. Moreover, discussion of

HRQOL information does not appear to increase the average length of medical consultations, perhaps because it focuses discussion on the topics of greatest importance to patients and results in a more efficient visit overall [205, 206, 216].

Assessment of HRQOL information is an important, initial step, but assessment alone is insufficient to affect change in health status or symptom burden [217–219]. By itself, assessment of HRQOL does not ensure patients will act on the results by communicating with their physicians about identified problems [218–220]. Assessment results without direct, immediate feedback to treating physicians may be inadequately utilized or may be monitored infrequently. Instead, researchers have suggested that, at a minimum, assessment results should be provided to physicians, who should be properly educated about how to effectively interpret the results [217, 219, 221]. This approach may be effective at positively impacting symptom burden and ultimately enhancing overall HRQOL for cancer patients and survivors.

One of the challenges of effectively monitoring and managing symptom burden is the treatment schedule for patients. For example, outpatient chemotherapy is often administered on a schedule that results in most symptoms emerging when patients are home, between scheduled clinic appointments, creating barriers for effective symptom management. Patient and provider barriers (described above) further compound the situation and deter efforts to appropriately monitor and manage symptoms secondary to chemotherapy [144, 211, 222]. Recognizing that some of these barriers can be partially addressed through the application of technology, a 4-year, multi-site randomized trial of the Symptom Monitoring and reporting system for advanced Lung cancer (SyMon-L) was conducted (PI: Yount, R01CA115361). The SyMon-L system used a combination of computer and interactive voice response technologies. Patients in the "intervention" and "control" arms called a toll-free number on a weekly basis for 12 weeks to complete a brief symptom measure, the FACT-Lung Symptom Index (FLSI) [223]. For "intervention" patients, symptom responses meeting a prespecified threshold warranting clinical attention generated real-time emails to their nurse, who then contacted the patient to manage their care in conjunction with the physician. Cumulative graphs of intervention patients' symptoms were generated for review during clinic visits (Fig. 15.3). Red symptom "alerts" were indicated on the graph when a score met the threshold of "quite a bit" or "very much" in an absolute sense or the score was two points worse than the previous week. Patients in the "control" arm completed the weekly symptom surveys by phone but their scores were not reported to the clinical team. The primary endpoint was overall symptom burden, as assessed by the Symptom Distress Scale (SDS) [143]. Preliminary results indicate that the intervention did not differentially reduce symptom burden in the intervention group; there were also no differences between the two arms in terms of HRQOL (FACT-G) [71]. The advent of electronic health records, with the opportunity to include patient symptoms and functioning directly into the medical record through patient portals, may help contribute to meaningful use of this information in treatment planning and outcome. Further research in this area is underway at several institutions.

HRQOL as an Endpoint for Randomized Controlled Trials

While some have suggested that psychological factors such as coping style or personality variables may contribute more to HRQOL compared to disease or treatment-related variables [224], it is generally accepted that psychological variables are highly correlated with treatment and disease-related variables. In fact, certain HRQOL domains may be independent predictors of important outcomes such as survival time [225]. Also, emotional symptoms affecting HRQOL, such as depression, appear to modulate functional abilities, such as swallowing in patients with head and neck cancer [226]. Therefore, HRQOL can serve as an important endpoint in randomized, clinical trials. To that end, the Institute of Medicine identified interventions aimed at improving

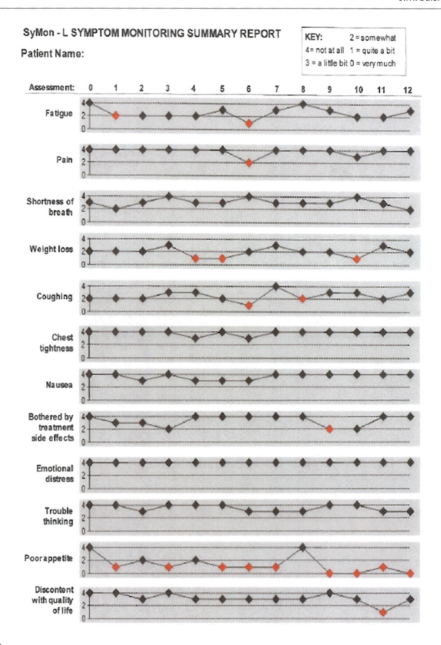

Fig. 15.3

HRQOL as an important target in cancer survivorship research [118].

The first call for HRQOL to be included as a parameter in clinical cancer research came over 20 years ago [174, 227]. The call for inclusion of HRQOL measurement into clinical trials has continued since that time [228]. Unfortunately, a recent review of randomized controlled trials (RCTs) published from 1994 to 2004 found that only 22% of these studies defined HRQOL or symptom control as a primary endpoint [229]. This study further stated that "current standards for analyzing HRQOL and symptom control in RCTs are poor" and urged further refinement of HRQOL measurement in the area of cancer clinical trials.

Another review [230] evaluated 159 RCTs and found a significant difference based on the time period during which the study was published. Specifically, only 39.3% of studies published 1990–2000 used "robust" HRQOL measures which were likely to support clinical decision-making, but the percentage was 64.3% of studies published after 2000. Optimistically, the study authors also concluded that there was no difference between industry sponsored trials and nonindustry sponsored trials in terms of the likelihood that HRQOL measurement was included.

Research has shown that validated and commonly used HRQOL instruments, even among disease-specific instruments, are not interchangeable, and it is important to consider the specific patient population in determining which instrument is most appropriate for measuring HRQOL [231]. It has become apparent that quality of life differs greatly based on stage of disease. For example, head and neck cancer patients who have higher T-stage (T3 and T4) and higher overall-stage (III and IV) have lower mean HRQOL scores [232]. Some HRQOL instruments and disease-specific modules (such as the EORTC) have been shown to have adequate sensitivity to differentiate between T3 and T4 staging among head and neck cancer patients [173], but more refinement is necessary and being undertaken [233]. Interest has therefore been generated to better assess HRQOL in late stage cancers using more specifically targeted instruments.

Similarly, researchers and clinicians alike can benefit through a better understanding of the role of minimally important differences (MIDs) when arriving at judgments about the meaningfulness of HRQOL scores. Much like the role effect sizes provide in facilitating determinations of clinical significance, an MID can be understood as "the smallest difference in score in the domain of interest which patients perceive as beneficial and which would mandate, in the absence of troublesome side effects and excessive cost, a change in the patient's management." [234] MIDs can be identified through both distribution- and anchor-based approaches. Distribution methods rely on statistical distributions of HRQOL scores, and include effect size, responsiveness index, reliable change index, and standard error of measurement (SEM). Anchor-based methods include cross-sectional or longitudinal differences in HRQOL scores that are compared or anchored to clinically familiar and relevant indicators (e.g., global rating of change, performance status). MIDs have been established for numerous scales and subscales in the FACIT measurement system [235] as well as for PROMIS Cancer scales when used with advanced stage cancer patients [236].

Incorporating Symptom-Specific Questionnaires into the FACT

Despite the existence of a number of well-validated, disease-specific HRQOL measures, groups such as the FDA have noted that these instruments may be of limited utility in detecting meaningful treatment changes and symptoms, given their multidimensional nature [4]. Moreover, the FDA Quality of Life Subcommittee of the Oncology Drug Advisory Committee has suggested that assessment of symptoms might represent a reasonable starting point in working toward a goal of more focused assessment of HRQOL domains [237–239]. An essential consideration in symptom assessment is that patient ratings of symptom importance may differ from those of oncology professionals such as nurses and physicians [240–242]. Therefore, it is important to have feedback and guidance from both oncology professionals as well as patients and to have more symptom-focused approaches to HRQOL assessment in a manner that is both clinically relevant and psychometrically acceptable.

In response to these needs, Cella et al. [243] have developed brief symptom indexes to address the most important symptoms and concerns across 11 different cancers (advanced bladder, brain, breast, colorectal, head and neck, hepatobiliary, kidney [244], lung [245], ovarian [246], and prostate cancers [247] and lymphoma). Guided by the combined input of providers (physicians, nurses) and patients, the investigators were able to compare responses and to retain the most frequently endorsed items for newly created priority symptom lists across 11 advanced cancers.

Indexes have been formatted by subscale, separating Disease-Related Symptom (DRS), Treatment Side Effect (TSE), and general Function and Well-Being (FWB) items for ease of use and scoring.

The development of these concise symptom indexes has the potential to benefit patient-centered care in a number of ways. First of all, each index has less than 25 items with a range of 16–24 items. They focus only on relevant symptoms and concerns thus minimizing response burden and maximizing potential utility in clinical practice evaluations. Second, because they were developed with the combined input from patients and providers, these indexes reflect patient- and provider-driven priorities for treatment. In this way, content validity is maximized. Third, the option of separate subscale scores for DRS, TSE, and general FWB, allows the investigators to examine potential disease-related vs. treatment-related sequelae. These symptom indexes may address concerns of medical oncology providers, patients being treated for advanced cancer, and regulatory agencies. Given their focus on patients' primary symptom concerns, rather than all potential concerns, their use in a regulatory setting may help minimize "claim expansiveness" in which a promotional claim goes beyond what was measured in the supporting study [243]. Further research should focus on the clinical utility of routine monitoring of these priority symptoms and their potential impact on decision-making, quality of care, and HRQOL.

Caregiver HRQOL

In 2009, nearly 66 million Americans (three in ten US households) reported at least one person providing unpaid care as a family caregiver [248]. Despite this fact, until recently, there has been a dearth of information about caregiver quality of life in cancer [249]. Studies have suffered from a number of methodologic flaws, including a lack of strong outcome evaluation, a reliance on descriptive and formative evaluations, reliance on small sample sizes and convenience samples,

widely varying interventions and confusion concerning the operationalization and measurement of major caregiver outcomes [250]. As survival rates have improved, the threat of cancer has changed in many cases from being a highly fatal illness to being a potentially chronic, manageable illness spanning the course of years or in some cases decades. While this clearly represents a positive change for patients, this has led to increased caregiver burden as patients' physical, functional, and emotional care needs span longer periods of time [251]. Interestingly, many studies have found that caregivers experience worse HRQOL than patients, even at terminal stages of illness [252].

Because there has historically been a lack of focus on caregiver needs, many of these needs may go unmet, and significantly affect psychological distress and HRQOL. A recent study of 223 family caregivers found that the mean number of unmet needs was significantly higher among women than men, other relatives than spouses, younger family members, those currently working and those of patients with metastatic disease [253]. In addition the presence of anxiety and depression was high (20–40%) in caregivers. Caregiver HRQOL has also been measured up to 5 years after diagnosis. It appears that at approximately 2 years post-diagnosis, cancer caregivers in general have HRQOL similar to that of the general population. Notably, caregivers report increased awareness of spirituality compared to pre-cancer diagnosis, and caregivers for patients who have poor mental and physical functioning are more likely to report impaired HRQOL [254].

At 5 years, three groups of caregivers remain: those continuing to care for a patient in active treatment, caregivers who are bereaved, and caregivers of patients in remission. Combining groups, caregiver HRQOL appears similar to the general population [255]; however, some notable differences exist between groups. In particular, current caregivers report the worst HRQOL. Bereaved caregivers have lower HRQOL than caregivers whose patients are currently in remission, and age and income appear significantly related to emotional well-being, with younger and poorer caregivers having higher levels of emotional distress. Among patients in remission, caregiver fear of recurrence has been linked to poorer HRQOL, and this in turn was linked to disease severity, with caregivers caring for a patient with more severe illness having the highest levels of fear of recurrence [256].

Another population of interest is parents whose children have been diagnosed with cancer. HRQOL appears worse in parents of children with cancer compared to parents whose children do not have cancer [257]. In addition, parents of children who have significant physical limitations, and also parents of children in active treatment, have the lowest HRQOL [258]. These clinical characteristics also appear to be mediated by caregiver burden and stress. The importance of screening for caregiver distress is highlighted by this still emerging literature.

A recent American Cancer Society consensus conference recommended the use of patient navigators to screen patient, but also caregiver HRQOL, and make appropriate referrals for psychosocial services [259]. Given the research cited above, interventions seem especially necessary in advanced cancer. A recent prospective, multi-institution, RCT attempted to do just this [260]. Patients and caregivers with advanced cancer who were enrolled on investigational trials participated in a standardized cognitive-behavioral problem-solving educational group. Interestingly, the intervention did not seem to have any effect on patients. However, the intervention appeared to slow declines in HRQOL in caregivers significantly compared to the no treatment arm.

In summary, caregiver quality of life is an important, and emerging, area of both clinical and research interest. Given what is known about declines in quality of life based on patient population, disease characteristics, and caregiver burden, more research should be done focusing on screening for distress in caregivers. Also, more research and clinical focus needs to be devoted to studying interventions aimed at stabilizing HRQOL in caregivers, or at the least impede HRQOL decline.

Conclusions and Future Research

HRQOL is a multidimensional concept that includes self-reported symptoms, functional abilities, and physical, mental, social, and spiritual health perceptions. HRQOL is measured with a variety of valid instruments. Global and specific approaches to assessing HRQOL may permit comparisons to healthy populations and within particular disease groups, respectively. HRQOL is increasingly accepted as an important endpoint in clinical trials and a key consideration when patients and providers are engaging in shared decision-making. Efforts to enhance and improve HRQOL measurement are ongoing with initiatives such as PROMIS providing increased brevity, precision, and flexibility for the assessment of HRQOL throughout the continuum of cancer care. Future research should focus on clinical applications of HRQOL outcomes, including benefits of symptom monitoring, impact on treatment decision-making, and relationship to clinical benchmarks and quality of care. Patient-centered outcomes research will likely benefit all.

References

1. National Cancer Institute. Estimated US cancer prevalence counts: who are our cancer survivors in the U.S.? http://cancercontrol.cancer.gov/ocs/prevalence/index.html. Accessed 16 Sept 2011.
2. American Cancer Society. Cancer facts & figures 2011. Atlanta: American Cancer Society; 2011.
3. Zafar S, Alexander S, Weinfurt K, Schulman K, Abernethy A. Decision making and quality of life in the treatment of cancer: a review. Support Care Cancer. 2009;17(2):117–27.
4. U. S. Department of Health and Human Services Food and Drug Administration, Center for Drug Evaluation and Research, Center for Biologics Evaluation and Research, Center for Devices and Radiological Health. Guidance for industry patient-reported outcome measures: use in medical product development to support labeling claims. 2009. http://purl.access.gpo.gov/GPO/LPS113413.
5. WHOQOL. Study protocol for the World Health Organization project to develop a quality of life assessment instrument (WHOQOL). Qual Life Res. 1993;2(2):153–9.

6. Morton RP, Izzard ME. Quality-of-life Outcomes in Head and Neck Cancer Patients. World J Surg. 2003;27(7):884–9.

7. Cella DF. Quality of life concepts and definition. J Pain Symptom Manage. 1994;9(3):186–92.

8. Cella DF. Methods and problems in measuring quality of life. Support Care Cancer. 1995;3(1):11–22.

9. Kornblith AB, Holland JC, Memorial Sloan-Kettering Cancer Center. Handbook of measures for psychological, social and physical function in cancer., Quality of life, vol. 1. New York: Memorial Sloan-Kettering Cancer Center; 1994.

10. Cella D. Quality of life. In: Breitbart W, Holland JC, Jacobsen PB, et al., editors. Psycho-oncology. New York, Oxford: Oxford University Press; 1998. p. 1135–46.

11. Ware Jr JE, Sherbourne CD. The MOS 36-item short-form health survey (SF-36). I. Conceptual framework and item selection. Med Care. 1992; 30(6):473–83.

12. Ware Jr J, Kosinski M, Keller SD. A 12-item short-form health survey: construction of scales and preliminary tests of reliability and validity. Med Care. 1996;34(3):220–33.

13. Ware JE, Snow KK, Kosinski M. SF-36 health survey: manual and interpretation guide. Lincoln, RI: QualityMetric Incorporated; 2000.

14. Stewart AL, Sherbourne CD, Hays R, et al. Summary and discussion of MOS measures. In: Stewart AL, Ware JE, editors. Measuring functioning and well-being: the medical outcomes study approach. Durham: Duke University Press; 1992. p. 345–71.

15. Bower JE, Ganz PA, Desmond KA, et al. Fatigue in long-term breast carcinoma survivors: a longitudinal investigation. Cancer. 2006;106(4):751–8.

16. Sarna L, Padilla G, Holmes C, Tashkin D, Brecht ML, Evangelista L. Quality of life of long-term survivors of non-small-cell lung cancer. J Clin Oncol. 2002;20(13):2920–9.

17. Alibhai SMH, Breunis H, Timilshina N, et al. Impact of androgen-deprivation therapy on physical function and quality of life in men with nonmetastatic prostate cancer. J Clin Oncol. 2010;28(34): 5038–45.

18. Hao Y, Stein K, Landrine H, Smith T, Kaw C, Corral I. Residential segregation and disparities in health-related quality of life among black and white cancer survivors. Health Psychol. 2011;30(2):137–44.

19. Hunt S, McKenna S, McEwen J, Williams J, Papp E. The Nottingham health profile: subjective health status and medical consultations. Soc Sci Med. 1981;55(2):301–11.

20. Franks PJ, Moffatt CJ. Health related quality of life in patients with venous ulceration: use of the Nottingham health profile. Qual Life Res. 2001; 10(8):693–700.

21. Jans MP, Schellevis FG, van Eijk JTM. The Nottingham health profile: score distribution, internal consistency and validity in asthma and COPD patients. Qual Life Res. 1999;8(6):501–7.

22. Joly F, Espie M, Marty M, Heron JF, Henry-Amar M. Long-term quality of life in premenopausal women with node-negative localized breast cancer treated with or without adjuvant chemotherapy. Br J Cancer. 2000;83(5):577–82.

23. Whynes DK, Neilson AR. Symptoms before and after surgery for colorectal cancer. Qual Life Res. 1997;6:61–6.

24. Ozalevli S, Ilgin D, Kul Karaali H, Bulac S, Akkoclu A. The effect of in-patient chest physiotherapy in lung cancer patients. Support Care Cancer. 2010;18(3):351–8.

25. Derogatis LR, Lopez MC. Psychosocial adjustment to illness scale: administration, scoring and procedures manual. Baltimore, MD: Johns Hopkins University School of Medicine; 1983.

26. Nishigaki M, Kazuma K, Oya M, et al. The influence of life stage on psychosocial adjustment in colorectal cancer patients. J Psychosoc Oncol. 2007;25(4): 71–87.

27. Lemieux J, Beaton D, Hogg-Johnson S, Bordeleau L, Hunter J, Goodwin P. Responsiveness to change to change due to supportive-expressive group therapy, improvement in mood and disease progression in women with metastatic breast cancer. Qual Life Res. 2007;16(6):1007–17.

28. Peppercorn J, Herndon J, Kornblith AB, et al. Quality of life among patients with Stage II and III breast carcinoma randomized to receive high-dose chemotherapy with autologous bone marrow support or intermediate-dose chemotherapy. Cancer. 2005;104(8):1580–9.

29. Fortner BV, Schwartzberg L, Tauer K, Houts AC, Hackett J, Stolshek BS. Impact of chemotherapy-induced neutropenia on quality of life: a prospective pilot investigation. Support Care Cancer. 2005;13(7):522–8.

30. Merluzzi TV, Sanchez MAM. Factor structure of the psychosocial adjustment to illness scale (self-report) for persons with cancer. Psychol Assess. 1997;9(3): 269–76.

31. Kornblith AB, Herndon JE, Zuckerman E, et al. Comparison of psychosocial adaptation of advanced stage Hodgkin's disease and acute leukemia survivors. Cancer and Leukemia Group B. Ann Oncol. 1998;9(3):297–306.

32. Bekkers MJ, van Knippenberg FC, van Dulmen AM, van den Borne HW, van Berge Henegouwen GP. Survival and psychosocial adjustment to stoma surgery and nonstoma bowel resection a 4-year follow-up. J Psychosom Res. 1997;42(3):235–44.

33. Olweny CL, Juttner CA, Rofe P, et al. Long-term effects of cancer treatment and consequences of cure: cancer survivors enjoy quality of life similar to their neighbours. Eur J Cancer. 1993;29A(6): 826–30.

34. Bergner M, Bobbitt RA, Carter WB, Gilson BS. The sickness impact profile: development and final revision of a health status measure. Med Care. 1981;19(8):787–805.

35. de Bruin AF, de Witte LP, Stevens F, Diederiks JP. Sickness impact profile: the state of the art of a generic functional status measure. Soc Sci Med. 1992;35(8):1003–14.

36. Pollard B, Johnston M. Problems with the sickness impact profile: a theoretically based analysis and a proposal for a new method of implementation and scoring. Soc Sci Med. 2001;52(6):921–34.

37. Blinderman CD, Homel P, Andrew Billings J, Tennstedt S, Portenoy RK. Symptom distress and quality of life in patients with advanced chronic obstructive pulmonary disease. J Pain Symptom Manage. 2009;38(1):115.

38. Ahlström G, Lindvall B, Wenneberg S, Gunnarsson LG. A comprehensive rehabilitation programme tailored to the needs of adults with muscular dystrophy. Clin Rehabil. 2006;20(2):132–41.

39. Selby PJ, Chapman JA, Etazadi-Amoli J, Dalley D, Boyd NF. The development of a method for assessing the quality of life of cancer patients. Br J Cancer. 1984;50(1):13–22.

40. Heitzmann CA, Merluzzi TV, Jean-Pierre P, Roscoe JA, Kirsh KL, Passik SD. Assessing self-efficacy for coping with cancer: development and psychometric analysis of the brief version of the Cancer Behavior Inventory (CBI-B). Psychooncology. 2011;20(3): 302–12.

41. Gielissen MF, Verhagen S, Witjes F, Bleijenberg G. Effects of cognitive behavior therapy in severely fatigued disease-free cancer patients compared with patients waiting for cognitive behavior therapy: a randomized controlled trial. J Clin Oncol. 2006;24(30):4882–7.

42. Vargas S, Wohlgemuth WK, Antoni MH, Lechner SC, Holley HA, Carver CS. Sleep dysfunction and psychosocial adaptation among women undergoing treatment for non-metastatic breast cancer. Psychooncology. 2010;19(6):669–73.

43. Spitzer WO, Dobson AJ, Hall J, et al. Measuring the quality of life of cancer patients: a concise QL-index for use by physicians. J Chronic Dis. 1981;34(12): 585–97.

44. Hird A, Wong J, Zhang L, et al. Exploration of symptoms clusters within cancer patients with brain metastases using the Spitzer quality of life index. Support Care Cancer. 2010;18(3):335–42.

45. Bonnetain F, Paoletti X, Collette S, et al. Quality of life as a prognostic factor of overall survival in patients with advanced hepatocellular carcinoma: results from two French clinical trials. Qual Life Res. 2008;17(6):831–43.

46. Scott C, Suh J, Stea B, Nabid A, Hackman J. Improved survival, quality of life, and quality-adjusted survival in breast cancer patients treated with efaproxiral (efaproxyn) plus whole-brain radiation therapy for brain metastases. Am J Clin Oncol. 2007;30(6):580–7. 510.1097/COC.1090b1013e3180653c3180650d.

47. Ganz PA, Schag CAC, Lee JJ, Sim MS. The CARES a generic measure of health-related quality of life for patients with cancer. Qual Life Res. 1992;1(1):19–29.

48. Schag CAC, Ganz PA, Heinrich RL. Cancer Rehabilitation Evaluation System-Short Form (CARES-SF): a cancer specific rehabilitation and quality of life instrument. Cancer. 1991;68(6): 1406–13.

49. Schag CA, Ganz PA, Polinsky ML, Fred C, Hirji K, Petersen L. Characteristics of women at risk for psychosocial distress in the year after breast cancer. J Clin Oncol. 1993;11(4):783–93.

50. Schag CA, Ganz PA, Wing DS, Sim MS, Lee JJ. Quality of life in adult survivors of lung, colon and prostate cancer. Qual Life Res. 1994;3(2):127–41.

51. Hawighorst S, Schoenefuss G, Fusshoeller C, et al. The physician-patient relationship before cancer treatment: a prospective longitudinal study. Gynecol Oncol. 2004;94(1):93–7.

52. Hjermstad MJ, Evensen SA, Kvaløy SO, Loge JH, Fayers PM, Kaasa S. The CARES-SF used for prospective assessment of health-related quality of life after stem cell transplantation. Psychooncology. 2003;12(8):803–13.

53. Casso D, Buist DS, Taplin S. Quality of life of 5-10 year breast cancer survivors diagnosed between age 40 and 49. Health Qual Life Outcomes. 2004; 2:25.

54. Clough-Gorr KM, Ganz PA, Silliman RA. Older breast cancer survivors: factors associated with change in emotional well-being. J Clin Oncol. 2007;25(11):1334–40.

55. Gotay CC, Moinpour CM, Unger JM, et al. Impact of a peer-delivered telephone intervention for women experiencing a breast cancer recurrence. J Clin Oncol. 2007;25(15):2093–9.

56. Ganz PA, Greendale GA, Petersen L, Zibecchi L, Kahn B, Belin TR. Managing menopausal symptoms in breast cancer survivors: results of a randomized controlled trial. J Natl Cancer Inst. 2000;92(13): 1054–64.

57. Aaronson NK, Ahmedzai S, Bergman B, et al. The European Organization for Research and Treatment of Cancer QLQ-C30: a quality-of-life instrument for use in international clinical trials in oncology. J Natl Cancer Inst. 1993;85(5):365–76.

58. Aaronson NK, Ahmedzai S, Bullinger M, Osoba D. The EORTC core quality of life questionnaire: interim results of an international field study. In: Osoba D, editor. Effect of cancer on quality of life. Boca Raton, FL: CRC Press, Inc.; 1991.

59. Osoba D, Aaronson NK, Muller M, et al. The development and psychometric validation of a brain cancer quality-of-life questionnaire for use in combination with general cancer-specific questionnaires. Qual Life Res. 1996;5(1):139–50.

60. Sprangers MA, Groenvold M, Arraras JI, et al. The European Organization for Research and Treatment of Cancer breast cancer-specific quality-of-life questionnaire module: first results from a three-country field study. J Clin Oncol. 1996;14(10):2756–68.

61. Greimel ER, Kuljanic Vlasic K, Waldenstrom AC, et al. The European Organization for Research and Treatment of Cancer (EORTC) quality-of-life questionnaire cervical cancer module: EORTC QLQ-CX24. Cancer. 2006;107(8):1812–22.

62. Sprangers MAG, te Velde A, Aaronson NK. The construction and testing of the EORTC colorectal cancer-specific quality of life questionnaire module (QLQ-CR38). Eur J Cancer. 1999;35(2):238–47.

63. Greimel E, Radisic VB, Daghofer F, et al. Psychometric validation of the European organisation for research and treatment of cancer quality of life questionnaire-endometrial cancer module (EORTC QLQ-EN24). Eur J Cancer. 2011;47(2):183–90.

64. Bjordal K, Hammerlid E, Ahlner-Elmqvist M, et al. Quality of life in head and neck cancer patients: validation of the European Organization for Research and Treatment of Cancer Quality of Life Questionnaire-H&N35. J Clin Oncol. 1999;17(3): 1008–19.

65. Bergman B, Aaronson NK, Ahmedzai S, Kaasa S, Sullivan M. The EORTC QLQ-LC13: a modular supplement to the EORTC Core Quality of Life Questionnaire (QLQ-C30) for use in lung cancer clinical trials. EORTC Study Group on Quality of Life. Eur J Cancer. 1994;30(5):635–42.

66. Stead ML, Brown JM, Velikova G, et al. Development of an EORTC questionnaire module to be used in health-related quality-of-life assessment for patients with multiple myeloma. European Organization for Research and Treatment of Cancer Study Group on Quality of Life. Br J Haematol. 1999;104(3):605–11.

67. Lagergren P, Fayers P, Conroy T, et al. Clinical and psychometric validation of a questionnaire module, the EORTC QLQ-OG25, to assess health-related quality of life in patients with cancer of the oesophagus, the oesophago-gastric junction and the stomach. Eur J Cancer. 2007;43(14):2066–73.

68. Greimel E, Bottomley A, Cull A, et al. An international field study of the reliability and validity of a disease-specific questionnaire module (the QLQ-OV28) in assessing the quality of life of patients with ovarian cancer. Eur J Cancer. 2003;39(10):1402–8.

69. Fitzsimmons D, Johnson CD, George S, et al. Development of a disease specific quality of life (QoL) questionnaire module to supplement the EORTC core cancer QoL questionnaire, the QLQ-C30 in patients with pancreatic cancer. EORTC Study Group on Quality of Life. Eur J Cancer. 1999;35(6):939–41.

70. Fossa SD, Aaronson NK, Newling D, et al. Quality of life and treatment of hormone resistant metastatic prostatic cancer. The EORTC Genito-Urinary Group. Eur J Cancer. 1990;26(11–12):1133–6.

71. Cella DF, Tulsky DS, Gray G, et al. The functional assessment of cancer therapy scale: development and validation of the general measure. J Clin Oncol. 1993;11(3):570–9.

72. Bonomi P, Kim K, Fairclough D, et al. Comparison of survival and quality of life in advanced non-small-cell lung cancer patients treated with two dose levels of paclitaxel combined with cisplatin versus etoposide with cisplatin: results of an Eastern Cooperative Oncology Group trial. J Clin Oncol. 2000;18(3): 623–31.

73. Cella DF, Tulsky DS. Quality of life in cancer: definition, purpose, and method of measurement. Cancer Invest. 1993;11(3):327–36.

74. Cella D. Measuring quality of life in palliative care. Semin Oncol. 1995;22(2 Suppl 3):73–81.

75. Dow KH, Ferrell BR, Leigh S, Ly J, Gulasekaram P. An evaluation of the quality of life among long-term survivors of breast cancer. Breast Cancer Res Treat. 1996;39(3):261–73.

76. Esper P, Mo F, Chodak G, Sinner M, Cella D, Pienta KJ. Measuring quality of life in men with prostate cancer using the functional assessment of cancer therapy-prostate instrument. Urology. 1997;50(6):920–8.

77. Esteve-Vives J, Batlle-Gualda E, Reig A. Spanish version of the health assessment questionnaire: reliability, validity and transcultural equivalency. Grupo para la Adaptacion del HAQ a la Poblacion Espanola. J Rheumatol. 1993;20(12):2116–22.

78. Lee WR, McQuellon RP, Case LD, deGuzman AF, McCullough DL. Early quality of life assessment in men treated with permanent source interstitial brachytherapy for clinically localized prostate cancer. J Urol. 1999;162(2):403–6.

79. Litwin M, Hays RD, Fink A, et al. Quality of life outcomes in men treated for localized prostate cancer. J Am Med Assoc. 1995;273:129–35.

80. Shrader-Bogen CL, Kjellberg JL, McPherson CP, Murray CL. Quality of life and treatment outcomes: prostate carcinoma patients' perspectives after prostatectomy or radiation therapy. Cancer. 1997;79(10): 1977–86.

81. Brady MJ, Cella DF, Mo F, et al. Reliability and validity of the Functional Assessment of Cancer Therapy-Breast (FACT-B) quality of life instrument. Behav Med. 1997;15(3):974–86.

82. Weitzner MA, Meyers CA, Gelke CK, Byrne KS, Cella DF, Levin VA. The Functional Assessment of Cancer Therapy (FACT) scale. Development of a brain subscale and revalidation of the general version (FACT-G) in patients with primary brain tumors. Cancer. 1995;75(5):1151–61.

83. Ward WL, Hahn EA, Mo F, Hernandez L, Tulsky DS, Cella D. Reliability and validity of the Functional Assessment of Cancer Therapy-Colorectal (FACT-C) quality of life instrument. Qual Life Res. 1999;8(3): 181–95.

84. Darling G, Eton D, Sulman J, Casson A, Cella D. Validation of the functional assessment of cancer therapy esophageal cancer. Cancer. 2006;107(4): 854–63.

85. List MA, D'Antonio LL, Cella DF, et al. The performance status scale for head and neck cancer patients and the functional assessment of cancer therapy-head and neck scale. A study of utility and validity. Cancer. 1996;77(11):2294–301.

86. Heffernan N, Cella D, Webster K, et al. Measuring health-related quality of life in patients with hepatobiliary cancers: the Functional Assessment of Cancer Therapy-Hepatobiliary questionnaire. J Clin Oncol. 2002;20(9):2229–39.

87. Cella DF, Bonomi AE, Lloyd SR, Tulsky DS, Kaplan E, Bonomi P. Reliability and validity of the Functional Assessment of Cancer Therapy-Lung (FACT-L) quality of life instrument. Lung Cancer. 1995;12(3):199–220.

88. Webster K, Chivington K, Shonk C, et al. Measuring quality of life (QOL) among patients with leukemia: the Functional Assessment of Cancer Therapy-Leukemia (FACT-L). Qual Life Res. 2002;11:678.

89. Pettengell R, Donatti C, Hoskin P, et al. The impact of follicular lymphoma on health-related quality of life. Ann Oncol. 2008;19(3):570–6.

90. Cormier JN, Ross M, Gershenwald J, et al. Prospective assessment of the reliability, validity, and sensitivity to change of the functional assessment of cancer therapy-melanoma questionnaire. Cancer. 2008;112(10):2249–57.

91. Tong MC, Lo PS, Wong KH, et al. Development and validation of the functional assessment of cancer therapy nasopharyngeal cancer subscale. Head Neck. 2009;31(6):738–47.

92. Basen-Engquist K, Bodurka-Bevers D, Fitzgerald MA, et al. Reliability and validity of the Functional Assessment of Cancer Therapy-Ovarian. J Clin Oncol. 2001;19(6):1809–17.

93. Janda M, Obermair A, Cella D, et al. The functional assessment of cancer-vulvar: reliability and validity. Gynecol Oncol. 2005;97(2):568–75.

94. Schipper H, Clinch J, McMurray A, Levitt M. Measuring the quality of life of cancer patients: the Functional Living Index-Cancer: development and validation. J Clin Oncol. 1984;2(5):472–83.

95. Eton DT, Lepore SJ. Prostate cancer and health-related quality of life: a review of the literature. Psychooncology. 2002;11(4):307–26.

96. Morrow GR, Lindke J, Black P. Measurement of quality of life in patients: psychometric analyses of the Functional Living Index-Cancer (FLIC). Qual Life Res. 1992;1(5):287–96.

97. Clinch JJ. The Functional Living Index – Cancer: ten years later. In: Spilker B, editor. Quality of life and pharmacoeconomics in clinical trials, vol. 2. Philadelphia: Lippincott-Raven Publishers; 1996. p. 215–25.

98. Laenen A, Alonso A. The Functional Living Index-Cancer: estimating its reliability based on clinical trial data. Qual Life Res. 2010;19(1):103–9.

99. Ganz PA, Coscarelli A, Fred C, Kahn B, Polinsky ML, Petersen L. Breast cancer survivors: psychosocial concerns and quality of life. Breast Cancer Res Treat. 1996;38(2):183–99.

100. Turner S, Gruenewald S, Spry N, Gebski V. Less pain does equal better quality of life following strontium-89 therapy for metastatic prostate cancer. Br J Cancer. 2001;84(3):297–302.

101. Siddiqui F, Kohl R, Swann S, Watkins-Bruner D, Movsas B. Gender differences in pretreatment quality of life in a prospective lung cancer trial. J Support Oncol. 2008;6(1):33–9.

102. Leake RL, Gurrin LC, Hammond IG. Quality of life in patients attending a low-risk gynaecological oncology follow-up clinic. Psychooncology. 2001;10(5):428–35.

103. Cohen SR, Mount BM, Strobel MG, Bui F. The McGill Quality of Life questionnaire: a measure of quality of life appropriate for people with advanced disease. A preliminary study of validity and acceptability. Palliat Med. 1995;9(3):207–19.

104. Cohen SR, Mount BM, Bruera E, Provost M, Rowe J, Tong K. Validity of the McGill Quality of Life Questionnaire in the palliative care setting: a multi-centre Canadian study demonstrating the importance of the existential domain. Palliat Med. 1997;11(1):3–20.

105. Cohen SR, Mount BM. Living with cancer: "good" days and "bad" days – what produces them? Can the McGill quality of life questionnaire distinguish between them? Cancer. 2000;89(8):1854–65.

106. Jones JM, McPherson CJ, Zimmermann C, Rodin G, Le LW, Cohen SR. Assessing agreement between terminally ill cancer patients' reports of their quality of life and family caregiver and palliative care physician proxy ratings. J Pain Symptom Manage. 2011;42(3):354–65.

107. Lowe SS, Watanabe SM, Baracos VE, Courneya KS. Associations between physical activity and quality of life in cancer patients receiving palliative care: a pilot survey. J Pain Symptom Manage. 2009;38(5):785–96.

108. Husain AF, Stewart K, Arseneault R, et al. Women experience higher levels of fatigue than men at the end of life: a longitudinal home palliative care study. J Pain Symptom Manage. 2007;33(4):389–97.

109. Sherman DW, Ye XY, McSherry C, Parkas V, Calabrese M, Gatto M. Quality of life of patients with advanced cancer and acquired immune deficiency syndrome and their family caregivers. J Palliat Med. 2006;9(4):948–63.

110. Ferrans CE, Powers MJ. Quality of life index: development and psychometric properties. Adv Nurs Sci. 1985;8(1):15–24.

111. Ferrans CE. Development of a quality of life index for patients with cancer. Oncol Nurs Forum. 1990;17(3 Suppl):15–9.

112. Ferrans CE, Powers MJ. Psychometric assessment of the Quality of Life Index. Res Nurs Health. 1992;15(1):29–38.

113. Lis C, Gupta D, Granick J, Grutsch J. Can patient satisfaction with quality of life predict survival in advanced colorectal cancer? Support Care Cancer. 2006;14(11):1104–10.

114. Sammarco A. Quality of life among older survivors of breast cancer. Cancer Nurs. 2003;26(6):431–8.

115. Gupta D, Granick J, Grutsch J, Lis C. The prognostic association of health-related quality of life scores

with survival in breast cancer. Support Care Cancer. 2007;15(4):387–93.

116. Warnecke RB, Ferrans CE, Johnson TP, et al. Measuring quality of life in culturally diverse populations. J Natl Cancer Inst Monogr. 1996;20:29–38.

117. Stein KD, Syrjala KL, Andrykowski MA. Physical and psychological long-term and late effects of cancer. Cancer. 2008;112(11 Suppl):2577–92.

118. Hewitt M, Greenfield S, Stovall E, Institute of Medicine (U.S.), American Society of Clinical Oncology. From cancer patient to cancer survivor: lost in transition. Washington, D.C.: National Academies Press; 2006.

119. Baker F, Denniston M, Zabora JR, Marcellus D. Cancer problems in living and quality of life after bone marrow transplantation. J Clin Psychol Med Settings. 2003;10(1):27–34.

120. Zhao L, Stein K, Smith T, Portier K, Baker F. Exploratory factor analysis of the cancer problems in living scale: a report from the American Cancer Society's studies of cancer survivors. J Pain Symptom Manage. 2009;37(4):676–86.

121. Baker F, Denniston M, Smith T, West MM. Adult cancer survivors: how are they faring? Cancer. 2005;104(S11):2565–76.

122. Smith T, Stein KD, Mehta CC, et al. The rationale, design, and implementation of the American Cancer Society's studies of cancer survivors. Cancer. 2007;109(1):1–12.

123. Zebrack BJ, Ganz PA, Bernaards CA, Petersen L, Abraham L. Assessing the impact of cancer: development of a new instrument for long-term survivors. Psychooncology. 2006;15(5):407–21.

124. Crespi CM, Ganz PA, Petersen L, Castillo A, Caan B. Refinement and psychometric evaluation of the impact of cancer scale. J Natl Cancer Inst. 2008; 100(21):1530–41.

125. Zebrack BJ, Yi J, Petersen L, Ganz PA. The impact of cancer and quality of life for long-term survivors. Psychooncology. 2008;17(9):891–900.

126. Crespi CM, Petersen L, Ganz PA, Smith SK, Zimmerman S. Measuring the impact of cancer: a comparison of non-Hodgkin lymphoma and breast cancer survivors. J Cancer Surviv. 2010;4(1):45–58.

127. Zebrack BJ, Donohue JE, Gurney JG, Chesler MA, Bhatia S, Landier W. Psychometric evaluation of the impact of cancer (IOC-CS) scale for young adult survivors of childhood cancer. Qual Life Res. 2010; 19(2):207–18.

128. Zebrack B. Developing a new instrument to assess the impact of cancer in young adult survivors of childhood cancer. J Cancer Surviv. 2009;3(3):174–80.

129. Wyatt GK, Friedman LL. Development and testing of a quality of life model for long-term female cancer survivors. Qual Life Res. 1996;5(3):387–94.

130. Wyatt G, Friedman LL. Long-term female cancer survivors: quality of life issues and clinical implications. Cancer Nurs. 1996;19(1):1–7.

131. Wyatt G, Kurtz ME, Friedman LL, Given B, Given CW. Preliminary testing of the Long-Term Quality

of Life (LTQL) instrument for female cancer survivors. J Nurs Meas. 1996;4(2):153–70.

132. Avis NE, Smith KW, McGraw S, Smith RG, Petronis VM, Carver CS. Assessing quality of life in adult cancer survivors (QLACS). Qual Life Res. 2005;14(4):1007–23.

133. Avis NE, Ip E, Foley KL. Evaluation of the quality of life in adult cancer survivors (QLACS) scale for long-term cancer survivors in a sample of breast cancer survivors. Health Qual Life Outcomes. 2006;4:92.

134. Ferrell BR, Dow KH, Grant M. Measurement of the quality of life in cancer survivors. Qual Life Res. 1995;4(6):523–31.

135. Ferrell BR, Dow KH, Leigh S, Ly J, Gulasekaram P. Quality of life in long-term cancer survivors. Oncol Nurs Forum. 1995;22(6):915–22.

136. Whedon M, Stearns D, Mills LE. Quality of life of long-term adult survivors of autologous bone marrow transplantation. Oncol Nurs Forum. 1995;22(10): 1527–35.

137. Zebrack B, Chesler M. A psychometric analysis of the quality of life-cancer survivors (QOL-CS) in survivors of childhood cancer. Qual Life Res. 2001; 10(4):319–29.

138. Litwin MS, Hays R, Fink A, Ganz PA, Leake B, Brook RH. The UCLA Prostate Cancer Index: development, reliability, and validity of health-related quality of life measure. Med Care. 1998;26(7): 1002–12.

139. Terrell JE, Nanavati KA, Esclamado RM, Bishop JK, Bradford CR, Wolf GT. Head and neck cancer-specific quality of life: instrument validation. Arch Otolaryngol Head Neck Surg. 1997;123(10): 1125–32.

140. Hollen PJ, Gralla RJ, Kris MG, Potanovich LM. Quality of life assessment in individuals with lung cancer: testing the Lung Cancer Symptom Scale (LCSS). Eur J Cancer. 1993;29A Suppl 1:S51–8.

141. Davidson-Homewood J, Norman A, Küchler T, Cunningham D, Watson M. Development of a disease specific questionnaire to supplement a generic tool for QoL in colorectal cancer. Psychooncology. 2003;12(7):675–85.

142. McCorkle R. The measurement of symptom distress. Semin Oncol Nurs. 1987;3(4):248–56.

143. McCorkle R, Young K. Development of a symptom distress scale. Cancer Nurs. 1978;1(5):373–8.

144. Cleeland CS, Mendoza TR, Wang XS, et al. Assessing symptom distress in cancer patients: the M.D. Anderson Symptom Inventory. Cancer. 2000;89(7):1634–46.

145. Chang VT, Hwang SS, Feuerman M. Validation of the Edmonton symptom assessment scale. Cancer. 2000;88(9):2164–71.

146. Portenoy RK, Thaler HT, Kornblith AB, et al. The Memorial Symptom Assessment Scale: an instrument for the evaluation of symptom prevalence, characteristics and distress. Eur J Cancer. 1994; 30A(9):1326–36.

147. De Haes JC, van Knippenberg FC, Neijt JP. Measuring psychological and physical distress in cancer patients: structure and application of the Rotterdam Symptom Checklist. Br J Cancer. 1990;62(6):1034–8.

148. Derogatis LR. SCL-90-R: administration, scoring, and procedures manual I for the revised version of the SCL-90. Baltimore, MD: Johns Hopkins University Press; 1977.

149. Derogatis LR, Spencer MS. The Brief Symptom Inventory (BSI): administration, scoring, and procedures manual. Baltimore: Johns Hopkins University School of Medicine, Clinical Psychometrics Research Unit; 1982.

150. Zabora J, BrintzenhofeSzoc K, Jacobsen P, et al. A new psychosocial screening instrument for use with cancer patients. Psychosomatics. 2001;42(3):241–6.

151. McNair DM, Lorr M, Droppleman LF. Profile of mood states (POMS). San Diego, CA: Educational and Industrial Testing Service; 1992.

152. Veit CT, Ware Jr JE. The structure of psychological distress and well-being in general populations. J Consult Clin Psychol. 1983;51(5):730–42.

153. Bradburn NM. The structure of psychological well-being. Chicago, IL: Aldine Publishing; 1969.

154. Bradburn NM, Caplovitz D. Reports on happiness: a pilot study of behavior related to mental health. Chicago, IL: Aldine; 1965.

155. Radloff LS. The CES-D scale: a self-report depression scale for research in the general population. Appl Psychol Measurement. 1977;1(3):385–401.

156. Zigmond AS, Snaith RP. The hospital anxiety and depression scale. Acta Psychiatr Scand. 1983;67(6): 361–70.

157. Spielberger CD, Gorsuch RL, Lushene RE. STAI manual for the state-trait anxiety inventory. Palo Alto, CA: Consulting Psychologists Press; 1970.

158. Horowitz M, Wilner N, Alvarez W. Impact of event scale: a measure of subjective stress. Psychosom Med. 1979;41(3):209–18.

159. Blanchard EB, Jones-Alexander J, Buckley TC, Forneris CA. Psychometric properties of the PTSD Checklist (PCL). Behav Res Ther. 1996;34(8): 669–73.

160. Mendoza TR, Wang XS, Cleeland CS, et al. The rapid assessment of fatigue severity in cancer patients: use of the brief fatigue inventory. Cancer. 1999;85(5):1186–96.

161. Cleeland CS, Ryan KM. Pain assessment: global use of the brief pain inventory. Ann Acad Med. 1994; 23(2):129–38.

162. Armstrong FD, Toledano SR, Miloslavich K, et al. The Miami pediatric quality of life questionnaire: parent scale. Int J Cancer Suppl. 1999;12:11–7.

163. Bhatia S, Jenney ME, Bogue MK, et al. The Minneapolis-Manchester quality of life instrument: reliability and validity of the adolescent form. J Clin Oncol. 2002;20(24):4692–8.

164. Bhatia S, Jenney ME, Wu E, et al. The Minneapolis-Manchester quality of life instrument: reliability and validity of the youth form. J Pediatr. 2004;145(1): 39–46.

165. Varni JW, Burwinkle TM, Katz ER, Meeske K, Dickinson P. The PedsQL in pediatric cancer: reliability and validity of the Pediatric Quality of Life Inventory Generic Core Scales, Multidimensional Fatigue Scale, and Cancer Module. Cancer. 2002; 94(7):2090–106.

166. Varni JW, Katz ER, Seid M, Quiggins DJ, Friedman-Bender A. The pediatric cancer quality of life inventory-32 (PCQL-32): I. Reliability and validity. Cancer. 1998;82(6):1184–96.

167. Varni JW, Katz ER, Seid M, Quiggins DJ, Friedman-Bender A, Castro CM. The Pediatric Cancer Quality of Life Inventory (PCQL). I. Instrument development, descriptive statistics, and cross-informant variance. J Behav Med. 1998;21(2):179–204.

168. Varni JW, Rode CA, Seid M, Katz ER, Friedman-Bender A, Quiggins DJL. The Pediatric Cancer Quality of Life Inventory-32 (PCQL-32). II. Feasibility and range of measurement. J Behav Med. 1999;22(4):397–406.

169. Goodwin DA, Boggs SR, Boggs SR, Graham-Pole J. Development and validation of the pediatric oncology quality of life scale. Psychol Assess. 1994;6(4):321–8.

170. Bijttebier P, Vercruysse T, Vertommen H, Gool SWV, Uyttebroeck A, Brock P. New evidence on the reliability and validity of the pediatric oncology quality of life scale. Psychol Health. 2001; 16(4):461.

171. Klassen A, Strohm S, Maurice-Stam H, Grootenhuis M. Quality of life questionnaires for children with cancer and childhood cancer survivors: a review of the development of available measures. Support Care Cancer. 2010;18(9):1207–17.

172. Trask PC, Hsu MA, McQuellon R. Other paradigms: health-related quality of life as a measure in cancer treatment: its importance and relevance. Cancer J. 2009;15(5):435–40.

173. Silveira AP, Gonçalves J, Sequeira T, et al. Patient reported outcomes in head and neck cancer: selecting instruments for quality of life integration in clinical protocols. Head Neck Oncol. 2010;2(32):1–9.

174. Aaronson NK. Quality of life: what is it? How should it be measured? Oncology. 1988;2(5):69–76.

175. Bergman B, Sullivan M, Sörenson S. Quality of life during chemotherapy for small cell lung cancer. II. A longitudinal study of the EORTC core quality of life questionnaire and comparison with the sickness impact profile. Acta Oncol. 1992;31(1): 19–28.

176. Boini S, Briancon S, Guillemin F, Galan P, Hercberg S. Impact of cancer occurrence on health-related quality of life: a longitudinal pre-post assessment. Health Qual Life Outcomes. 2004;2(1):4.

177. Andrykowski MA, Brady MJ, Hunt JW. Positive psychosocial adjustment in potential bone marrow transplant recipients: cancer as a psychosocial transition. Psychooncology. 1993;2(261):276.

178. Lee L, Chung C-W, Chang Y-Y, et al. Comparison of the quality of life between patients with non-small-cell lung cancer and healthy controls. Qual Life Res. 2011;20(3):415–23.

179. Anastasi A, Urbina S. Psychological testing. Upper Saddle River, NJ: Prentice Hall; 1997.

180. Lord FM. Applications of item response theory to practical testing problems. Hillsdale, NJ: Lawrence Erlbaum; 1980.

181. Richardson M. The relation between the difficulty and the differential validity of a test. Psychometrika. 1936;1(2):33–49.

182. Streiner DL, Norman GR. Health measurement scales: a practical guide to their development and use. Oxford, New York: Oxford University Press; 1995.

183. Cella D, Riley W, Stone A, et al. The Patient Reported Outcomes Measurement Information System (PROMIS) developed and tested its first wave of adult self-reported health outcome item banks: 2005–2008. J Clin Epidemiol. 2010;63(11):1179–94.

184. Liu H, Cella D, Gershon R, et al. Representativeness of the PROMIS internet panel. J Clin Epidemiol. 2010;63(11):1169–78.

185. Rothrock N, Hays R, Spritzer K, Yount SE, Riley W, Cella D. Relative to the general US population, chronic diseases are associated with poorer health-related quality of life as measured by the Patient-Reported Outcomes Measurement Information System (PROMIS). J Clin Epidemiol. 2010;63(11):1195–204.

186. Cella D, Yount S, Rothrock N, et al. The Patient-Reported Outcomes Measurement Information System (PROMIS): progress of an NIH roadmap cooperative group during its first two years. Med Care. 2007;45(5 Suppl 1):S3–11.

187. DeWalt DA, Rothrock N, Yount S, Stone AA, PROMIS Cooperative Group. Evaluation of item candidates: the PROMIS qualitative item review. Med Care. 2007;45(5 Suppl 1):S12–21.

188. Reeve BB, Hays RD, Bjorner JB, et al. Psychometric evaluation and calibration of health-related quality of life item banks: plans for the Patient-Reported Outcomes Measurement Information System (PROMIS). Med Care. 2007;45(5 Suppl 1):S22–31.

189. Wilkie DJ, Huang HY, Berry DL, et al. Cancer symptom control: feasibility of a tailored, interactive computerized program for patients. Fam Community Health. 2001;24(3):48–62.

190. Cleeland CS. Cancer-related symptoms. Semin Radiat Oncol. 2000;10(3):175–90.

191. Passik SD, Kirsh KL, Donaghy K, et al. Patient-related barriers to fatigue communication: initial validation of the fatigue management barriers questionnaire. J Pain Symptom Manage. 2002;24(5):481–93.

192. Beckman HB, Frankel RM. The effect of physician behavior on the collection of data. Ann Intern Med. 1984;101(5):692–6.

193. Dalton JA, Blau W, Carlson J, et al. Changing the relationship among nurses' knowledge, self-reported behavior, and documented behavior in pain management:

does education make a difference? J Pain Symptom Manage. 1996;12(5):308–19.

194. Schuit KW, Sleijfer DT, Meijler WJ, et al. Symptoms and functional status of patients with disseminated cancer visiting outpatient departments. J Pain Symptom Manage. 1998;16(5):290–7.

195. Whelan TJ, Mohide EA, Willan AR, et al. The supportive care needs of newly diagnosed cancer patients attending a regional cancer center. Cancer. 1997;80(8):1518–24.

196. Thomason TE, McCune JS, Bernard SA, Winer EP, Tremont S, Lindley CM. Cancer pain survey: patient-centered issues in control. J Pain Symptom Manage. 1998;15(5):275–84.

197. Cleeland CS. Barriers to the management of cancer pain. Oncology. 1987;1(2 Suppl):19–26.

198. Riddell A, Fitch MI. Patients' knowledge of and attitudes toward the management of cancer pain. Oncol Nurs Forum. 1997;24(10):1775–84.

199. Twycross R, Lack S. Symptom control in far advanced cancer: pain relief. London: Raven Pitman; 1984.

200. Diekmann JM, Engber D, Wassem R. Cancer pain control: one state's experience. Oncol Nurs Forum. 1989;16(2):219–23.

201. Ward SE, Goldberg N, Miller-McCauley V, et al. Patient-related barriers to management of cancer pain. Pain. 1993;52(3):319–24.

202. von Roenn JH, Cleeland CS, Gonin R, Hatfield AK, Pandya KJ. Physician attitudes and practice in cancer pain management. A survey from the Eastern Cooperative Oncology Group. Ann Intern Med. 1993;119(2):121–6.

203. Jacox A, Carr DB, Payne R. New clinical-practice guidelines for the management of pain in patients with cancer. N Engl J Med. 1994;330(9):651–5.

204. Fortner BV, Schwartzberg LS, Stepanski EJ, Houts AC. Symptom burden for patients with metastatic colorectal cancer treated with first-line FOLFOX or FOLFIRI with and without Bevacizumab in the community setting. Support Cancer Ther. 2007;4(4):233–40.

205. Detmar SB, Aaronson NK. Quality of life assessment in daily clinical oncology practice: a feasibility study. Eur J Cancer. 1998;34(8):1181–6.

206. Velikova G, Brown JM, Smith AB, Selby PJ. Computer-based quality of life questionnaires may contribute to doctor-patient interactions in oncology. Br J Cancer. 2002;86(1):51–9.

207. Carlson LE, Speca M, Hagen N, Taenzer P. Computerized quality-of-life screening in a cancer pain clinic. J Palliat Care. 2001;17(1):46–52.

208. Davis K, Cella D, Yount S, et al. Computer technology as a platform for weekly symptom monitoring of patients with advanced lung cancer. Lung Cancer. 2003;41(S2):S266.

209. Detmar SB, Muller M, Wever LD, Schornagel JH, Aaronson NK. Patient-Physician communication during outpatient palliative treatment visits: an observational study. J Am Med Assoc. 2001;285(10): 1351–7.

210. Taenzer P, Speca M, Atkinson M, et al. Computerized quality of life screening in an oncology clinic. Cancer Pract. 1997;5(3):168–75.
211. Naughton M, Homsi J. Symptom assessment in cancer patients. Curr Oncol Rep. 2002;4:256–63.
212. Brown V, Sitzia J, Richardson A, Hughes J, Hannon H, Oakley C. The development of the Chemotherapy Symptom Assessment Scale (C-SAS): a scale for the routine clinical assessment of the symptom experiences of patients receiving cytotoxic chemotherapy. Int J Nurs Stud. 2001;38:497–510.
213. Detmar SB, Aaronson N, Wever LD, Muller M, Schornagel JH. How are you feeling? Who wants to know? Patients' and oncologists' preferences for discussing health-related quality of life issues. J Clin Oncol. 2000;18(18):3295–301.
214. Montazeri A, Gillis CR, McEwen J. Measuring quality of life in oncology: is it worthwhile? Experiences from the treatment of cancer. Eur J Cancer Care. 1996;5(3):168–75.
215. Street RL, Gold WR, McDowell T. Using health surveys in medical consultations. Med Care. 1994;32(7):732–44.
216. Detmar SB, Muller MJ, Wever LD, Schornagel JH, Aaronson NK. The patient-physician relationship. Patient-physician communication during outpatient palliative treatment visits: an observational study. JAMA. 2001;285(10):1351–7.
217. Detmar SB, Muller MJ, Schornagel JH, Wever LD, Aaronson NK. Health-related quality-of-life assessments and patient-physician communication: a randomized controlled trial. JAMA. 2002;288(23):3027–34.
218. Rosenbloom S, Victorson D, Hahn E, Peterman A, Cella D. Assessment is not enough: a randomized controlled trial of the effects of HRQL assessment on quality of life and satisfaction in oncology clinical practice. Psychooncology. 2007;16(12):1069–79.
219. Velikova G, Booth L, Smith AB, et al. Measuring quality of life in routine oncology practice improves communication and patient well-being: a randomized controlled trial. J Clin Oncol. 2004;22(4):714–24.
220. Mooney KH, Beck SL, Friedman RH, Farzanfar R. Telephone-linked care for cancer symptom monitoring: a pilot study. Cancer Pract. 2002;10(3):147–54.
221. Taenzer P, Bultz BD, Carlson LE, et al. Impact of computerized quality of life screening on physician behavior and patient satisfaction in lung cancer outpatients. Psychooncology. 2000;9(3):203–13.
222. VonRoenn J, Cleeland CS, Gonin R, Hatfield AK, Pandya KJ. Physician attitudes and practice in cancer pain management. A survey from the Eastern Cooperative Oncology Group. Ann Intern Med. 1993;119:121–6.
223. Cella D, Paul D, Yount S, et al. What are the most important symptom targets when treating advanced cancer? A survey of providers in the National Comprehensive Cancer Network (NCCN). Cancer Invest. 2003;21(4):526–35.
224. Aarstad AKH, Aarstad HJ, Beisland E, Osthus AA. Distress, quality of life, neuroticism and psychological coping are related in head and neck cancer patients during follow-up. Acta Oncol. 2011;50(3):390–8.
225. Meyer F, Fortin A, Gelinas M, et al. Health-related quality of life as a survival predictor for patients with localized head and neck cancer treated with radiation therapy. J Clin Oncol. 2009;27(18):2970–6.
226. Chan JYK, Lua LL, Starmer HH, Sun DQ, Rosenblatt ES, Gourin CG. The relationship between depressive symptoms and initial quality of life and function in head and neck cancer. Laryngoscope. 2011;121(6):1212–8.
227. Aaronson NK, Bullinger M, Ahmedzai S. A modular approach to quality-of-life assessment in cancer clinical trials. Recent Results Cancer Res. 1988;111:231–49.
228. Au H-J, Ringash J, Brundage M, Palmer M, Richardson H, Meyer RM. Added value of health-related quality of life measurement in cancer clinical trials: the experience of the NCIC CTG. Expert Rev Pharmacoecon Outcomes Res. 2010;10(2):119–28.
229. Joly F, Vardy J, Pintilie M, Tannock IF. Quality of life and/or symptom control in randomized clinical trials for patients with advanced cancer. Ann Oncol. 2007;18(12):1935–42.
230. Efficace F, Osoba D, Gotay C, Sprangers M, Coens C, Bottomley A. Has the quality of health-related quality of life reporting in cancer clinical trials improved over time? Towards bridging the gap with clinical decision making. Ann Oncol. 2007;18(4):775–81.
231. Gotay CC. Assessing cancer-related quality of life across a spectrum of applications. J Natl Cancer Inst Monogr. 2004;33:126–33.
232. Dwivedi R, St. Rose S, Chisholm E, et al. Evaluation of factors affecting post-treatment quality of life in oral and oropharyngeal cancer patients primarily treated with curative surgery: an exploratory study. Eur Arch Otorhinolaryngol. 2012;269(2):591–9.
233. Tschiesner U, Becker S, Berghaus A, et al. Content validation of the International Classification of Functioning, Disability and Health core sets for head and neck cancer: a multicentre study. J Otolaryngol Head Neck Surg. 2010;39(6):674–87.
234. Jaeschke R, Singer J, Guyatt GH. Measurement of health status. Ascertaining the minimal clinically important difference. Control Clin Trials. 1989;10(4):407–15.
235. Yost KJ, Eton DT. Combining distribution- and anchor-based approaches to determine minimally important differences: the FACIT experience. Eval Health Prof. 2005;28(2):172–91.
236. Yost KJ, Eton DT, Garcia SF, Cella D. Minimally important differences were estimated for six Patient-Reported Outcomes Measurement Information System-Cancer scales in advanced-stage cancer patients. J Clin Epidemiol. 2011;64(5):507–16.

237. Beitz J. Quality-of-life end points in oncology drug trials. Oncology. 1999;13(10):1439.

238. U. S. Food and Drug Administration, Center for Drug Evaluation and Research. Meeting of the Quality of Life Subcommittee of the Oncologic Drugs Advisory Committee. 2000. http://www.fda. gov/ohrms/dockets/ac/cder00.htm#Oncologic%20 Drugs%20Advisory%20Committee. Accessed 1 Jul 2010.

239. Leidy NK, Revicki DA, Geneste B. Recommendations for evaluating the validity of quality of life claims for labeling and promotion. Value Health. 1999; 2(2):113–26.

240. Brunelli C, Costantini M, Di Giulio P, et al. Quality-of-life evaluation: when do terminal cancer patients and health-care providers agree? J Pain Symp Manage. 1998;15(3):151–8.

241. Stephens RJ, Hopwood P, Girling DJ, Machin D. Randomized trials with quality of life endpoints: are doctors' ratings of patients' physical symptoms interchangeable with patients' self- ratings? Qual Life Res. 1997;6(3):225–36.

242. Stromgren AS, Groenvold M, Sorensen A, Andersen L. Symptom recognition in advanced cancer. A comparison of nursing records against patient self-rating. Acta Anaesthesiol Scand. 2001;45(9):1080–5.

243. Cella D, Rosenbloom SK, Beaumont JL, et al. Development and validation of 11 symptom indexes to evaluate response to chemotherapy for advanced cancer. J Natl Compr Canc Netw. 2011;9(3):268–78.

244. Rao D, Butt Z, Rosenbloom S, et al. A comparison of the renal cell carcinoma symptom index (RCC-SI) and the functional assessment of cancer therapy – kidney symptom index (FKSI). J Pain Symptom Manage. 2009;38(2):291–8.

245. Yount S, Beaumont J, Rosenbloom S, et al. A brief symptom index for advanced lung cancer. Clin Lung Cancer. 2012;13(1):14–23.

246. Jensen SE, Rosenbloom SK, Beaumont JL, et al. A new index of priority symptoms in advanced ovarian cancer. Gynecol Oncol. 2011;120(2):214–9.

247. Victorson DE, Beaumont JL, Rosenbloom SK, Shevrin D, Cella D. Efficient assessment of the most important symptoms in advanced prostate cancer: the NCCN/FACT-P symptom index. Psychooncology. 2011;20(9):977–83.

248. Collins LG, Swartz K. Caregiver care. Am Fam Physician. 2011;83(11):1309–17.

249. Kim Y, Given BA. Quality of life of family caregivers of cancer survivors: across the trajectory of the illness. Cancer. 2008;112(11):2556–68.

250. Trask PC, Pearman T. Depression. In: Feuerstein M, editor. Handbook of cancer survivorship. New York, N.Y: Springer; 2007. p. 173–90.

251. Kim Y, Baker F, Spillers RL. Cancer caregivers' quality of life: effects of gender, relationship, and appraisal. J Pain Symptom Manage. 2007;34(3): 294–304.

252. Song JI, Shin DW, Choi JY, et al. Quality of life and mental health in family caregivers of patients with terminal cancer. Support Care Cancer. 2011;19(10): 1519–26.

253. Fridriksdottir N, Saevarsdottir P, Halfdanardottir SI, et al. Family members of cancer patients: needs, quality of life and symptoms of anxiety and depression. Acta Oncol. 2011;50(2):252–8.

254. Kim Y, Wellisch D, Spillers R, Crammer C. Psychological distress of female cancer caregivers: effects of type of cancer and caregivers' spirituality. Support Care Cancer. 2007;15(12):1367–74.

255. Kim Y, Spillers RL. Quality of life of family caregivers at 2 years after a relative's cancer diagnosis. Psychooncology. 2010;19(4):431–40.

256. Kim Y, Carver C, Spillers R, Love-Ghaffari M, Kaw C-K. Dyadic effects of fear of recurrence on the quality of life of cancer survivors and their caregivers. Qual Life Res. 2012;21(3):517–25.

257. Eyigor S, Karapolat H, Yesil H, Kantar M. The quality of life and psychological status of mothers of hospitalized pediatric oncology patients. Pediatr Hematol Oncol. 2011;28(5):428–38.

258. Litzelman K, Catrine K, Gangnon R, Witt W. Quality of life among parents of children with cancer or brain tumors: the impact of child characteristics and parental psychosocial factors. Qual Life Res. 2011;20(8):1261–9.

259. Palos GR, Hare M. Patients, family caregivers, and patient navigators. Cancer. 2011;117(S15): 3590–600.

260. Meyers FJ, Carducci M, Loscalzo MJ, Linder J, Greasby T, Beckett LA. Effects of a Problem-Solving Intervention (COPE) on quality of life for patients with advanced cancer on clinical trials and their caregivers: Simultaneous Care Educational Intervention (SCEI): linking palliation and clinical trials. J Palliat Med. 2011;14(4):465–73.

Exercise for Cancer Patients: Treatment of Side Effects and Quality of Life

Karen M. Mustian, Lisa K. Sprod, Michelle Janelsins,
Luke Peppone, Jennifer Carroll, Supriya Mohile,
and Oxana Palesh

Introduction

The American Cancer Society (ACS) estimates that nearly 1.5 million Americans will be diagnosed with cancer and almost 600,000 Americans will die from cancer in 2011 [1]. Despite the large number of cancer cases and deaths, the 5-year survival rate for *all* cancer types has increased to 68% in the second decade of the twenty-first century [1]. While the odds of cancer survival have increased due to improved screening and treatments, cancer patients and survivors endure acute (arising during treatment and resolving within days, weeks, or months), chronic or long-term (arising during treatment and persisting for months or years), and late (arising weeks or months after treatments have been completed) side effects from their cancer and its treatments.

K.M. Mustian, Ph.D., M.P.H., A.C.S.M, F.S.B.M. (✉)
L.K. Sprod, Ph.D., A.C.S.M. • M. Janelsins, Ph.D.
L. Peppone, Ph.D., M.P.H. • J. Carroll, M.D., M.P.H.
S. Mohile, M.D., M.P.H.
Physical Exercise, Activity and Kinesiology (PEAK)
Laboratory, Department of Radiation Oncology,
James P. Wilmot Cancer Center, University of Rochester
School of Medicine and Dentistry, 265 Crittenden
Boulevard, Rochester, NY 14642, USA
e-mail: Karen_Mustian@urmc.rochester.edu

O. Palesh, Ph.D., M.P.H.
Department of Psychology, Stanford Cancer Institute,
Stanford University, Palo Alto, CA, USA

These side effects negatively impact cancer patients during treatment and survivors in the years following treatment completion. Exercise plays a significant role in managing some of these side effects and improving quality of life (QOL) before, during, and after treatments. The purpose of this chapter is to provide an overview of the exercise oncology literature supporting the use of exercise as an effective intervention for helping cancer patients to cope with their diagnosis and treatments, improving some of the most prevalent side effects experienced by cancer patients, and increasing QOL.

Cancer Treatment-Related Side Effects

The news of a cancer diagnosis and the subsequent, life-saving treatments for cancer, such as surgery, chemotherapy, radiation therapy, and hormone therapy, lead to impaired QOL and mental and physical side effects that interfere with a patient's ability to cope with and complete treatments and the ability to function independently and complete essential activities of daily living. Cancer-related fatigue, other mental side effects, and physical dysfunction such as impaired muscular and cardiorespiratory function are common cancer treatment-related side effects that impair a cancer patient's ability to complete treatments, and to recover from the cancer and its treatments.

B.I. Carr and J. Steel (eds.), *Psychological Aspects of Cancer*,
DOI 10.1007/978-1-4614-4866-2_16, © Springer Science+Business Media, LLC 2013

Cancer-Related Fatigue

Cancer-related fatigue (CRF) is one of the most frequently reported and troublesome side effects reported by cancer patients [2–8]. Cancer patients report CRF throughout the entire cancer experience from the point of diagnosis, throughout treatments, and in many cases for years after treatments are complete [2–7]. Cancer patients often describe CRF as more distressing than other cancer-related side effects including vomiting, nausea, pain, and depression [3–7] due to its influence on activities of daily living and QOL. As many as 100% of cancer survivors undergoing treatment report CRF, with almost half indicating severe CRF [3–7]. Over two-thirds of cancer survivors report chronic or long-term CRF following treatment completion, with up to 38% indicating that this chronic CRF is severe at 6 months and beyond after completing treatment [3–7]. Patients who receive a combination of treatment modalities are more likely to report CRF and have severe CRF and to develop chronic CRF compared to patients treated with a single modality [3–7]. CRF differs from the fatigue experienced by individuals without cancer in its severity, impact on function and QOL and persistence, and inability to be alleviated by rest alone [3–7]. Recovery from cancer and its treatments is impaired when CRF persists and its negative effects on function and QOL continue to increase. [3–7] One of the most troubling aspects of CRF for cancer patients is the lack of effective remedies to prevent or alleviate this side effect adding to the distress they endure. CRF commonly co-occurs with many additional mental and physical side effects. While we do not know whether these co-occurring side effects are implicated in the development of CRF, they also impair a cancer survivor's recovery and QOL [3–7].

Mental Health Side Effects

Impairments in mental health are common in cancer survivors. Ten to 25% of cancer patients report depression [9]. Between 30 and 50% of cancer patients have sleep disruption [10]. Sleep dysfunction is exacerbated in patients who spend a significant amount of time napping during the day, usually in an effort to relieve negative side effects, because this leads to night sleep time being disrupted by periods of wakefulness and movement [11]. Forty five to 59% of cancer patients report pain [12]. Approximately half of cancer patients report anxiety, and 20% meet the clinical criteria for an anxiety disorder [13]. As many as 80% of cancer patients have cognitive problems, such as impaired memory and concentration [14]. Cancer patients also have a difficult time working, participating in leisure and social activities and in activities with their families, and sustaining meaningful relationships, and they often experience negative outcome expectancies and hopelessness during and after treatment [2, 3, 6, 7].

Muscle and Bone Loss

Muscle atrophy and muscle weakness frequently occur as a result of cancer and its treatments, particularly hormonal therapies [4, 6, 15–19]. Adenosine triphosphate (ATP) is a key mediator in generating muscle mass and in contractile function which is directly related to muscle strength/weakness. As such, decreased ATP synthesis may play a significant role in the development of CRF and other side effects [15] as well as impaired functional independence and QOL. In addition to premature sarcopenia and other muscle-related problems, chemotherapy, radiation therapy, and hormonal therapy lead to diminished bone mineral density. Chemotherapy often leads to premature menopause and a rapid loss in bone resulting from the sudden lack of endogenous estrogen production [20]. Primary or prophylactic oophorectomy in premenopausal women also reduces estrogen production and subsequently leads to decreases in bone mineral density [21]. Aromatase inhibitors also significantly increase rates of bone loss due to reduced estrogen production [22]. This cancer treatment-induced bone loss, ultimately, results in increased fracture risks for breast cancer survivors.

Cardiopulmonary Toxicity

Certain chemotherapeutic agents can lead to cardiotoxicity and impaired respiratory function [2, 3, 6, 7]. The anthracyclines, for example, have been widely recognized as having the potential to lead to cardiomyopathy. Although the exact mechanisms of anthracycline-induced cardiotoxicity have not been fully established, myocyte cell deaths resulting from apoptosis and necrosis are likely contributors. These effects can occur during treatment but may not manifest until years after treatment completion [23]. Trastuzumab and other kinase-targeting agents, which improve cancer survival, may also adversely affect cardiac function in some patients. Chemotherapy-induced cardiotoxicity is dose dependent and higher cumulative doses increase the risk of cardiac dysfunction [24, 25]. Cardiac dysfunction can manifest as left ventricular dysfunction, pericarditis, congestive cardiomyopathy, valvular disease, sinus tachycardia, supraventricular arrhythmias, and conduction abnormalities [7, 24, 25]. Chest irradiation can synergistically increase the risk of cardiotoxicity when given concurrent with cardiotoxic chemotherapy [7, 24, 25]. Radiation can cause acute damage to cardiac tissue through vascular inflammation and dilation, increased capillary permeability, and interstitial edema [7, 24, 25]. CRF is one of the earliest preclinical indicators of cardiac damage [7]. As cardiac function worsens, the heart is placed under greater stress, and CRF becomes more severe [7]. Methotrexate and bleomycin are used to treat certain types of cancer and both treatments are known to lead to pulmonary toxicity. Shortness of breath is a common side effect when lung function is impaired [26, 27].

Exercise as a Promising Therapy for Cancer Side Effects

Cancer survivors suffer from a wide range of side effects and side effect severity can vary greatly between survivors [4, 6]. This heterogenous response to treatment is the result of numerous factors including differences in cancer diagnosis, such as the type and stage of disease,

the types of treatment used to treat the cancer, and the underlying health status of the individual [4–6]. Therefore, it is important to develop interventions that can be used by a wide range of cancer survivors that are capable of reducing numerous side effects simultaneously [4–6]. Exercise can be individually tailored and shows great promise as an intervention capable of improving side effects such as CRF, cardiotoxicity, bone loss, psychosocial symptoms, impaired immune function, neurotoxicity, and neuroendocrine dysfunction [4–7]. Exercise can be performed using a variety of modes, such as aerobic exercise, resistance training, and mindfulness-based exercise, all of which have been found to reduce various side effects from cancer and its treatment [4–7].

Exercise

Side effects of cancer treatments can be acute, chronic, or late and evidence supports the use of exercise to minimize each of these types of side effects [4–7]. Recent reviews have summarized data indicating that exercise can improve CRF, sleep disruption, cognitive function, depression, anxiety, self-esteem, cardiopulmonary function, body composition, muscular strength, and flexibility in cancer survivors during and after treatment [4–7, 28–43].

Aerobic Exercise

Aerobic exercise is a type of exercise that utilizes large muscle groups for prolonged periods of time within a range of intensity levels with the largest physical conditioning effects seen in the cardiorespiratory and pulmonary systems [44]. Running, cycling, swimming, and walking are modes of aerobic exercise [44]. Researchers have found aerobic exercise to be a valuable intervention for the reduction of many cancer- and treatment-related side effects such as CRF, sleep disruption, depression, anxiety, and nausea while improving cardiopulmonary function and QOL [4–7, 28–43, 45].

Researchers have found that exercise can be beneficial when performed during treatment. Summaries of a few of these studies are highlighted. Mock and colleagues reported that during chemotherapy and radiation for breast cancer, patients who performed home-based walking at a moderate intensity (50–70% of maximum heart rate) reported reductions in CRF, sleep disruption, depression, anxiety, and nausea with improvements in cardiopulmonary function and QOL. Home-based walking was performed for 10–45 min per day, 4–6 days per week, for 1–6 months [46–49]. Colorectal cancer patients undergoing chemotherapy treatments who participated in a moderate-intensity walking (65–75% maximum heart rate) and flexibility program 20–30 min per day, 3–5 days per week reported greater functional, physical, and emotional well-being, QOL, and satisfaction with life and lower levels of CRF, depression, and anxiety when compared to wait-list controls. In addition, aerobic capacity and flexibility improved in colorectal patients undergoing exercise [50]. Prostate cancer patients receiving radiation treatments who participated in a moderate-intensity (60–70% maximum heart rate) home-based walking program for 30 min a day, 3 days a week for 10 weeks also reported improvements in CRF compared to usual care controls. Additionally, the exercises improved aerobic capacity [51]. Female breast cancer survivors undergoing chemotherapy concurrent with participation in an aerobic exercise intervention which was progressive in nature, beginning with 15 min per session at 60% of VO_2peak for three sessions per week and progressing to 45-min sessions at 80% of VO_2peak, using a treadmill, cycle ergometer, or elliptical trainer showed improvements in anxiety [45].

Cycle ergometer interventions have also been found to reduce side effects in patients undergoing cancer treatments [52, 53]. In a study by Dimeo and colleagues, cancer patients who had undergone surgery for lung or gastrointestinal tumors were prescribed a stationary cycle intervention which consisted of cycling for 30 min, 5 days per week, for 3 weeks. Patients in the cycle ergometer arm improved in CRF, physical performance, and global health [52]. In another study

by Dimeo and colleagues, cancer patients who were receiving high-dose chemotherapy followed by autologous peripheral blood stem cell transplantation were prescribed an exercise intervention which included a moderately intense bed cycle ergometer interval program which consisted of 1-min intervals at 50% of heart rate reserve and 1 min of rest, for a total of 30 min, 7 days per week. Compared to usual care controls, patients who exercised reported less CRF and psychological stress [53]. Courneya and colleagues also found that breast cancer patients who were undergoing chemotherapy treatments were able to tolerate a higher relative dosage of chemotherapy treatment if performing aerobic exercise [45].

Aerobic exercise also has beneficial effects following treatment. A study of breast cancer survivors who had completed treatment and were given a moderate-intensity home-based walking exercise intervention in which they walked 2–5 days per week for 12 weeks at 55–65% of maximum heart rate. Compared to control group participants, the exercise group reported improvements in CRF, mood, vigor, and body esteem [54].

Resistance Exercise

Resistance training exercises have been found to benefit cancer survivors by reducing side effects of cancer treatment when performed during and following cancer treatment [4–7, 28–43, 45]. Resistance training involves muscle contraction against resistance with the largest physical conditioning effects seen in the muscular and skeletal systems [44]. Resistance can come in many forms, including dumbbells, therapeutic resistance bands, or even body weight [44].

Highlights from a few of these studies follow. During chemotherapy treatment for breast cancer, performing resistance training that consisted of two sets of 8–12 repetitions, three times per week, for the duration of chemotherapy resulted in an increase in self-esteem, upper and lower body strength, and lean body mass when compared to a usual care control group [55]. Segal and colleagues also found benefits from resistance training in prostate cancer survivors who were receiving androgen deprivation therapy. The resistance training program included two sets of 8–12 repetitions 3 days per week for 12 weeks. Participants that underwent the exercise intervention reported improved CRF, cognitive function, and QOL with additional improvements in muscular strength [56]. Courneya and colleagues also found that breast cancer patients who were undergoing chemotherapy treatments were able to tolerate a higher relative dosage of chemotherapy treatment if performing resistance exercise [45].

Schmitz and colleagues studied the safety and efficacy of resistance training in breast cancer survivors who had recently completed primary treatment. The twice-weekly resistance training for 6–12 months was safe and resulted in decreased body fat and increased lean body mass [57]. Similarly, Ahmed and colleagues assessed the safety of resistance training for breast cancer survivors who had recently completed treatment. Six months of twice-weekly resistance training did not result in any change in arm circumference in participants [58]. A progressive, moderate-intensity resistance training and impact training (jump exercises), preformed three times per week for 1 year, has been found to preserve bone mineral density in the lumbar spine of breast cancer survivors who are taking aromatase inhibitors, when compared to a control condition [59].

also demonstrated the benefits of performing aerobic and resistance exercise during radiation treatment. A 4-week individually tailored, home-based aerobic and resistance training program resulted in improved CRF, QOL, sleep, aerobic capacity, strength, and immune function [11, 61]. Sprod and colleagues found that breast and prostate cancer patients receiving radiation treatments who exercised for 4 weeks using the home-based aerobic and resistance training program developed by Dr. Mustian exhibited greater improvements in sleep quality than non-exercising controls. Associations between interleukin-6 and sleep efficiency and duration were demonstrated suggesting that improvements in sleep due to exercise may be mediated by cytokines [11]. Despite undergoing radiation treatments, participants were able to progressively increase the number of steps walked per day from 5,000 to nearly 12,000 [11, 61]. Researchers have found that a combined resistance and aerobic exercise intervention performed two times per week for 12 weeks can result in improved muscle mass, muscular strength, physical function, and balance in prostate cancer survivors undergoing androgen suppression therapy [62]. Milne and colleagues also used an exercise intervention that combined aerobic and resistance training for 12 weeks that resulted in improved muscular strength and aerobic fitness in breast cancer survivors who had completed treatment [63].

Combined Aerobic and Resistance Exercise

Researchers have also assessed the benefits of exercise programs that combine aerobic exercise and resistance training on cancer- and treatment-related side effects [4–7, 28–43, 45]. A select few of these studies are highlighted.

Early-stage breast cancer survivors receiving chemotherapy and/or radiation who participated in an aerobic and resistance exercise intervention 2 days a week for 12 weeks reported improvements in CRF, QOL, satisfaction with life, and also physical function compared to usual care [58, 60]. Mustian and colleagues [11, 61] have

Mindfulness-Based Exercise

Mindfulness-based exercise modes such as Tai Chi Chuan and Yoga provide substantial benefits for cancer patients by relieving side effects, improving physical function, and increasing QOL. For example, Mustian and colleagues [64–68] demonstrated that a community-based 12-week, 15-move, Yang Style Short-Form of Tai Chi Chuan improved aerobic capacity, strength, flexibility, body composition, self-esteem, QOL, bone formation and resorption, and immune function among breast cancer patients post treatment.

Joseph and colleagues [69] showed improvements in sleep, QOL, treatment tolerance, mood, appetite, and bowel function among cancer patients participating in yoga as part of a study comparing yoga, support therapy, and meditation interventions among cancer patients receiving radiation therapy. The yoga intervention consisted of simple yoga postures and breathing and visualization exercises two times a week for 90 min for 8 weeks. Cohen and colleagues [70] showed lower sleep disturbance among lymphoma cancer patients participating in yoga as part of a study comparing the effectiveness of a Tibetan yoga exercise program to that of a waitlist control for improving sleep, fatigue, and psychological adjustment. The patients were receiving treatment or within 12 months post treatment. The Tibetan yoga intervention consisted of one yoga session a week for 7 weeks, with foci on yoga postures, visualization, breathing, and mindfulness.

Recommendations for Exercise in Cancer Survivors

Providing Information on Exercise

Most cancer patients indicate that they do not discuss initiating or continuing an exercise program with their treating oncologist or primary care physician during throughout their cancer experience [5, 71–73]. Research shows that cancer patients want their oncologists to initiate discussion about exercise [74]. Research has shown that cancer patients would prefer to receiving information on exercise and discuss it during the time period in which they are receiving treatments (i.e., during chemotherapy and during radiation therapy); specifically they prefer receiving this information shortly after they have initiated treatments and prior to completion [75].

Medical Clearance and Contraindications for Exercise

When first initiating a conversation with cancer patients about exercise, oncologists need to discuss with cancer survivors how they can *safely* begin an exercise program during and after treatments

and to inform survivors of any potential contraindications (e.g., orthopedic, cardiopulmonary, oncologic) that can affect their exercise tolerance [76, 77]. Although a medical evaluation should not be a barrier to participating in exercise and a large number of cancer patients will be able to initiate an exercise program with the goal of achieving the public health recommended levels of exercise safely, a medical assessment prior to exercise testing, prescription, and participation is recommended for individuals at greater risk for increased side effect burden (either via number or severity or the combination), long-term or chronic side effects, late effects, and increased burden from multiple concomitant co-morbidities [76, 77]. An evaluation to determine musculoskeletal morbidities and peripheral neuropathies for all cancer survivors and assessment of fracture risk for survivors who have received hormonal treatments is recommended [76, 77]. Cancer patients with bone metastasis and survivors with cardiac toxicity need to be evaluated to determine whether or not exercise is safe at all and what the recommended exercise prescription should be for relevant cancer-related outcomes (mental and physical) [76, 77].

Referrals to Exercise Professionals

In addition to providing information on how to safely begin exercising, cancer patients want their oncologists to be able to provide referrals and resources to aid in obtaining safe and effective exercise prescriptions they can do before, during, and after their treatments [72]. Cancer patients who receive exercise prescriptions and/or referrals from their physician return to exercise more quickly during and after treatment and have better cancer treatment adherence [78–80]. Cancer patients also benefit from an oncology referral to a *qualified* exercise specialist, specifically an oncology-certified exercise professional [76, 77]. The majority of cancer patients want to receive exercise counseling and prescription from a qualified and experienced exercise professional affiliated with the cancer center in which they receive treatment [71]. Exercise professionals that would have the minimum qualifications and necessary knowledge to work with the unique needs of cancer patients include individuals with formal education at the Bachelor's level or higher in accredited exercise science or kinesiology programs [76, 77]. Certification by the American College of Sports Medicine with the Oncology Specialty is preferable because it ensures that the exercise professional has the minimum competencies required to safely and effectively prescribe exercise for cancer patients [76, 77]. This certification, which can be obtained by individuals with varied educational backgrounds (e.g., exercise physiologists, physical therapists, nurses), provides a very useful professional competency benchmark [44, 76, 77, 81].

Exercise Prescription Guidelines for Cancer Survivors

Following the exercise guidelines established by the ACS for cancer prevention may prove beneficial for cancer survivors [81]. The ACS guidelines are aimed at adopting an active lifestyle and recommend that adults participate in at least 30 min of physical activity, ideally 45–60 min, at least 5 days per week, at a moderate to vigorous intensity [81]. More recently, the American College of Sports Medicine published their first "Exercise Guidelines for Cancer Survivors." The ACSM guidelines are the first to be developed through an extensive review of the extant scientific evidence by a team of expert exercise oncology researchers [76, 77]. The ACSM guidelines for exercise participation by cancer survivors are based on the US Department of Health and Human Services Physical Activity Guidelines for Americans [82]. These guidelines recommended individuals participate in 150 min of moderate-intensity or 75 min of vigorous-intensity aerobic physical exercise along with strength training two to three times per week and regular stretching to achieve mental and physical health benefits [76, 77, 82–84]. These guidelines also suggest that individuals with chronic conditions should participate in physical exercise to the extent that they are able, even if they are unable to achieve the recommended levels [76, 77, 82–84].

Evidence from current research also suggests that cancer survivors are a heterogenous group and because of this exercise prescriptions for cancer survivors should be individualized and tailored considering the health status, disease trajectory, previous and/or current treatment, and individual's current fitness level along with past and present exercise participation and preferences in order to be safe and effective [76, 77, 82]. The ACSM guidelines for cancer survivors also recommend starting patients at a low to moderate level of physical exercise and slowly increasing the frequency, intensity, and duration over a period of weeks [44, 76, 77]. When considering individualized exercise prescriptions the American College of Sports Medicine Guidelines for Exercise Testing and Prescription provide an excellent resource as a starting point [44]. In addition, information from specific clinical trials that focus on the use of exercise for improving cancer-related outcomes is helpful. For example, research suggests that exercise interventions involving moderately intense (55–75 % of heart rate maximum—corresponding to a rating of perceived exertion between 11 and 14 [85]) aerobic exercise ranging from 10 to 90 min in duration, 3–7 days/week are consistently effective at managing side effects and improving QOL among cancer survivors with an early-stage diagnosis (i.e., non-metastatic disease) [6, 61, 86, 87]. Stationary cycling may be a useful mode of physical exercise for survivors with impairments such as ataxia or balance difficulties [6, 61, 86, 87]. Short bouts of activity (3–10 min) accompanied by periods of rest culminating in a total of 30 min daily can also be effective at reducing side effects and improving QOL [6, 61, 86, 87]. Preliminary research suggests that progressive resistance exercise (e.g., therapeutic resistance bands, dumbbells, fixed weight systems) performed three times a week at a moderate to vigorous intensity (60–90 % of 1-repetition maximum) progressively increasing up to two to four sets ranging from 8 to 15 repetitions is effective at reducing side effects and improving QOL among cancer survivors. Research also suggests that mindfulness-based modes of exercise such as Yoga and Tai Chi Chuan performed one to three times a week for 60–90 min at a moderate intensity level can reduce side effects and improve QOL.

Studies have also demonstrated that low-intensity exercise is safe and well tolerated by survivors with metastatic disease. To decrease the risk of lymphedema, compression sleeves should be worn when appropriate, but recent research suggests that resistance training does not result in increased incidence of lymphedema [6, 58, 61, 76, 77, 86, 87]. It is also prudent to advise cancer survivors to avoid excessive high-intensity exercise which can potentially compromise the immune system and interfere with treatment and recovery [6, 61, 86, 87].

Summary

The current exercise and cancer control literature provides consistent support for the efficacy of exercise interventions in managing cancer- and treatment-related side effects as well as QOL. However, this body of literature is still in its infancy and limitations do exist. Small sample sizes, a lack of consistency in the type and amounts of exercise utilized, and methodological concerns make it difficult to generalize the findings to the diverse cancer survivor population. Additionally, making comparisons based on dose and exercise mode is challenging due to a lack of appropriate statistical and follow-up analyses (e.g., intent-to-treat analyses in randomized controlled trials) [6, 7, 28–32, 61]. Despite these limitations, preliminary evidence consistently suggests that that physical activity is not only safe but also advantageous for cancer survivors in managing multiple side effects associated with cancer and cancer treatments. Overall, research suggests that aerobic activity, resistance training, a combination of both, and mindfulness forms of exercise such as yoga and Tai Chi are effective in helping cancer patients cope with their disease and recover.

References

1. American Cancer Society. Cancer facts & figures 2011. Atlanta, GA: American Cancer Society; 2011.
2. Hofman M, Ryan JL, Figueroa-Moseley CD, Jean-Pierre P, Morrow GR. Cancer-related fatigue: the scale of the problem. Oncologist. 2007;12 Suppl 1:4–10.
3. Morrow GR. Cancer-related fatigue: causes, consequences, and management. Oncologist. 2007; 12 Suppl 1:1–3.
4. Mustian KM, Peppone LJ, Palesh O, Janelsins MC, Purnell JQ, Darling T. Exercise and cancer-related fatigue. US Oncol. 2010;6:20–3.
5. Mustian KM, Griggs JJ, Morrow GR, et al. Exercise and side effects among 749 patients during and after treatment for cancer: a University of Rochester Cancer Center Community Clinical Oncology Program Study. Support Care Cancer. 2006;14(7):732–41.
6. Mustian KM, Morrow GR, Carroll JK, Figueroa-Moseley CD, Jean-Pierre P, Williams GC. Integrative nonpharmacologic behavioral interventions for the management of cancer-related fatigue. Oncologist. 2007;12(1):52–67.
7. Mustian K, Adams MJ, Schwartz R, Lipshultz S, Constine L. Cardiotoxic effects of radiation therapy in Hodgkin's lymphoma and breast cancer survivors and the potential mitigating effects of exercise. In: Rubin P, Constine L, Marks L, Okunieff P, editors. Cancer survivorship research and education: late effects on normal tissues. Berlin: Springer; 2008. p. 103–15.
8. Sprod LK. Considerations for training cancer survivors. Strength Cond J. 2009;31(1):39–47.
9. Pirl WF, Roth AJ. Diagnosis and treatment of depression in cancer patients. Oncology (Williston Park). 1999;13(9):1293–301.
10. Savard J, Morin CM. Insomnia in the context of cancer: a review of a neglected problem. J Clin Oncol. 2001;19(3):895–908.
11. Sprod LK, Palesh OG, Janelsins MC, et al. Exercise sleep quality and mediators of sleep in breast and prostate cancer patients receiving radiation therapy. Community Oncol. 2010;7(10):463–71.
12. Chang VT, Hwang SS, Feuerman M, Kasimis BS. Symptom and quality of life survey of medical oncology patients at a veterans affairs medical center: a role for symptom assessment. Cancer. 2000;88(5):1175–83.
13. Stark D, Kiely M, Smith A, Velikova G, House A, Selby P. Anxiety disorders in cancer patients: their nature, associations, and relation to quality of life. J Clin Oncol. 2002;20(14):3137–48.
14. Bower JE, Bower JE. Behavioral symptoms in patients with breast cancer and survivors [Review] [135 refs]. J Clin Oncol. 2008;26(5):768–77.
15. Ryan JL, Carroll JK, Ryan EP, Mustian KM, Fiscella K, Morrow GR. Mechanisms of cancer-related fatigue. Oncologist. 2007;12(1):22–34.
16. Tischler ME, Slentz M. Impact of weightlessness on muscle function [Review] [37 refs]. ASGSB Bull. 1995;8(2):73–81.
17. Tisdale MJ. Cachexia in cancer patients [Review] [94 refs]. Nat Rev Cancer. 2002;2(11):862–71.
18. Tisdale MJ, Tisdale MJ. The 'cancer cachectic factor'. Support Care Cancer. 2003;11(2):73–8.
19. Mustian KM, Palesh O, Heckler CE, et al. Cancer-related fatigue interferes with activities of daily living among 753 patients receiving chemotherapy: a URCC CCOP study. J Clin Oncol. 2008;26(20 suppl):abstr 9500.

20. Bruning PF, Pit MJ, de Jong-Bakker M, van den Ende A, Hart A, van Enk A. Bone mineral density after adjuvant chemotherapy for premenopausal breast cancer. Br J Cancer. 1990;61(2):308–10.

21. Shuster LT, Gostout BS, Grossardt BR, Rocca WA. Prophylactic oophorectomy in premenopausal women and long-term health. Menopause Int. 2008;14(3): 111–6.

22. Howell A, Cuzick J, Baum M, et al. Results of the ATAC (Arimidex, Tamoxifen, Alone or in Combination) trial after completion of 5 years' adjuvant treatment for breast cancer. Lancet. 2005;365(9453):60–2.

23. Yeh ETH. Cardiotoxicity induced by chemotherapy and antibody therapy. Annu Rev Med. 2006;57(1): 485–98.

24. Schneider CM, Dennehy CA, Carter SD. Exercise and cancer recovery. Champaign, IL: Human Kinetics; 2003.

25. Schneider CS, Hsieh CC, Sprod LK, Carter SD, Hayward R. Exercise training manages cardiopulmonary function and fatigue during and following cancer treatment in male cancer survivors. Integer Cancer Ther. 2007;6(3):235–41.

26. Cottin V, Tébib J, Massonnet B, Souquet PJ, Bernard JP. Pulmonary function in patients receiving long-term low-dose methotrexate. Chest. 1996;109: 933–8.

27. Mustian KM, Hofman M, Morrow GR, Griggs JJ, Jean-Pierre P, Kohli S, Roscoe JA, Simondet J, Bushunow P. Cancer-Related Fatigue (CRF) and Shortness of Breath (SOB) among survivors: A prospective URCC CCOP study. NCI Cancer Survivorship Annual Meeting: Embracing the Future, Bethesda, MD. Presentation; 2006.

28. Galvao DA, Newton RU. Review of exercise intervention studies in cancer patients. J Clin Oncol. 2005;23(4):899–909.

29. Knols R, Aaronson N, Uebelhart D, Fransen J, Aufdemkampe G. Physical exercise in cancer patients during and after medical treatment: a systematic review of randomized and controlled clinical trials. J Clin Oncol. 2005;23(16):3830–42.

30. Stevinson C, Lawlor D, Fox K. Exercise interventions for cancer patients: systematic review of controlled trials. Cancer Causes Control. 2004;15:1035–56.

31. Schmitz KH, Holtzman J, Courneya KS, Masse LC, Duval S, Kane R. Controlled physical activity trials in cancer survivors: a systematic review and meta-analysis [Review] [64 refs]. Cancer Epidemiol Biomarkers Prev. 2005;14(7):1588–95.

32. McNeely ML, Campbell KL, Rowe BH, Klassen TP, Mackey JR, Courneya KS. Effects of exercise on breast cancer patients and survivors: a systematic review and meta-analysis. CMAJ. 2006;175(1): 34–41.

33. Pekmezi DW, Demark-Wahnefried W. Updated evidence in support of diet and exercise interventions in cancer survivors [Review]. Acta Oncol. 2011;50(2): 167–78.

34. Duijts SF, Faber MM, Oldenburg HS, et al. Effectiveness of behavioral techniques and physical exercise on psychosocial functioning and health-related quality of life in breast cancer patients and survivors–a meta-analysis [Review]. Psychooncology. 2011;20(2):115–26.

35. De WS, Van BS, De Waele S, Van Belle S. Cancer-related fatigue [Review]. Acta Clin Belg. 2010;65(6):378–85.

36. Arnold M, Taylor NF, Arnold M, Taylor NF. Does exercise reduce cancer-related fatigue in hospitalised oncology patients? A systematic review [Review]. Onkologie. 2010;33(11):625–30.

37. Friedenreich CM, Friedenreich CM. Physical activity and breast cancer: review of the epidemiologic evidence and biologic mechanisms [Review]. Recent Results Cancer Res. 2011;188:125–39.

38. Knols RH, de Bruin ED, Shirato K, et al. Physical activity interventions to improve daily walking activity in cancer survivors [Review]. BMC Cancer. 2010;10:406.

39. Pinto BM, Ciccolo JT, Pinto BM, Ciccolo JT. Physical activity motivation and cancer survivorship [Review]. Recent Results Cancer Res. 2011;186:367–87.

40. Lowe SS, Lowe SS. Physical activity and palliative cancer care [Review]. Recent Results Cancer Res. 2011;186:349–65.

41. Schmitz K, Schmitz K. Physical activity and breast cancer survivorship [Review]. Recent Results Cancer Res. 2011;186:189–215.

42. Cramp F, James A, Lambert J, Cramp F, James A, Lambert J. The effects of resistance training on quality of life in cancer: a systematic literature review and meta-analysis [Review]. Support Care Cancer. 2010;18(11):1367–76.

43. Jones LW, Peppercom J, Scott JM, et al. Exercise therapy in the management of solid tumors [Review]. Curr Treat Options Oncol. 2010;11(1–2):45–58.

44. American College of Sports Medicine. ACSM's Guidelines for exercise testing and prescription. 8th ed. Baltimore, MD: Lippincott Williams & Wilkins; 2010.

45. Courneya KS, Segal RJ, Gelmon K, et al. Six-month follow-up of patient-rated outcomes in a randomized controlled trial of exercise training during breast cancer chemotherapy. Cancer Epidemiol Biomarkers Prev. 2007;16(12):2572–8.

46. Mock V, Burke MB, Sheehan P, et al. A nursing rehabilitation program for women with breast cancer receiving adjuvant chemotherapy. Oncol Nurs Forum. 1994;21(5):899–907.

47. Mock V, Pickett M, Ropka ME, et al. Fatigue and quality of life outcomes of exercise during cancer treatment. Cancer Pract. 2001;9:119–27.

48. Mock V, Dow KH, Meares CJ, et al. Effects of exercise on fatigue, physical functioning, and emotional distress during radiation therapy for breast cancer. Oncol Nurs Forum. 1997;24(6):991–1000.

49. Mock V, Frangakis C, Davidson N, et al. Exercise manages fatigue during breast cancer treatment: a randomized controlled trial. Psychooncology. 2005;14:464–77.

50. Courneya KS, Friedenreich CM, Quinney HA, Fields AL, Jones LW, Fairey AS. A randomized trial of exercise and quality of life in colorectal cancer survivors. Eur J Cancer Care (Engl). 2003;12(4):347–57.

51. Windsor PM, Nicol KF, Potter J. A randomized, controlled trial of aerobic exercise for treatment-related fatigue in men receiving radical external beam radiotherapy for localized prostate carcinoma. Cancer. 2004;101(3):550–7.

52. Dimeo F, Thomas F, Raabe-Menssen C, Propper F, Mathias M. Effect of aerobic exercise and relaxation training on fatigue and physical performance of cancer patients after surgery. A randomised controlled trial. Support Care Cancer. 2004;12:774–9.

53. Dimeo FC, Stieglitz RD, Novelli-Fischer U, Fetscher S, Keul J. Effects of physical activity on the fatigue and psychologic status of cancer patients during chemotherapy. Cancer. 1999;85(10):2273–7.

54. Pinto BM, Goldstein MG, Ashba J, Sciamanna CN, Jette A. Randomized controlled trial of physical activity counseling for older primary care patients. Am J Prev Med. 2005;29(4):247–55.

55. Courneya KS, Segal RJ, Gelmon K, et al. Six-month follow-up of patient-rated outcomes in a randomized controlled trial of exercise training during breast cancer chemotherapy. Cancer Epidemiol Biomarkers Prev. 2007;16(12):2572–8.

56. Segal RJ, Reid RD, Courneya KS, et al. Resistance exercise in men receiving androgen deprivation therapy for prostate cancer [comment]. J Clin Oncol. 2003;21(9):1653–9.

57. Schmitz K, Ahmed R, Hannan P, Lee D. Safety and efficacy of weight training in recent breast cancer survivors to alter body composition, insulin and insulin-like growth factor axis proteins. Cancer Epidemiol Biomarkers Prev. 2005;14(7):1588–95.

58. Ahmed RL, Thomas W, Yee D, Schmitz KH. Randomized controlled trial of weight training and lymphedema in breast cancer survivors. J Clin Oncol. 2006;24(18):2765–72.

59. Winters-Stone KM, Dobek J, Nail L, et al. Strength training stops bone loss and builds muscle in postmenopausal breast cancer survivors: a randomized, controlled trial. Breast Cancer Res Treat. 2011;127(2):447–56.

60. Campbell A, Mutrie N, White F, McGuire F, Kearney N. A pilot study of a supervised group exercise program as a rehabilitation treatment for women with breast cancer receiving adjuvant treatment. Eur J Oncol Nurs. 2005;9(1):56–63.

61. Mustian KM, Peppone L, Darling T, Palesh O, Heckler C, Morrow GR. A 4-week home-based aerobic and resistance exercise program during radiation therapy: a pilot randomized clinical trial. J Support Oncol. 2009;7:158–67.

62. Galvao DA, Taaffe DR, Spry N, et al. Combined resistance and aerobic exercise program reverses muscle loss in men undergoing androgen suppression therapy for prostate cancer without bone metastases: a randomized controlled trial. J Clin Oncol. 2010; 28(2):340–7.

63. Milne HM, Wallman KE, Gordon S, Courneya KS. Effects of a combined aerobic and resistance exercise program in breast cancer survivors: a randomized controlled trial. Breast Cancer Res Treat. 2008; 108(2):279–88.

64. Mustian KM, Katula JA, Gill DL, Roscoe JA, Lang D, Murphy K. Tai Chi Chuan, health-related quality of life and self-esteem: a randomized trial with breast cancer survivors. Support Care Cancer. 2004;12(12):871–6.

65. Mustian KM, Katula JA, Zhao H. A pilot study to assess the influence of tai chi chuan on functional capacity among breast cancer survivors. J Support Oncol. 2006;4(3):139–45.

66. Mustian KM, Palesh OG, Flecksteiner SA. Tai Chi Chuan for breast cancer survivors. Med Sport Sci. 2008;52:209–17.

67. Peppone LJ, Mustian KM, Janelsins MC, et al. Effects of a structured weight-bearing exercise program on bone metabolism among breast cancer survivors: a feasibility trial. Clin Breast Cancer. 2010;10:224–9.

68. Janelsins MC, Davis PD, Widemean L, et al. Effects of Tai Chi Chuan on insulin and cytokine levels in a pilot randomized and controlled study on breast cancer survivors. Clin Breast Cancer. 2011;11:161–70.

69. Joseph CD. Psychological supportive therapy for cancer patients. Indian J Cancer. 1983;20:268–70.

70. Cohen LW. Psychological adjustment and sleep quality in a randomized trial of the effects of a Tibetan yoga intervention in patients with lymphoma. Cancer. 2004;100(10):2253–60.

71. Jones LW, Courneya KS. Exercise counseling and programming preferences of cancer survivors. Cancer Pract. 2002;10(4):208–15.

72. Jones LW, Courneya KS. Exercise discussions during cancer treatment consultations. Cancer Pract. 2002;10(2):66–74.

73. Sabatino SA, Coates RJ, Uhler RJ, Pollack LA, Alley LG, Zauderer LJ. Provider counseling about health behaviors among cancer survivors in the United States. J Clin Oncol. 2007;25(15):2100–6.

74. Yates JS, Mustian KM, Morrow GR, et al. Prevalence of complementary and alternative medicine use in cancer patients during treatment. Support Care Cancer. 2005;13(10):806–11.

75. Sprod LK, Peppone LJ, Palesh OG, et al. Timing of information on exercise impacts exercise behavior during cancer treatment (N=748): a URCC CCOP protocol. J Clin Oncol. 2010;28(15):9138.

76. Schmitz KH, Courneya KS, Matthews C, et al. American College of Sports Medicine roundtable on exercise guidelines for cancer survivors. Med Sci Sports Exerc. 2010;42(7):1409–26.

77. Schmitz KH, Courneya KS, Matthews C, et al. American College of Sports Medicine roundtable on exercise guidelines for cancer survivors [Erratum appears in Med Sci Sports Exerc. 2011 Jan;43(1):195]. Med Sci Sports Exerc. 2010;42(7):1409–26.

78. Segar ML, Katch VL, Roth RS, et al. The effect of aerobic exercise on self-esteem and depressive and anxiety symptoms among breast cancer survivors. Oncol Nurs Forum. 1998;25(1):107–13.

79. Courneya KS, Mackey JR, Jones LW. Coping with cancer: can exercise help? Phys Sportsmed. 2000;28: 49–73.

80. Jones LW, Courneya KS, Fairey AS, Mackey JR. Effects of an oncologist's recommendation to exercise on self-reported exercise behavior in newly diagnosed breast cancer survivors: a single-blind, randomized controlled trial. Ann Behav Med. 2004;28(2):105–13.

81. Doyle C, Kushi LH, Byers T, et al. Nutrition and physical activity during and after cancer treatment: an American Cancer Society guide for informed choices. CA Cancer J Clin. 2006;56(6):323–53.

82. Secretary of Health and Human Services. Physical Activity Guidelines Advisory Committee report, 2008. Part A: executive summary. Nutr Rev. 2009; 67(2):114–20.

83. Haskell WL, Lee IM, Pate RR, et al. Physical activity and public health: updated recommendation for adults from the American College of Sports Medicine and the American Heart Association. Med Sci Sports Exerc. 2007;39(8):1423–34.

84. Haskell WL, Lee IM, Pate RR, et al. Physical activity and public health: updated recommendation for adults from the American College of Sports Medicine and the American Heart Association. Circulation. 2007;116(9):1081–93.

85. Borg GA. Psychophysical bases of perceived exertion. Med Sci Sports Exerc. 1982;14(5):377–81.

86. Holmes MD, Chen WY, Feskanich D, Kroenke CH, Colditz GA. Physical activity and survival after breast cancer diagnosis. JAMA. 2005;293(20):2479–86.

87. Courneya KS, Segal RJ, Mackey JR, et al. Effects of aerobic and resistance exercise in breast cancer patients receiving adjuvant chemotherapy: a multicenter randomized controlled trial. J Clin Oncol. 2007;25(28):4396–404.

Use of the Classic Hallucinogen Psilocybin for Treatment of Existential Distress Associated with Cancer

17

Charles S. Grob, Anthony P. Bossis, and Roland R. Griffiths

This chapter will review the potential of a treatment approach that uses psilocybin, a novel psychoactive drug, to ameliorate the psychospiritual distress and demoralization that often accompanies a life-threatening cancer diagnosis. Early research with classic hallucinogens in the 1950s had a major impact on the evolving field of psychiatry, contributing to early discoveries of basic neurotransmitter systems and to significant developments in clinical psychopharmacology. While published reports of therapeutic breakthroughs with difficult to treat and refractory patient populations were initially met with mainstream professional enthusiasm, by the late 1960s and early 1970s the growing association of hallucinogens with widespread indiscriminate use led to the temporary abandonment of this promising psychiatric treatment model. After a hiatus lasting several decades, however, regulatory and scientific support has grown for the resumption of clinical research investigations exploring the safety and

efficacy of a treatment model utilizing the classic hallucinogen, psilocybin, in a subject population that had previously demonstrated positive therapeutic response, patients with existential anxiety due to a life-threatening cancer diagnosis.

Psilocybin

Psilocybin is a naturally occurring compound that is an active constituent of many species of mushrooms, including the genera Psilocybe, Conocybe, Gymnopilus, Panaeolus, and Stropharia. Psilocybin containing mushrooms grow in various parts of the world, including the United States and Europe, but until recently they have been consumed primarily in Mexico and Central America, where they were called by the ancient Aztec name of *teonanacatl* (flesh of the gods). In addition to psilocybin, other naturally occurring classic hallucinogens include mescaline from peyote and dimethyltryptamine (DMT) from various plants. All three of these substances have a long history of ceremonial use by indigenous people for religious and healing purposes. Following the arrival of Europeans in the New World in the sixteenth and seventeenth centuries, however, the use of plant hallucinogens by native people was harshly condemned and punished under the strict laws of the Spanish Inquisition, and forced to go underground. This suppression was so effective that hallucinogenic mushroom use was eventually assumed to be nonexistent, until the discovery by amateur mycologist,

C.S. Grob, M.D.(✉)
Department of Psychiatry,
Harbor-UCLA Medical Center, Box 498
1000W, Carson St., Torrance, CA 90509, USA
e-mail: cgrob@labiomed.org

A.P. Bossis, Ph.D.
Department of Psychiatry, New York University School of Medicine, New York, NY, USA

R.R. Griffiths, Ph.D.
Departments of Psychiatry and Neuroscience,
Johns Hopkins University School of Medicine,
Baltimore, MD, USA

R. Gordon Wasson, of their extant ceremonial use by indigenous Mazatec people of Oaxaca, in the central Mexican highlands. Invited to participate in a healing ritual using mushrooms as a psychoactive sacrament, Wasson published his observations in the popular American press in 1957, catalyzing both popular and professional interest [65, 85]. Subsequently, the eminent Swiss natural products chemist, Albert Hofmann, succeeded in isolating the active tryptamine alkaloid, psilocybin, from samples of the hallucinogenic mushrooms from Mexico sent to him by Wasson.

Psilocybin is 4-phosphoryloxy-N,N-dimethyltryptamine and possesses a chemical structure similar to the neurotransmitter serotonin (5-hydroxytryptamine). Psilocybin is rapidly metabolized to psilocin, which is a highly potent agonist at serotonin 5-HT-2A and 5-HT-2C receptors [79, 80]. Research suggests that the primary site of action for the psychoactive effects of psilocybin is the 5-HT-2A receptor [73, 98]. During the 1960s psilocybin was subjected to psychopharmacological investigation, and found to be active orally at around 10 mg, with stronger effects at higher doses, and to have a 4–6-h duration of experience. Psilocybin was also determined to be thirty times stronger than mescaline and approximately 1/100–150 as potent as lysergic acid diethylamide (LSD) [44]. Compared to LSD, psilocybin was considered to be more strongly visual, less emotionally intense, more euphoric, and with fewer panic reactions and less likelihood of inducing paranoia [78]. Similar to other classic hallucinogens, psilocybin was observed to produce an altered state of consciousness that was characterized by changes in perception, cognition, and mood in the presence of an otherwise clear sensorium, along with visual illusions and internal visionary experience (though rarely frank hallucinations), states of ecstasy, dissolution of ego boundaries, and the experience of union with others and with the natural world.

In the late 1990s, psilocybin was subjected to renewed examination by contemporary investigators, including Franz Vollenweider and colleagues at the Heffter Research Center and the University of Zurich, in Switzerland. Careful medical and laboratory evaluations conducted there identified a relatively safe physiological range of action in normal volunteer subjects [36, 94]. Positron emission tomographic (PET) studies also demonstrated that psilocybin induces a global increase in cerebral metabolic rate of glucose, most markedly in the frontomedial and frontolateral cortex, anterior cingulate and temporomedial cortext [97]. In another recent study, at the University of Arizona, Francisco Moreno examined the use of psilocybin in the treatment of severe, refractory obsessive-compulsive disorder, observing that psilocybin appeared to be safe, well tolerated, and capable of inducing "robust acute reductions" in OCD symptoms [67]. Further investigations of psilocybin in normal volunteers were conducted at the Johns Hopkins University exploring the emergence of psychospiritual states of consciousness following psilocybin administration [30] (see section below). The Johns Hopkins group also published a set of recommended guidelines for safe conduct of high-dose research with classic hallucinogens [47].

Psychiatric Research with Classic Hallucinogens: Historical Perspective

Hallucinogens consist of a diverse group of biologically active compounds. Hallucinogens in plant form are thought to have been utilized by prehistoric and early civilizations as essential features of their religious, initiation, and healing rituals. Ethnobotanists have catalogued more than one hundred species of plant hallucinogens, the majority in the Western hemisphere, where they played a vital role within indigenous ceremonial practices [91]. In the late nineteenth Century, interest in psychoactive plants was catalyzed by discoveries of anthropologists studying native people around the world, who shipped specimens to leading European pharmacologists of that era, including Arthur Heffter and Louis Lewin, who succeeded, respectively, in isolating mescaline from the southwest American cactus peyote, *Lophophora williamsii*, and harmine from *banisteriopsis caapi*, one of the plants brewed to create the Amazonian plant hallucinogen decoction, ayahuasca.

The classic hallucinogens can be divided structurally into two classes of alkaloids: the tryptamines, including psilocin and psilocybin (constituents of Psilocybe and several other mushroom genera), DMT (constituent of the plant admixture ayahuasca and other hallucinogenic preparations), and D-LSD, and the phenethylamines, including mescaline (constituent of peyote) and various synthetic compounds. The primary pharmacological effects of these substances are mediated at 5-HT$_{2A}$ receptors where they function as agonists. The first classic hallucinogen to be characterized pharmacologically was mescaline, which was discovered in 1896 and synthesized de novo in the laboratory in 1919 [45]. While some attention was given in the early twentieth Century to potential medicinal applications of hallucinogens and there were preliminary efforts to formally classify and analyze visions induced by alkaloids discovered in particular plants [1, 55], widespread medical and psychiatric interest did not emerge until the mid-twentieth Century, following Albert Hofmann's serendipitous discovery of LSD at the Sandoz Laboratories in Basel, Switzerland, in 1943 [40].

From the 1950s, when formal study of the range of effect of hallucinogens and their potential in treatment models was initiated, until the early 1970s, when cultural and political turmoil led to the termination of studies, over 1,000 clinical and research reports were published in the medical and psychiatric literature describing the response to hallucinogen administration of approximately 40,000 research subjects and patients [33]. While initial research focused on the presumed capacity of hallucinogens to induce psychotic-like experience, interest in this psychotomimetic model waned [2, 32]. By the late 1950s and into the 1960s, however, significant new research activity was catalyzed by studying potential treatment applications of hallucinogens, most notably for several notoriously difficult-to-treat clinical conditions, including alcoholism, drug addiction, obsessive-compulsive disorder, chronic post-traumatic stress disorder, antisocial disorder, infantile autism, and the overwhelming existential anxiety often experienced in the presence of terminal cancer. Two discrete treatment models were proposed, involving the administration of lower versus higher dosages of hallucinogens and the application of different theoretical

mechanisms of action for their observed therapeutic effect. The initial treatment structure investigated, the psycholytic model, called for the administration of relatively low dosages of hallucinogens, with the postulated goal of facilitating the release of repressed psychic material, particularly in anxiety states and obsessional neuroses. Using this approach, some clinicians claimed to have achieved breakthroughs in reducing the duration and improving the outcome of psychotherapeutic treatment, presumably by facilitating ego regression, uncovering early childhood memories, and inducing an affective release [10].

As investigators began to explore the effects of higher dosages of hallucinogens on clinical subjects and patients, however, they began to appreciate that hallucinogens were capable of occasioning entirely new and novel dimensions of consciousness. Humphrey Osmond, a Canadian alcoholism researcher, noted that this high-dose hallucinogen, or *psyche-delic* (translated from the ancient Greek as "mind revealing") treatment model, appeared to free up the mind from its habitual moorings and allow it to access states of consciousness resembling spontaneous psychospiritual epiphanies. Osmond observed that even after the effects of the administered drug had worn off, individuals were still left with a deeply positive and therapeutic impact from having had a mystical level transcendent experience [74]. With certain conditions in particular, including alcoholism and other addictive disorders, the mysticomimetic capacity of the hallucinogen experience often appeared to have induced remissions from intractable psychological conditions to a greater degree unique than conventional treatment modalities. While the low-dose psycholytic model usually involved active discourse between patient and psychotherapist in the service of analyzing underlying neurotic complexes, the high-dose psychedelic model involved the development of an alternative treatment structure, with the subject lying down, wearing eyeshades and listening to preselected music throughout much of the session. During the session, the patient was encouraged to go deeply into the experience, with the facilitator maintaining an active presence but generally not engaging in verbal dialogue until the concluding phase of the treatment session.

One patient population that demonstrated positive response to the hallucinogen treatment model were individuals with advanced cancer with overwhelming anxiety in reaction to their terminal illness. Beginning with the observations of internal medicine investigators in the late 1950s at the Chicago Medical School [51, 52] and UCLA [15], and extending by the mid 1960s to psychiatrists and psychologists at the University of Maryland [35, 77, 84] and UCLA [23], a growing consensus within the field of hallucinogen investigations was achieved that patients with advanced-stage cancer treated with this novel approach frequently sustained significant improvements of their psychospiritual status. Moving accounts were reported of patient experiences, including reduced physical pain and lessened need for narcotic medication, improved quality of life, and greater acceptance of the inevitable and in some cases imminent end of their lives. Of particular interest, the most positive therapeutic outcomes, reflected in lowered anxiety, demoralization, and fear of death, and in improved mood and quality of meaningful interpersonal relations, were in patients who during the course of what was often their only hallucinogen treatment session experienced a deeply felt mystical state of consciousness. Unfortunately, these promising observations were terminated prematurely, largely in response to public and political concern about the misuse of these compounds in the 1960s.

Contemporary Psilocybin Research in Patients with Life-Threatening Cancer

Following decades of inactivity, it has been possible in recent years to obtain the regulatory approval and funding necessary to resurrect this long neglected treatment model. While improvements in caring for patients at the end of life have occurred in the intervening years, including the development of the hospice movement and the field of palliative medicine, it is still clear that even with these innovative approaches many individuals still go through the final phase of their life with high levels of anxiety, depression, and demoralization. Given the pressing need for more effective therapeutic interventions in individuals struggling with cancer and reactive existential crisis, along with the promising preliminary findings of the hallucinogen treatment model from the previous generation of research in patients with terminal medical illness, it is not surprising that this has become a prominent focus for current research efforts as well. Indeed, in recent years three investigations have been approved in the United States that have examined the use of psilocybin treatment for anxiety and demoralization in patients with a life-threatening cancer diagnosis—at Harbor-UCLA Medical Center, Johns Hopkins University, and New York University.

In 2004 the Harbor-UCLA psilocybin treatment protocol for anxiety in patients with advanced cancer was initiated. A total of 12 patients were recruited for a double-blind, placebo-controlled investigation, using a moderate dose (0.2 mg/kg) of psilocybin. All patients were screened to meet inclusion and exclusion criteria, which included a diagnosis of advanced-stage cancer but still functional enough to undergo full screening, preparation for the psilocybin sessions, and participation in two all-day sessions spaced several weeks apart, one active drug and the other placebo. Support with integration of the experience and collection of follow-up reports and quantitative data analyses continued with each patient for at least 6 months. Recruitment for all patients into the study, their participation in both psilocybin and placebo treatment sessions, and collection of data concluded in early 2008. At the time of the writing of this chapter, in 2011, 11 of the 12 participants have died.

The report describing the rationale for the investigation, methodology employed, and findings up to 6 months after treatment was published in the *Archives of General Psychiatry* [34]. All patients tolerated the psilocybin experience well, and there were no medical or psychological crises. Repeated administration of quantitative rating scales revealed improved mood and lessened anxiety, reaching significance at some monthly data collection points. Overall, patients reported their participation in the psilocybin treatment as having been a very valuable experience, allowing them to improve their quality of life and augmenting their capacity to withstand the psychological stressors of their medical condition. While the Harbor-UCLA research investigation has been completed, both the Johns

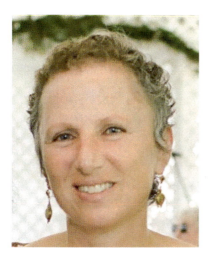

gation has been completed, both the Johns Hopkins and NYU projects are currently ongoing. The Johns Hopkins and NYU studies, initiated in 2006 and 2009, respectively, both approved to use a significantly higher dose than the Harbor-UCLA protocol, which will likely allow for more exploration of the psychospiritual dimension of the experience. These studies also offer more flexibility for subject inclusion, and allow for the entry of early-stage cancers that are nonetheless considered potentially life threatening. It is strongly hoped that additional research groups will also initiate treatment protocols exploring the utility of the psilocybin treatment model with medical patients encountering existential crisis and demoralization at the end of life.

Comments from Annie L, a 53-year-old woman with a diagnosis of metastatic ovarian cancer, 6 months after her participation in a Harbor-UCLA psilocybin cancer-anxiety study:

> "I had lost my faith because of anxiety, and I was just terrified. I was so anxious that it was hard to think about anything else. I didn't think I was so worried about death as I was about the process of dying. About suffering and being in pain and having all kinds of medical procedures. I was becoming so irritable with my husband. I was just so anxious... My intention (for participation in the study) was to be able to control my anxiety so

I could enjoy the rest of my life. I was not enjoying my life at all.

> As soon as it (the psilocybin) started working I knew I had nothing to be afraid of... It connected me with the universe... It was very gentle... And there were people (the treatment team) right there if I got upset... Everything looked absolutely beautiful. I didn't see things that weren't there. With my eyes closed I saw patterns, and visions and faces. I thought about being involved with people I loved, things I would do with people I knew, things I would tell them... I had an amazing spiritual experience. It re-connected me to the universe.

Comments from her husband 4 months after her death:

> "Annie's mood remained greatly improved for some time after the treatment. She also had much less anxiety, and her fear of getting sicker and her fear of the dying process also diminished a great deal. Beyond that, she and I got along much better after her psilocybin treatment ... I have no doubt that the treatment Annie went through was of great value to her ..."

Overview and Prevalence of Emotional Distress in Advanced Cancer

For many cancer patients, the advanced stage of illness is fraught with a significant degree of emotional suffering. As the illness trajectory progresses from diagnosis through medical treatment and eventually to the prospect of dying, the patient may be faced with considerable psychological distress and despair. In recent years, there has been a growing focus on the prevalence and clinical treatment of psychological distress in patients with advanced cancer that are facing the end of life [20, 48, 50, 57, 86]. Emotional suffering in advanced illness has been characterized as "severe distress associated with events that threaten the intactness of the person" ([9], p. 640).

The occurrence of psychological distress in cancer patients has been well documented with the highest prevalence rates among advanced cancer and end-of-life patients. While some cancer patients may cope effectively with the challenges of the disease, others experience a broad range of psychological stressors and symptoms. The prevalence of psychiatric disorders in cancer patients has been reported at approximately 50 %

[17, 61, 71] with the presence of any depressive or anxiety disorder at 24 % [102]. The prevalence of major depression has been reported at 15 % [41, 42, 101] with a range of all depressive disorders in cancer patients at 20 [102] to 26 % [19, 27]. Anxiety spectrum disorders have been documented at 14 % [102] with the prevalence of any anxiety symptoms at 21 % [17]. The prevalence of suicide in advanced and end-stage cancer is twice as high as that found in the general population [11] and an increased desire for hastened death in terminal patients has been established [5]. Kelly and colleagues [53] found that 22 % of advanced cancer patients had a desire for hastened death.

Focus on Spiritual and Existential Distress in Palliative Care

With a growing awareness of emotional suffering at the end of life, palliative care has increasingly focused on the specific domain of spiritual and existential distress as a significant component of quality of life in cancer and end-of-life cancer patients [16, 20, 66, 70, 88]. In palliative care, outcomes are no longer focused solely on biomedical or physical measures such as tumor or disease progression, but have expanded to include quality of life, now considered a central focus. Spiritual and existential factors are currently regarded as determinants of quality of life in advanced cancer and end-of-life patients. Distress in cancer and palliative care patients is viewed as a "multifactorial unpleasant emotional experience of a psychological, social, and/or spiritual nature" that impacts patients' capacity to effectively cope with the myriad challenges of cancer [71].

Existential or spiritual pain of terminal cancer patients has been defined as "the extinction of the being and meaning of the self due to the approach of death. It can be explained as meaninglessness of life, loss of identity, and worthlessness of living that are derived from deprivation of the future, others, and autonomy of people as beings founded on temporality, beings in relationship, and beings with autonomy" [69]. An individual's search for spiritual and existential meaning is frequently triggered by a diagnosis of cancer.

The alleviation of spiritual and existential distress is a primary objective of palliative and end-of-life care. A report by the Institute of Medicine listed spiritual well-being as an essential influence on quality of life and one of the six domains of quality supportive care of the dying [22]. Similarly, a report by the Consensus Conference in association with the National Consensus Project for Quality Palliative Care identified spiritual and existential issues as two of the eight core essential domains of quality palliative care [81]. The World Health Organization describes palliative care as "an approach that improves the quality of life of patients and their families facing the problems associated with life-threatening illness, through the prevention and relief of suffering by means of early identification and impeccable assessment and treatment of pain and other problems, physical, psychosocial and spiritual" [103].

Religion vs. Spirituality

Despite the overlap and ambiguity that have existed between the concepts of religion and spirituality, a consensus in the research literature has begun to emerge regarding the distinction between these two research constructs. Religion has been defined as structured belief systems that address universal questions and may provide a framework for making sense of ultimate questions of meaning and for expressing spirituality [93]. Spirituality tends to be a broader, more inclusive category than religion. It can be defined as "that which allows a person to experience transcendent meaning in life" [82] and "a personal search for meaning and purpose in life, which may or may not be related to religion" [95].

Whereas religion may be commonly viewed as a structured framework of beliefs and rituals that may include an expression of spirituality, spirituality may be experienced without the context of an organized religious system as a search for transcendence, meaning, and connection to ultimate meaning, nature, or to how an individual defines or experiences the concept of God. The Report of the Consensus Conference on spirituality in palliative care suggested the following definition (National Consensus Panel Report):

Spirituality is the aspect of humanity that refers to the way individuals seek and express meaning and purpose and the way they experience their connectedness to the moment, to self, to others, to nature, and to the significant or sacred [81].

Spiritual Well-Being and Psychological Distress

The domain of spiritual and existential well-being is now widely accepted as an important determinant in the quality of life in palliative care and end-stage cancer [16, 21, 39, 60, 66, 92]. Coping with terminal cancer is a multifactorial and variable process. Enhanced spiritual well-being and the ability to attain meaning when facing end-stage cancer appears to be a key factor in effectively coping with advanced disease. Psychosocial factors in advanced cancer associated with heightened existential and spiritual distress include anxiety and depression [26, 72], anger, alienation, hopelessness, loss of meaning, loss of dignity, vulnerability, isolation, fear, and shock [39, 99, 100]. Chochinov and colleagues [12] identified specific psychosocial correlates of spiritual and existential suffering in advanced cancer patients that include loss of will to live, loss of a sense of dignity, hopelessness, and feeling as a burden to others. Impaired spiritual well-being has also been associated with a poorer tolerance of physical symptoms whereas an enhanced sense of meaning and spirituality has been shown to increase an individual's tolerance levels for physical symptoms [3]. Myriad health care domains and outcomes have been associated with existential distress including quality of life, symptom and disease progression, psychological distress, depression [86], interpersonal functioning [16, 102], suicidal ideation [63], and demoralization syndrome, defined as "a psychiatric state in which hopelessness, helplessness, meaningless, and existential distress are the core phenomena" (p. 13. [54]).

Demoralization is defined by Kissane et al. [54] as a syndrome characterized by hopelessness, loss of meaning, and existential distress. This syndrome, which is delineated as a separate construct, has been identified as a primary risk factor for depression in advanced cancer patients. A desire for hastened death in advanced cancer patients has also been identified with this syndrome. Observed in palliative care and advanced cancer populations, this syndrome is associated with chronic medical illness, fear of loss of dignity, social isolation, and the sense of being a burden on others [54]. Kissane and colleagues propose that for targeted psychotherapies or interventions to be effective, they must aim to explore and restore meaning and hope within the context of advancing disease and impending death.

A desire for hastened death has been associated with lower levels of spiritual well-being [4, 86, 87]. A growing number of studies have presented evidence supporting a model that depression and hopelessness are chief determinants and predictors of a desire for hastened death (Rodin et al., 2008; [5, 48]). For example, in a study exploring the relationships among depression, hopelessness, and desire for hastened death, Breitbart and colleagues [5] identified depression as a robust predictor of desire for hastened death. In this study, patients with major depression were four times more likely to have a desire for hastened death.

Enhanced Spiritual Well-Being as a Buffer Against Emotional Distress

While there has been a documented relationship between lack of spiritual well-being and elevated psychosocial distress, there is increasing evidence to support the hypothesis that *enhanced* spiritual or existential well-being is associated with *improved* psychological functioning and might even prove to be a buffer against psychological syndromes associated with the end of life. Exploring the relationship between spiritual well-being, depression, and psychological distress in end-of-life cancer patients, a growing body of research has shown that higher levels of spiritual well-being are correlated with lower levels of emotional distress and serve as a buffer against depression, desire for hastened death, loss of will to live, and hopelessness as well as provide an increase in quality of life [5, 21, 50, 63, 72]. Individuals with an enhanced sense of spiritual well-being are also emotionally equipped to cope more effectively with the physical challenges of advanced and end-stage cancer [3].

The concept of meaning has received considerable attention in palliative care and psycho-oncology research as an important construct related to improved quality of life. Cultivating a sense of meaning in advanced cancer has been shown to improve spiritual well-being and overall quality of life while reducing levels of psychological distress [60, 64, 68]. For some patients, the search for meaning in end-of-life cancer, while a psychologically and spiritually complex, arduous, and courageous process, may provide them with a sense of peace and acceptance. Viktor Frankl, in *Man's Search for Meaning*, wrote that "man is not destroyed by suffering; he is destroyed by suffering without meaning" ([24], p. 135). Although not written about the end-of-life struggle with cancer or life-threatening disease, Frankl's landmark book was written from his personal experience of survival during his 3 years in Auschwitz and other concentration camps. His struggle to derive personal meaning in the face of horror and death has resulted in universal life lessons for those facing severe suffering or existential distress. In *The Will to Meaning: Foundations and Applications of Logotherapy* [25], Frankl wrote, "Meaning can be found in life literally up to the last moment, up to the last breath, in the face of death" (p. 76).

Meaning-enhancing interventions have been demonstrated to improve quality of life in palliative care and decrease wishes for euthanasia and for hastened death [6, 102]. Dame Cicely Saunders, who gave rise to the hospice movement and emphasized spiritual and psychological factors in palliative and hospice care, introduced the concept of "total pain" of the terminal patient that emphasizes psychospiritual as well as physical aspects of care and distress. Influenced by Frankl, she believed that the "total pain" of the terminal patient was related to a "lack of meaning" [89, 90]. In a quantitative thematic analysis [96] of all published literature on spirituality in palliative care, the most cited themes were meaning and purpose followed by self-transcendence and transcendence.

With an increasing body of evidence [5, 50, 63, 72] supporting the premise that enhanced spiritual well-being provides protection against depression, hopelessness, and desire for hastened death among other psychosocial forms of suffering, there is growing interest in interventions that enhance or improve psychological well-being and provide meaning in terminal patients. In recent years, there have been published reviews of interventions targeted at improving end-of-life psychological well-being and reducing various aspects of psychiatric distress [13, 38, 58, 92]. Interventions aimed at enhanced spiritual well-being, meaning, and dignity in advanced cancer patients are now being developed and studied for effectiveness [6, 14, 38].

Despite the growing awareness of spiritual and existential distress among end-of-life cancer patients and the impact on quality of life, there remains a paucity of psychotherapeutic approaches and interventions to directly address this suffering. In a study evaluating spiritual and existential needs among cancer patients, Moadel and colleagues [66] found that from 21 to 51 % of patients reported unmet spiritual or existential needs. The unmet spiritual or existential needs cited by patients were overcoming fears (51 %), finding hope (42 %), finding meaning in life (40 %), and finding spiritual resources (39 %).

Breitbart (2010) [6] notes that while some interventions are aimed at improved mood, none examine the effect of spiritual well-being and few interventional studies are directed at advanced or end-stage cancer patients. Furthermore, aside from hallucinogen-induced mystical experience (discussed below), none provide the means for a direct intensive alteration in consciousness with the potential for a transformative experience directly related to the sacred or to broad spiritual and existential phenomena. Blinderman and Cherny [7] note, "It has been observed that existential distress is the least studied domain of patient distress. Given the paucity of research in this area, additional qualitative and quantitative studies are needed to help further understand this domain of suffering and the possible areas of intervention by health care professionals" (p. 380). Lethborg et al. [59] suggest that "the specific techniques most effective in enhancing meaning and connection (in advanced cancer) are yet to be defined, and such clarification would require intervention-focused research that, in order to appropriately demonstrate change, would need to be longitudinal" (p. 387).

Uniqueness of Psilocybin Mystical Experience Treatment Model

The hallucinogen treatment model, which has been shown to generate a mystical or spiritual experience [30], offers a highly unique and novel therapeutic approach to promote transcendence, meaning, and reduction in anxiety for terminal cancer patients [34]. It is the only approach with the dying of its kind in medicine, psychiatry, and the behavioral sciences. Reviews of the literature on the importance of spirituality in end-of-life suffering [83, 96] identify transcendence and meaning as the most common factors. Of the few spiritual well-being-enhancing interventions for end-of-life patients currently available, the hallucinogen treatment model is the only approach that potentially facilitates a radical shift in consciousness yielding a transpersonal, transcendent, spiritual, and mystical experience.

Access to the transpersonal and transcendent non-ordinary dimensions of consciousness is an integral aspect of the enhanced spiritual well-being generated by the hallucinogen-induced mystical experience. Eric Cassell, the distinguished internist who has contributed considerably to the conversation on dying in America and who has written extensively about the nature of suffering, medicine, and the compassionate and ethical treatment of the terminally ill, writes in his classic article *The Nature of Suffering and The Goals of Medicine*, "Transcendence is probably the most powerful way in which one is restored to wholeness after an injury to personhood. When experienced, transcendence locates the person in a far larger landscape. The suffering is not isolated by pain but is brought closer to a transpersonal

source of meaning and to the human community that shares those meanings. Such an experience need not involve religion in any formal sense; however, in its transpersonal dimension, it is deeply spiritual" [9]. Meaning and transcendence, Cassell suggests, provide unique avenues for the amelioration of suffering at the end of life.

Access to the transpersonal realm has the potential to alter a terminal cancer patient's perspective to his or her existential suffering. Transpersonal psychology "is concerned with the study of humanity's highest potential, and with the recognition, understanding, and realization of unitive, spiritual, and transcendent states of consciousness" (p. 91, [56]). For Aldous Huxley [43], the British writer who dedicated attention to comparative spirituality and to the application of hallucinogens in the dying, the hallucinogen-induced mystical experience may reveal the individual to the "perennial philosophy." This *philosophia perennis* is the philosophical concept which states that all the world's religions and philosophical traditions share a single truth. Mystical, numinous, and peak states of consciousness have been written about extensively throughout history by observers and investigators of philosophy, religion, and consciousness including Carl Jung [49], Abraham Maslow [62], Rudolph Otto [75], William James [46], and Richard Bucke [8], and appear within the canon of the major religious and wisdom traditions.

For many cancer patients, the mystical experience of consciousness provides a profound ontological shift. This ontological or paradigm shift in awareness has the capability to alter and transform a cancer patient's assumptions and beliefs regarding the nature of being, the self, the body, disease, and death itself. Often, for the patient who has had this awareness, the body and cancer are experienced as separate (i.e., "I am not my cancer"). The self-experience or self-image of the patient may be recalibrated into a broader existential view where the meaning of cancer and even death itself may be transformed and may no longer be a profoundly anxiety-provoking experience as it was before. The terror of death may be altered as an individual experiences connection to the transpersonal realm, to others, to nature

Table 17.1 Phenomenological features of a mystical type experience—either naturally occurring or occasioned by a classical hallucinogen

- *Unity*: A core feature—a strong sense of the interconnectedness of all people and things—All is one—sometimes a sense of pure consciousness or a sense all things are alive
- *Sacredness*: Reverence, awe, or holiness
- *Noetic quality*: A sense of encountering ultimate reality
- *Transcendence of time and space*: A sense of timelessness, when past and future collapse into the present moment—an infinite realm with no space boundaries
- *Deeply felt positive mood*: Universal love, joy, peace, tranquility
- *Ineffability and paradoxicality*: A sense that the experience cannot be adequately described in words—a sense of the reconciliation of paradoxes

itself, or to the sacred. Often, the patient may experience consciousness as continuing indefinitely, thereby dramatically modifying or transforming the concept of death of the self.

The primary characteristics of a mystical experience, which are summarized in Table 17.1, appear directly related to the potential for a reduction in existential and psychospiritual distress. The potential primary effects or benefits of mystical or peak consciousness states in cancer patients are (1) improved psychological, spiritual, and existential well-being; (2) ability to cognitively or emotionally reframe the impact of cancer, dying, and death; (3) increased capacity for appreciation of time living; (4) increased appreciation and experience of connectedness to sacredness, nature, relationships, and family; (5) ability to attend to unfinished business; (6) the possibility to conceptualize death as "not the end" but a transition of some manner in continuing consciousness; (7) increased sense of meaning and purpose; and (8) increased acceptance and peace with death.

Johns Hopkins Studies of Psilocybin-Occasioned Mystical Type Experience

Building on observations made in a study conducted in early 1960s in seminary students at Harvard [18, 76], two recent double-blind studies

conducted at Johns Hopkins [29–31] have demonstrated that under carefully controlled conditions, high doses of psilocybin occasion profound personally and spiritually meaningful experiences in the majority of healthy, normal healthy participants. One study [30, 31] involved 36 volunteers who participated in 2 or 3 day-long sessions during which they received, on separate sessions, a high dose of psilocybin (30 mg/70 kg) or a dose of methylphenidate hydrochloride. The design of the study effectively obscured to volunteers and study staff who monitored the sessions exactly what drug conditions were being tested. A subsequent study [29] involved 18 participants who received, in mixed order, a range of psilocybin doses (placebo, 5, 10, 20, and 30 mg/70 kg) over five sessions. The participants in both studies had a mean age of 46 years and were well educated and high functioning. All but one was hallucinogen naïve. Study monitors met individually with each participant for a total of 8 h before the first session and for 2 h between sessions to help develop rapport and trust, which are believed to minimize the risk of adverse reactions to classic hallucinogens. The 8-h drug sessions were conducted in an aesthetic living room-like environment designed specifically for the study (Fig. 17.1). Two monitors were present throughout the session. For most of the time during the session, participants were encouraged to lie on the couch and use an eye mask and headphones. Participants were encouraged to focus their attention on their inner experiences throughout the session. Details and rationale for screening, preparing volunteers, and managing sessions and aftercare were similar to those described by Johnson et al. [47].

As expected, psilocybin produced increases in measures previously shown to be sensitive to hallucinogenic drugs, including perceptual changes (e.g., visual illusions), greater emotionality (e.g., increased joy and peacefulness and, less frequently, fear and anxiety), and cognitive changes (e.g., changes in a sense of meaning, sometimes suspiciousness). But perhaps the most interesting effect was that psilocybin produced large increases on extensively studied, well-validated questionnaires that were designed to measure naturally occurring mystical type experiences as described

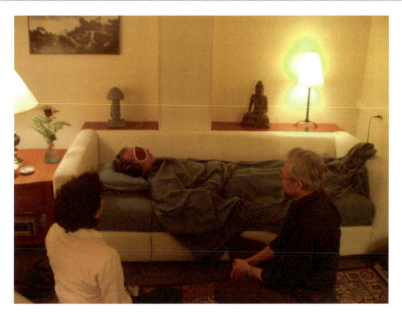

Fig. 17.1 The living room-like session room used in the Johns Hopkins psilocybin research studies. Comfortable, aesthetic environments free of unnecessary medical or research equipment, in combination with careful volunteer screening, volunteer preparation, and interpersonal support from two or more trained monitors, help to mini- mize the probability of acute psychological distress dur- ing sessions. The use of eyeshades and headphones (through which supportive music is played) may contrib- ute to safety by reducing distractions as well as social pressure to verbally interact with research personnel (reprinted from [47])

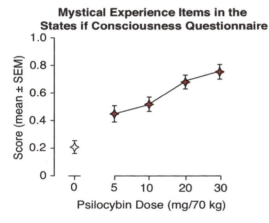

Fig. 17.2 Post-session ratings on a questionnaire designed to assess mystical experience. Psilocybin pro- duced orderly dose-related increases, with most partici- pants fulfilling the criteria for having had a "complete" mystical experience (data from [29])

sure of mystical experience obtained at the end of the session day [29]. "Complete" mystical experiences were those in which volunteers met a priori criteria on all six phenomenological dimen- sions of the mystical experience (Table 17.1). The percentage of volunteers who fulfilled criteria for having had a "complete" mystical experience was an increasing function of dose: 0 %, 5.6 %, 11.1 %, 44.4 %, and 55.6 % at 0 mg/70 kg, 5 mg/70 kg, 10 mg/70 kg, 20 mg/70 kg, and 30 mg/70 kg, respectively. Seventy-two percent of volunteers had "complete" mystical experiences at either or both the 20 and 30 mg/70 kg session. On retro- spective questionnaires completed 1 or 2 months after the psilocybin session and 14 months after the last session, volunteers reported sustained positive changes in attitudes, mood, altruism, behavior, and life satisfaction. Figure 17.3 shows that most participants considered the experience to be among the five most spiritually significant experiences of their lives, including single most. Participants also endorsed various domains of change that suggest increased self-efficacy (e.g., increased self-confidence and sense of inner

by mystics and religious figures worldwide and throughout the ages, including measures not previously used to assess changes after a drug experience. Figure 17.2 shows that psilocybin produced orderly dose-related increases in a mea-

Top 5 Most Spiritually Significant Experiences

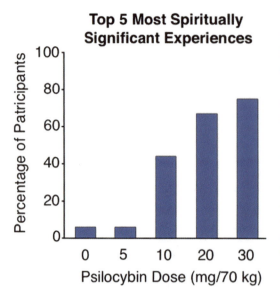

Fig. 17.3 Retrospective ratings of the spiritual significance of the psilocybin experience 1 month after sessions. Not shown, at 14 months after the last session, 94 % of participants rated the experience during the 20 and/or 30 mg/70 kg sessions to be among the top five most spiritually significant experiences of their lives, including single most (data from [29])

authority) and decreased perceived stress (e.g., decreased nervousness, increased inner peace, and ability to tolerate frustration). Ratings of the volunteers' behavior by community observers (friends, family members, colleagues at work) who were blind to drug condition were consistent with the volunteer self-ratings, indicating that the changes were real rather than imagined.

Of further relevance to the use of psilocybin in palliative treatment of existential anxiety associated with terminal illness, Griffiths et al. [29] also showed that the religious subscale of the Death Transcendence Scale was significantly increased over screening levels at both 1- and 14-month follow-up. This is notable, because questions on this scale assess a sense of continuity after death (i.e., Death is never just an ending but part of a process; Death is a transition to something even greater in this life; My death does not end my personal existence; I believe in life after death; There is a Force or Power that controls and gives meaning to both life and death).

Clinical Case Vignette of a Patient in an Ongoing Psilocybin Cancer-Anxiety Study

Roy is a 53-year-old white, American-born male. He is married, has no children, and is a college graduate. Roy is a warm, well-related, highly intelligent man with no psychiatric history or mental status alterations aside from existential distress, anxiety, and depressive affects associated with living with cancer. Both his parents are deceased, his father of cancer. Roy's sister-in-law died of cancer. He reports a fulfilling and very happy relationship with his wife that was evident when they were together in the preliminary research meetings. He cited that one of the primary sources of emotional distress in contemplating the progression and possibility of eventually dying of cancer is losing time and a future with his wife. In August 2007, Roy was diagnosed with cholangiocarcinoma, a cancer of the bile ducts involving malignant growths in the ducts that carries bile from the liver to the small intestine. In September of that same year, he underwent a partial Whipple and liver resection. His gallbladder, major bile ducts, parts of the duodenum and pancreas, and the right lobe of his liver were removed. Surgery was followed by 6 months of chemotherapy. In November 2008, a CT scan showed metastasis to the lungs.

Since February 2009, chemotherapy was implemented biweekly. He reported that this biweekly intensive chemotherapy had been extraordinarily difficult causing extreme fatigue, cognitive "cloudiness," pain, overall body aches, discomfort, and psychological distress. He required assistance during weeks when chemotherapy was administered. He has chemotherapy-induced neuropathy in the hands and feet. After 3 years of contending with the physical and psychological effects of cancer along with the debilitating effects of chemotherapy, Roy had grown increasingly anxious and depressed at which point he inquired about the psilocybin research study at New York University School of Medicine and Bluestone Center for Clinical Research.

The patient had two research study sessions, one with psilocybin and the other with placebo. Both the patient and the study monitors were blinded to the study drug administration. During one of the experimental study sessions, presumably the psilocybin session, Roy swallowed the capsule and sat on the couch listening to soft classical music and viewing picture books with images of nature. Two clinical researchers, male and female, were present throughout the session. Thirty minutes after taking the capsule, the patient was encouraged to lie down on a couch prepared like a bed with sheets, pillows, and blankets. Throughout the session, it was recommended that the patient wear eyeshades and headphones. The music played was mostly classical and instrumental. The room replicates a warm and nicely furnished living area with paintings, Asian area rug, soft lighting, flowers, books, and personal items from the patient.

At 2 h post ingestion and following a period of silence, the patient stated, "Birth and death is a lot or work" repeating it twice and began to cry softly. Over the course of the session, which lasted approximately 6 h, Roy alternated between crying softly, smiling, and laughing. For long periods of time, he lay completely still and silent sometimes uttering short sentences, sometimes with a look of awe on his face. During a 2-h period while lying completely still he stated, "it's really so simple, it's really so simple." All this occurred with eyeshades and headphones on and only with minimal interaction from the monitors. Statements that Roy made during those 2 h which when compared to his written journal and post-session interviews suggest that he had a "complete" mystical experience by fulfilling all of the major criteria for such an experience (see Table 17.1). He later said to the monitors that, during this period, he experienced himself as completely safe—the safest he had ever felt—and he had an intense experience of maximal love. He indicated that he experienced existence or consciousness as continuing infinitely and it was all filled with love, it *was* love, there was neither death nor a beginning. He reported that these insights and experience gave him enormous comfort and meaning. He appeared at complete peace, but as if engaged in an active internal scene.

Approximately 5 h after he took the capsule, he sat up as the experience began to wane in its intensity. He reported that the experience was "life changing" and he was motivated to live more fully in the present moment. He repeated that the message was "so simple, it is love, it's all about the purity of love, energy of love." He felt as if his cancer and the prospect of dying lost significance with this new "knowledge" or awareness. He stated that he experienced love that was of indescribable intensity—"like nothing I've experienced here." At one point during the experience, he reported, "I went into my lungs and saw two spots" (referring to the nodules identified by medical imaging), and said he felt "they were no big deal," that the "cancer is not important, the important stuff is love." He continued to discuss his newfound perspective on cancer that grew from the experience stating, "cancer is nothing to fear," and "cancer wasn't very important." He stated the most important "ingredient" in life is "the purity and simplicity of love." His wife rejoined him in the session room. They hugged, cried, and the patient stated to her, "'It was amazing, amazing, I saw, I touched … the face of God."

Roy has continued to report and present with sustained and marked positive changes in attitude, coping, and mood 18 weeks after the session. He has characterized this experience as the most important life experience he has had second only to his marriage. Despite his cancer and uncertain future, he remarked, "I am the luckiest man on earth" and that "my quality of life is dramatically improved." He has begun a meditation practice since this experience. He stated that "I experienced infinity that lasts forever and that is love" and that this insight and awareness have stayed with him and shaped his attitude towards others, his wife, his disease, and the world. Despite the continuing difficult chemotherapy schedule and struggling with sickness for days at a time and additional surgical procedures, he is coping in a highly effective manner. He still feels that "the cancer is irrelevant" within the context of his new awareness, although he remains highly committed and involved in his medical treatments and decisions. Weeks after the session he stated that "this is the best I've felt in years" and that he felt "the happiest in his life." While realistic about his diagnosis and prognosis, he remains committed to cultivating a positive attitude and has been able to remain emotionally connected to the imagery and existential insights of the psilocybin research session. In the end, he states that the overwhelming message was that of "love, warmth, acceptance" and connection to something greater, eternal, and sacred. The experience of transcendence and the cultivation of meaning appear to be the primary factors contributing to his insight, to the awareness drawn from the session, and to his coping with the existential and spiritual challenges of cancer.

The following are excerpts from a journal entry the patient wrote on the evening and in the days following his experience:

> From here on love was the only consideration. Everything that happened, anything and everything that was seen or heard centered on love. It was and is the only purpose. Love seemed to emanate from a single point of light … It was so pure. The sheer joy … the bliss was indescribable. And in fact there are no words to accurately capture my experience … my state … this place. I know I've had no earthly pleasure that's ever come close to this feeling … no sensation, no image of beauty, nothing during my time on earth has felt as pure and joyful and glorious as the height of this journey … I felt very warm but pleasantly so …
>
> I was beginning to wonder if man spent too much time and effort at things unimportant … trying to accomplish so much … when really, it was all so simple. No matter the subject, it all came down to the same thing. Love. Earthly matters such as food, music, architecture, anything, everything … aside from love, seemed silly and trivial. I was convinced in that moment that I had figured it all out (or it was figured out for me) … it was right there in front of me … love … the only thing that mattered. This was now to be my life's cause. I announced, "OK, I get it! You can all punch out now … our work is done!" But quickly I realized that no … our work … our existence … our energy … is never done … it goes on and on without end.
>
> I thought about my cancer ….I took a tour of my lungs. I could see some things but it was more a matter of feeling the inside of my lungs. I remember breathing deeply to help facilitate the "seeing." There were nodules but they seemed rather unimportant … I was being told (without words) to not worry about the cancer … it's minor in the scheme of things … simply an imperfection of your humanity and that the more important matter … the real work to be done is before you. Again love.

> [On the day after the experience] …I felt spectacular … both physically and mentally! It had been a very long time since I'd felt that good … a serene sense of balance … a level of contentedness, peace and happiness that lasted all day and into the evening. Undoubtedly, my life has changed in ways I may never fully comprehend. But I now have an understanding … an awareness that goes beyond intellect … that my life, that every life, and all that is the universe, equals one thing … love.

Conclusion: Psilocybin Treatment Implications for Palliative Care and Psycho-Oncology

While living with advanced cancer may for some patients be a process of depression, despair, and increased distress, for others it can provide an opportunity for personal meaning, enhanced interpersonal relationships, spiritual growth, clarity, and acceptance. Frequently, a life-threatening cancer triggers a search for meaning and transcendence and an awakening of spirituality. A growing body of literature now substantiates the importance and relevance of spiritual well-being and spirituality in palliative and hospice care. For many patients, the search for meaning that is frequently triggered by end-of-life-stage cancer is a courageous and difficult journey. Ideally, dying should be viewed, not as a medical problem, but as an important and vital part of life experience with potential for discovery and meaning.

Researchers from several decades ago reported encouraging results from their early efforts developing a hallucinogen treatment model with patients suffering from the psychospiritual distress and demoralization often associated with advanced-stage cancer. More recent efforts to reexplore the judicious application of hallucinogen treatment with patients struggling with existential anxiety in the face of a life-threatening cancer diagnosis have similarly observed significant amelioration of psychological suffering. While valuable knowledge can be gleaned from clinical studies conducted from the 1950s to the early 1970s, it is necessary to conduct modern investigations utilizing state-of-the-art research methodologies in order to definitively establish the safety and efficacy of this novel treatment. To date, contemporary studies conducted at three academic medical centers are producing positive results. While still preliminary, these encouraging reports will hopefully facilitate the development of additional investigations with the hallucinogen treatment model, particularly in patient populations refractory to conventional therapeutic approaches [28].

A unique aspect of utilizing a classic hallucinogen (e.g., psilocybin) to treat the severe psychological demoralization and existential anxiety seen in life-threatening medical illness is its seeming capacity to facilitate powerful states of spiritual transcendence that exert in the patient a profound therapeutic impact with often dramatic improvements in psychological well-being. Recently conducted research at Johns Hopkins University has demonstrated that, under carefully structured conditions in normal volunteer subjects, induction of such transcendent and mystical states of consciousness occurs in most subjects studied. This is a critical advancement in the field because, for the first time, a specific treatment has been developed that is able to reliably facilitate the emergence of a transpersonal level of consciousness that appears to have significant therapeutic value. For a patient population struggling with often overwhelming levels of existential anxiety and demoralization, such a therapeutic intervention may have the capacity to reinfuse a sense of meaning and purpose into their lives. The hallucinogen treatment model therefore offers a novel and potentially valuable approach for addressing the existential crisis often observed in cancer patients, with the potential of significantly improving overall quality of life and psychospiritual well-being for the time that remains in their lives.

References

1. Berringer K. Der mescalinrausch. Berlin: Springer; 1927.
2. Bleuler M. Comparison of drug-induced and endogenous psychoses in man. In: Breatly PB, Deniker R, Raduco-Thomas D, editors. Proceedings of the first international congress of neuropsychopharmacology. Amsterdam: Elsevier; 1958.
3. Brady MJ, Peterman AH, Fitchett G, Mo M, Cella D. A case for including spirituality in quality of life measurement in oncology. Psychooncology. 1999;8:417–28.
4. Breitbart W, Gibson C, Chochinov HM. Palliative care. In: Levenson JL, editor. The American psychiatric publishing textbook of psychosomatic medicine. Washington, DC: American Psychiatric Publisher; 2005.
5. Breitbart W, Rosenfeld B, Pessin H, Kaim M, Funesti-Esch J, Galietta M, Nelson CJ, Brescia R. Depression, hopelessness, and desire for hastened death in terminally ill patients with cancer. J Am Med Assoc. 2000;284:2907–11.
6. Breitbart W, Rosenfeld B, Gibson C, Pessin H, Poppito S, Nelson C, Tomarken A, Kosinski A, Berg A, Jacobson C, Sorger B, Abbey J, Olden M. Meaning-centered group psychotherapy for patients with advanced cancer: a pilot randomized controlled trial. Psychooncology. 2010;19:21–8.
7. Blinderman C, Cherny N. Existential issues do not necessarily result in existential suffering: lessons from cancer patients in Israel. Palliat Med. 2005;19:371–80.
8. Bucke RM. Cosmic consciousness. Philadelphia, PA: Innes & Sons; 1901.
9. Cassel EJ. The nature of suffering and the goals of medicine. N Engl J Med. 1982;306:639–45.
10. Chandler AL, Hartman MA. Lysergic acid diethylamide (LSD-25) as a facilitating agent in psychotherapy. Arch Gen Psychiatry. 1960;2:286–9.
11. Chochinov HM, Wilson KG, Lander S. Depression, hopelessness, and suicidal ideation in the terminally ill. Psychosomatics. 1998;39:336–70.
12. Chochinov HM, Hack T, Hassard T, Krisjanson L, McClemont S, Harlos M. Understanding the will to live in patients nearing death. Psychosomatics. 2005;46:7–10.
13. Chochinov HM, Cann BJ. Interventions to enhance the spiritual aspects of dying. J Palliat Med. 2005;8(Supplement 1):S103–15.
14. Chochinov HM, Hack T, Hassard T, Kristjanson LJ, McClemont S, Harlos M. Dignity therapy: a novel psychotherapeutic intervention for patients near the end of life. J Clin Oncol. 2005;23:5520–5.
15. Cohen S. LSD and the anguish of dying. Harper's. 1965 Sept: 69–78
16. Cohen SR, Mount BM, Tomas JN, Mount LF. Existential well-being is an important determinant of quality of life. Cancer. 1996;77:576–86.
17. Derogatis LR, Morrow GR, Fetting J, Penman D, Piasetsky C, Schmale AM, Henrichs M, Carnicke CL. J Am Med Assoc. 1983;249:751–7.
18. Doblin R. Pahnke's Good Friday experiment: a long-term follow-up and methodological critique. J Transpersonal Psychol. 1991;23:1–28.
19. Durkin I, Kearney M, O'Siorain L. Psychiatric disorder in a palliative care unit. Palliat Med. 2003;17:212–8.
20. Edwards A, Pang N, Shiu V, Chan C. The understanding of spirituality and the potential role of spiritual care in end-of-life and palliative care: a

meta-study of qualitative research. Palliat Med. 2010;24(8):753–70.

21. Fernsler J, Klemm P, Miller M. Spiritual well-being and demands of illness in people with colorectal cancer. Cancer Nurs. 1999;22:134–40.

22. Field M, Cassel C, editors. Approaching death: improving care at the end-of-life. Washington, DC: National Academy Press; 1997.

23. Fisher G. Psychotherapy for the dying: principles and illustrative cases with special reference to the use of LSD. Omega. 1970;1:3–15.

24. Frankl VE. Man's search for meaning. Boston, MA: Beacon; 1984.

25. Frankl VF. The will to meaning: foundations and applications of logotherapy. New York: Penguin; 1988.

26. Galfin JM, Walkins ER, Harlow T. Psychological distress and rumination in palliative care patients and their caregivers. J Palliat Med. 2010;13: 1345–8.

27. Greenberg L, Lantz MS, Likourezos A, Burack OR, Chichin E, Carter J. Screening for depression in nursing home palliative care patients. J Geriatr Psychiatry Neurol. 2004;17:212–8.

28. Griffiths RR, Grob CS. Hallucinogens as medicine. Sci Am. 2010;303(December):77–9.

29. Griffiths RR, Johnson MW, Richards WA, Richards BD, McCann U, Jesse R. Psilocybin occasioned mystical-type experiences: immediate and persisting dose-related effects. Psychopharmacology (Berl). 2011;218:649–65.

30. Griffiths RR, Richards WA, McCann U, Jesse R. Psilocybin can occasion mystical experiences having substantial and sustained personal meaning and spiritual significance. Psychopharmacology (Berl). 2006;187:268–83.

31. Griffiths RR, Richards WA, Johnson MW, McCann U, Jesse R. Mystical-type experiences occasioned by psilocybin mediate the attribution of personal meaning and spiritual significance 14 months later. J Psychopharmacol. 2008;22(6):621–32.

32. Grinspoon L, Bakalar JB. Psychedelic drugs reconsidered. New York: Basic Books; 1979.

33. Grinspoon L, Bakalar JB. Can drugs be used to enhance the psychotherapeutic process? Am J Psychother. 1986;40:393–404.

34. Grob CS, Danforth AL, Chopra GS, Hagerty M, McKay CR, Halberstadt AL, Greer G. Pilot study of psilocybin treatment for anxiety in patients with advanced-stage cancer. Arch Gen Psychiatry. 2011;68:71–8.

35. Grof S, Goodman LE, Richards WA, Kurland AA. LSD-assisted psychotherapy in patients with terminal cancer. Int Pharmacopsychiatry. 1973;8:129–44.

36. Hasler F, Grimberg U, Benz MA, Huber T, Vollenweider FX. Acute psychological and physiological effects of psilocybin in healthy humans: a double-blind, placebo-controlled dose effects study. Psychopharmacology (Berl). 2004;172:145–56.

37. Henoch I, Danielson E. Existential concerns among patients with cancer and interventions to meet them: an integrative literature review. Psychooncology. 2009;18:225–36.

38. Henry M, Cohen R, Lee V, Sauthier P, Provencher D, Drouin P, Gauthier P, Gotlieb W, Lau S, Drummond N, Gilbert L, Stanimir G, Sturgeon J, Chasen M, Mitchell J, Nixon Huang L, Ferland M, Mayo N. The meaning making intervention (MMi) appears to increase meaning in life in advanced ovarian cancer: a randomized controlled pilot study. Psychooncology. 2010;19:1340–7.

39. Hills J, Paice JA, Cameron JR, Shott S. Spirituality and distress in palliative care consultation. J Palliat Med. 2005;8:782–8.

40. Hofmann A. LSD—my problem child: reflections on sacred drugs, mysticism and science. Los Angeles, CA: J.P. Tarcher; 1985.

41. Hotoph M, Chidgey J, Addington-Hall J, Ly KL. Depression in advanced disease: a systematic review. Part 1. Prevalence and case finding. Palliat Med. 2002;16:81–97.

42. Hotopf M, Price A. Palliative care psychiatry. Psychiatry. 2009;8:212–5.

43. Huxley A. The perennial philosophy. New York: Harper & Brothers; 1945.

44. Isbell H. Comparison of the reactions induced by psilocybin and LSD-25 in man. Psychopharmacologia. 1959;1:29–38.

45. Jacob P, Shulgin AT. Structure-activity relationships of the classic hallucinogens and their analogs. NIDA Res Monogr. 1994;146:74–91.

46. James W. The varieties of religious experience. New York: Longman's Green, and Co.; 1919.

47. Johnson MW, Richards WA, Griffiths RR. Human hallucinogen research: guidelines for safety. J Psychopharmacol. 2008;22:603–20.

48. Jones JM, Huggins MA, Rydall AC, Rodin GM. Symptomatic distress, hopelessness, and the desire for hastened death in hospitalized cancer patients. J Psychosom Res. 2003;55:411–8.

49. Jung C. Psychology and religion. New Heaven, CT: Yale University Press; 1938.

50. Kandasamy A, Chaturvedi S, Desai G. Spirituality, distress, depression, anxiety, and quality of life in patients with advanced cancer. Indian J Cancer. 2011;48:55–8.

51. Kast EC. The measurement of pain, a new approach to an old problem. J New Drugs. 1962;2:344–51.

52. Kast EC, Collins VJ. Lysergic acid diethylamide as an analgesic agent. Anesth Analg. 1964;43:285–91.

53. Kelly B, Burnett P, Pelusi D, Badger S, Varghese F, Robertson M. Terminally ill cancer patients' wish to hasten death. Palliat Med. 2002;16:339–45.

54. Kissane D, Clarke DM, Street AF. Demoralization syndrome-A relevant psychiatric diagnosis for palliative care. J Palliat Care. 2001;17:12–21.

55. Kluver H. Mescal: the 'Divine' plant and its psychological effects. London: Keegan Paul; 1928.

56. Lajoie DH, Shapiro SI. Definitions of transpersonal psychology: the first twenty-three years. J Transpersonal Psychol. 1992;24:79–98.

57. Lee V. The existential plight of cancer: meaning making as a concrete approach to the intangible search for meaning. Support Care Cancer. 2008;16:779–85.

58. LeMay K, Wilson KG. Treatment of existential distress in life threatening illness: a review of manualized interventions. Clin Psychol Rev. 2008;28: 472–93.

59. Lethborg C, Aranda S, Cox S, Kissane D. To what extent does meaning mediate adaptation to cancer? The relationship between physical suffering, meaning in life, and connection to others in adjustment to cancer. Palliat Support Care. 2007;5:377–88.

60. Lin HR, Bauer-Wu SM. Psycho-spiritual well-being in patients with advanced cancer: an integrative review of the literature. J Adv Nurs. 2003;44:69–80.

61. Massie MJ. Prevalence of depression in patients with cancer. J Natl Cancer Inst Monogr. 2004;32:57–71.

62. Maslow AH. Religions, values, and peak experience. Columbus, OH: Ohio State University Press; 1964.

63. McClain CS, Rosenfeld B, Breitbart W. Effect of spiritual well-being on end-of-life despair in terminally-ill cancer patients. Lancet. 2003;361:1603–7.

64. McMillan SC, Weitzner M. How problematic are various aspects of quality of life in patients with cancer at the end of life? Oncol Nurs Forum. 2000;27:817–23.

65. Metzner R. Teonanacatl: sacred mushroom of visions. Verona, CA: Four Trees Press; 2004.

66. Moadel A, Morgan C, Fatone A, Grennan J, Carter J, Laruffa G, Skummy A, Dutcher J. Seeking meaning and hope: self-reported spiritual and existential needs among an ethnically-diverse cancer population. Psychooncology. 1999;8:378–85.

67. Moreno FA, Wiegand CB, Taitano K, Delgado PL. Safety, tolerability and efficacy of psilocybin in patients with obsessive-compulsive disorder. J Clin Psychiatry. 2006;67:1735–40.

68. Morita T, Tsunoda J, Inoue S, Chihara S. An exploratory factor analysis of existential suffering in Japanese terminally ill cancer patients. Psychooncology. 2000;9:164–8.

69. Murata H. Spiritual pain and its care in patients with terminal cancer: construction of a conceptual framework by philosophical approach. Palliat Support Care. 2003;1:15–21.

70. National Institute for Clinical Excellence. Improving supportive and palliative care for adults with cancer. London: National Institute for Clinical Excellence; 2004.

71. The National Comprehensive Cancer Network: Distress Management Clinical Practice Guidelines in Oncology. www.NCCN.org (2009; 2010)

72. Nelson CJ, Rosenfeld B, Breitbart W, Galietta M. Spirituality, religion, and depression in the terminally ill. Psychosomatics. 2002;43:213–20.

73. Nichols DE. Hallucinogens. Pharmacol Ther. 2004;101:131–81.

74. Osmond H. A review of the clinical effects of psychotomimetic agents. Ann N Y Acad Sci. 1957;66:418–34.

75. Otto R. The idea of the holy. London: Oxford University Press; 1923.

76. Pahnke W. Drugs and mysticism: an analysis of the relationship between psychedelic drugs and the mystical consciousness. Thesis presented to the President and Fellows of Harvard University for the Ph.D. in Religion and Society; 1963

77. Pahnke WN. The psychedelic mystical experience in the human encounter with death. Harvard Theol Rev. 1969;62:1–21.

78. Passie T. A history of the use of psilocybin in psychotherapy. In: Metzner R, editor. Teonanacatl: sacred mushroom of vision. El Verano, CA: Four Trees Press; 2004.

79. Passie T, Seifert J, Schneider U, Emrich HM. The pharmacology of psilocybin. Addict Biol. 2002;7:357–64.

80. Presti DE, Nichols DE. Biochemistry and neuropharmacology of psilocybin mushrooms. In: Metzner R, editor. Teonanacatl: sacred mushroom of vision. El Verano, CA: Four Trees Press; 2004.

81. Puchalski C, Ferrell B, Virani R, Otis-Green S, Baird P, Bull J, Chochinov M, Handzo G, Nelson-Becker H, Prince-Paul M, Pugliese K, Sulmasy D. Improving the quality of spiritual care as a dimension of palliative care: the report of the consensus conference. J Palliat Med. 2009;12:885–904.

82. Puchalski CM, Romer AL. Taking a spiritual history allows clinicians to understand patients more fully. J Palliat Med. 2000;3:129–37.

83. Puchalski CM, Kilpatrick SD, McCullough ME, Larson DB. A systematic review of spiritual and religious variables in Palliative Medicine, American Journal of Hospice and Palliative Care, Hospice Journal, Journal of Palliative Care, and Journal of Pain and Symptom Management. Palliat Support Care. 2003;1:7–13.

84. Richards WA, Rhead JC, DiLeo FB, Yensen R, Kurland AA. The peak experience variable in DPT-assisted psychotherapy with cancer patients. J Psychedelic Drugs. 1977;9:1–10.

85. Riedlinger TJ. The sacred mushroom seeker: essays for R. Gordon Wasson. Portland, OR: Dioscorides Press; 1990.

86. Rodin G, Lo C, Mikulincer M, Donner A, Gagliese L, Zimmermann C. Pathways to distress: the multiple determinants of depression, hopelessness, and the desire for hastened death in metastatic cancer patients. Soc Sci Med. 2009;68:562–9.

87. Rodin G, Zimmermann C, Rydall A, Jones J, Shepherd FA, Moore M, Fruh M, Donner A, Gagliese L. The desire for hastened death in patients with metastatic cancer. J Pain Symptom Manage. 2007;6: 661–75.

88. Rousseau P. Spirituality and the dying patient. J Clin Oncol. 2000;18:2000–2.

89. Saunders CM. The management of terminal malignant disease. London: Edward Arnold; 1978.

90. Saunders C. Spiritual pain. J Palliat Care. 1988;4: 29–32.

91. Schultes RE, Hofmann A. Plants of the gods: their sacred, healing and hallucinogenic powers. Rochester, VT: Healing Arts Press; 1992.

92. Sinclair S, Pereira J, Raffin S. A thematic review of the spirituality literature within palliative care. J Palliat Med. 2006;9:464–79.

93. Storey P, Knight CF. UNIPAC Two: alleviating psychological and spiritual pain in the terminally ill. Gainesville, FL: American Academy of Hospice and Palliative Medicine; 1997.

94. Studerus E, Gamma A, Vollenweider FX. Psychometric evaluation of the altered states of consciousness rating scale (OAV). PLoS One. 2010;5: 1–19.

95. Tanyi RA. Towards clarification of the meaning of spirituality. J Adv Nurs. 2002;39:500–9.

96. Vachon M, Fillion L, Achille M. A conceptual analysis of spirituality at the end of life. J Palliat Med. 2009;12:53–7.

97. Vollenweider FX, Leenders KL, Scharfetter C, Maguire P, Stadelmann O, Angst J. Positron emission tomography and fluorodeoxyglucose studies of metabolic hyperfrontality and psychopathology in the psilocybin model of psychosis. Neuropsychopharmacology. 1997;16:357–72.

98. Vollenweider FX, Vollenweider-Scherpenhuyzen MF, Bäbler A, Vogel H, Hell D. Psilocybin induces schizophrenia-like psychosis in humans via a serotonin-2 agonist action. Neuroreport. 1998;9: 3897–902.

99. Weisman AD. Early diagnosis of vulnerability in cancer patients. Am J Med Sci. 1976;271:187–96.

100. Weisman AD, Worden JW. The existential plight in cancer: significance of the first 100 days. Int J Psychiatry Med. 1976;7:1–15.

101. Wilson KG, Chochinov HM, de Faye BJ, Breitbart W. Diagnosis and management of depression in palliative care. In: Chochinov HM, Breitbart W, editors. Handbook of psychiatry in palliative medicine. New York: Oxford University Press; 2000. p. 25–49.

102. Wilson KG, Chochinov HM, Skirko MG, Allard P, Chary S, Gagnon PR, Macmillan K, De Luca M, O'Shea F, Kuhl D, Fainsinger RL, Clinch JJ. Depression and anxiety disorders in palliative cancer care. J Pain Symptom Manage. 2007;33:118–29.

103. World Health Organization: WHO definition of palliative care. www.who.int/cancer/palliative/definition.en/ (2011). Accessed Feb 2011

The Placebo and Nocebo Effects in Cancer Treatment

18

Franziska Schuricht and Yvonne Nestoriuc

Looking at the Placebo and Nocebo Effects in Cancer Treatment

Resulting from the growing scientific knowledge and research on the placebo effect over the last few decades, the less popular counterpart, the nocebo effect, has also received increasing attention. Therefore, a theory on the existence of an active psychobiological placebo and nocebo responses is becoming more defined. Moreover, precise study designs and neuroimaging methodologies allow us to begin developing models about the underlying mechanisms. Understanding the placebo and nocebo effects will help us to gain new insights in the interaction of psychological and physiological processes in health and disease [1]. The potential power of placebo and nocebo phenomena to advance therapeutic effects by increasing desired effects and reducing wearing effects, respectively, also makes them meaningful in the context of cancer treatment [2]. This chapter presents an overview of empirical evidence of the placebo and nocebo effects in cancer patients. Moreover, current knowledge on placebo and nocebo mechanisms in oncology is reviewed and clinical implications with regard to ethical issues are discussed. First of all, we

provide a definition of the terms placebo, placebo and nocebo effects, and placebo and nocebo responses.

Definition and Conceptual Background

Placebo: "I Shall Please"

The term placebo usually refers to an inert substance, sham agent or procedure that is not expected to have any direct physiological effect. In clinical trials, placebos are routinely used to provide baselines against which the effects of active interventions are evaluated. In some clinical studies, however, active placebos are used. These do not produce any direct therapeutic effects but rather mimic the side effect profile of the active pharmacological substance [3]. This supports the recipient's belief in actually receiving the active drug, and thus, increases the placebo effect because positive expectations are one of the basic mechanisms thought to underly the placebo effect (see "Patient Expectations"). By subtracting the effects in the placebo group from the overall response in treatment group, information about the size of the specific treatment effect can be obtained. Historically, placebos have been used to treat harmful symptoms for thousands of years [1]. In this manner, placebos are not just used to "please" the patient as the standard etymology of the word placebo suggests [4] but rather to procure real health benefits.

F. Schuricht • Y. Nestoriuc, Ph.D. (✉)
Clinical Psychology and Psychotherapy,
Deparment of Psychology, Philipps University Marburg,
Gutenbergstrasse 18 35037, Marburg, Germany
e-mail: yn@staff.uni-marburg.de

B.I. Carr and J. Steel (eds.), *Psychological Aspects of Cancer*,
DOI 10.1007/978-1-4614-4866-2_18, © Springer Science+Business Media, LLC 2013

Viewing both the clinical and the historical conceptualizations of placebo raises the question of how something that is thought to be inert can actually cause desired effects. Confrontation with this paradox leads to changes in the conceptualization of placebo, shifting the focus away from the inert content of the placebo agent, and rather examining the therapeutic context surrounding the administration of a placebo [5]. Today, a whole body of research studies the conglomeration of beneficial effects that the therapeutic context can have on the patient's treatment experience and health outcome. The therapeutic context includes characteristics of the individual patient, the clinician, the treatment environment and their interactions. These factors lead to different endogenous processes involved in the patient [6]. The extent to which these processes differ from those in an untreated natural history group constitutes the *placebo response*. The *placebo effect* is thought to result from these endogenous placebo responses and describes all the improvements in outcome measures that can directly be observed in the placebo group [1]. The comparison to a no treatment baseline condition is desirable to disentangle unspecific changes that contribute to the overall improvements from the true placebo responses and placebo effects, respectively. Examples for these unspecific changes are: spontaneous remission, natural symptom fluctuation of a disease, and regression to the mean [7]. It has to be noted that most clinical trials, however, are conducted to evaluate an active treatment in comparison to a placebo treatment rather than to evaluate a placebo treatment against a non-treatment group. Whether or not information from these trails can be used to determine the true placebo effects and placebo responses depends in large part on their specific design and thus the range of alternative explanations for treatment effects (e.g., whether the natural history of the examined condition is established or not) [1].

However, with regard to recent placebo conceptualizations it became clear that the explicit administration of a placebo is not necessary to examine the placebo effect. Placebo effects can also be observed by an experimental variation in the context of active treatments [6] (e.g., open versus hidden administration of medication). Thus, critical challenges for placebo research are first, to clearly determine the true placebo effect, and second, to reveal its modulation by interacting factors of the psychosocial context in which a treatment appears.

For the purpose of this chapter, we use the term *placebo* to refer to substances or treatments that per se have no known direct beneficial effect on a given condition. The term *placebo response* refers to the psychophysiological processes attributed to the context of treatment administration including both cases: placebo and active treatments. *Placebo effect* is used to refer to the true improvements in outcome measures that result from the placebo responses and can be directly observed [1]. Thus, according to the logic of a clinical trial, placebo effects can be estimated by either subtracting the unspecific changes occurring in a non-treatment group from the overall changes in the placebo group or through a systematic manipulation of the treatment context (see Fig. 18.1).

Nocebo: "I Shall Harm"

The term nocebo was introduced to distinguish the beneficial effects of a placebo or an active treatment from the distressing effects that it may cause [8]. Nocebo refers to the administration of an inert substance (i.e., placebo) along with the suggestion or expectation to get worse [9]. Furthermore, the term nocebo-related effect is used when symptom worsening follows negative expectations from active treatments without placebo administration (i.e., non-specific medication side effects [10]). According to Hahn [11], a nocebo effect occurs when a person who expects to experience adverse effects from a specific treatment, subsequently actually does. In addition to expectation, conditioning and prior experience (own or witnessed) with adverse effects of treatments are further potential pathways of nocebo effects [10, 12].

The incidence of patients in a placebo group reporting adverse side effects (i.e., nocebo effects) is with a percentage of about 25 % considerable high [10, 13] and even increases when structured

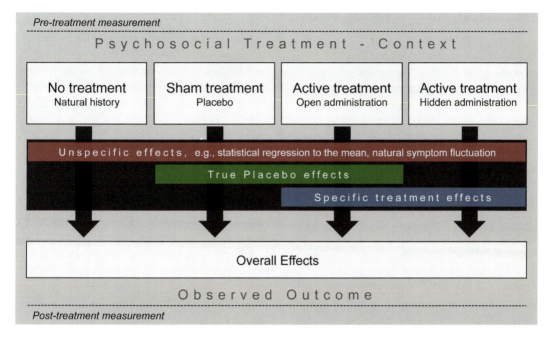

Fig. 18.1 Unraveling the "black box" between pre- and post-treatment measurements in clinical trials: true placebo effects can be obtained by comparisons between a placebo and a no treatment arm; specific intervention effects are determined by comparisons between the active treatment and a placebo. Furthermore, it is shown that comparisons of different treatment applications, e.g., hidden versus open, provide alternative options to gain information about the true placebo effect

methods are used to assess side effects [14]. Discontinuation rates due to adverse effects have been shown to be equally high in drug and placebo groups [15]. Furthermore, side effect profiles in placebo groups of different active drugs for the same condition (e.g., antidepressants or antimigraine drugs) have been shown to depend on the expected side effect profile of the active drug [14, 16]. Taken together, there is considerable evidence for the clinically relevant incidence and specificity of nocebo effects.

Only a minority of the side effects reported in clinical trials or routine care are, in fact, specifically attributable to the pharmacological action of a drug [10]. Side effects not associated with a known treatment are called non-specific side effects or nocebo-related effects [9] and as such are ideally suited to study the underlying nocebo responses. Non-specific side effects often appear as generalized and diffuse symptoms such as fatigue, difficulties in concentrating, headache, or insomnia, they occur mostly dose independent, and are partly explained by the nocebo phenomenon [10].

To summarize, the *nocebo effect* considered in this chapter refers to the adverse events that have no known pharmacological relation to a given treatment, but are attributed to the treatment (placebo or active) by the patient. The endogenous processes associated with these negative expectations and the nocebo effects are called *nocebo responses*.

The Placebo and Nocebo Effects in Oncology

Within the last decades, there has been an extensive increase in innovative attempts to cancer treatment and the management of symptoms that are related to the disease and its treatment. Placebo-controlled randomized clinical trials that evaluate the efficacy of new interventions also provide a useful tool to get insights into the influence placebo and nocebo effects may have in oncology. This section discusses this potential role of the placebo and nocebo effects in oncology. Exemplary studies are reviewed and effects are grouped into symptom categories.

Subjective Measures in Placebo Groups

In the context of cancer, the examination of placebo or nocebo effects applies mainly to the symptoms that can be problematic at the time of diagnosis, during and after cancer treatment, rather than to the tumor itself. Cancer-related fatigue, nausea and vomiting, cancer pain, and vasomotor symptoms are some of the most common bothersome symptoms experienced by cancer patients. These symptoms are typically assessed by the patients themselves referring to the subjective quality of their conscious experiences.

Cancer-related Fatigue

The National Comprehensive Cancer Network defines cancer-related fatigue (CRF) as "a distressing persistent, subjective sense of physical, emotional and/or cognitive tiredness or exhaustion related to cancer or cancer treatment that is not proportional to recent activity and interferes with usual functioning" [17]. CRF is highly prevalent with up to 90 % of sufferers in cancer patients receiving active treatment and up to 75 % in cancer survivors [18]. A variety of both pharmacological and non-pharmacological treatment attempts for the management of CRF are provided [17, 19]. Nevertheless, due to the complex nature of CRF the underlying mechanisms are not yet fully understood [20], which makes it difficult to treat appropriately. In a retrospective analysis of two clinical trials on CRF treatments, de la Cruz et al. [21] examined the frequency and predictors of placebo and nocebo effects in patients with advanced cancer suffering from severe CRF. Patients were randomly assigned to receive either a pharmacological agent (methylphenidate in a first trial, donepezil in a second trial) or a placebo for 7 days. As specified by the authors, patients were considered to be placebo responders if they revealed a defined improvement in fatigue measure scores between baseline and end of the study, and they were considered nocebo responders if they reported more than two side effects from the placebo.

According to these definitions, more than half of the 105 patients receiving placebo actually showed a positive placebo response and almost three-quarters experienced nocebo effects. Factors associated with the beneficial effects in the placebo group were worse anxiety, physical well-being and fatigue scores at baseline, whereas worse baseline pain, drowsiness, and sleep were associated with a more frequent side effect reporting. The response rates for placebo and nocebo appear surprisingly high and the authors provide different explanations. For example, they discuss the subjective nature of the examined symptoms, and effects of regression to the mean that might have been relevant especially in patients with worse baseline measures [21]. Furthermore, the two trials neither assessed expectations necessary to prove the nocebo hypotheses according to Hahn [11] nor was a non-treatment natural history group analyzed to control for several non-specific effects that may have lead to improved outcome measures in the placebo groups. Thus, the high magnitude of beneficial as well as distressing effects in the placebo groups might have been due to many different reasons in addition to placebo and nocebo effects. However, as CRF is established to be a persisting symptom, and the duration of the study was with 7 days quite short, it is not likely that the high magnitude of beneficial effect is mainly caused by symptom fluctuation. With regard to the high rates of side effects (e.g., 79 % insomnia, 53 % anorexia, 38 % nausea, and 34 % restlessness), the authors discuss the role of a list with all potential side effects of the active drug that has been provided to the patients. These lists might have contributed to heightened negative expectations about treatment outcome. Even though expectations were not measured, this is a plausible explanation for the high rates of side effects in the placebo groups, and besides, would be in line with the nocebo hypotheses [11].

In summary, there is evidence for placebo and nocebo effects occurring in clinical trials of advanced cancer patients with CRF. In the placebo groups of two randomized controlled trials almost half of the patients showed symptom improvement (i.e., placebo effects), while two thirds of the patients experienced adverse symptoms (i.e., nocebo effects). The depicted response rates in the placebo groups also point to the relevance of placebo- and nocebo-related effects in the active treatment groups (e.g., relevance of patient expectations). Future studies that systematically vary the context in which the active and placebo treatments are given (e.g., with or without full information about the desired and potential undesired effects of the active treatment) could provide more information to unravel specific treatment effects/side effects and placebo/nocebo effects (see Fig. 18.1). The mechanisms underlying CRF, yet, are poorly understood [20] and well-designed controlled clinical trials are needed all the more to unravel the promising influence the placebo effect may have in successful CRF management.

Chemotherapy-induced Nausea and Vomiting

Chemotherapy-induced nausea and vomiting (CINV) constitutes another serious problem encountered by up to three quarters of all cancer patients [22]. Despite several advances in the management of CINV, there are many patients who do either not respond to antiemetic therapies or experience additional adverse drug reactions when receiving antiemetics [2]. Taking this into consideration, Zhang et al. [2] call the researchers' attention to the potential of the placebo effect in preventing CINV. Referring to 11 randomized, double-blind placebo-controlled clinical trials the authors argue that a wide range in antiemetic response rates do not only occur in active drug treatment (17–100 %) but also in placebo treatment (0–74 %). Even though antiemetic drugs are overall superior compared to placebo in the control of emesis, these findings suggest that to a certain extent appropriate symptom relief can also be achieved with placebos. Thus, Zhang et al. [2] hypothesize that in some cases active drugs can be replaced by placebos, thereby preventing additional risk for adverse drug interactions. Especially for patients receiving polypharmic chemotherapy, additional medications should be reduced whenever possible. Thereby, the authors highlight the importance of further research examining the appropriate use of placebos [2].

A precise detection of predictors of placebo effects is crucial for the hypothesized application of placebos as adjuncts or even alternatives to active medication. There is a wide range of response variation in both the pharmacological and the placebo treatment. Thus, the influence of the treatment context in interaction with demographical, physical, and psychological variables, however challenging methodically, needs to be investigated. Hence, the discussed clinical applications of placebo research in the prevention of CINV still remain challenging suggestions and, furthermore, raise ethical issues (see "The Ethical Dilemma of Intervention").

Cancer-related Pain

Chronic pain associated with the cancer treatments is getting more into the focus of research interest. Pain can occur in different terms such as postmastectomy pain syndrome as one example for postsurgical sequelae, chronic neuropathic pain following radiotherapy, or radiation-induced brachial plexopathy. The standard cancer pain management mostly implies biomedical approaches. Despite the good analgesic effects, the available drugs often raise the patients' concerns about potential side effects [23, 24]. Robb et al. [23] conducted a randomized controlled trial to examine innovative non-pharmacological approaches to cancer pain management. They compared the effectiveness of transcutaneous electrical nerve stimulation (TENS), transcutaneous spinal electro analgesia (TSE), and a sham TSE (placebo) in 41 women with chronic pain following breast cancer treatment. Both TENS and TSE devices used electricity to ease pain. The placebo devices had disabled wires but apart from that were identical to the active machines. The researchers found improved worst and average pain scores in all the three intervention groups throughout a 3-week trial. Furthermore, patients exhibited significantly lower anxiety scores after TENS and placebo use. There were no significant differences between the conditions neither regarding pain nor anxiety. Of the six women who completed the long term-term follow up of the trial, four and two reported still benefits from using the placebo machine at 3 and 12 months, respectively [23].

The study allowed no comparison with standard pharmacological treatments or a non-treatment natural history group, and therefore no clear statement about the magnitude of the specific effects, found in both the TENS/TSE treatment groups and the placebo treatment groups, can be obtained. However, natural symptom fluctuation is an unlikely cause given the high chronicity of the symptom and the short duration of the study with 3 weeks total. Furthermore, as there were no significant differences in the efficacy of the active TENS, TSE, and the sham TSE, the beneficial effects cannot be a result of the specific mechanism of the active devices. Thus, underlying placebo responses should be taken into consideration when interpreting the results of Robb et al. [23]. Besides pain reduction, the finding of significant decrease in anxiety scores is interesting. Anxiety and pain seem to be related, and due to this pathway the occurrence of placebo effects may be predictable in some cases (see "Links to Neurobiological and Immunological Responses").

In 2003, Chvetzoff and Tannock [25] published a systematic review of placebo and nocebo effects not only regarding cancer symptom management but also tumor response in a variety of tumors (see "Tumor Responses"). The researchers reviewed the patients' responses to placebo in 37 randomized controlled trials as well as the patients' responses to best supportive care in 10 randomized controlled trials. Thereby, some of the trials examined individual responses while other trails looked at average group responses. Regarding subjective measures, significant improvements in pain (and appetite), both on individual and average levels, were found. In five of six trials that reported individual evaluation of pain, 4–21 % of altogether 149 patients indicated a reduction in pain or decreased their use of analgesic medication (8–27 % of patients reported improvements in appetite). An average overall improvement of pain in placebo groups was reported in two of six trials (for appetite in one of seven trials); in the four other trials pain levels remained stable. Patients in the pharmacologic treatment arms showed higher response rates regarding pain reduction on individual level; with the exception of one Etidronate trial. Looking at average group changes, there was an overall pain improvement in three of six trials, with two of these showing substantial improvements. Interestingly, these were also the trials for which the improvement in

the placebo arm was reported. No improvement in pain, however, appeared in any of the two best supportive care arms.

Taken together, the findings of Robb et al. [23] and Chvetzoff and Tannock [25] support the hypothesis that placebo and nocebo effects play a vital role in the field of cancer associated pain. Most placebo research has been conducted with pain and pain treatment for many conditions, thus, providing a variety of reasonable models to explain the analgesic placebo effects and hyperalgesic nocebo effects. Thereby, the role of emotional states is discussed as one important mediating factor [26] (see "Links to Neurobiological and Immunological Responses"). The results of Robb et al. [23] also point to a potential link between decreased anxiety and pain relief. As the cancer disease and its treatment often are accompanied with anxiety and insecurity, helping patients to cope with these emotional states constitutes a promising therapeutic attempt. Furthermore, the finding that improvements in pain were significantly more likely for patients in the placebo groups than in the best supportive care groups [25] suggests that receiving a specific treatment, regardless whether it is active or placebo, rather than receiving regular care, promotes analgesic effects. To confirm this hypothesis further studies that systematically compare the effects of active, placebo, and best supportive care arms are needed. Thereby, investigation of the mediating role of the patients' expectations about the benefits of a treatment might be helpful to develop symptom predicting models and therapeutic interventions for symptom prevention.

Vasomotor Symptoms in Cancer Treatment

Another subject relevant in the context of cancer treatment especially for breast and prostate cancers is vasomotor symptoms, most commonly, hot flashes. A hot flash is defined as "a subjective sensation of heat that is associated with objective signs of cutaneous vasodilation and a subsequent drop in core temperature" [27]. It is one of the symptoms that occur with considerable frequency during endocrine therapy. Endocrine breast and prostate cancer therapies are one of the major adjuvant medical treatment modalities to decrease the risk of local and distant relapse [28].

In numerous placebo-controlled randomized clinical trials of interventions to decrease hot flashes a substantial placebo response has been shown [29]. Sloan et al. [30] reviewed the data of 375 patients in seven placebo-controlled randomized trials. They found that 4 weeks of placebo treatment could reduce the frequency and intensity of hot flashes by about 25 % [30]. With single exceptions of studies that even showed a trend for greater improvement in the placebo than in the treatment group, placebos and active treatment showed in most cases equal effects in the treatment of hot flashes, when complementary interventions (such as phytoestrogens, homeopathy) were evaluated. For pharmacological interventions (e.g., progestagens, clonidine hydrochloride, selective serotonin reuptake inhibitors) predominantly significant effects of drug over placebo treatments were shown [29].

Especially with regard to pharmacological interventions, desired effects partly were accompanied by increased occurrence of undesired adverse events. For example, Pandya et al. [31] demonstrated a reduction of hot flashes by about 37 and 38 % after treatment with oral clonidine for 4 and 8 weeks, respectively, in women with a history of breast cancer. In comparison, in the placebo arm, hot flashes decreased by about 20 % after 4 weeks and by about 24 % after 8 weeks. However, patients taking clonidine reported significantly more difficulties sleeping than patients in the placebo group [31].

These findings point out the challenge to compare and contrast not only the desired effects in active and placebo treatments, but also the risk of undesired side effects. Better knowledge about baseline symptom profiles would help to judge the course of symptom increases and decreases following either placebo or (variations of) active treatments and thus, support further clinical decision making about the most effective symptom management. Future studies should systematically assess and take into account the baselines for primary outcome measures such as hot flashes in addition to measures of the general health states.

Adverse Events in Placebo Groups

Adverse events were reported in most of the included trials in the review of Chvetzoff and Tannock [25]. Ten to sixty percent of patients in placebo conditions experienced distressing symptoms that were quite similar among trials, including nausea and vomiting, abdominal pain, lethargy, dry mouth, and diarrhea. An association could be found between the incidence and type of negative effects in the placebo groups and side effects in the treatment groups, thus pointing to the potential role of specific expectations about adverse symptom profiles in the development of nocebo effects. The authors discuss two potential mechanisms for the documented high rates of adverse effects in the placebo arms: First, they might have been accessory symptoms of the cancer itself (e.g., fatigue) that had been misattributed as adverse side effects of the treatment by the patients. Second, the authors consider the frequent occurrence of adverse events as a result of side effect anticipation [25], which would support the nocebo hypotheses [11]. A clear differentiation between these two suggestions is difficult because specific adverse event profiles are not reported. However, the subjective, more generalized character of most of the reported symptoms as well as the fact that these symptoms were experienced almost independently from the type of cancer is in line with the explanation of nocebo effects that might have contributed to the high incidence of adverse events in the placebo groups. Thus, in order to be able to clearly separate the alternative hypotheses, further studies are needed that assess both adverse events and patients' expectations of treatment effects in all trial arms.

Objective Measures in Placebo Groups

Changes in symptoms and in physiological parameters that are evident to the observer are categorized as more objective measures. In the context of cancer treatment, symptoms such as weight gain and improvement in performance status as well as tumor responses are examples for objective measures.

Weight Gain and Performance Status

Cancer-related anorexia and cachexia can have different physiological and psychological causes, and are associated with poor outcomes including reduced quality of life and poor performance [32]. Hence, many cancer treatments include weight gain as an objective to improve patients overall health status and health-related quality of life. The assessment of the patients' performance status is often used as an additional measure to quantify the subjective patient self-ratings of general well-being and health-related quality of life from a more objective perspective. Different scoring systems are available for operationalization, most commonly the Karnofsky performance status and the Eastern Cooperative Oncology Group scales [33].

In their review of placebo groups in cancer trials, Chvetzoff and Tannock [25] included 11 trials that had weight gain as one of their outcome measures. Thereby, different cut off criteria were used to define the effect in weight gain (e.g., weight gain of at least 5 % or at least 2 kg). Most of the altogether 678 and 544 assessable patients in the active treatment group and in the placebo group, respectively, suffered from advanced cancer. On the individual level, 7–17 % of the patients in the placebo arms of five trials met the respective criterion. On average group level, which was reported in six of the reviewed trials, there was net weight loss in the placebo arms. For comparison, in the active (most frequently: Megestrol acetate) treatment arms individual response rates ranged from 6 to 28 %. On average levels, weight improved in two, decreased in one, and remained stable in three trials for patients receiving pharmacological treatment. In one trial that compared active treatment with best supportive care, weight gain in 18 % of the 50 patients with non-small-cell lung cancer could be observed in the best supportive care arm [25].

Regarding physician -rated performance status, 6 and 14 % of 35 and 31 patients, respectively, showed improvement in the placebo arms of two trials that assessed individual response rates. Average levels of performance status remained either stable (six trials) or decreased (three trials). The same response pattern was found for the average performance level in the pharmacological treatment arms. Looking at the individual level (slightly) higher improvements in performance status were observed in patients receiving medication: 18 and 12 % of 72 and 87 patients, respectively. Performance status was also evaluated in five trials with a best supportive care control arm. On individual level, 4–19 % of altogether 238 patients were reported to have improved performance status. On average, there was a decrease in mean of performance status for the group receiving best supportive care in one trial [25].

Taken together, Chvetzoff and Tannock [25] show that on individual level improvements in weight gain and performance status can be observed with a placebo treatment. Response rates in the placebo and the best supportive care arms were quite similar and slightly but not substantial below the individual response rates in the pharmacological treatment arm. First, these results highlight the importance of a control arm to separate for drug specific and unspecific effects. Second, they raise the question about the underlying factors that actually contributed to the comparable individual improvements in both types of control arms. Receiving a pill alone can be excluded as the main factor as this would have lead to advantage of the placebo compared to the best supportive care arms. The supportive management, in turn, may itself have introduced placebo effects through the positive effects of the psychosocial context associated with the intent of controlling symptoms. On average level, there were no improvements in any of the included placebo or best supportive care arms. However, also patients receiving active treatment rarely improved neither in weight gain nor in performance status. Thus, there seem to be single individuals that benefit from receiving a drug, a placebo, or best supportive care while others experience worsening or do not response at all. This leads to the conclusion that, at least for the reviewed trials, there has not been any substantial specific treatment effect to improve weight gain and performance status.

Table 18.1 Symptom-improvement in randomized placebo-controlled cancer trials on individual and average level

Symptom [reference]	Treatment arm		Placebo arm	
	Trials	Response	Trials	Response
	Individual level (% patients)			
Fatigue [21]	Not specified		1	59 %
Nausea and vomiting [2]	11	17–100 %	11	0–74 %
Pain [25]	6	7–55 %	6	0–21 %
Weight gain [25]	5	6–28 %	5	7–17 %
Performance status [25]	2	12–18 %	2	6–14 %
Tumor responses [25]	10	0–37 %	10	0–7 %
	Group average level (number of trials)			
Pain [25]	6	2↑↑ 2↑ 2→	6	0↑↑ 2↑ 4→
Weight gain [25]	6	2↑ 3→ 1↓	6	0↑ 0→ 6↓
Performance status [25]	9	6→ 2↓ 1↓↓	9	6→ 3↓ 0↓↓

↑↑ overall measure improved substantially, ↑ overall measure improved, → overall measure remained stable, ↓ overall measure decreased, ↓↓ overall measure decreased rapidly

Tumor Responses

Ten of the randomized controlled clinical trials reviewed by Chvetzoff and Tannock [25] examined primarily objective tumor responses, which were either defined as a decreased tumor size according to the World Health Organization criteria (in seven trails), as a 50 % reduction of tumor diameter (in one trial), or as a reduction in levels of a serum marker for at least 50 % (two trials). In five trials, response rates following these criteria were reported in the placebo arms, ranging from 2 to 7 %; in the other five trials no placebo responses were shown. Thereby, the 7 % response rate that appeared in a trial for renal cell cancer was even higher than the response rate in the active treatment group with only 4 %. This trial, however, was excluded due to spontaneous regression that is known to occur in this type of tumor. Thus, the overall response rate to placebo decreased to 1.4 % of patients in placebo groups. Response rates in the active treatment groups using different medications were quite heterogeneous ranging from 2 to 37 %, with five additional

trials showing zero response. In one trial with best supportive care an objective tumor response was only observed in one of 191 patients [25].

To conclude, it appears that tumor responses are unusual in groups receiving placebo or best supportive care. This implies that higher response rates in controlled trials are more likely to be viewed as resulting from pharmacologic as placebo effects, especially if studies are double-blinded [7]. To further prove this hypothesis, the comparison of placebo versus treatment responses of several trials using the same pharmacological agent (more than one or two as it was the case in the reviewed results) would be helpful. In addition, the examination of systematic variations in the way agents are applied (e.g., with or without extra information about the desired effects or about the mode of pharmacological action) would be interesting, and besides, ethically justified (see "The Ethical Dilemma of Intervention") to test for placebo effects in tumor responses. An overview of the reviewed results is given in Table 18.1.

Psychological Mechanisms Underlying the Placebo and Nocebo Effects

A profound understanding of the mechanisms underlying the placebo and nocebo effects is crucial for the prediction of the conditions under which placebo and nocebo responses may occur. This in turn is essential to provide actual applications for daily health care. Various research results demonstrate evidence for two central mechanisms that are likely to play important roles in cancer research and across domains: expectations and classical conditioning.

Classical Conditioning

In the typical process of classical conditioning, a neutral stimulus, which on its own elicits no overt response, is presented along with a stimulus of some significance, the unconditioned stimulus (US), which normally evokes a certain response called unconditioned response (UCR). If the two stimuli are repeatedly paired, they eventually become associated. The previously neutral stimulus then constitutes a conditioned stimulus (CS) that also evokes a response: the conditioned response (CR) [34].

According to the nature of the context in which this form of associative learning occurs, it may result in both placebo and nocebo effects. For example, in case of medication one person may primarily associate positive experiences of symptom relief while another mainly has had stressful experiences of undesired side effects. These associations may be learned, activated outside of the individual's consciousness, and accompanied by changes in physiological processes, including both placebo and nocebo responses. Thereby, not only single features of the treatment but the whole therapeutic context and more generalized associations can serve as the conditions stimulus [1]. For example, about one-third of chemotherapy patients suffer from severe nausea just by meeting the infusion nurse or upon entering a room painted in the same color as the infusion room. Thus, previously neutral stimuli have been asso-

ciated with the aversive side effects of the chemotherapy [10].

Following the model of classical conditioning [34], the brain is not just able to automatically learn an association between the UCR and a CS but also to extinct the association if that pathway is neutralized. Thus, if a blue colored coffee bar used to cause nausea during the period of chemotherapy because the infusion room was colored in the same blue, this effect should subside some time after the chemotherapy has been finished. In fact, neither nocebo nor placebo responses do always fit these pattern. The occurrence of placebo and nocebo effects can remain far longer than extinction theories predict. On the other hand, an association that has been formed by frequent experiences can be reversed immediately just by a change of instruction [1].

Thus, although there is empirical support for classical conditioning to contribute to the placebo and nocebo effects, more complex cognitive processes also seem to be involved. Cognitive factors, such as patients' expectations about the potential beneficial and adverse treatment effects as well as their interaction with conditioning and learning experiences with prior treatments, need to be considered.

Patient Expectations

In the therapeutic context, treatment expectations refer to the cognitive representations of the desired and undesired effects related to a specific treatment. These internal beliefs and expectations are thought to accompany changes in endogenous processes associated with the placebo or the nocebo response. Thereby, they actually raise the probability of the treatment outcomes the patient had hoped for or had been afraid of [35].

Within the self-regulation model of health [36], expectations about illness and treatment have been shown to predict illness behavior and medication adherence in breast cancer [37]. In addition to conscious expectations, automatic processes are especially relevant to side effect reporting [38]. Response expectations reflect automatic processes that are specific for unvolitional outcome (e.g., the expectation that one will become nauseated) [39]. Robust associations between response expectations and side effects have recently been demonstrated in cancer patients, with highest correlations for pain ($r=0.58$), followed by fatigue ($r=0.46$) and nausea ($r=0.32$) [40].

Several studies present empirical evidence for the role of patients' expectations in the development of post chemotherapy nausea [41–44]. Patients who expect to suffer from nausea following chemotherapy are significantly more likely to experience nausea than patients who did not anticipate such symptoms. Age, gender, and education level seem to influence these treatment side effect expectations. Patients aged younger than 60 years, female patients and patients with higher education expect more symptoms than older patients, male patients, and patients with lower education level [45]. Thereby, it has been shown that the association between expected and experienced nausea seems not to depend on the specific characteristics of the chemotherapy treatment [44].

Negative expectations of treatment appear to raise the individual's attention to the cues he or she is being afraid of. This in turn can lead to the tendency to misinterpret preexisting, ambiguous somatic sensations adversely, and to attribute them to the medication, while changes that might actually be positive remain unnoticed [10, 46]. In analogy, positive expectations are likely to shape perception focused on cues related to symptom relief and healing [35]. This biased somatic focus can be seen as a kind of feedback that supports factors underlying placebo and nocebo responding [5]. Therefore, the degree of somatic focus is assumed to have a moderating influence on the role of expectations in health [47].

Conditioning versus Expectation: An Integrative Point of View

It is difficult to determine the relative contributions of expectation and conditioning for placebo or nocebo effects, because they are unlikely to operate independently. It seems rather plausible

that conditioning processes and expectation are somehow entangled within placebo and nocebo effects [48]. In one possible view, conditioning may be defined as a process that contributes to the generation of expectations [49], for example through prior own or witnesses experiences with the positive and adverse effects of specific treatments of medication. In this case, a person who feels sick in an infusion room, because the features of this room have been associated with the specific side effects of the infusion, may expect to have this symptom in this context in future. In another model, conditioning may be seen as a result of expectation-induced effects: the higher a person's actual expectation with regard to a specific context, the greater is the expectation effect, and the greater are the potential future conditioning effects that are associated with the context [48]. With regard to the latter example, a patient might expect to feel sick during infusion because somebody told her before, and thereby, becomes more likely to actually feel sick (see Fig. 18.2).

Links to Neurobiological and Immunological Responses

Not all physiological processes are equally likely to be affected by conditioning and expectation. Depending on the pharmacological agent used for preconditioning, different placebo or nocebo responses can be produced [48]. Variations in hormone secretion [50] and suppressive effects on immunological parameters [51] are typical examples of physiological responses associated with conditioned placebo and nocebo effects, respectively. It appears that these endocrine and immunological changes cannot be manipulated by verbally induced expectations. In contrast, verbal suggestions have been shown to affect and even reverse conditioned outcomes that can be directly experienced by the individual such as variation in pain and motor performance [50]. These findings lead to the assumption that conditioning is more significant in mediating placebo and nocebo effects when unconscious physiological functions are the primary outcome, whereas expectations

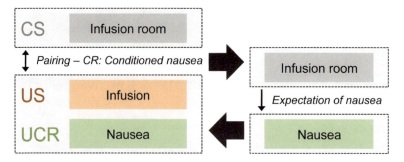

Fig. 18.2 The two central mechanisms of conditioning and expectation may be entangled within placebo and nocebo effects. For example, to feel nauseated just by entering the chemotherapy-infusion room initially could be a result of either conditioning (*left-hand side*) or expectation (*right-hand side*). Interaction of both processes in the further development and maintaining of the symptom is likely

may play the dominant role for placebo- and nocebo-related effects to occur if outcome measures can be directly perceived [35, 50].

Since verbally induced analgesic responses have been shown to be naloxone sensitive [52], a strong role of opioids in expectation-based placebo effects is suggested. Recent results of neuroimaging research indicate that placebo treatment has broad effects on opioid activity in cortical and subcortical regions as well as on their functional connectivity [53]. Furthermore, verbally induced hyperalgesic effects have been found to be associated to hyperactivity of the hypothalamic-pituitary-adrenal (HPA) axis. This nocebo effect has shown to be blocked by the application of benzodiazepine diazepam and the cholecystokinin (CCK) antagonist proglumide. Thereby, diazepam antagonized both HPA hyperactivity and hyperalgesia, whereas proglumide did not affect HPA axis but still blocked nocebo hyperalgesia. These findings indicate that the CCK antagonist is not likely to operate on the direct pathway of nocebo-induced anxiety but rather affects anxiety-induced hyperalgesia, whereas the anxiolytic drug is assumed to directly act on nocebo-induced anxiety [26]. However, these results support the existence of a CCK-dependent link between anticipatory anxiety and pain [10, 26]. The hypothesis that nocebo hyperalgesia is primarily produced through an affective–cognitive pain pathway could be confirmed by the findings of a recent neuroimaging study that examined neuronal correlates of expectancy-induced hyperalgesic effects.

Many brain regions observed in this study either belonged to the pain network or are known to play an important role in processing the affective components of pain [54].

Besides opioids and CCK, the role of the neurotransmitter dopamine in placebo and nocebo responses has received increasing attention. Dopamine release in the nucleus accumbens, a region associated with reward processing, correlates with opioid release in anticipation of pain under placebo treatment [1]. Therefore, it also plays a role in placebo analgesia. On the contrary, a deactivated dopamine release in the nucleus accumbens has been found during nocebo hyperalgesia [48]. To determine if or how exactly dopaminergic mechanisms are involved in the placebo and nocebo responses across domains, more research is needed. However, if placebo and nocebo responses are actually associated with dopaminergic reward pathways, the examination of the degree of how outcomes can be modified by changes in affective and motivational states may help in a priori decision whether placebo treatments will be effective or not [1].

To conclude, several physiological processes are identified to be associated with the placebo and nocebo effects, respectively. Until now, the central pain-modulating circuits are in the focus of the placebo and nocebo researches and provide reliable results using neuroimaging methodologies more recently. Studies that investigate the physiological correlates of placebo and nocebo effects explicitly in cancer patients have—to our best knowledge—not been conducted until today. Pain, however, also plays a major role in cancer treatment (see "Cancer-related Pain"). A better understanding of the physiological underpinnings of placebo and nocebo effects in the field of pain, thus, is also relevant in oncology. The neurochemical substrates assumed to be mainly involved in the placebo- and nocebo-related analgesic and hyperalgesic effects, respectively, are endogenous opioids, CCK, and dopamine. To examine not only one of these neurophysiological correlates, but to look at their interacting processes resulting from (changes of) the treatment context and associated psychological mechanisms may help to shed more light on the interindividual differences of placebo and nocebo responding, and thus, allow a more adaptive (cancer) treatment approach.

Clinical Relevance of Placebo and Nocebo in Cancer Treatment

The Role of Information and Personal Interaction

The information a patient receives about a treatment can modify his or her expectations of the treatment outcome and therefore affect his or her response [55]. Verbal instructions that can alter expectations may either be hopeful and trust-inducing or fearful and stress-inducing [56]. In the former case the placebo effect is supported by positive expectations, in the latter negative expectations increase the likelihood of nocebo effects (see Fig. 18.3). However, if negative expectations can contribute to the experience of adverse effects and affect health negatively, how then should patients be informed regarding the possibility of specific side effects without causing harm?

First of all it has to be noted that the instructions by the provider usually do not constitute the only source of information. The mass media, the Internet, or advertisement of pharmaceuticals provides a wide range of opportunities to receive treatment information [10]. This may be quite helpful and supporting for patients who are able to single out relevant details of interest. But in order to handle the potential overload of facts from an objective point of view, patient's actually needs some kind of specific expertise. This can enable the patient not just to evaluate and integrate the pieces of information different sources may provide, but also to value the quality of the informational source itself. A lot of patients are not in that position. Sometimes, they hear about their type of diseases or the recommended treatment for the first time of their life. In these cases, incorrect or biased information, misunderstandings, and uncertainty may contribute to anxiety, doubts, and suspicions about the treatment. This in turn can cause a sense of vulnerability and further increase the likelihood of nocebo responses such as reviewed above. In a study that examined the efficacy of TENS versus TSE in a placebo-controlled trial in women with chronic pain following breast cancer treatment (reviewed under "Cancer-related Pain") [23], the majority of women reported great benefit just from the opportunity to discuss their pain problems in detail. Thereby, the researchers identified an important clinical need especially as most of the women reported to be dissatisfied with prior consultations and the amount of received information about the potential causes of their pain and treatment options. Since the two active treatment arms did not differ in reduced pain report and anxiety scores, nor did the placebo arm, the personal interaction including the therapeutic value of getting the pain problems validated is discussed as one plausible reason for overall improvements [23].

As some patients may feel uneasy to express suspicions about their treatment by themselves, the physicians or therapists should encourage the patients explicitly to openly discuss the results of their own research including hopes, wishes but also their concerns. The goal should be to provide a clear and realistic understanding of a given condition and the treatment recommended. With regard to negative messages including potential side effects of cancer therapy, the way in which they are framed may affect the overall outcome [10]. Understanding which side effects may appear and why, for example in the context of pharmacological responses, may change the patients appraisal of side effects. Furthermore, the way

Fig. 18.3 Information
about a treatment can
affect treatment response
due to placebo and nocebo
effects, respectively. Hope
and trust in treatment are
associated with a positive
health outcome and are
thought to be mediated by
different physiological
pathways like neuronal
increase of opioids and
dopamine. Anxiety and
insecurity, on the
conotrary, are associated
with a CCK-ergic
facilitaion of pain and
increases in cortisol that
may lead to more negative
health outcomes. *CCK*
cholecystokinin

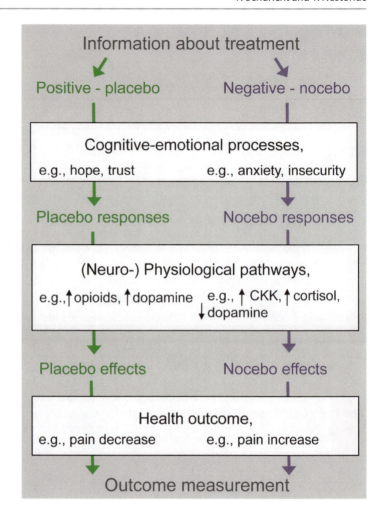

how bad news about the cancer diagnosis is disclosed to the patients has been shown to have major impact on several clinical outcomes [57], including the patients' level of hopefulness [58] and subsequent psychological adjustment [59, 60]. In a recent study of our research group in Marburg [61] we used a systematic measure according to the SPIKES-Protocol (Six-Step Protocol for Delivering Bad News) [57] to ask 370 patients with prior diagnosed cancer about their main preferences with regard to "breaking the bad news" of their cancer diagnosis. We found that factors such as to understand the diagnosis, to have adequate time to talk to the doctor, the possibility to ask questions, and to be reassured and feel understood are most important to the patients. Less than half of the patients reported

to be satisfied with how the diagnosis of cancer had been communicated to them, and significant differences between the patients' wishes and the experienced reality could be shown. These results point out the huge gap between the way diagnosis are communicated and the patients' preferences [61].

Providing objective information about cancer treatment also implicates an education regarding the desired effects for which a treatment is actually recommended. In order to induce positive expectations in patients, it is relevant to choose clear and understandable instructions. Certain expectations of therapeutic benefit have in turn been associated with larger placebo responses compared to uncertain expectations [62]. Furthermore, it has also been shown that negative treatment-related expectations in patients induced by their providers are associated with subsequent clinical worsening and nocebo effects [63].

Thus, a verbally induced belief regarding the therapeutic outcome likely seems to trigger the mechanisms underlying the placebo and nocebo effects, respectively, and thereby actually contributes to either positive or negative outcomes. As many patients probably see their health care providers as one basic authority in who they do trust, both the quality of information given to the patients and the way of how it is given obtain an important role.

The Ethical Dilemma of Intervention

A randomized controlled design is the gold standard to examine the safety and effectiveness of a new intervention. Thereby, either an active control or a placebo is used in the control arm. In oncology, placebos have been applied far less frequently compared to other therapeutic areas. This is mostly due to ethical concerns associated with placebo use in cancer trials [64]. Some groups of cancer physicians, patients, and ethicists consider placebo-controlled trials unethical whenever any active treatment is available. Other fractions argue to permit placebo controls if certain methodologic and ethical criteria are both fulfilled. Daugherty et al. [64] provide an overview of guidelines regarding the appropriate use of placebos in cancer clinical trials.

First of all, from a methodological point of view, placebos may be only justified to control for unspecific effects that may bias information regarding the efficacy of the intervention. In conditions where high placebo response rates, high symptom fluctuation, or spontaneous remissions are unlikely to occur, single-arm trials may be adequate. A significant tumor response rate, for example, is more considered as a direct effect of the treatment and probably less likely to be influenced by placebo effects (see "Tumor Responses") [7, 64].

Second, under the given circumstances of no available effective standard treatment for a given cancer diagnoses, the use of placebos seems more acceptable. For these cancer patients, the risk-benefit ratio may be reasonable, and is in line with clinical equipoise. Equipoise means not to be sure about which of two or more interventions is most safe and effective, and is viewed as the most widely accepted ethical justification for randomized controlled trials [64, 65]. Additional for the trial to be ethical, patients in the placebo arm must also receive best supportive care. On the contrary, when a treatment is available that is likely to prevent serious harm the use of placebo controls is generally unethical. Daughtery et al. [64] point to the placebo-controlled trials in the late 1980s and early 1990s as such an "ethical dilemma" because with metoclopramide there had already been an effective treatment available.

Third, in some trial designs patients become unblinded to the intervention they receive if their disease takes progress, and get changed to the active intervention when they had been receiving placebo before. This procedure provides an attempt to reduce concerns especially of the patients with their decision to participate in the randomized placebo-controlled trial or not. Potential participants, as a fourth point, always have to be fully disclosed regarding the usage of a placebo control in the trial [64].

Ethical issues not only arise with the usage of placebos in the control-arms of randomized trials. It is even more critical to provide clear advice for the explicit use of placebos for treatment without deception. Finnis et al. [48] discuss the option of full disclosure which would be fulfilled by telling the patient that a placebo is given, that the placebo has no active drug in it, but is thought to be working through psychological mechanisms that are likely to promote symptom relief. How such a kind of placebo disclosure may affect placebo responses is still mostly unclear [48].

Summary, Recommendations, and Conclusions

The field of placebo research is both challenging and promising at the same time. In this chapter, we first pointed out the importance of well-designed controlled trials to actually differentiate the true placebo and nocebo effects from unspecific influences. In clinical research, however, biasing influences can hardly be eliminated completely. Taking this into consideration, it is necessary to control for potential biases. One rather effective strategy to control for potential biases is to try to match the respective treatment arms with respect to all possible factors apart from the active substance or procedure under evaluation. For example, this can be done by applying same best supportive care in all trial arms with additional placebo and active pill application in the placebo and the pharmacologic treatment arm, respectively, and no additional application in the best supportive care arm. Thereby, the influences of attention and patient–caretaker interaction time can be controlled.

In some cases, however, potential biases can hardly to be controlled. This is for example due to the ethical need to inform every patient in a clinical trial about the likelihood of receiving the active or the control treatment. This may a priory decrease the strength of positive expectations compared to double-blinded laboratory trials [66]. Therefore, it might be helpful to assess the patients' treatment expectations independently from the study design. Furthermore, we pointed out that the patients' concerns about their disease and its treatment should be openly discussed to reduce negative emotional states. Anxiety, for example, has been shown to be likely involved in placebo responding.

Effects in placebo groups of cancer trials have been predominantly found with the more subjective symptoms, like pain, nausea, and fatigue. Especially placebo analgesic effects become more and more established. It seems that regarding these subjective outcomes the influence of expectations, one of the basic placebo and nocebo mechanisms, is more powerful because conscious expectation may likely form conscious symptom experiences. For study objectives that are not directly accessible to the patients' perception, such as immunological changes, conditioning as the second central mechanism may be more meaningful. With account to the reviewed trials examining tumor responses, there have been no significant effects in the placebo arms. It has to

be noted, however, that no long-term changes have been reported for any of the trial arms including active treatments. Thus, future studies are needed to evaluate long-term health developments and, furthermore, to investigate the benefit-risk ratios of different treatment options for cancer-related symptoms and tumor responses.

Taken together we conclude that especially with more subjective conditions there is evidence that indicates the potential role the placebo and nocebo effects can have in the context of cancer treatment. However, further well-designed clinical studies are needed to confirm these first findings. As the interpretation of effects in placebo groups is often limited by methodological and ethical aspects, researcher are to be encouraged to use alternative paradigms, focusing more on the possible variations of the treatment context. Thereby, we believe understanding of the placebo and nocebo effects in cancer patients can be advanced, with the primary aim of enhancing placebo while decreasing nocebo effects, and thus, improve patient care and quality of life.

References

1. Atlas LY, Wager TD, William PB. The placebo response. Encyclopedia of consciousness. Oxford: Academic Press; 2009:201–16.
2. Zhang Z, Wang Y, Wang Y, Xu F. Antiemetic placebo: reduce adverse drug interactions between chemotherapeutic agents and antiemetic drugs in cancer patients. Med Hypotheses. 2008;70(3):551–5.
3. Edward SJL, Stevens AJ, Braunholtz DA, Lilford RJ, Swift T. The ethics of placebo-controlled trials: a comparison of inert and active placebo controls. World J Surg. 2005;29(5):610–4.
4. Aronson J. Please, please me. BMJ. 1999; 318(7185):716.
5. Price DD, Finniss DG, Benedetti F. A comprehensive review of the placebo effect: recent advances and current thought. Annu Rev Psychol. 2008;59(1):565–90.
6. Miller FG, Kaptchuk TJ. The power of context: reconceptualizing the placebo effect. J R Soc Med. 2008;101(5):222–5.
7. Temple RJ. Implications of effects in placebo groups. J Natl Cancer Inst. 2003;95(1):2.
8. Kennedy WP. The nocebo reaction. Med World. 1961;95:203–5.
9. Enck P, Benedetti F, Schedlowski M. New insights into the placebo and nocebo responses. Neuron. 2008;59(2):195–206.

10. Barsky AJ, Saintfort R, Rogers MP, Borus JF. Nonspecific medication side effects and the nocebo phenomenon. JAMA. 2002;287:622–7.

11. Hahn RA. The nocebo phenomenon: concept, evidence, and implications for public health. Prev Med. 1997;26:607–11.

12. Colloca L, Petrovic P, Wager TD, Ingvar M, Benedetti F. How the number of learning trials affects placebo and nocebo responses. Pain. 2010;151(2):430–9.

13. Shepherd M. The placebo: from specificity to the non-specific and back. Psychol Med. 1993;23(03):569–78.

14. Rief W, Nestoriuc Y, von Lilienfeld-Toal A, et al. Differences in adverse effect reporting in placebo groups in SSRI and tricyclic antidepressant trials: a systematic review and meta-analysis. Drug Saf. 2009;32:1041–56.

15. Rief W, Avorn J, Barsky AJ. Medication-attributed adverse effects in placebo groups: implications for assessment of adverse effects. Arch Intern Med. 2006;166(2):155–60.

16. Amanzio M, Corazzini LL, Vase L, Benedetti F. A systematic review of adverse events in placebo groups of anti-migraine clinical trials. Pain. 2009;146(3):261–9.

17. National Comprehensive Cancer Network. Cancer related fatigue. Clinical practice guidelines in oncology. Fort Washington, PA: National Comprehensive Cancer Network; 2011.

18. Cella D, Davis K, Breitbart W, Curt G. Cancer-related fatigue: prevalence of proposed diagnostic criteria in a United States sample of cancer survivors. J Clin Oncol. 2001;19(14):3385.

19. Minton O, Richardson A, Sharpe M, Hotopf M, Stone PC. Psychostimulants for the management of cancer-related fatigue: a systematic review and meta-analysis. J Pain Symptom Manage. 2011;41(4):761–7.

20. Wagner LI, Cella D. Fatigue and cancer: causes, prevalence and treatment approaches. Br J Cancer. 2004;91(5):822–8.

21. de la Cruz M, Hui D, Parsons HA, Bruera E. Placebo and nocebo effects in randomized double-blind clinical trials of agents for the therapy for fatigue in patients with advanced cancer. Cancer. 2010;116(3):766–74.

22. Schwartzberg L. Chemotherapy-induced nausea and vomiting: state of the art in 2006. J Support Oncol. 2006;4(2 Suppl 1):3–8.

23. Robb KA, Newham DJ, Williams JE. Transcutaneous electrical nerve stimulation vs transcutaneous spinal electroanalgesia for chronic pain associated with breast cancer treatments. J Pain Symptom Manage. 2007;33(4):410–9.

24. Eija k, Tiina T, Pertti J N. Amitriptyline effectively relieves neuropathic pain following treatment of breast cancer. Pain. 1996;64(2):293–302.

25. Chvetzoff Gl, Tannock IF. Placebo effects in oncology. J Natl Cancer Inst. 2003;95(1):19–29.

26. Benedetti F, Amanzio M, Vighetti S, Asteggiano G. The biochemical and neuroendocrine bases of the hyperalgesic nocebo effect. J Neurosci. 2006;26(46): 12014–22.

27. Finck G, Barton DL, Loprinzi CL, Quella SK, Sloan JA. Definitions of hot flashes in breast cancer survivors. J Pain Symptom Manage. 1998;16(5):327–33.

28. Kaplan M, Mahon S, Cope D, Keating E, Hill S, Jacobson M. Putting evidence into practice: evidence-based interventions for hot flashes resulting from cancer therapies. Clin J Oncol Nurs. 2011;15(2):149–57.

29. Boekhout AH, Beijnen JH, Schellens JHM. Symptoms and treatment in cancer therapy-induced early menopause. Oncologist. 2006;11(6):641.

30. Sloan JA, Loprinzi CL, Novotny PJ, Barton DL, Lavasseur BI, Windschitl H. Methodologic lessons learned from hot flash studies. J Clin Oncol. 2001;19(23):4280–90.

31. Pandya KJ, Raubertas RF, Flynn PJ, et al. Oral clonidine in postmenopausal patients with breast cancer experiencing tamoxifen-induced hot flashes: a University of Rochester Cancer Center Community Clinical Oncology Program study. Ann Intern Med. 2000;132(10):788.

32. Inui A. Cancer anorexia cachexia syndrome: current issues in research and management. CA Cancer J Clin. 2002;52(2):72–91.

33. Conill C, Verger E, Salamero M. Performance status assessment in cancer patients. Cancer. 1990;65(8): 1864–6.

34. Pavlov IP. Conditional reflexes. an investigation of the psychological activity of the cerebral cortex. London: Oxford University Press; 1927.

35. Colloca L, Miller FG. Role of expectations in health. Curr Opin Psychiatry. 2011;24(2):149.

36. Leventhal H, Nerenz D, Steele DJ. Illness representations and coping with health threats. In: Baum A, Taylor SE, Singer JE, editors. Handbook of Psychology and Health. Volume IV. Social Psychology aspects of health. Hillsdale, NJ: Erlbaum; 1984. p. 219–52.

37. Rozema H, Völlink T, Lechner L. The role of illness representations in coping and health of patients treated for breast cancer. Psychooncology. 2009;18(8): 849–57.

38. Roscoe JA, Jean-Pierre P, Shelke AR, Kaufman ME, Bole C, Morrow GR. The role of patients' response expectancies in side effect development and control. Curr Problem Cancer. 2006;30(2):40–98.

39. Kirsch I. Response expectancy theory and application: a decennial review. Appl Prev Psychol. 1997;6: 69–79.

40. Sohl SJ, Schnur JB, Montgomery GH. A meta-analysis of the relationship between response expectancies and cancer treatment-related side effects. J Pain Symptom Manage. 2009;38(5):775–84.

41. Hitckok JT, Roscoe JA, Morrow GR. The role of patients expectations in the developement of anticipatory nausea related to chemotherapy for cancer. J Pain Symptom Manage. 2001;22(4):843–50.

42. Colagiuri B, Roscoe JA, Morrow GR, Atkins JN, Giguere JK, Colman LK. How do patient expectancies, quality of life, and postchemotherapy nausea interrelate? Cancer. 2008;113(3):654–61.

43. Higgins S, Montgomery G, Bovbjerg D. Distress before chemotherapy predicts delayed but not acute nausea. Support Care Cancer. 2007;15(2):171–7.

44. Roscoe JA, Hickok JT, Morrow GR. Patient expectations as predictor of chemotherapy-induced nausea. Ann Behav Med. 2000;22(2):121–6.

45. Hofman M, Morrow GR, Roscoe JA, et al. Cancer patients' expectations of experiencing treatment-related side effects. Cancer. 2004;101(4):851–7.

46. Rief W, Broadbent E. Explaining medically unexplained symptoms-models and mechanisms. Clin Psychol Rev. 2007;27(7):821–41.

47. Geers AL, Weiland PE, Kosbab K, Landry SJ, Helfer SG. Goal activation, expectations, and the placebo effect. J Pers Soc Psychol. 2005;89(2):143.

48. Finniss DG, Kaptchuk TJ, Miller F, Benedetti F. Biological, clinical, and ethical advances of placebo effects. Lancet. 2010;375(9715):686–95.

49. Colloca L, Sigaudo M, Benedetti F. The role of learning in nocebo and placebo effects. Pain. 2008; 136(1–2):211–8.

50. Benedetti F, Pollo A, Lopiano L, Lanotte M, Vighetti S, Rainero I. Conscious expectation and unconscious conditioning in analgesic, motor, and hormonal placebo/nocebo responses. J Neurosci. 2003;23(10):4315–23.

51. Goebel MU, Trebst AE, Steiner JAN, et al. Behavioral conditioning of immunosuppression is possible in humans. FASEB J. 2002;16(14):1869.

52. Levine J, Gordon N, Fields H. The mechanisms of placebo analgesia. Lancet. 1978;312(8091):654–7.

53. Wager TD, Scott DJ, Zubieta J-K. Placebo effects on human Î¼-opioid activity during pain. Proc Natl Acad Sci. 2007;104(26):11056–61.

54. Kong J, Gollub RL, Polich G, et al. A functional magnetic resonance imaging study on the neural mechanisms of hyperalgesic nocebo effect. J Neurosci. 2008;28(49):13354–62.

55. Flaten MA, Simonsen T, Olsen H. Drug-related information generates placebo and nocebo responses that modify the drug response. Psychosom Med. 1999;61(2):250–5.

56. Moerman DE, Jonas WB. Deconstructing the placebo effect and finding the meaning response. Ann Intern Med. 2002;136(6):471–6.

57. Baile WF, Buckman R, Lenzi R, Glober G, Beale EA, Kudelka AP. SPIKES – a six-step protocol for delivering bad news: application to the patient with cancer. Oncologist. 2000;5(4):302–11.

58. Sardell AN, Trierweiler SJ. Disclosing the cancer diagnosis. Procedures that influence patient hopefulness. Cancer. 1993;72(11):3355–65.

59. Roberts CS, Cox CE, Reintgen DS, Baile WF, Gibertini M. Influence of physician communication on newly diagnosed breast patients' psychologic adjustment and decision making. Cancer. 1994; 74(S1):336–41.

60. Last BF, Van Veldhuizen AMH. Information about diagnosis and prognosis related to anxiety and depression in children with cancer aged 8–16 years. Eur J Cancer. 1996;32(2):290–4.

61. Stumpenhorst M, Seifart C, Seifart U, Rief W. Breaking bad news badly? -Wie Krebsdiagnosen Patienten vermittelt werden. Poster presented at the 7th Workshopcongress of the German Psychological Society (Clinical Psychology and Psychotherapy Section), Berlin, Germany; 2011.

62. Pollo A, Amanzio M, Arslanian A, Casadio C, Maggi G, Benedetti F. Response expectancies in placebo analgesia and their clinical relevance. Pain. 2001; 93(1):77–84.

63. Benedetti F, Lanotte M, Lopiano L, Colloca L. When words are painful: unraveling the mechanisms of the nocebo effect. Neuroscience. 2007;147(2):260–71.

64. Daugherty CK, Ratain MJ, Emanuel EJ, Farrell AT, Schilsky RL. Ethical, scientific, and regulatory perspectives regarding the use of placebos in cancer clinical trials. J Clin Oncol. 2008;26(8):1371–8.

65. Freedman B. Equipoise and the ethics of clinical research. Bioethics Anthol. 1999;317(3):45.

66. Rief W. Lessons to be learned from placebo groups in clinical trials. Pain. 2011;152(8):1693–94.

Psychological Factors and Survivorship: A Focus on Post-treatment Cancer Survivors

19

Ellen Burke Beckjord, Kerry A. Reynolds, and Ruth Rechis

Psychological Factors and Survivorship: A Focus on Post-treatment Cancer Survivors

Since a "war on cancer" was declared in the 1970s, research and clinical services focused on psychological factors in cancer have followed closely behind medical and epidemiological advances in cancer prevention and control. The field of psycho-oncology, developed to specifically address the "human experience" of cancer (including psychological and emotional experiences), emerged about 10 years after the "war on cancer" began, and has been an extremely active area of empirical study and clinical care ever since [1, 2]. Over the past decade in particular, as the number of people alive in the United States with a personal history of cancer surpassed the 10 million mark, psycho-oncology research and practice has increasingly focused on the *post-treatment* phase of the cancer trajectory [3–5]. Figure 19.1 shows the growth in the number of cancer survivors alive in the United States today

over the first decade of the new millennium [6], with a sample of key events that have occurred in psycho-oncology emblematic of the increase in attention paid to life after cancer treatment ends.

The events highlighted in Fig. 19.1 represent significant progress in understanding the experiences of post-treatment cancer survivors, and the variety of research and clinical efforts that are underway to ensure that our health care system is prepared to meet the needs of this population of nearly 12 million (and growing) people. The Biennial Cancer Survivorship conferences held by the National Cancer Institute's (NCI) Office of Cancer Survivorship [7], in collaboration with the American Cancer Society (ACS), the Centers for Disease Control and Prevention (CDC), and LIVE*STRONG* (the Lance Armstrong Foundation) have created a consistent setting for showcasing cutting-edge research and care practices devoted to post-treatment cancer survivors. The LIVE*STRONG* Survivorship Centers of Excellence represent a platform of diverse cancer centers from which we will derive new knowledge about best practices in post-treatment survivorship care [8]. Peer-reviewed publications, including *Journal of Clinical Oncology* and *Journal of Cancer Survivorship*, have been created or devoted entire special issues to survivorship care, with an emphasis on the post-treatment period [9, 10]. Surveillance research to document the experiences of post-treatment cancer survivors has been established by LIVE*STRONG* [11, 12]; ACS [13], and the CDC, with the inclusion of a cancer survivorship module in the

E.B. Beckjord, Ph.D., M.P.H. (✉)
Department of Psychiatry, Biobehavioral Medicine in Oncology Program, University of Pittsburgh, Pittsburgh, PA, USA

K.A. Reynolds, Ph.D.
RAND Corporation, Santa Monica, CA, United States

R. Rechis, Ph.D.
Evaluation and Research, LIVESTRONG, Austin, TX, USA

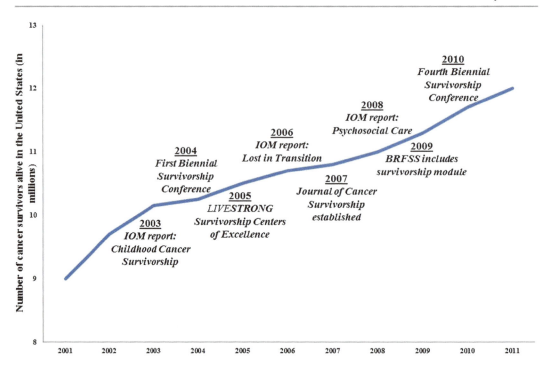

Fig. 19.1 Key post-treatment survivorship events of the past decade

annual Behavioral Risk Factors and Surveillance System survey starting in 2009 [14]. Finally, in the past decade, three landmark reports were released by the Institute of Medicine (IOM): one focused on post-treatment survivorship for pediatric cancers [15]; one devoted exclusively to the transition out of primary treatment for cancer and into post-treatment survivorship [16]; and the third focused on the need for psychosocial care across the cancer trajectory, including the post-treatment survivorship phase [17].

One broad conclusion from the past decade of work devoted to understanding the post-treatment experiences of cancer survivors is that there are numerous physical, emotional, and practical challenges encountered in the post-treatment period [5, 11]; that these challenges are distinct from the experiences people have earlier in the cancer trajectory, near time of diagnosis or during treatment [16, 18]; and require further study to adequately characterize and clinically address [4, 19, 20]. Indeed, even for cancers such as breast cancer—which has been extensively studied from psychological and psychosocial perspectives—we know much more about the psycho-oncology of time near diagnosis and during treatment compared to what we understand about the post-treatment period [21].

This chapter is focused on the psychological experiences of adult post-treatment cancer survivors, which are not as well described or understood in the literature as the physical long-term and late effects of cancer and its treatment [22]. The psychological component of post-treatment cancer survivorship has been referred to by a variety of terms, including psychological health (e.g., [23]); quality of life (e.g., [22]); mental health-related quality of life (e.g., [24, 25]); psychosocial factors (e.g., [21]); depression (e.g., [26]); and broader characterizations of symptoms of depression, anxiety, and post-traumatic stress disorder (PTSD) (e.g., [27]). Here, we will consider a broad range of "psychological factors," certainly not restricted to psychological or psychiatric disorders, but more generally a range of emotionally relevant experiences that may cause stress, distress, or disruption in the post-treatment period. As such, we will use terms like "psychological concerns," "distress," "emotional disruption," and the like interchangeably.

At this point, it is worth noting two areas that will not be included in this chapter. There is evidence that *positive* psychological experiences in post-treatment cancer survivorship, such as post-traumatic growth, will not be reviewed in this chapter, though do represent important psychological factors in cancer survivorship [23, 28] and are commonly encountered in the post-treatment phase. Kornblith et al. [29] found that 75 % of post-treatment ovarian cancer survivors reported that cancer had had at least one positive impact on their life. Bellizzi et al. [30] found about the same percentage of survivors of non-Hodgkin lymphoma (NHL) reported the same. Yet Bellizzi et al. [30] also found that a similar percentage of post-treatment NHL survivors said cancer had been responsible for at least one negative impact, and that this, rather than positive impact, was associated with (poorer) HRQOL. Other studies have found different results with associations between post-traumatic growth and more positive psychological outcomes for cancer survivors (e.g., [31]). Overall, we have a better understanding of psychopathology and negative psychological experiences in the context of cancer than we do for positive psychological experiences, and continued methodological and psychometric research is needed to advance what we know about positive psychological outcomes associated with cancer, and in particular, how to promote positive psychological experiences in the post-treatment period [32].

Second, the literature reviewed and data presented will focus on post-treatment survivors of cancers diagnosed in adulthood. Post-treatment survivors of childhood cancers certainly encounter psychological challenges—particularly survivors of central nervous system tumors (compared to hematological malignancies)—and with some evidence that post-treatment psychological adjustment is worse among women, survivors who were treated with cranial radiation therapy, or who were diagnosed at younger ages [15, 33]. Because the epidemiology of cancer and its treatment for pediatric oncology is relatively distinct from cancers diagnosed during adulthood, this review will focus on post-treatment survivors of adult cancer diagnoses.

Though post-treatment survivorship is an evolving field of inquiry and clinical care [34], there is evidence that psychological concerns are under-addressed in the post-treatment phase [4, 16, 17, 21, 35], with estimates indicating that as many as half of post-treatment cancer survivors do not receive the help they need for emotional or psychological concerns (e.g., [29]). Understanding the psychological experiences of post-treatment cancer survivors is critical to ensuring that our health care system can better respond to the needs of this growing group. This chapter is divided into three sections: first, we briefly review the literature on the psychological, emotional, and psychosocial experiences of post-treatment cancer survivors, a literature comparatively smaller than studies focused on individuals newly diagnosed or in-treatment (beyond the scope of this chapter). Second, we describe methods and results of a unique data source, the 2010 LIVE*STRONG* Survey for People Affected by Cancer, which provides one of the largest samples of post-treatment cancer survivors' emotional concerns. Finally, we turn to the 2006 and 2008 IOM reports [16, 17] to derive recommendations for addressing psychological factors in survivorship, given the results of the literature to date and the new data provided by the LIVE*STRONG* survey.

Psychological Factors in Post-treatment Cancer Survivorship: A Brief Review

What Do We Know About the Types and Levels of Psychological Distress Encountered in Post-treatment Survivorship?

It is important to begin any review of psychological factors in post-treatment cancer survivorship with an overarching conclusion that has been revealed in numerous studies on the topic: there is no evidence that most post-treatment cancer survivors experience clinically significant levels of emotional distress (i.e., meet diagnostic criteria for a psychiatric disorder) [4, 22–24, 27–29, 35–37]. Further, it is important to qualify this broad conclusion with two other commonly encountered results: there are a not-insignificant number of post-treatment cancer survivors who, though a minority, encounter psychological, psychosocial, and emotional concerns in the post-treatment period that are disruptive and cause for concern [11, 38–43] and the trajectories of psychological experiences of post-treatment cancer survivors are highly idiographic; that is, highly variable and related to a number of pre-morbid, disease, treatment, and post-treatment factors [19, 35, 36].

Estimates of emotional distress, such as moderate to severe symptoms of anxiety and depression, among post-treatment cancer survivors of multiple cancer types range from in the neighborhood of 15–20 % (e.g., [40]); to 20–30 % (e.g., [39, 41, 44, 45]); and even as high as greater than 40 % (e.g., [42]). Emotional issues typically rank high in lists of post-treatment survivors' unmet needs; in a study of post-treatment ovarian cancer survivors, Kornblith et al. found that 30 % of women reported that their emotional needs were not fully met, second only to their needs regarding sexual dysfunction [29]. A few studies have used an age-matched control design to determine whether post-treatment cancer survivors have more psychological or emotional problems than their healthy same-aged peers. The results of these studies have been mixed; using nationally representative data from the National Health Interview Survey, Mao et al. [46] found that distress was higher among people with a personal history of cancer (26 % reported emotional distress) compared to age-matched controls with no history of cancer (16 % reported emotional distress). In a study of individuals enrolled in a managed care organization, post-treatment cancer survivors were statistically significantly more likely to have a psychiatric diagnosis (34 %) than age-matched controls (30 %), driven largely by higher rates of anxiety or sleep disorders (not including PTSD) among members with a personal history of cancer [47]. In contrast, in a study of post-treatment breast cancer survivors, Ganz et al. showed that HRQOL did not differ between women with a history of breast cancer and age-matched controls, though menopausal symptoms and problems with sexual function were more common in the women with a history of cancer [24]. Other studies have used instruments to measure emotional outcomes among post-treatment cancer survivors that have normative data available for comparison. These studies have generally found that the outcomes for post-treatment cancer survivors are as good as or better than population norms (e.g., [21, 29]).

In addition to symptoms of general anxiety and depression, studies have also specifically examined symptoms of PTSD, which has been shown to be the most commonly diagnosed psychiatric condition among newly diagnosed cancer patients [48]. Clinically significant levels of PTSD symptoms have been estimated at lower levels than anxiety and depression, usually at levels between 10 and 20 % (e.g., [27]). However, in a recent study of NHL survivors who were at least 7 years post-diagnosis, PTSD symptoms had persisted or worsened over a period of 5 years after treatment for more than one-third of survivors [49]. In a sample of cancer survivors 1-year post-stem cell transplant, Rusiewicz et al. [42] found that symptoms of PTSD were not universally common. In fact, in their sample, some survivors reported high levels of emotional distress and symptoms of PTSD while others reported high levels of emotional distress with no symptoms of PTSD (i.e., symptoms of more general anxiety and/or depression), suggesting that symptoms of PTSD may represent a distinct psychological experience in the post-treatment period.

In contrast to symptoms of depression, anxiety, or PTSD, a psychological experience that is often found to be prevalent among post-treatment cancer survivors is fear of recurrence [4, 50, 51]. Estimates of the percentage of post-treatment survivors who report fears of recurrence range upwards of 30 % [22, 23, 28, 36, 39, 52]. Fears of recurrence are more common among post-treatment survivors with other psychological concerns, such as symptoms of anxiety and depression, but interestingly, fears of recurrence have not always been shown to significantly disrupt quality of life [44]. This may be, in part, due to fears of recurrence occurring in conjunction with follow-up tests and treatments, thereby leaving long stretches of time when post-treatment cancer survivors may be able to keep fears of recurrence successfully at bay [16, 44].

Finally, the length of time that psychological disruptions last for post-treatment survivors varies significantly. There is some evidence that emotional concerns resolve at a slow pace over the first year post-treatment [21]; other studies suggest that distress remains for longer, between 1 and 2 years after treatment ends [38]. Long-term studies of post-treatment cancer survivors have documented the typical 20–30 % of participants with emotional problems as far out as 4 years post-diagnosis [27]. We explore the relationship between time since diagnosis and psychological distress more fully in the next section of this review, where we consider the correlates of psychological disruption in post-treatment survivorship.

What Disease and Sociodemographic Factors Are Associated with Psychological Disruption in the Post-treatment Period?

With an understanding of the nature of psychological problems encountered in the post-treatment period, it is reasonable next to consider under what circumstances such problems are most likely to present. A useful framework, introduced by Andrykowski et al. [23], identifies a necessary balance or match between the stress and burden associated with cancer and the resources that one has available to cope with or respond to that stress and burden as a critical factor in preventing psychological distress. When these factors are not matched or balanced, either due to an increase in stress or burden, a decrease in resources, or both, psychological problems are likely to occur.

Evidence for this framework's validity in the post-treatment period can be found across a variety of studies involving numerous types of cancer. Regarding factors that increase the stress and burden of cancer and that have been associated with more psychological problems in the post-treatment period, multiple studies have shown that

survivors who are experiencing more physical symptoms or problems are more likely to experience more emotional problems as well [4, 23, 46]. The most commonly encountered physical problems in the post-treatment period are fatigue, cardiovascular disorders, fertility, and second malignancies [53]; a full review of these and other physical long-term and late effects is beyond the scope of this chapter, but it is worth noting that a challenge in diagnosing and treating psychological issues in post-treatment survivorship is that commonly encountered physical issues (e.g., fatigue) are also symptoms of psychiatric disorder (e.g., major depressive disorder [26]). There is some evidence that physical problems that have significant and direct impact on function or physical appearance are more likely to be associated with worse psychological outcomes (e.g., surgical treatment for cancer that results in disfigurement or loss of a specific bodily function [36]). Further, while the relationship between physical and emotional problems is not unique to the cancer experience, it may be particularly important in the context of post-treatment survivorship. In their study of cancer survivors and age-matched healthy controls, Mao et al. found that more physical problems were associated with higher levels of emotional distress only among cancer survivors, but not for those without a history of the disease [46].

Also related to the stress and burden of the cancer experience are treatment received and time since diagnosis. A significant amount of evidence has indicated that cancer survivors who undergo systemic treatment with chemotherapy are more likely to experience psychological problems in the post-treatment period [22, 35, 36, 49]. Additional, though not direct, support for this hypothesis can be found in a study by Rusiewicz et al. [42], who showed that 43 % of cancer survivors 1-year post-stem cell transplant reported clinically significant levels of emotional distress, a percentage that is arguably higher than what is typically observed. This may, in part, be due to the severity of the treatment experience of stem cell transplant that is also more intense than typically experienced in other types of cancer. Still, the association between receipt of systemic treatment and poorer psychological outcomes is not universal: a recent publication by Ganz et al. found no significant difference in psychosocial recovery for breast cancer survivors who did and who did not receive chemotherapy (though did note that for women who did receive chemotherapy, symptoms tended to be more severe and to persist somewhat longer [21]). Other results suggest that survivors' recalled experiences of symptom severity during treatment are better predictors of long-term psychological outcomes, as compared to treatment received per se [44]. This result underscores the idiographic nature of the cancer experience and the relationship between treatment and emotional outcomes—the "emotional fallout" of cancer and its treatment [36] for two people affected by cancer who experience the same type of treatment very differently is likely to be different as well. For time since treatment ended, though there is some reasonable support for the assertion that emotional distress subsides in the first year or two post-treatment (e.g., [4, 35, 52]), other studies have observed no relationship between time since diagnosis or when treatment ends and emotional outcomes [46], or observe relatively high percentages of post-treatment survivors reporting emotional concerns far into the post-treatment period (e.g., [27]).

Andrykowski's framework [23] suggests that resources are required to prevent the stress and burden posed by cancer and its treatment from negatively affecting psychological outcomes. "Resources" can be interpreted fairly broadly, but should at least include premorbid psychological distress (which would presumably reduce resources available for dealing with the stress and burden of cancer) and a variety of psychosocial and environmental resources that may provide support during the cancer experience as well. Indeed, individuals with a history of psychiatric disorders have been found to be more likely to experience higher levels of emotional distress during their cancer experience [48], including the post-treatment period [4, 28, 36]. It is worth noting that the percentage of cancer survivors who have a history of a psychiatric disorder has been shown to be comparable to the percentage of the general population with such a history, at a lifetime prevalence rate of about

50 % [48, 54]. Other resources associated with better psychological outcomes in the post-treatment period include external and internal factors such as having a spouse or partner (e.g., [22]) or adequate social support [27, 36]; higher socioeconomic status evidenced by level of education attained and annual income [22, 27, 46, 49]; and personality or trait-like variables such as dispositional optimism [4, 44].

Finally, there are some sociodemographic characteristics associated with emotional outcomes in the post-treatment period that do not easily fit into the "stress or burden" or "resource" categories are age and gender. Female post-treatment survivors have consistently reported more emotional concerns in the post-treatment period as compared to men (e.g., [38, 45, 46]), and younger survivors report more psychological disruption as well [22, 25, 36–39, 45, 46]. For example, though Mao et al. found that individuals with a history of cancer reported, on average, higher levels of emotional distress compared to age-matched healthy controls, they found that this difference was largest for cancer survivors under age 44 [46]. The increased distress among younger post-treatment cancer survivors may be a function of a sense of social isolation, as more than 50 % of all cancer diagnoses occur in individuals age 65 and older [3]. Finally, race and ethnicity have not consistently been associated with psychological outcomes in the post-treatment period, though in one study [22] was found to moderate an association between physical and emotional concerns, wherein African American prostate cancer survivors reported more emotional distress than Whites experiencing the same levels of sexual dysfunction in the post-treatment period.

Summary

While clinically significant levels of emotional distress may not be common in a majority of post-treatment cancer survivors, a variety of psychological concerns are encountered in the post-treatment period, some more common than others (e.g., fear of recurrence), and are more likely to occur for individuals who experience stress and burden associated with cancer in excess of resources available to cope with that stress. Given the idiographic nature of psychological factors in post-treatment cancer survivorship, it would be particularly useful to examine a variety of emotional concerns in a large sample of individuals in the post-treatment period who are asked to reflect on the experience of emotional concerns that are specifically new to them since completing their treatment for cancer. Though framing the question of emotional concerns in this way is not free from problems of potential recall bias (i.e., will survivors accurately recall whether a specific emotional concern did or did not have a pre-treatment onset?), asking about new emotional concerns since treatment ended across a variety of areas and examining the correlates of emotional concerns, their relationship with physical concerns, and patterns of care received for emotional concerns would significantly advance our understanding of the post-treatment emotional landscape. The 2010 LIVE*STRONG* Survey for People Affected by Cancer provides such a data source, and will be examined here.

The Emotional Concerns of Post-treatment Cancer Survivors: Evidence from the 2010 LIVESTRONG Survey for People Affected by Cancer

Participants and Procedures

The 2010 LIVE*STRONG* Survey for People Affected by Cancer built upon the 2006 LIVE*STRONG* Survey for Post-Treatment Cancer Survivors [12]. The 2006 survey instrument was designed through a process that engaged both cancer survivors and experts in the field of survey methodology and oncology through peer review, focus groups, and a pilot test. The majority of the 2010 survey content was focused on the physical, emotional, and practical concerns of post-treatment cancer survivors; however, there were additional areas of the survey aimed at survivors currently in treatment and individuals affected by cancer who did not have a personal history of cancer. The results shown here are focused on the

3,682 post-treatment cancer survivors who completed the 2010 survey. Post-treatment cancer survivors included individuals who had been diagnosed with cancer and who reported that they were currently finished with treatment or were managing cancer as a chronic condition.

The survey was fielded online and opened on 20 June 2010, in conjunction with the release of Parade Magazine's issue devoted to cancer survivorship. The survey was available on LIVESTRONG.org as well as LIVESTRONGespanol.org. LIVESTRONG constituents, including cancer patient and survivors, were notified about the survey by email and through Twitter and Facebook. Additionally, LIVE*STRONG* reached out to many of its community, national and international partner organizations and all state cancer coalitions to provide information about the survey, and to assist these organizations in reaching potential respondents. LIVE*STRONG* also collaborated with Comprehensive Cancer Centers, such as members of the LIVE*STRONG* Survivorship Center of Excellence Network, to share the survey with their constituents. The study was reviewed and approved by the Western Institutional Review Board.

Measures

Physical and emotional concerns. The goal of the LIVE*STRONG* survey program is to gather surveillance data from large groups of people affected by cancer, with an emphasis on post-treatment cancer survivors. The surveys assess whether or not survivors are currently experiencing specific concerns, the degree to which those concerns cause functional impairment, and whether or not care is received to help alleviate their concerns. As such, symptom checklists or multi-item measures of physical health or emotional outcomes were not well suited for the LIVE*STRONG* survey efforts; rather, *LIVESTRONG* research staff developed content for the survey (in collaboration with subject matter experts and with feedback from their constituency) that would allow respondents to indicate if they were experiencing a particular physical or emotional concern in the post-treatment period (practical concerns were assessed as well, though will not be addressed here; please see Ref. [11] for a full description of the 2006 and 2010 LIVE*STRONG* surveys).

Post-treatment cancer survivors were asked about physical and emotional concerns that had a post-treatment onset; that is, they were asked to endorse physical and emotional concerns that they were experiencing in the post-treatment period that they had not experienced before their treatment began. Physical and emotional concerns were organized into groups of related items, which will be referred to as "collections." For example, one emotional concern collection contained four items related to sadness and depression (e.g., "I have felt blue or depressed"). If a respondent endorsed any item in a collection, then they were counted as having endorsed the concern category. Fourteen collections focused on physical concerns (e.g., incontinence; sexual dysfunction; pain); eight focused on emotional concerns (for a full copy of the survey and complete list of the physical concerns queried, please see Ref. [11]).

The eight emotional concerns considered in the 2010 survey were fear of recurrence (three item collection; e.g., "I have been preoccupied with concerns about cancer"); sadness and depression (seven item collection; e.g., "I have felt blue or depressed"); grief and identity issues (four item collection; e.g., "I have felt that I have lost a sense of my identity"); family member cancer risk (three item collection; e.g., "I have worried that my family members were at risk of getting cancer"); personal appearance (three item collection; e.g., "I have felt unattractive"); cancer-related stigma (four item collection; e.g., "I have felt ashamed because I have had cancer"); personal relationships (five item collection; e.g., "I have been reluctant to start new relationships"); and faith and spirituality (two item collection; e.g., "I have felt that I have lost a sense of my faith or spirituality").

Functional impairment. If a respondent endorsed any item in an emotional concern collection, they were counted as having endorsed that emotional concern and were further asked to what degree

the concern impaired their daily functioning (*a lot, a little, not at all, do not know*).

Receipt of care. Finally, if a respondent endorsed an emotional concern collection, they were asked whether they had received care for the concern (*yes, no*).

Sociodemographic and medical variables. A number of sociodemographic and medical variables are included in the current study, based on variables that have been associated with psychological factors in post-treatment survivorship and that represent indices of the stress and burden of cancer as well as resources to cope with cancer. These include age, gender, race/ethnicity, level of education, marital status, annual income, time since treatment ended, and type of treatment received.

Data Analysis

Data were analyzed using SPSS 16.0. Descriptive statistics were used to summarize the emotional concerns of post-treatment cancer survivors and their sociodemographic and medical characteristics. Bivariate statistics (*t*-tests; bivariate correlation; analysis of variance) were used to examine associations between number of emotional concerns and sociodemographic and medical variables, including number of physical concerns reported. We used logistic regression to model the endorsement of each of the emotional concern categories separately, where each model included the same independent variables (sociodemographic characteristics; medical variables; and number of physical concerns). Linear regression was used to model the total number of emotional concerns reported in the context of sociodemographic and medical variables and number of physical concerns reported. Finally, we used logistic regression to look at the correlates of having received care for any emotional or physical concern, where dependent variables included sociodemographic characteristics; medical variables; number of physical concerns; and number of emotional concerns. Due to the high

Table 19.1 Sample description ($n = 3,682$)

Current age	49.9 years (SD = 12.2)
Gender	65.2 % female
Race/ethnicity	93.3 % White
Level of education	High school or less: 8.5 %
	Some college: 36.4 %
	College degree: 31.7 %
	Post-college degree: 23.4 %
Annual income	$60K or less: 28.4 %
	$61K to ≤$100K: 24.7 %
	$100K or more: 27.3 %
	Prefer not to answer: 19.6 %
Marital status	66.8 % married
Age at diagnosis	43.4 years (SD = 13.9)
Time since last treatment	4.37 years (SD = 5.85)
Type of cancer	Breast: 27.5 %
	Testicular: 6.4 %
	Non-Hodgkin lymphoma: 5.6 %
	Hodgkin lymphoma: 4.7 %
	Prostate: 6.9 %
	Other (includes more than 50 types of cancer, each reported by less than 5 % of respondents): 48.9 %
Type of treatment	Chemotherapy, radiation, and surgery: 26.3 %
	Chemotherapy plus radiation or surgery: 23.8 %
	Only chemotherapy: 8.7 %
	No chemotherapy: 41.3 %
Number of emotional concerns	3.67 (SD = 1.9) (range = 0–8)
Number of physical concerns	3.56 (SD = 2.6) (range = 0–14)

number of statistical tests conducted, we chose to conservatively evaluate statistical significance at a level of $p < 0.01$.

Results

Sample characteristics. Table 19.1 shows the sociodemographic and medical characteristics of the 3,682 post-treatment cancer survivors who responded to the 2010 LIVE*STRONG* Survey for People Affected by Cancer.

The sample was relatively young, with an average age under 50 years, and more than half were female. The vast majority reported White race/ethnicity, and most (about 55 %) had at least a college degree or more education. More than one-quarter had an annual income of more than $100,000 per year (though about 20 % preferred not to answer the income query). About 70 % of the sample were married or living with a partner.

On average, more than 4 years had passed since respondents' last treatment for cancer, and the average age at diagnosis for the sample was 43 years old. A wide variety of cancer types were represented, the largest being breast cancer survivors (27.5 %), though no other cancer type included more than 10 % of the sample. Respondents had endured a lot of treatment for their cancer: more than half had received chemotherapy as part of their treatment regimen, and within that group, most received at least on other treatment (surgery, radiation, or both) as well. Finally, respondents reported an average of almost four post-treatment emotional and physical concerns.

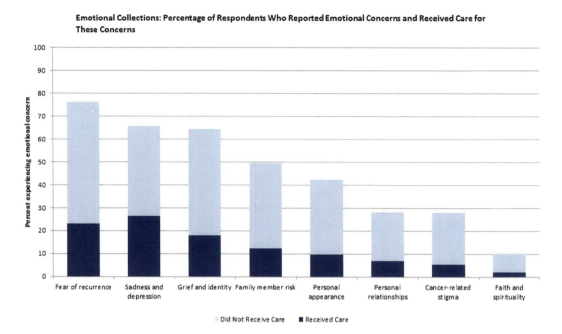

Emotional Collections: Percentage of Respondents Who Reported Emotional Concerns and Received Care for These Concerns

Fig. 19.2 Prevalence of emotional concerns and care received for each

Emotional concerns. Figure 19.2 shows the percent of respondents who endorsed each emotional concern.

Overall, 95 % of respondents endorsed at least one emotional concern. Fear of recurrence was most common, with more than 70 % of respondents endorsing that concern. Half or more of the sample reported sadness and depression, grief and identity concerns, and concerns about family member risk for cancer. More than one-third endorsed having new concerns since treatment ended about personal appearance, personal relationships, and dealing with cancer-related stigma; a small number (10 %) reported concerns about faith and spirituality.

Though many survey respondents endorsed these emotional concerns, few reported that the concerns caused "a lot" of functional impairment. Less than 10 % of respondents who endorsed any concern said that it caused "a lot" of functional impairment, except for those reporting concerns about personal appearance (10 % reported "a lot" of functional impairment); personal relationships (16 % reported "a lot" of functional impairment); and concerns about faith and spirituality (12 % reported "a lot" of functional impairment).

In fact, though fears of recurrence were the most commonly endorsed emotional concern, it was ranked sixth out of eight concerns in terms of functional impairment (only 6 % reported that fears of recurrence caused "a lot" of functional impairment), whereas concerns about faith and spirituality were least common, but ranked second in terms of functional impairment.

Figure 19.2 also shows, for each group of respondents who reported an emotional concern, the percentage who reported to receive care for the concern. The results here are fairly alarming, given that fewer than half of any group of post-treatment cancer survivors reporting an emotional concern said that they received care for the concern, though in light of the functional impairment data, it may be that for most survivors with emotional concerns, the concerns do not disrupt their lives to a degree that they believe warrants treatment. Further, receipt of care was higher when looking across all emotional concerns: overall, 66 % of respondents who reported at least one emotional concern said that they received care for an emotional concern.

In bivariate analyses (data not shown; all $p < 0.01$), more emotional concerns were associated with younger age; female gender; not having a spouse or partner; and by those with annual incomes of $60,000 per year or less (compared to those making $100,000 or more). Regarding medical variables, longer times since treatment ended were associated with fewer emotional concerns; respondents who had received the most treatment (chemotherapy plus radiation and surgery) reported the most emotional concerns; and respondents who reported more physical concerns reported more emotional concerns as well (bivariate correlation = 0.47).

Who reports which concerns? Multivariate logistic models of each concern category. To examine whether specific sociodemographic and medical characteristics were differentially associated with each of the eight emotional concerns queried in the survey, we used multivariate logistic regression to model the odds of endorsing each concern category separately (Table 19.2). Two variables were consistently associated with higher odds of endorsing each emotional concern: younger age (except for the concern of family member risk of cancer, which was not associated with age) and reporting more physical concerns (all $p < 0.01$). Education, race/ethnicity, and annual income were not reliably associated with any emotional concerns, except survivors who preferred not to report their annual income had significantly lower odds of reporting concerns about their physical appearance, compared to those who reported less than $60,000 per year (OR = 0.57; 95 % CI = 0.44, 0.74; $p < 0.01$).

Compared to men, women had higher odds of reporting fear of recurrence (OR = 1.43; 95 % CI = 1.19, 1.72); concerns about family member risk of cancer (OR = 1.44; 95 % CI = 1.23, 1.68); concerns about personal appearance (OR = 2.65; 95 % CI = 2.21, 3.12), and cancer-related stigma (OR = 1.33; 95 % CI = 1.01, 1.60; all $p < 0.01$). Respondents without a spouse or partner were significantly less likely to endorse concerns about family member risk of cancer (OR = 0.68; 95 % CI = 0.57, 0.81), but were more likely to report concerns about personal relationships (OR = 2.69; 95 % CI = 2.21, 3.27) and cancer-related stigma (OR = 1.32; 95 % CI = 1.08, 1.61; all $p < 0.01$).

Finally, for medical variables, respondents who received less treatment had lower odds of endorsing some emotional concerns compared to post-treatment survivors who had received chemotherapy, radiation, and surgery. Survivors who only received chemotherapy had lower odds of reporting concerns about family member cancer risk (OR = 0.65; 95 % CI = 0.49, 0.87) and survivors who did not receive chemotherapy had lower odds of reporting concerns about personal appearance (OR = 0.61; 95 % CI = 0.50, 0.76) but higher odds of reporting concerns about personal relationships (OR = 1.53; 95 % CI = 1.21, 1.93; all $p < 0.01$). Longer times since treatment ended was associated with fewer emotional concerns, including lower odds of reporting fears of recurrence; concerns about personal appearance; personal relationships; or cancer-related stigma (all ORs = 0.99; $p < 0.01$); however, longer times since treatment ended were associated with slightly higher odds of reporting concerns about family member risk of cancer (OR < 1.01; $p < 0.01$).

Who Reports the Most Concerns? Multivariate Linear Regression Model of Number of Emotional Concerns

In looking at the sociodemographic and medical characteristics associated with number of emotional concerns reported (Table 19.3), only younger age ($B = -0.19$), female gender ($B = 0.11$), and reporting more physical concerns ($B = 0.44$) were associated with reporting more emotional concerns (all $p < 0.01$).

Longer times since treatment ended were marginally associated with fewer emotional concerns ($B = -0.04$; $p = 0.02$) as was preferring not to report annual income (as compared to reporting $60,000 or less per year; $B = -0.05$; $p = 0.02$).

Who is most likely to receive care for concerns? Finally, we used multivariate logistic regression to examine associations between sociodemographic characteristics, medical variables, and emotional and physical concerns with odds of receiving care for emotional or physical concerns for respondents who reported at least one

Table 19.2 Logistic regressions modeling endorsement of each emotional concern separately

Study variables		Fear of recurrence	Sadness and depression	Grief and identity	Family member risk
		OR (95 % CI)	OR (95 % CI)	OR (95 % CI)	OR (95 % CI)
Age		0.98 (0.97, 0.98)*	0.98 (0.97, 0.99)*	0.98 (0.98, 0.99)*	0.99 (0.99, 1.00)
Gender	Male	(reference)	(reference)	(reference)	(reference)
	Female	1.43 (1.19, 1.72)*	1.09 (0.93, 1.29)	1.18 (1.00, 1.40)	1.44 (1.23, 1.68)*
Race/ethnicity	White	(reference)	(reference)	(reference)	(reference)
	Other	0.66 (0.47, 0.92)	0.85 (0.62, 1.16)	0.78 (0.57, 1.07)	1.05 (0.78, 1.41)
Education	College or more	(reference)	(reference)	(reference)	(reference)
	College graduate	0.87 (0.68, 1.10)	1.10 (0.89, 1.36)	0.98 (0.79, 1.21)	1.10 (0.91, 1.34)
	Some college	0.79 (0.62, 0.99)	1.01 (0.82, 1.24)	0.84 (0.69, 1.04)	1.16 (0.95, 1.41)
	≤High school	0.56 (0.41, 0.83)	1.05 (0.75, 1.45)	1.00 (0.71, 1.39)	1.27 (0.94, 1.73)
Marital status	Married/partnered	(reference)	(reference)	(reference)	(reference)
	Other	0.82 (0.67, 1.00)	0.87 (0.72, 1.04)	0.89 (0.74, 1.07)	0.68 (0.57, 0.81)*
Annual income	<$60K	(reference)	(reference)*	(reference)	(reference)
	$61K to ≤$100K	1.07 (0.84, 1.37)	0.93 (0.74, 1.15)	1.01 (0.80, 1.27)	0.93 (0.75, 1.14)
	$100K or more	1.19 (0.92, 1.54)	1.33 (1.06, 1.69)	0.93 (0.74, 1.17)	0.97 (0.78, 1.20)
	Prefer not to answer	1.08 (0.83, 1.41)	1.11 (0.87, 1.41)	1.02 (0.80, 1.31)	0.84 (0.67, 1.06)
Type of treatment	Chemo, radiation, and surgery	(reference)	(reference)	(reference)*	(reference)*
	Chemo and radiation OR surgery	1.08 (0.86, 1.37)	1.08 (0.87, 1.36)	1.01 (0.81, 1.26)	0.78 (0.64, 0.96)
	Chemotherapy only	1.00 (0.71, 1.42)	1.30 (0.94, 1.80)	1.16 (0.85, 1.60)	0.65 (0.49, 0.87)*
	No chemotherapy	1.08 (0.86, 1.37)	1.02 (0.83, 1.25)	0.83 (0.67, 1.02)	0.98 (0.81, 1.19)
Time since treatment ended		0.99 (1.09, 0.99)*	1.00 (0.99, 1.00)	1.00 (0.99, 1.01)*	1.00 (1.00, 1.01)*
Number of physical concerns		1.13 (1.09, 1.18)*	1.25 (1.21, 1.30)*	1.28 (1.23, 1.32)*	1.11 (1.08, 1.14)*

Study variables		Personal appearance	Personal relationships	Cancer-related stigma	Faith and spirituality
		OR (95 % CI)	OR (95 % CI)	OR (95 % CI)	OR (95 % CI)
Age		0.97 (0.97, 0.98)*	0.98 (0.98, 0.99)*	0.96 (0.96, 0.97)*	0.98 (0.97, 0.98)*
Gender	Male	(reference)	(reference)	(reference)	(reference)
	Female	2.65 (2.21, 3.12)*	0.99 (0.81, 1.20)	1.33 (1.01, 1.60)*	0.88 (0.68, 1.13)
Race/ethnicity	White	(reference)	(reference)	(reference)	(reference)
	Other	0.75 (0.54, 1.04)	0.97 (0.68, 1.37)	0.85 (0.60, 1.21)	1.10 (0.71, 1.71)

Education				
College or more	(reference)	(reference)	(reference)	(reference)
College graduate	1.21 (0.97, 1.51)	0.95 (0.75, 1.21)	0.86 (0.68, 1.09)	0.79 (0.58, 1.07)
Some college	1.03 (0.83, 1.28)	0.80 (0.63, 1.01)	0.82 (0.65, 1.03)	0.65 (0.48, 0.89)
≤High school	1.09 (0.78, 1.53)	0.96 (0.67, 1.37)	0.57 (0.39, 0.83)	0.49 (0.29, 0.84)
Marital status				
Married/partnered	(reference)	(reference)	(reference)	(reference)
Other	1.04 (0.86, 1.26)	2.69 (2.21, 3.27)*	1.32 (1.08, 1.61)*	1.10 (0.85, 1.44)
Annual income				
<$60K	(reference)*	(reference)	(reference)	(reference)
$61K to ≤$100K	0.91 (0.72, 1.14)	0.82 (0.65, 1.05)	1.04 (0.81, 1.32)	0.89 (0.65, 1.23)
$100K or more	0.90 (0.71, 1.14)	0.71 (0.55, 0.92)	0.90 (0.70, 1.16)	0.84 (0.60, 1.17)
Prefer not to answer	0.57 (0.44, 0.74)*	0.70 (0.53, 0.92)	0.91 (0.70, 1.20)	0.73 (0.49, 1.06)
Type of treatment				
Chemo, radiation, and surgery	(reference)*	(reference)*	(reference)	(reference)*
Chemo and radiation OR surgery	0.86 (0.69, 1.07)	0.89 (0.70, 1.13)	0.90 (0.71, 1.14)	0.74 (0.54, 1.02)
Chemotherapy only	0.71 (0.52, 0.97)	1.19 (0.85, 1.67)	0.98 (0.70, 1.36)	0.57 (0.34, 0.94)
No chemotherapy	0.61 (0.50, 0.76)*	1.53 (1.21, 1.93)*	1.23 (0.98, 1.56)	1.14 (0.89, 1.54)
Time since treatment ended	0.99 (0.99, 0.99)*	0.99 (0.99, 1.00)*	0.99 (0.98, 0.99)*	1.00 (0.99, 1.00)
Number of physical concerns	1.34 (1.30, 1.39)*	1.41 (1.35, 1.46)*	1.20 (1.16, 1.24)*	1.18 (1.13, 1.24)*

*$p<0.01$

Table 19.3 Linear regression modeling total number of emotional concerns (model adjusted $R2 = 0.28$)

Study variables		Standardized β (beta)	p
Age		**−0.19**	**<0.01**
Gender	Male	(reference)	
	Female	**0.11**	**<0.01**
Race/ethnicity	White	(reference)	
	Other	−0.03	0.10
Education	College or more	(reference)	
	College graduate	0.00	0.98
	Some college	−0.03	0.23
	≤High school	−0.03	0.09
Annual income	<$60K	(reference)	
	$61K to ≤$100K	−0.02	0.42
	$100K or more	−0.02	0.32
	Prefer not to answer	−0.05	0.02
Marital status	Married/partnered	(reference)	
	Other	0.03	0.09
Type of treatment	Chemo, radiation, and surgery	(reference)	
	Chemo and radiation OR surgery	−0.03	0.06
	Chemotherapy only	−0.01	0.66
	No chemotherapy	−0.01	0.43
Time since treatment ended		−0.04	0.02
Number of physical concerns		**0.44**	**<0.01**

emotional concern ($n = 2,869$). In the model of receipt of care for emotional concerns (Table 19.4), we found that women were more likely to have received care for emotional concerns compared to men (OR = 1.64; 95 % CI = 1.36, 1.97). Longer times since diagnosis were associated with slightly higher, though significant, odds of receiving care for emotional concerns (OR = 1.00; 95 % CI = 1.00, 1.01) and compared to survivors who received chemotherapy, surgery, and radiation, those who received chemotherapy with surgery OR radiation had significantly lower odds of receiving care for emotional concerns (OR = 0.64; 95 % CI = 0.51, 0.81). Finally, more physical and more emotional concerns were associated with higher odds of receiving care for emotional concerns [ORs = 1.19 (1.12, 1.24) and 1.21 (1.13, 1.28), respectively, all $p < 0.01$].

In an exploratory analysis (data not shown), we also modeled odds of receiving care for physi-

cal concerns for respondents who reported at least one physical concern ($n = 3,199$). Overall, 69 % of post-treatment survivors who reported at least one physical concern received care. Odds of receiving care for physical concerns were lower among respondents who received chemotherapy without additional treatment or with only one additional treatment compared to survivors who received chemotherapy, surgery, and radiation [ORs = 0.48 (0.33, 0.70) and 0.59 (0.45, 0.78), respectively]. Similar to the results of the model of receiving care for emotional concerns, longer times since treatment ended and reporting more physical concerns were both associated with higher odds of receiving care for physical concerns [ORs = 1.00 (1.00, 1.01) and 1.87 (1.74, 2.01) respectively, all $p < 0.01$]. However, respondents who reported more emotional concerns had lower odds of receiving care for physical concerns (OR = 0.92; 95 % CI = 0.87, 0.98; $p = 0.01$).

Table 19.4 Logistic regression modeling receipt of care for emotional concerns (for respondents who reported at least one emotional concern; $n = 2,869$)

Study variables		OR (95 % CI)
Age		0.99 (0.98, 1.00)
Gender	Male	(reference)
	Female	1.64 (1.36, 1.97)*
Race/ethnicity	White	(reference)
	Other	0.81 (0.56, 1.15)
Education	College or more	(reference)
	College graduate	0.99 (0.79, 1.25)
	Some college	0.89 (0.71, 1.12)
	≤High school	0.62 (0.43, 0.90)
Marital status	Married/partnered	(reference)
	Other	1.07 (0.88, 1.31)
Annual income	<$60K	(reference)
	$61K to ≤$100K	1.20 (0.94, 1.54)
	$100K or more	1.06 (0.83, 1.37)
	Prefer not to answer	1.35 (1.03, 1.77)
Type of treatment	Chemo, radiation, and surgery	(reference)*
	Chemo and radiation OR surgery	0.64 (0.51, 0.81)*
	Chemotherapy only	0.71 (0.51, 0.99)
	No chemotherapy	0.85 (0.68, 1.08)
Time since treatment ended		1.00 (1.00, 1.01)*
Number of physical concerns		1.19 (1.12, 1.24)*
Number of emotional concerns		1.21 (1.13, 1.28)*

$*p < 0.01$

Addressing the Emotional Needs of Post-treatment Cancer Survivors

The results of the 2010 LIVE*STRONG* survey suggest that emotional concerns among post-treatment cancer survivors are exceedingly common, and that individuals often encounter new emotional challenges after cancer treatment ends that they had not experienced in earlier phases of their cancer journey. The LIVE*STRONG* survey asked about emotional concerns in a way that is different from other investigations of post-treatment cancer survivors, using a format that allowed for a variety of emotional concerns to be fielded to respondents, offering a more in-depth and nuanced picture of the emotional landscape of the post-treatment period. The consistency of the results with previous studies—that younger survivors reported more emotional concerns; that

emotional and physical concerns were strongly associated—suggests that the survey structure offered a valid means for assessing cancer survivors' post-treatment concerns.

Also consistent with previous research (e.g., [24, 44]) was the result that while emotional concerns were common, reports of emotional concerns were usually not accompanied by high levels of functional impairment. This finding may ease some of the concern over the difference between the percentage of survivors who reported an emotional concern and the percentage who received care for the concern (95 % reported at least one emotional concern; only 66 % received care for any emotional concern). It may be that the post-treatment survivors in the study sample did not judge their emotional concerns to be at a level requiring intervention, if their concerns were not consistently and significantly causing functional impairment.

However, the difference between reports of emotional concerns and receipt of care was striking, particularly when considering the results for each concern separately, and other studies have found that there are significant numbers of post-treatment cancer survivors who do not receive psychological or psychosocial care that they need (e.g., [29, 45]). Post-treatment survivors may not be aware of available psychosocial care [27], underscoring the need for psychosocial services to be more fully integrated into routine cancer care [17].

How might this be accomplished? Some have argued for routine screening to provide early identification of distress [2, 17, 23, 55]. Such early identification of distress could have benefits in the post-treatment period as well, as there is evidence that untreated distress during cancer treatment predicts poorer psychological adjustment in the post-treatment period [56]. This approach is also congruent with the most recent conceptualizations of cancer survivorship, which emphasize prevention, in recognition of the increased numbers of people affected by cancer who will go on to live the balance of their full life expectancy [3]. However, it is worth noting that screening for distress in cancer patients is not without risks or burden. There is evidence that screening does not lead to adequate enough numbers of survivors who need psychological services but are not getting them to offset the burden of false-positive screens [57]. Some have suggested that screening should not be aimed at identification of distress, but identification of unmet needs [45]. This approach is consistent with the results of this study and the larger literature on psychological experiences of post-treatment cancer survivors, which suggests that survivors may experience a number of concerns in the post-treatment period without having these concerns significantly disrupt their mood or quality of life. Further, a recent study by Arora et al. [58] showed that many post-treatment cancer survivors do not feel that their follow-up care providers have an adequate understanding of the ways that cancer has impacted their QOL. The results of routine screening to capture survivors' unmet needs might serve to facilitate better patient–provider communication on these issues.

Andrykowski [59] has recently called for a more tailored approach to psycho-oncological intervention, suggesting that we can do a better job of matching our intervention approaches to the specific needs of people affected by cancer. Indeed, the results of this study suggest that there are patterns of relationships between sociodemographic and medical variables and emotional concerns in the post-treatment period: compared to men, women were more likely to report concerns of an interpersonal nature, such as concerns about appearance, cancer-related stigma, and family member cancer risk. Post-treatment survivors who had been treated with chemotherapy were more likely to have concerns about appearance than those who did not; fears of recurrence, concerns about appearance, and problems with personal relationships were all more common closer to the time when treatment ends. Screening for needs related to these areas before the end of treatment would enable supportive care providers to deliver more personalized pyscho-oncology interventions to patients as they transition into the post-treatment period.

Increases in the use of survivorship care plans (SCPs) may improve the degree to which cancer survivors receive the psychosocial services they need in the post-treatment period. The SCP can contain follow-up recommendations derived from the results of routine psychosocial screening or care received during treatment, thereby helping to integrate psychosocial services into routine care pathways when primary cancer treatment ends [5, 17, 60]. In this way, the SCP may also serve to decrease the stigma that still accompanies psychosocial care [61], which can pose a real barrier to receipt of treatment, particularly if an individual is coping with cancer-related stigma as well (reported by nearly one-third of post-treatment survivors in our study).

SCPs were specifically called for by the 2006 IOM report [16] and the inclusion of psychosocial elements of care into the SCP was defined in the 2008 report [17]. A recent study of the LIVE*STRONG* Survivorship Centers of Excellence overviews the challenges of implementing SCPs in survivorship care [60]: all of the Centers failed to meet at least 75 % concordance with IOM guidelines in their SCPs or treatment summaries, and regarding psychosocial issues specifically, less than half of SCPs were concordant with IOM recommendations regarding the inclusion of psychosocial elements in the SCP. Additionally, the creation and provision of SCPs were found to be extremely time consuming for clinical care providers. It may be that increased use of electronic health records and other health information technology applications serve to facilitate the efficient and effective provision of SCPs [62], which in turn can serve as a platform from which to engage in better patient–provider communication about psychosocial issues in post-treatment survivorship [58]. SCPs may also serve to empower cancer survivors by providing them with information they need to reduce emotional concerns related to fears about recurrence or family member risk of cancer [28], both of which were observed in half or more of survivors in this study.

Another function of SCPs is to facilitate receipt of follow-up cancer care and care for symptom management. The results regarding receipt of care in the LIVE*STRONG* data were intriguing; in particular, the association between reports of concerns and receipt of care. For receipt of care for emotional concerns, more emotional concerns and more physical concerns were both associated with higher odds of receiving care, suggesting that post-treatment survivors with higher emotional and physical symptom burdens are more likely to seek care for emotional concerns. However, we observed a different result for receipt of care for physical concerns: here, more physical concerns were associated with higher odds of receiving care for physical concerns, but more emotional concerns were associated with lower odds of receiving care for physical concerns.

This result is worth further study, as we cannot draw inferential conclusions from this cross-sectional, observational data. One hypothesis is that higher levels of emotional distress, evidenced by more emotional concerns, create a barrier to engaging in physical health care. This has been observed in studies of people with mental illness, who are less likely to engage in preventive health care, in

part as a function of the ways that psychiatric symptoms may prevent behavioral activation needed to engage in care (e.g., [63]).

There is a large and involved literature on the role of psychological factors in physical health, and in cancer, this topic has been particularly controversial and debated for several decades (e.g., [64–66]). It is beyond the scope of this chapter to address this debate, which is more often focused on the ways that psychological factors may affect biobehavioral mediators of health outcomes (e.g., [67]) than on how psychological factors affect health care seeking behavior. However, it is worth noting that, given the results of the LIVE*STRONG* survey, the degree to which emotional disruption in the post-treatment period interferes with receipt of follow-up cancer care is an area of investigation that requires further study.

Limitations

There are a number of limitations to the current assessment of psychological factors in post-treatment survivorship and the data presented from the LIVE*STRONG* survey. As noted earlier, we did not include research focused on positive psychological developments in the wake of cancer, nor did we include the experiences of post-treatment survivors of cancers diagnosed in childhood in our review. The respondents to the LIVE*STRONG* survey are a self-selected group of Internet-using cancer survivors, and do not represent the majority of cancer survivors alive in the United States today with respect to age, type of cancer, race/ethnicity, or socioeconomic status. The survey did not include measurement of trait-like variables shown to be associated with adjustment in the post-treatment period, such as optimism (e.g., [44]). Finally, it was beyond the scope of this chapter to include results from the LIVE*STTRONG* survey on the practical concerns (e.g., concerns about employment) of post-treatment cancer survivors, though these concerns are certainly relevant to psychosocial experiences in the post-treatment phase.

Summary

Despite these limitations, the LIVE*STRONG* data do offer a large sample of post-treatment cancer survivors, and our results confirm and extend previous work on psychological factors in post-treatment survivorship. Considering Andrykowski's framework that identifies a balance between the stress and burden of cancer against resources available as key to the prevention of psychological disruption [23], given the lack of evidence to suggest that stress and burden significantly increase in the post-treatment period, but that the resources provided by the health care system at time of diagnosis and during treatment significantly decrease when treatment ends [20], the results shown here are congruent with a conceptualization of the post-treatment period as being one in which new stressors and burdens related to cancer emerge, but resolve at a pace that is slower than the one at which the resources provided by the health care system disappear when treatment ends. In this way, SCPs may serve as a function to help post-treatment survivors remain aware of and stay connected to the resources provided by their cancer care team, enabling them to avoid significant psychosocial disruption during the post-treatment period.

References

1. Dolbeault S, Szporn A, Holland JC. Psycho-oncology: where have we been? Where are we going? Eur J Cancer. 1999;35(11):1554–8.
2. Holland JC, Alici Y. Management of distress in cancer patients. J Support Oncol. 2010;8(1):4–12.
3. Rowland JH, Bellizzi KM. Cancer survivors and survivorship research: a reflection on today's successes and tomorrow's challenges. Hematol Oncol Clin North Am. 2008;22(2):181–200, v.
4. Alfano CM, Rowland JH. Recovery issues in cancer survivorship: a new challenge for supportive care. Cancer J. 2006;12(5):432–43.
5. Ganz PA. Survivorship: adult cancer survivors. Prim Care. 2009;36(4):721–41.
6. Altekruse SF, Kosary CL, Krapcho M, Neyman N, Aminou R, Waldron W, Ruhl J, Howlader N, Tatalovich Z, Cho H, Mariotto A, Eisner MP, Lewis DR, Cronin K, Chen HS, Feuer EJ, Stinchcomb DG, Edwards BK, editors. SEER Cancer Statistics Review, 1975–2008, Editor 2010. Bethesda, MD: National Cancer Institute.
7. National Cancer Institute. Office of cancer survivorship website. 2011. http://dccps.cancer.gov/ocs/index. html. Accessed March 2011
8. Rechis R, Eargle E, Dutchover Y, Berno D. Defining survivorship care: lessons learned from the LIVESTRONG Survivorship Center of Excellence Network: a LIVESTRONG report. Austin, TX: LIVESTRONG; 2010.
9. Feuerstein M. Defining cancer survivorship. J Cancer Surviv. 2007;1(1):5–7.
10. Rowland JH, Hewitt M, Ganz PA. Cancer survivorship: a new challenge in delivering quality cancer care. J Clin Oncol. 2006;24(32):5101–4.
11. Rechis R, Reynolds KA, Beckjord EB, Nutt S, Burns RM, Schaefer JS. "I Learned to Live With It" is not good enough: challenges reported by post-treatment cancer survivors in the LIVESTRONG surveys. Austin, TX: LIVESTRONG; 2011.
12. Rechis R, Boerner L, Nutt S, Shaw K, Berno D, Duchover Y. How cancer has affected post-treatment survivors: a LIVESTRONG report. Austin, TX: LIVESTRONG; 2010.
13. Smith T, et al. The rationale, design, and implementation of the American Cancer Society's studies of cancer survivors. Cancer. 2007;109(1):1–12.
14. Centers for Disease Control and Prevention. Behavioral risk factor surveillance system webpage. 2011. http://www.cdc.gov/brfss/. Accessed March 2011
15. Institute of Medicine. Childhood cancer survivorship: improving care and quality of life. Washington, DC: Institute of Medicine; 2003.
16. Institute of Medicine. From cancer patient to cancer survivor: lost in transition. Hewitt M, Greenfield S, Stovall E, editors. Washington, DC: Editor 2006, National Acadamies; 2006
17. Institute of Medicine. Cancer care for the whole patient: meeting psychosocial health needs, Adler N, Page AEK, editors. Washington, DC: Editor 2008, National Acadamies; 2008.
18. Phillips JL, Currow DC. Cancer as a chronic disease. Collegian. 2010;17(2):47–50.
19. Stanton AL, Revenson TA, Tennen H. Health psychology: psychological adjustment to chronic disease. Annu Rev Psychol. 2007;58:565–92.
20. Stanton AL, et al. Promoting adjustment after treatment for cancer. Cancer. 2005;104(11 Suppl):2608–13.
21. Ganz PA, et al. Physical and psychosocial recovery in the year after primary treatment of breast cancer. J Clin Oncol. 2011;29(9):1101–9.
22. Bloom JR, Petersen DM, Kang SH. Multi-dimensional quality of life among long-term (5+ years) adult cancer survivors. Psychooncology. 2007;16(8):691–706.
23. Andrykowski MA, Lykins E, Floyd A. Psychological health in cancer survivors. Semin Oncol Nurs. 2008;24(3):193–201.
24. Ganz PA, et al. Life after breast cancer: understanding women's health-related quality of life and sexual functioning. J Clin Oncol. 1998;16(2):501–14.

25. Smith SK, et al. The impact of cancer and quality of life for post-treatment non-Hodgkin lymphoma survivors. Psychooncology. 2010;4:45–8.
26. Bottomley A. Depression in cancer patients: a literature review. Eur J Cancer Care. 1998;7:181–91.
27. Mehnert A, Koch U. Psychological comorbidity and health-related quality of life and its association with awareness, utilization, and need for psychosocial support in a cancer register-based sample of long-term breast cancer survivors. J Psychosom Res. 2008;64(4):383–91.
28. Stein KD, Syrjala KL, Andrykowski MA. Physical and psychological long-term and late effects of cancer. Cancer. 2008;112(11 Suppl):2577–92.
29. Kornblith AB, et al. Long-term adjustment of survivors of ovarian cancer treated for advanced-stage disease. J Psychosoc Oncol. 2010;28(5):451–69.
30. Bellizzi KM, et al. Positive and negative life changes experienced by survivors of non-Hodgkin's lymphoma. Ann Behav Med. 2007;34(2):188–99.
31. Lelorain S, Bonnaud-Antignac A, Florin A. Long term posttraumatic growth after breast cancer: prevalence, predictors and relationships with psychological health. J Clin Psychol Med Settings. 2010;17(1):14–22.
32. Gorin SS. Theory, measurement, and controversy in positive psychology, health psychology, and cancer: basics and next steps. Ann Behav Med. 2010;39(1):43–7.
33. Lund LW, et al. A systematic review of studies on psychosocial late effects of childhood cancer: structures of society and methodological pitfalls may challenge the conclusions. Pediatr Blood Cancer. 2011;56(4):532–43.
34. Shapiro CL, et al. The LIVESTRONG Survivorship Center of Excellence Network. J Cancer Surviv. 2009;3(1):4–11.
35. Stanton AL. Psychosocial concerns and interventions for cancer survivors. J Clin Oncol. 2006;24(32):5132–7.
36. Meyerowitz BE, Kurita K, D'Orazio LM. The psychological and emotional fallout of cancer and its treatment. Cancer J. 2008;14(6):410–3.
37. Zebrack BJ, et al. The impact of cancer and quality of life for long-term survivors. Psychooncology. 2008;17(9):891–900.
38. Brant JM, et al. Symptom trajectories in posttreatment cancer survivors. Cancer Nurs. 2011;34(1):67–77.
39. Foster C, et al. Psychosocial implications of living 5 years or more following a cancer diagnosis: a systematic review of the research evidence. Eur J Cancer Care (Engl). 2009;18(3):223–47.
40. Gao W, et al. Psychological distress in cancer from survivorship to end of life care: prevalence, associated factors and clinical implications. Eur J Cancer. 2010;46(11):2036–44.
41. Harrington CB, et al. It's not over when it's over: long-term symptoms in cancer survivors – a systematic review. Int J Psychiatry Med. 2010;40(2): 163–81.
42. Rusiewicz A, DuHamel KN, Burkhalter J, Ostroff J, Winkel G, Scigliano E, Papadopoulos E, Moskowitz C, Redd W. Psychological distress in long-term survivors of hematopoietic stem cell transplantation. Psychooncology. 2008;17:329–37.
43. Zabora J, et al. The prevalence of psychological distress by cancer site. Psychooncology. 2001;10(1): 19–28.
44. Deimling GT, et al. Cancer-related health worries and psychological distress among older adult, long-term cancer survivors. Psychooncology. 2006;15(4): 306–20.
45. van Scheppingen C, et al. Does screening for distress efficiently uncover meetable unmet needs in cancer patients? Psychooncology. 2011;20(6):655–63.
46. Mao JJ, et al. Symptom burden among cancer survivors: impact of age and comorbidity. J Am Board Fam Med. 2007;20(5):434–43.
47. Earle CC, Neville BA, Fletcher R. Mental health service utilization among long-term cancer survivors. J Cancer Surviv. 2007;1(2):156–60.
48. Dausch B, Compas BE, Beckjord E, Luecken L, Anderson-Hanley C, Sherman M, Grossman C. Rates and correlates of DSM-IV diagnoses in women newly diagnosed wtih breast cancer. J Clin Psychol Med Settings. 2004;11(3):159–69.
49. Smith SK, et al. Post-traumatic stress symptoms in long-term non-Hodgkin's lymphoma survivors: does time heal? J Clin Oncol. 2011;29(34):4526–33.
50. Thewes B, et al. Fear of cancer recurrence: a systematic literature review of self-report measures. Psychooncology, 2011;21(6):571–87.
51. McGinty HL, Goldenberg JL, Jacobsen PB. Relationship of threat appraisal with coping appraisal to fear of cancer recurrence in breast cancer survivors. Psychooncology, 2010;21(2):203–10.
52. Baker F, et al. Adult cancer survivors: how are they faring? Cancer. 2005;104(11 Suppl):2565–76.
53. Fosså SD, Vassilopoulou-Sellin R, Dahl AA. Long term physical sequelae after adult-onset cancer. J Cancer Surviv Res Pract. 2008;2(1):3–11.
54. Kessler RC, McGonagle KA, Zhao S, Nelson CB, Hughes M, Esheman S, et al. Lifetime and 12-month prevalence of DSM-III-R psychiatric disorders in the United States. Arch Gen Psychiatry. 1994;51:8–19.
55. Velikova G. Patient benefits from psychosocial care: screening for distress and models of care. J Clin Oncol. 2010;28(33):4871–3.
56. Lam WW, et al. Distress trajectories at the first year diagnosis of breast cancer in relation to 6 years survivorship. Psychooncology, 2010;21(1):90–9.
57. Palmer SC, et al. Is screening effective in detecting untreated psychiatric disorders among newly diagnosed breast cancer patients? Cancer. 2011;118(10):2735–43.
58. Arora NK, et al. Assessment of quality of cancer-related follow-up care from the cancer survivor's perspective. J Clin Oncol. 2011;29(10):1280–9.
59. Andrykowski MA. Refining the fundamental question in intervention research in psycho-oncology: perhaps Godot has already arrived? Psychooncology. 2011; 20(3):335–6.

60. Stricker CT, et al. Survivorship care planning after the Institute of Medicine recommendations: how are we faring? J Cancer Surviv. 2011;5(4):358–70.

61. Holland JC, Kelly BJ, Weinberger MI. Why psychosocial care is difficult to integrate into routine cancer care: stigma is the elephant in the room. J Natl Compr Canc Netw. 2010;8(4):362–6.

62. Hesse BW, Suls JM. Informatics-enabled behavioral medicine in oncology. Cancer J. 2011;17(4): 222–30.

63. Lord O, Malone D, Mitchell AJ. Receipt of preventive medical care and medical screening for patients with mental illness: a comparative analysis. Gen Hosp Psychiatry. 2010;32(5):519–43.

64. Coyne JC, Stefanek M, Palmer SC. Psychotherapy and survival in cancer: the conflict between hope and evidence. Psychol Bull. 2007;133(3):367–94.

65. Coyne JC, Tennen H. Positive psychology in cancer care: bad science, exaggerated claims, and unproven medicine. Ann Behav Med. 2010;39(1):16–26.

66. Giese-Davis J, et al. Decrease in depression symptoms is associated with longer survival in patients with metastatic breast cancer: a secondary analysis. J Clin Oncol. 2011;29(4):413–20.

67. Andersen BL, et al. Biobehavioral, immune, and health benefits following recurrence for psychological intervention participants. Clin Cancer Res. 2010; 16(12):3270–8.

Complementary Mind–Body Therapies in Cancer

Daniel A. Monti and Andrew B. Newberg

Introduction

The term "complementary and alternative medicine" (CAM) refers to the broad range of health systems, modalities, and practices that are not part of the conventional and politically dominant health system [1, 2]. Functionally defined, CAM refers to those interventions that are neither taught widely in medical schools nor generally available in US hospitals. Several practices that are considered CAM in the United States include complex traditional health systems from other cultures, such as traditional Chinese medicine, as well as components of these systems that are practiced as distinct entities, such as acupuncture [3]. The National Center for Complementary and Alternative Medicine categorizes CAM in the following domains: whole medical systems such as homeopathy and ayurveda; mind–body medicine such as meditation and art therapy; biologically based practices such as herbs and dietary supplements; manipulative and body based practices such as chiropractic and massage; and energy medicine such as biofield therapies and magnets [4]. The use of CAM treatments in the United States is substantial, especially among those with chronic medical problems, including cancer. Eisenberg et al. published the first national survey on the use of CAM in 1993, which revealed that one in three respondents had used an unconventional or CAM treatment in the previous year [2]. Follow-up studies confirmed CAM use rates at least that high [5, 6], and most studies suggested that people use these treatments in addition to conventional medical care. Recent data confirm that CAM use continues to be particularly high among those with chronic diseases such as cancer [7]. Studies have indicated that many people do not disclose their use of CAM treatments to their conventional physicians, with many reporting that they perceive their doctors as unreceptive to the issue [6].

One possible explanation for the patient–physician communication gap on this topic is the limited information most physicians have about CAM, especially given its historical absence as a covered subject in conventional Western medical training. In addition, despite a recent surge of interest in CAM from the medical community, including some form of CAM curriculum at a growing number of medical schools [8], there is currently a limited evidence base on the topic.

The field of cancer survivorship research has been steadily growing along with the number of

D.A. Monti, M.D. (✉)
Department of Psychiatry and Emergency Medicine,
Myrna Brind Center of Integrative Medicine,
Thomas Jefferson University and Hospital, 925 Chestnut Street, Suite 120, Philadelphia, PA 19107, USA
e-mail: Daniel.monti@jefferson.edu

A.B. Newberg
Department of Radiology and Emergency Medicine,
Myrna Brind Center of Integrative Medicine
e-mail: andrew.newberg@jefferson.edu

cancer survivors in the US. When the National Cancer Act was passed in 1971, there were three million cancer survivors. Since that time, the number of cancer survivors has more than tripled. There are currently approximately 10.8 million survivors in the US [9].

One of the arenas in which there has been substantial interest in the use of CAM modalities is in the field of oncology, both during active treatment and in the post-treatment survivorship phase [10–15]. The use of CAM interventions is a growing area of interest in cancer survivorship research. CAM can be a challenging issue for oncologists, primary care physicians, and other mainstream medical professionals caring for cancer survivors, especially given that survivors are exposed to reams of information on the Internet and in the media that can cause them to stray into territory that may trigger discomfort and concern from their physicians.

Motivations for CAM use are multidimensional, including improvement of quality of life [16], enhancement of immune function [17], coping with pain [18, 19], and to decrease anxiety and other psychological symptoms [15, 20]. In regard to this last category, even though there is a large number of cancer survivors with high stress levels [21], and unmet psychosocial needs [22, 23], uptake of conventional supportive programs often is low [24]. For a myriad of reasons, CAM modalities may be seen as desirable options for some survivor groups to address unmet needs [25]. Issues related to CAM use may be particularly relevant to diverse groups with culturally based health beliefs, the underserved, and those who experience health disparities in the mainstream health care system [26]. As the number of cancer survivors increases, it includes more diverse groups who may be utilizing CAM, so it becomes even more important to understand why particular subgroups of survivors are using CAM, what forms of CAM they are using, and whether this is being integrated into the rest of their care [27]. Although at this point there has been little formal assessment of the patterns and predictors of CAM use among cancer survivors from diverse ethnic groups, there is some data to suggest that CAM use is overall similarly high across ethnic

groups, with subgroup variations in patterns of use [25, 28]. For example, even though use of mind–body therapies is consistently high on the list of commonly used CAM modalities overall, it is particularly high in some minority subgroups such as African Americans [25].

There are potential advantages for practitioners to be able to discuss CAM with their patients and in some cases integrate it with their conventional care [26]. One way of facilitating meaningful discussion would be for oncologists to have a positive platform from which to establish some "common ground" with the CAM-oriented patient. We previously have suggested that particular mind–body therapies with an evidence base could provide such a platform and serve as a bridge to connect potentially beneficial supportive interventions to patients, while also opening a general dialogue about CAM and the needs particular patients might be attempting to address with CAM approaches [29]. The end result could be an improved physician–patient relationship and overall improved patient care [26]. Mind–body therapies are a chosen platform because several have at least some positive supportive data, and many target stress reduction, which is a tangible endpoint that is associated with improved quality of life and better health outcomes. Moreover, such interventions generally are not practiced as an "alternative" to regular oncological care; hence, they can be integrated into the overall cancer survivorship treatment plan with relatively low risk [29].

Psychosocial Stress and Cancer

A report of cancer incident rates between 1992 and 2004 showed increases in some cancer types and decreases in others, with an overall slight decline of cancer incidence between both sexes [30]. At the same time, the mortality rates continue to decline [9, 30]. Thus, for increasing numbers of people, the diagnosis of cancer means coping with a chronic illness that has a variable course for an undetermined amount of time. Given the numerous stressful challenges involved with having a cancer diagnosis [31], it is not surprising that as many as one-third of cancer survivors report high stress levels [32, 33]. Stress can manifest in a variety of psychological symptoms, such as anxiety and depression [34–39], intrusive cancer-related thoughts (i.e., traumatic stress symptoms) [40–43], and/or physical symptoms, such as fatigue [33, 43], increased pain [44], and impaired sleep [45–47]. Amplified stress in cancer patients has been associated with increased morbidity and mortality [23, 48, 49], decreased immune function [50–53], increased relapse [52], and decreased health-related quality of life [54, 55]. Given the known negative impact of stress on cancer patients, stress has become a priority issue in cancer treatment and research [55, 56]. Targeting stress-related variables with psychosocial interventions has been an important emphasis in cancer care models [57–65]. Moreover, recent pre-clinical data have suggested possible direct effects of stress on tumor cell biology [66, 67] and potential indirect effects through increased oxidative stress [68], underscoring the importance of addressing stress across survivor populations.

Although the conventional standard for addressing distress in cancer survivors has largely been through supportive group programs, there are significant challenges in recruiting participants to these programs, despite availability, particularly in hard-to-reach populations [24]. In addition, it has been well established that there are widespread health disparities that impact on cancer prevention, treatment, and survivorship and palliative care [69]. In the field of cancer survivorship research, there is an emerging body of literature acknowledging such disparities and supporting the development of interventions that are sensitive to social, cultural, and economic differences, particularly as these factors influence quality of life [70–72]. Some of the selected findings from this research suggest that the survivorship experience varies by ethnicity, gender, and age [73–75]. For example, population studies suggest that ethnic groups that are low utilizers of conventional supportive group interventions may be relatively high utilizers of CAM [25, 28].

As the field of cancer survivorship and health disparities grows, it will be important to access hard-to-reach and underserved populations. Therefore, there is a need to continue exploring novel interventions and options for support for the growing and diverse population of cancer survivors. Although the evidence base for most CAM treatments is not clearly established, many of the mind–body therapies that have been used to support cancer patients generally are regarded as safe. We focus our discussion on a few modalities that have a promising evidence basis to serve as adjunctive interventions for supporting the psychosocial needs of cancer survivors.

Conceptual Framework

There are several theoretical models for understanding the concepts of stress, distress, coping, and stress reduction. Self-regulation is one such construct that appears to be applicable to a wide variety of psychosocial interventions, whether they are conventional or CAM. It has been shown that measuring self-regulation is reliable and may be a useful predictor of cancer patients' ability to find benefits in their cancer experience [76]. In a broader context, self-regulation theory is a framework for conceptualizing psychosocial stress and it provides an explanation for observed therapeutic effects. Although this framework cannot be seen as complete for any intervention, we propose self-regulation theory as a common ground for considering the effects of the mind–body interventions to be discussed.

Self-regulation theory [77, 78] provides a foundation for understanding reactions to perceptions of physical and emotional well-being. Functionally defined, self-regulation theory explains how people cope with and adapt to, stressful situations such as health problems or threats (e.g., a cancer diagnosis). The model reflects two aspects of information processing: (1) the objective data, such as a laboratory result or tumor stage, and (2) subjective appraisal of that data, such as fear or anger. An essential component to this theory is the personal schema that is formed from the combined objective and subjective aspects of the health threat. The schema can be characterized as the lens through which all subsequent health-related information and cues are perceived, and hence the determining factor for coping behaviors. The schema and resultant coping behaviors form a feedback loop, where one impacts the other. Hence, techniques that affect subjective appraisal of health-related information will affect coping behaviors related to that information; likewise, techniques that modulate coping responses can affect the schema itself. The ability to negotiate subjective appraisals of health threats and resulting coping responses both directly affect stress levels [79].

Mind–body therapies may affect self-regulation by either targeting the schema, the coping responses, or both. For example, some therapies teach techniques that may modify appraisals of the health-related data (e.g., mindfulness), others may provide methods to dampen or alter physiological responses to the data (e.g., biofeedback), while others may directly alter perception of the data itself (e.g., hypnosis).

Complementary Mind–Body Therapies

The term "Mind–Body Therapies" is a somewhat ambiguous categorization that generally refers to a collection of treatments that recognize the bidirectional nature of psyche and soma. Many of these modalities are classified as CAM, mostly because they are not currently part of a dominant conventional therapeutic paradigm. Alleviating stress through various mental and physical exercises tends to be a focus of these interventions. There are numerous mind–body techniques; below is a brief description of a few of those classified as CAM that may have particular relevance to cancer survivors, based upon available supportive data and relative safety.

Hypnosis

Franz Anton Mesmer (1734–1815) captivated the public in the eighteenth century when he introduced a form of hypnosis, which he called "animal magnetism" [80]. Mesmer made such an

impact that his technique came to be known as "mesmerism," a word that is still sometimes used to describe a hypnotic-like trance. The word "hypnosis" (from the Greek root *hypnos*, meaning sleep) is misleading in some ways because the phenomenon to which it refers is not a form of sleep; rather, it is a complex process of attentive, receptive concentration. This state, also called a "trance," is characterized by a modified sensorium, an altered psychological state and characteristically minimal motor functioning. In addition to achieving deep relaxation, the hypnotic treatment may include direct suggestions for specific changes in physiology and cognition [81]. Guided imagery is often an integral part of hypnotic technique.

There are data suggesting that hypnosis may be efficacious for a variety of mental health problems [82, 83] and physical disorders that are exacerbated by stress, including pain [83]. A NIH Technology Assessment Panel [18] concluded that there was strong evidence for the use of hypnosis in alleviating chronic pain conditions, including pain associated with cancer. Hypnosis has been shown to be particularly helpful for a variety of acute and chronic cancer pain issues in children [84], and there is evidence to suggest that children may have better responsiveness to hypnosis than adults [85]. Studies have demonstrated that hypnosis can be an effective means for some cancer patients to alleviate nausea and vomiting associated with chemotherapy [86]. Hypnotic effects are thought to occur through three primary mechanisms: muscle relaxation, perceptual alteration, and cognitive distraction [87]. Hence, learning new ways of perceiving an experience and developing coping strategies to negotiate the experience are important self-regulatory aspects of hypnosis.

Meditation Practices

Many common forms of meditation are extracted from traditional Eastern systems that encompass lifestyle issues beyond the meditative techniques. For example, Yoga is an ancient Eastern Indian system of health that prescribes a multiphasic approach to living, including proper diet, behavior, physical exercise, and sleep hygiene. Likewise, Qigong meditation practices often are derived from complex traditional Chinese medicine practices. A recently released report from the Agency for Healthcare Research and Quality, Department of Health and Human Services [88] comprehensively reviewed and synthesized the state of research on a variety of meditation practices. Although cancer was not the focus, the report reviewed encouraging data suggesting therapeutic benefits from several meditation practices for a variety of health conditions, but the authors were unable to translate that data into firm conclusions due to the poor quality of many of the studies. Below we focus on a few meditation-based practices that are commonly used by cancer survivors and have at least some substantive supportive evidence for use.

Mindfulness-based stress reduction (MBSR) is a standardized, 8 week intervention that incorporates mindfulness meditation, Hatha Yoga practices, and other techniques for the purposes of stress reduction and improvement of quality of life [89]. MBSR is the most studied meditation intervention, with suggested therapeutic benefits in several illness populations, including cancer [90–96]. Speca et al. [94] published the first randomized, controlled study of MBSR in a mixed group of cancer patients, demonstrating significant improvements in mood disturbances and decreased stress as compared to wait-list controls. These improvements were maintained at 6-month follow-up [95]. Another report showed that breast ($n=33$) and prostate cancer ($n=9$) patients who received the 8-week MBSR program had shifts in their immune profiles (reduction in Th1 pro-inflammatory to Th2 anti-inflammatory environment) associated with decreased depressive symptomology [96]. These trends continued at 1-year follow up [97].

A primary goal of MBSR is to develop the capacity to be relaxed and aware in each moment, while maintaining a non-judgmental attitude [89]. In this regard, thoughts and emotions are not viewed as wrong or faulty but rather as events. Together, this allows for conscious observation of both the actual experience (objective data) and the emotional response to it (subjective appraisal), which may facilitate improved self-regulation and more healthful coping strategies.

Qigong practices involve slow body movements and meditation, with or without imagery and breathing techniques. Common forms of qigong emphasize self-regulation of emotion (e.g., maintaining a peaceful, calm mood) and focused attention. In China there was a huge resurgence in qigong after the Great Cultural Revolution in China during the mid-1970s, which has since extended to the Western world, including the United States [19]. Yet, the majority of studies on the topic have been performed in China. A review of 50 Chinese studies on the use of qigong in cancer patients showed that although there was some indication that qigong had a positive impact on several parameters of cancer survivorship, the results cannot be considered conclusive given the poor design of most of the studies [98]. Outside of China the majority of studies are done on healthy volunteers. One study showed that qigong practice lowered cortisol levels with concomitant changes in numbers of cytokine-secreting peripheral blood cells in a group of 19 healthy volunteers [99]. These biological indicators suggest stress reduction, which was not directly measured. Positive results from a well-designed study in patients with late-stage complex regional pain syndrome provide potential support for the consideration of qigong as a complementary intervention for management of stress-related symptoms in cancer patients. This randomized, placebo-controlled clinical trial found that qigong training was associated with short-term pain reduction and long-term anxiety reduction [100].

Tai Chi is characterized by a set of exercises that emphasize a series of postures and movements along with controlled breathing. Also derived from TCM, the movements are designed to balance chi, which refers to the body's energy or life force. Tai Chi is sometimes referred to as "moving meditation" because the exercises are paired with training the mind to be calm and relaxed. The variety and patterning of the movements are slow, gentle and light, requiring focused concentration. The movements may facilitate self-regulation by their intention to foster a sense of inner and outer harmony as the movements become more fluid, yet controlled, and the mind more alert, yet peaceful [101].

There is some data to suggest cardiovascular benefits from Tai Chi, such as lowered blood pressure and heart rate [102], indirectly suggesting stress reduction and improved self-regulation. A Japanese study of older adults found significantly higher scores in health-related quality of life, particularly in the domains of physical functioning and vitality, in older adults who practiced Tai Chi as compared to age-matched national standards [103]. Although Tai Chi is common use, the data on cancer populations are limited. A recent systematic review of controlled clinical trials of Tai Chi as a supportive therapy for cancer patients searched the literature using 19 databases from their respective inceptions through October 2006, without language restrictions [104]. Of the 27 potentially relevant studies, only four met the criteria of "controlled clinical trial", and all four assessed patients with breast cancer. Two of these were considered well designed and they both reported significant differences in psychological and physiological symptoms as compared to psychosocial support control [105]. Hence, the data to support the use of Tai Chi are encouraging but limited and inconclusive.

Art therapy

Art therapy facilitates self-regulation by providing concrete tasks for expressing representations in a tangible and personally meaningful manner. A recent qualitative study of women with breast cancer suggests that the process of art making and art therapy provides unique opportunities to address psychosocial needs [106]. Research with cancer survivors and with other populations supports the use of tasks that allow for focused expression of unpleasant emotions, which can lead to a reduction in medical symptoms, such as pain, and an increased sense of well-being [107–110]. Although there are numerous published case and qualitative studies from the field of art therapy, including the widely reported and beneficial use of art therapy with cancer popula-

tions in both individual and group formats [111–114], few controlled studies exist. One particularly well-done clinical trial of an art therapy intervention with hospitalized children with post-traumatic stress disorder demonstrated that the use of specific art tasks was associated with stress reduction [115]. Recent reports in the cancer literature include the utilization of art therapy in a largely qualitative study of children with cancer, which resulted in enhanced communication and expression of emotional appraisals of the cancer experience [116]. In addition, significant reductions of anxiety were reported in a pre-post assessment of caregivers of persons with cancer ($n = 69$) who received a brief art therapy intervention [117]. Most recently, a controlled trial of art therapy demonstrated improved depression scores and fatigue levels in a group of cancer patients in active chemotherapy [118].

Mindfulness-based Art Therapy

Mindfulness-based art therapy (MBAT) was developed to engender health promoting skills and behaviors in a heterogeneous group format that can include patients with a variety of cancer types [119]. The two main components of MBAT, art therapy and MBSR, are paired with the purpose of facilitating both verbal and non-verbal information processing. Art therapy tasks are designed to meaningfully complement the MBSR curriculum, which may enhance the non-verbal process of negotiating subjective appraisals of health-related information and advance more adaptive coping. This combined intervention is new and there is limited available data. In a recently published RCT of MBAT [119], 111 women with a variety of cancer diagnoses were paired by age and randomized to either an 8-week MBAT intervention group or a wait list control group. As compared to controls, the MBAT group demonstrated significant decreases in symptoms of distress and significant improvements in key aspects of health-related quality of life. A recent follow-up to this study showed similar outcomes, and in addition, a subgroup from the cohort received pre- and post-intervention FMRI assessments that revealed changes in caudate activation from baseline and decreased cingulated activation in response to a stressful cue [29]. Another report of a group of prostate survivors showed improvements from the MBAT intervention consistent with the RCT of women [120].

Multi-modal interventions have gained in popularity likely because of the potential for an additive therapeutic effect. A recent study of women with breast cancer used a multi-modal format that included several of the elements of the MBAT intervention, showing increased emotional regulation and psychological adjustment [121]. The disadvantage of multi-modal interventions from a research standpoint is the inability to distinguish the relative contribution of the components in regard to observed effects.

Music Therapy

Music therapy is an increasingly popular adjunctive intervention for supporting the psychosocial needs of cancer survivors. Music therapy may facilitate self-regulation and enhanced coping by providing a soothing stimulus to counter distressing ones, using either music alone or music combined with guided imagery. The utility of music therapy to evoke relaxation was assessed in a meta-analysis of 22 music therapy trials that had quantitative outcomes, with overall findings suggesting decreased stress-based arousal [122]. Although specific data in cancer populations are quite limited, a recent report surveyed the coping strategies of 192 cancer outpatients; 43 % reported using music as a coping strategy, second only to prayer [123]. In a group of autologous stem cell transplant recipients ($n=62$), those receiving music therapy as compared to controls had significantly lower mood disturbance [124]. In a randomized trial of cancer patients receiving radiation therapy ($n=63$), non-significant trends in stress reduction were observed in the music condition as compared to controls who did not receive music [125]. Significant results were seen in a randomized clinical trial ($n=80$) comparing terminal cancer patients receiving hospice care in

their homes who were assigned to a music therapy intervention or to usual hospice care [126]. In that study, those who received repeated sessions of music therapy showed significant improvement in quality of life scores, while those not receiving music therapy showed decreased quality of life scores.

Neuroemotional Technique

A relative newcomer to the cancer survivorship literature, the neuroemotional technique (NET) pairs standard psychological approaches, such as addressing cognitive distortions, and desensitization procedures (e.g., relaxed breathing while visualizing distressing cues), with elements of traditional Chinese medicine, such as utilizing acupuncture pulse points [19]. This is mainly accomplished by having the patient touch particular pulse points while visualizing emotionally distressing experiences. Although there is limited data, NET may be applicable to cancer survivors as an intervention to alleviate traumatic stress symptoms [80]. Full post-traumatic stress disorder is rather uncommon in cancer survivors, but subsyndromal traumatic stress symptoms related to the cancer illness experience can be seen in as many as one third of survivors, causing significant impairment and distress [21, 41]. A recently published pilot study of NET in seven female cancer survivors with cancer-related traumatic stress symptoms compared pre-/post-intervention changes in response to recalling a distressing cancer-related event. The results showed encouraging decreases in physiologic reactivity to the distressing event and decreases in subjective ratings of distress related to the event [127]. A few other small studies suggest an anti-anxiety effect of the intervention [19]. Although there is no current evidence that the CAM component (acupressure) of NET adds to the effectiveness of the psychological aspects of the technique, the combination may appeal to survivor subpopulations that are attracted to CAM treatments. Improved self-regulation from NET may occur from modulating the character and intensity of subjective appraisals.

Exploring Mechanisms of Self-Regulation through Neuroimaging

Meditation practices are among the most common mind–body therapies used by cancer patients and survivors. In the past 30 years, researchers have been able to explore the biological effects and mechanism of meditation in much greater detail, largely due to the development of more advanced imaging technologies. Initial studies measured changes in autonomic activity, such as heart rate and blood pressure, as well as electroencephalographic changes. More recent studies have explored changes in hormonal and immunological functions associated with meditation. Functional neuroimaging has opened a new window into the investigation of meditative states by exploring the neurological correlates of these experiences. A growing number of neuroimaging studies of mindfulness and other meditation practices are currently available in the literature. The neuroimaging techniques include positron emission tomography (PET) [128, 129], single photon emission computed tomography (SPECT) [130], and functional magnetic resonance imaging (FMRI) [131]. Each of these techniques provides different advantages and disadvantages in the study of meditation. In terms of the larger topic of meditation, in addition to MM, the most common other type involves purposeful attention on a particular object, image, phrase, or word. This form of meditation is designed to lead to a subjective experience of absorption with the object of focus—a dissolution of the differentiation of self and object. There is another distinction in which meditation is guided by following along with a leader who verbally directs the practitioner, either in person or on tape. Others merely practice the meditation on their own volition. We might expect that this difference between volitional and guided meditation should also be reflected in specific differences in cerebral activation. Phenomenological analysis suggests that the end result of many practices of meditation is similar, although this result might be described using different characteristics depending on the culture and individual. Therefore, it seems reasonable that while the initial neurophysiological activation occurring during any given practice may differ, there should eventually be a convergence of data.

For example, brain imaging studies suggest that willful acts and tasks that require sustained attention are initiated via activity in the prefrontal cortex (PFC), particularly in the right hemisphere [25, 132–136]. The cingulate gyrus has also been shown to be involved in focusing attention, probably in conjunction with the PFC [136]. Since many meditation practices require intense focus of attention, it seems appropriate that meditation would be associated with activation of the PFC (particularly the right), as well as the cingulate gyrus. This notion is supported by the increased activity observed in these regions on several of the brain imaging studies of volitional types of meditation [128, 130, 131]. Activation of the PFC can result in increased thalamic activity which may either activate or inhibit neuronal activity in other structures. For example, several studies have demonstrated an increase in GABA, the primary inhibitory neurotransmitter, during meditation [137]. This inhibition may help with focused attention as well as have an impact on feelings of stress and anxiety. It should also be noted that the dopaminergic system, via the basal ganglia, is believed to participate in regulating the glutamatergic system and the interactions between the prefrontal cortex and subcortical structures. A PET study utilizing 11C-Raclopride to measure the dopaminergic tone during Yoga Nidra meditation demonstrated a significant increase in dopamine levels during the meditation practice [138]. They hypothesized that this increase may be associated with the gating of cortical–subcortical interactions that lead to an overall decrease in readiness for action that is associated with this particular type of meditation.

In addition to the complex cortical-thalamic activity, meditation might also be expected to alter activity in the limbic system given its impact on emotions. It has also been reported that stimulation of limbic structures is associated with experiences similar to those described during various meditation states [139, 140]. The results of the FMRI study by Lazar et al. support the notion of increased activity in the regions of the amygdala and hippocampus during meditation [131]. On the other hand, studies of mindfulness meditation in particular have reported enhanced PFC activity in conjunction with decreased activity in the amygdala which corresponds with diminished reactivity to emotional stimuli [141, 142]. Thus, different types of meditation practices may result in different activity levels in the limbic structures depending on whether emotional responses are enhanced or diminished.

Activity in the right lateral amygdala has been shown to modulate activity in the ventromedial portion of the hypothalamus which can result in either excitation or stimulation of the peripheral parasympathetic system [143]. Increased parasympathetic activity should be associated with the subjective sensation first of relaxation, and eventually, of a more profound quiescence. Activation of the parasympathetic system would also cause a reduction in heart rate and respiratory rate. All of these physiological responses have been observed during meditation [144]. In accord with the Indo-Tibetan tradition of self-healing, one study narrowed its analysis of MM specifically to that of mindfulness-based stress reduction; meditators experienced a notable reduction of stress levels, along with the secretion of hormones (such as cortisol) associated with stress response [145]. In fact, there are typically marked changes in autonomic nervous system activity. Several studies have demonstrated predominant parasympathetic activity during meditation associated with decreased heart rate and blood pressure, decreased respiratory rate, and decreased oxygen metabolism [48]. However, a recent study of two separate meditative techniques suggested a mutual activation of parasympathetic and sympathetic systems by demonstrating an increase in the variability of heart rate during meditation [146]. The increased variation in heart rate was hypothesized to reflect activation of both arms of the autonomic nervous system.

Thus, the physiological changes associated with practices such as meditation are varied and significant. Depending on the particular issues associated with a patient, different types of practices may be of more or less benefit. However, more studies are needed to better assess how meditation and other CAM practices produce their clinical effects.

Conclusions

In the past decade or more, there has been an ongoing increase in both the overall number of cancer survivors and the percentage of cancer survivors utilizing CAM treatments. Although it is important for oncology providers to be aware of CAM modalities their patients are using, patient disclosure and communication about the topic remains problematic. Mind–body therapies categorized as CAM could potentially serve as a positive platform from which providers could discuss CAM and even link survivor subgroups to services that might at least partially address unmet psychosocial needs. This would be especially relevant for survivor subgroups that have a cultural bias towards CAM. The mind–body therapies reviewed have some supportive evidence and a rationale for use in cancer survivors. Self-regulation could be a useful framework to contextualize the goals and outcomes of mind–body therapies. Recent advances in neuroimaging and other techniques have begun to provide some initial understanding of potential effects of some mind–body interventions, particularly meditation practices. Although the data on efficacy and mechanisms of action are incomplete and nonconclusive, the potential benefits of using complementary mind–body therapies in survivor care plans warrant consideration.

References

1. O'Connor BB, Lazar JS. Talking with patients about their use of alternative therapies. Prim Care Clin Off Pract. 1997;24(4):699–714.
2. Eisenberg DM, Kessler RC, Foster C, et al. Unconventional medicine in the United States: prevalence, costs, and patterns of use. New Engl J Med. 1993;328(4):246–52.
3. Eskinazi D. Policy perspectives: factors that shape alternative medicine. JAMA. 1998;328(4): 246–52.
4. NCCAM 2007. Publication No. D347, Updated February, 2007. http://nccam.nih.gov/health/whatiscam/ NCCAM. Accessed August 2012
5. Eisenberg DM, Davis RB, Ettner SL, et al. Trends in alternative medicine use in the United States, 1990–1997: results of a follow-up national survey. JAMA. 1998;280(18):1569–75.

6. Elder N, Gillcrist A, Minz R. Use of alternative health care by family practice patients. Arch Fam Med. 1997;6:181–4.

7. Saydah S, Eberhardt M. Use of complementary and alternative medicine among adults with chronic diseases: United States 2002. J Altern Complement Med. 2006;12(8):805–12.

8. Wetzel MS, Eisenberg DM, Kaptchuk TJ. Courses involving complementary and alternative medicine at US medical schools. JAMA. 1998;280:784–7.

9. Ries LAG, Melbert D, Krapcho M, et al. (editors). SEER cancer statistics review, 1975–2004. Bethesda, MD: National Cancer Institute. http://seer.cancer.gov/csr/1975_2004. Accessed May 2012

10. Ernst E, Cassileth BR. The prevalence of complementary/alternative medicine in cancer: a systematic review. Cancer. 1997;83(4):777–82.

11. Goldstein MS. Complementary and alternative medicine: its emerging role in oncology. J Psychosoc Oncol. 2003;21(2):1–21.

12. Cassileth BR, Deng G. Complementary and alternative therapies for cancer. Oncologist. 2004;9:80–9.

13. Kronenberg F, Mindes J, Jacobson JS. The future of complementary and alternative medicine for cancer. Cancer Invest. 2005;223:420–6.

14. Verhoef MJ, Balneaves LG, Boon HS, Vroegindewey BN. Reasons for and characteristics associated with complementary and alternative medicine use among adult cancer patients: a systematic review. Integr Cancer Ther. 2005;4(4):274–86.

15. Matthews AK, Sellergren MA, Dezheng H, List M, Fleming G. Complementary and alternative medicine use among breast cancer survivors. J Altern Complement Med. 2007;13(5):555–62.

16. Burstein HJ. Discussing complementary therapies with cancer patients: what should we be talking about? J Clin Oncol. 2000;18:2501–4.

17. Boon H, Stewart M, Kennard MA, et al. Use of complementary/alternative medicine by breast cancer survivors in Ontario: prevalence and perceptions. J Clin Oncol. 2000;18:2515–21.

18. National Institutes of Health (NIH), Technology Assessment Panel on Integration of Behavioral and Relaxation Approaches into the Treatment of Chronic Pain and Insomnia. Special Communication; 1996.

19. Monti DA, Yang J. Complementary medicine in chronic cancer care. Semin Oncol. 2005;32(2): 225–31.

20. Burstein HJ, Gelber S, Guadagnoli E, Weeks JC. Use of alternative medicine by women with early stage breast cancer. N Engl J Med. 1999;22:1733–9.

21. Butler LD, Koopman C, Classen C, Spiegel D. Traumatic stress, life events, and emotional support among women with advanced breast cancer. Health Psychol. 1999;18:555–60.

22. Spiegel D, Giese-Davis J. Depression and cancer: mechanisms and disease progression. Biol Psychiatry. 2003;54(3):269–82.

23. Brown KW, Levy R. Psychological distress and cancer survival: a follow-up 10 years after diagnosis. Psychosom Med. 2003;65:636–43.

24. Owen JE, Goldstein JS, Lee JH, Breen N, Rowland JH. Use of health-related and cancer-specific groups among adult cancer survivors. Cancer. 2007; 109(12):2580–9.

25. Mackenzie E, Taylor L, Bloom BS, et al. Ethnic minority use of complementary and alternative medicine (CAM): a national probability survey of CAM utilizers. Altern Ther Health Med. 2003;9(4):50–6.

26. Sufian M. Cultural context of treatment. In: Spiera H, Oreskes I, editors. Rheumatology for the health care professional. St. Louis: Warren H. Green; 1991.

27. Miller MF, Bellizzi KM, Sufian M, Goldstein MS, Ballard-Barbash R. Use of dietary supplements among ethnically diverse cancer survivors in California. J Am Diet Assoc. (in press).

28. Hsiao A-F, Wong WD, Goldstein MS, et al. Variations in complementary and alternative medicine (CAM) use across racial/ethnic groups and the development of ethnic-specific measures of CAM use. J Altern Complement Med. 2006;12(3):281–90.

29. Monti DA, Sufian M, Peterson C. Potential role of mind–body therapies in cancer survivorship. Cancer. 2008;112(11):2607–16.

30. Espey DK, Wu X, Swan J, et al. Annual report to the nation on the status of cancer, 1975–2004, featuring cancer in American Indians and Alaska natives. Cancer. 2007. doi:10.1002/cncr.23044.

31. Jacobsen P, Holland J. The stress of cancer: psychological responses to diagnosis and treatment. In: Cooper C, Watson M, editors. Cancer and stress: psychological, biological, and coping mechanisms. Chichester: John Wiley & Sons; 1991. p. 147–69.

32. Goodkin K, Antoni MH, Helder L, Sevin B. Psychoneuroimmunological aspects of disease progression among women with human papilloma virus-associated cervical dysplasia and human immunodeficiency virus type 1 co-infection. Int J Psychiatry Med. 1993;23:119–48.

33. Carlson L, Angen M, Cullum J, et al. High levels of untreated distress and fatigue in cancer patients. Br J Cancer. 2004;90(12):2297–304.

34. Derogatis LR, Morrow GR, Fetting J, et al. The prevalence of psychiatric disorders among cancer patients. J Am Med Assoc. 1983;249(6):751–7.

35. Massie MJ, Popkin MK. Depressive disorders. In: Holland J, editor. Psycho-oncology. New York: Oxford University Press; 1998. p. 518–40.

36. McDaniel JS, Musselman DL, Porter MR, et al. Depression in patients with cancer: diagnosis, biology and treatment. Arch Gen Psychiatry. 1995;52:89–99.

37. Massie M, Shakin E. Management of depression and anxiety in cancer patients. In: Breitbart W, Holland J, editors. Psychiatric aspects of symptom management in cancer patients. Washington, D.C.: American Psychiatric Press; 1993. p. 1–22.

38. Kunkel EJ. The assessment and management of anxiety in the patient with cancer. New Dir Ment Health Serv. 1993;57:61–9.

39. Kissane DW, Grabsch B, Love A, Clarke DM, Bloch S, Smith C. Psychiatric disorder in women with early stage and advanced breast cancer: a comparative analysis. Aust N Z J Psychiatry. 2004;38(5):320–6.

40. McGarvey EL. Evidence of acute stress after diagnosis of cancer. South Med J. 1998;91:864–6.

41. Koopman C, Butler LD, Classen C, et al. Traumatic stress symptoms among women with recently diagnosed primary breast cancer. J Trauma Stress. 2002;15:277–87.

42. Brewin C, Watson M, McCarthy S, Hyman P, Dayson D. Intrusive memories and depression in cancer patients. Behav Res Ther. 1998;36(12):1131–42.

43. Bennett B, Goldstein D, Lloyd A, et al. Fatigue and psychological distress – exploring the relationship in women treated for breast cancer. Eur J Cancer. 2004;40:1689–95.

44. Breibart W, Payne DK. Pain. In: Holland J, editor. Psycho-oncology. New York: Oxford University Press; 1998. p. 450–67.

45. Savard J, Simard S, Blanchet J, et al. Prevalence, clinical characteristics and risk factors for insomnia in the context of breast cancer. Sleep. 2001;24:583–90.

46. Lavie P. Sleep disturbance in the wake of traumatic events. N Engl J Med. 2001;345:1825–32.

47. Palesh O, Collie K, Batiuchok D. A longitudinal study of depression, pain, and stress as predictors of sleep disturbance among women with metastatic breast cancer. Biol Psychiatry. 2007;75(1):37–44.

48. Cohen M, Kunkel E, Levenson J. Associations between psychological stress and malignancy. In: Hubbard J, Workman E, editors. Handbook of stress medicine: an organ system approach. Boca Raton: CRC Press; 1998. p. 205–28.

49. Ell K, Nishimoto R, Mediansky J, Hamovitch M. Social relations, social support and survival among patients with cancer. J Psychosom Res. 1992;36(6):531–41.

50. Fawzy I, Fawzy N, Hyun C, et al. Malignant melanoma: effects of an early structured psychiatric intervention, coping and affective state on recurrence and survival 6 years later. Arch Gen Psychiatry. 1993;50:681–9.

51. Spiegel D, Bloom J, Kraemer H, Gottheil E. Effect of psychosocial treatment on survival of patients with metastatic breast cancer. Lancet. 1989;2:889–90.

52. Uchino B, Cacioppo J, Kiecoult-Glaser J. The relationship between social support and physiological processes: a review with emphasis on underlying mechanisms and implications for health. Psychol Bull. 1996;119(3):488–531.

53. Carlson LE, Speca M. Mindulfness-based stress reduction in relation to quality of life, mood, symptoms of stress, and immune parameters in breast and prostate cancer outsubjects. Psychosom Med. 2003;65:571–81.

54. Zabora JR, Blanchard CG, Smith ED, et al. Prevalence of psychological distress among cancer patients across the disease continuum. J Psychosoc Oncol. 1997;15(2):73–87.

55. Hewitt M, Rowland JH. Mental health service use among adult cancer survivors: analyses of the National Health Interview Survey. J Clin Oncol. 2002;20(23):4581–90.

56. Sanson-Fisher R, Girgis A, Boyes A, Bonevski B, Burton L, Cook P. The unmet supportive care needs of cancer patients. Cancer. 2000;88(1):226–37.

57. Myer TJ, Mark MM, Wood R. Effects of psychosocial interventions with adult cancer patients: a meta-analysis of randomized experiments. Health Psychol. 1995;14(2):101–8.

58. Fobair P. Cancer support groups and group therapies: part I: historical and theoretical backgrounds and research on effectiveness. J Psychosoc Oncol. 1997;15(1):63–81.

59. Spiegel D, Bloom J, Yalom I. Group support for patients with metastatic breast cancer: a randomized prospective outcome study. Arch Gen Psychiatry. 1981;38:527–33.

60. Goodwin PJ, Leszcz MD. The effect of group psychosocial support on survival in metastatic breast cancer. New Engl J Med. 2001;345(24):1719–26.

61. Shrock D, Palmer R, Taylor B. Effects of a psychosocial intervention on survival among patients with stage I breast and prostate cancer: a matched case control study. Altern Ther Health Med. 1999;5(3):49–55.

62. Jacobsen P, Hann D. Cognitive-behavioral Interventions. In: Holland J, editor. Psychooncology. New York: Oxford University Press; 1998. p. 717–29.

63. Classen C, Sephton S, Diamond S, Spiegel D. Studies of life-extending psychosocial interventions. In: Holland J, editor. Psychooncology. New York: Oxford University Press; 1998. p. 730–42.

64. Spiegel D, Moore R. Imagery and hypnosis in cancer patients. Oncology. 1997;11(8):1179–95.

65. Spiegel D, Sephton S, Terr A, Stites D. Effects of psychosocial treatment in prolonging cancer survival may be mediated by neuroimmune pathways. Ann N Y Acad Sci. 1998;840:674–83.

66. Yang EV, Kim SJ, Donovan EL, Chen M, Gross AC, Webster Marketon JI, et al. Norepinephrine upregulates VEGF, IL-8 and IL-6 expression in human melanoma tumor cell lines: implications for stress-related enhancement of tumor progression. Brain Behav Immun. 2009;23:267–75.

67. Lee JW, Shahzad MM, Lin YG, Armaiz-Pena G, Mangala LS, Han HD, et al. Surgical stress promotes tumor growth in ovarian carcinoma. Clin Cancer Res. 2009;15:2695–702.

68. Martinez-Outschoorn UE, Balliet RM, Rivadeneira DB, Chiavarina B, Pavlides S, Wang C, et al. Oxidative stress in cancer associated fibroblasts drives tumor-stroma co-evolution. A new paradigm for understanding tumor metabolism, the field effect and genomic instability in cancer cells. Cell Cycle. 2010;9(16):3256–76

69. Institute of Medicine (IOM). The unequal burden of cancer: an assessment of NIH research and programs for ethnic minorities and the medically underserved. Washington, DC: National Academy Press; 1999.

70. Aziz NM, Rowland JH. Cancer survivorship research among ethnic minority and medically underserved groups. Oncol Nurs Forum. 2002;29(5):789–801.

71. Campbell LC, Keefe FJ, McKee DC, et al. Prostate cancer in African Americans: relationship of patient and partner self-efficacy to quality of life. J Pain Symptom Manage. 2004;28(5):433–44.

72. Hamilton JB, Sandelowski M. Types of social support in African Americans with cancer. Oncol Nurs Forum. 2004;31(4):792–800.

73. Deimling GT, Bowman KF, Sterns S, Wagner LJ, Kahana B. Cancer-related health worries and psychological distress among older adult, long-term survivors. Psychooncology. 2006;15(4):306–20.

74. Demark-Wahnefried W, Clipp EC, Morey MC, et al. Lifestyle intervention development study to improve physical function in older adults with cancer: outcomes from Project LEAD. J Clin Oncol. 2006;24(21):3465–73.

75. Penedo FJ, Molton I, Dahn JR, et al. Ethnicity and determinants of quality of life after prostate cancer treatment. Urology. 2006;67(5):1022–7.

76. Graves KD, Carter CL. Outcome expectations and self-regulation in cancer patients: reliability, initial factor structure, and relationships with benefit finding. Palliat Support Care. 2005;3(3):209–19.

77. Leventhal H, Diefenbach M, Leventhal EA. Illness cognition: using common sense to understand treatment adherence and affect cognitions interactions. Cogn Ther Res. 1992;16:43–163.

78. Leventhal H, Zimmerman R, Gutmann M. Compliance: a self-regulation perspective. In: Gentry D, editor. Handbook of behavioral medicine. New York: Guilford Press; 1984. p. 369–436.

79. Folkman S. Personal control and stress and coping processes: a theoretical analysis. J Pers Soc Psychol. 1984;46(4):839–52.

80. Monti DM, Stoner M. Complementary and alternative medicine. In: Kornstein SG, Clayton AH, editors. Women's mental health. New York: Guilford; 2002. p. 344–56.

81. Spiegel H, Greenleaf M, Speigel D. Hypnosis. In: Saddock BJ, Saddock VA, editors. Kaplan and Saddock's comprehensive textbook of psychiatry. Philadelphia, PA: Lippincott Williams & Wilkins; 2000. p. 2128–45.

82. Stanton HE. Using hypnotherapy to overcome examination anxiety. Am J Clin Hypn. 1993;35(3): 198–204.

83. Marks IM, Gelder MG, Edwards G. Hypnosis and desensitization for phobics: a controlled prospective trial. Br J Psychiatry. 1968;114:1263–74.

84. Liossi C, Hatira P. Clinical hypnosis in the alleviation of procedure-related pain in pediatric oncology patients. Int J Clin Exp Hypn. 2003(1); 51:4–28.

85. Wakeman RJ, Kaplan JZ. An experimental study of hypnosis in painful burns. Am J Clin Hypn. 1978;21:3–12.

86. Genuis ML. The use of hypnosis in helping cancer patients control anxiety, pain, and emesis: a review of empirical studies. Am J Clin Hypn. 1995;37: 316–25.

87. Spiegel H, Spiegel D. Trance and treatment: clinical uses of hypnosis. New York: Basic Books; 1978.

88. Ospina MB, Bond K, Karkhaneh M, et al. Meditation practices for health: state of the research. AHRQ Agency for Healthcare Research and Quality, Evidence Report/Technology Assessment Number 155. Prepared for Agency for Healthcare Research and Quality Contract No. 290-02-0023. Prepared by University of Alberta Evidence-based Practice Center, Edmonton, Alberta, Canada. AHRQ Publication No. 07-E010; 2007. http://www.ahrq.gov/clinic/tp/medittp.htm. Accessed June 2007

89. Santorelli SF, Kabat-Zinn J (editors). Mindfulness-based stress reduction professional training: mindfulness-based stress reduction curriculum guide and supporting materials, Masschusetts: University of Masschusetts Medical School; 2007.

90. Kabat-Zinn J, Massion AO, Kristeller J, et al. Effectiveness of a meditation-based stress reduction program in the treatment of anxiety disorders. Am J Psychiatry. 1992;149:936–43.

91. Kabat-Zinn J, Lipworth L, Burney R, et al. Four-year follow-up of a meditation-based program for self-regulation of chronic pain: treatment outcomes and compliance. Clin J Pain. 1987;2:159–73.

92. Reibel D, Greeson J, Brainard G. Mindfulness-based stress reduction and health-related quality of life in a heterogeneous patient population. Gen Hosp Psychiatry. 2001;23:183–92.

93. Coker KH. Meditation and prostate cancer. Semin Urol Oncol. 1999;17:111–8.

94. Speca M, Carlson L, Goodey E, Angen M. A randomized wait-list controlled clinical trial: the effects of a mindfulness-based stress reduction program on mood and symptoms of stress in cancer patients. Psychosom Med. 2000;62:613–22.

95. Carlson L, Ursuliak Z, Goodey E, Angen M, Speca M. The effects of mindfulness meditation-based stress reduction program on mood and symptoms of stress in cancer outpatients: 6-month follow-up. Support Care Cancer. 2001;9:112–3.

96. Carlson LE, Speca M, Patel KD, Goodey E. Mindfulness-based stress reduction in relation to quality of life, mood, symptoms of stress and levels of cortisol, dehydroepiandrosterone sulfate (DHEAS) and melatonin in breast and prostate cancer outpatients. Psychoneuroendocrinology. 2004;29(4):448–74.

97. Carlson LE, Speca M, Patel KD, Faris P. One year pre-post intervention follow-up of psychological, immune, endocrine and blood pressure outcomes of mindfulness-based stress reduction (MBSR) in breast and prostate cancer outpatients. Brain Behav Immun. 2007;21(8):1038–49.

98. Chen K, Yeung R. Exploratory studies of qigong therapy for cancer in China. Intergr Cancer Ther. 2002;1:345–70.

99. Jones BM. Changes in cytokine production in healthy subjects practicing Guolin qigong: a pilot study. BMC Complement Altern Med. 2001;1(8): 1472–9.

100. Wu WH, Bandilla E, Ciccone DS, et al. Effects of Qigong on late-stage complex regional pain syndrome. Altern Ther Health Med. 1999;5:45–54.

101. Li F, Fisher KJ, Harmer P, et al. A simpler eight-form easy tai chi for elderly adults. J Aging Phys Activ. 2003;11(2):206–18.

102. Jones AY, Dean E, Scudds RJ. Effectiveness of a community-based tai chi program and implications for public health initiatives. Arch Phys Med Rehabil. 2005;86(4):619–25.

103. Kin S, Toba K, Orimo H. [Health-related quality of life (HRQOL) in older people practicing Tai Chi – comparison of the HRQOL with the national standards for age-matched controls]. [Japanese] Nippon Ronen Igakkai Zasshi Jpn J Geriatr. 2007;44(3):339–44.

104. Lee MS. Pittler MH. Ernst E. Is Tai Chi an effective adjunct in cancer care? A systematic review of controlled clinical trials. [Review] [24 refs]. Support Care Cancer. 2007;15(6):597–601.

105. Woo J, Hong A, Lau E, Lynn H. A randomized controlled trial of Tai Chi and resistance exercise on bone health, muscle strength and balance in community-living elderly people. Age Aging. 2007;36(3):262–8.

106. Collie K, Long BC. Considering meaning in the context of breast cancer. J Health Psychol. 2005;10(6): 843–53.

107. Shakin E, Rowland J, Holland J. Psychological aspects of breast cancer: one nation's approach to an international problem. In: Hoogstraten B, Burn I, Bloom H, editors. Breast cancer. Heidelberg: Springer; 1989. p. 89–99.

108. Smyth JM. Written emotional expression: effect sizes, outcome types and moderating variables. J Consult Clin Psychol. 1998;66:174–84.

109. Pennebaker JW, Mayne TJ, Francis ME. Linguistic predictors of adaptive bereavement. J Pers Soc Psychol. 1997;72:864–71.

110. Stanton AL, Danoff-Burg S, Cameron C, et al. Emotionally expressive coping predicts psychological and physical adjustment in breast cancer. J Consult Clin Psychol. 2000;68(5):875–82.

111. Gabriel B, Bromberg E, Vandenbovenkamp J, Kornblith AB, Luzzatto P. Art therapy with adult bone marrow transplant patients in isolation: a pilot study. Psychooncology. 2001;10(2):114–23.

112. Deane K, Fitch M, Carman M. An innovative art therapy program for cancer patients. Can Oncol Nurs J. 2000;10(4):147–51, 152–57.

113. Luzzatto P. From psychiatry to psycho-oncology: personal reflections on the use of art therapy with cancer patients. In: Pratt M, Wood M, editors. Art therapy in palliative care. New York: Rutledge, New York; 1998. p. 169–75.

114. Malchiodi C (editor). Medical art therapy with adults. Philadelphia: Jessica Kingsley Publishers; 1999. p. 13–20.

115. Chapman L, Morabito D, Ladakakos C, et al. The effectiveness of an art therapy intervention in reducing post-traumatic stress disorder (PTSD) symptoms in pediatric trauma patients. J Am Art Ther Assoc. 2001;18(2):100–4.

116. Rollins JA. Tell me about it: drawing as a communication tool for children with cancer. J Pediatr Oncol Nurs. 2005;22(4):203–21).

117. Walsh SM, Radcliffe RS, Castillo LC, Kumar AM, Broschard DM. A pilot study to test the effects of art-making classes for family caregivers of patients with cancer. Oncol Nurs Forum. 2007;34(1):38.

118. Bar-Sela G, Atid L, Danos S, Gabay N, Epelbaum R. Art therapy improved depression and influenced fatigue levels in cancer patients on chemotherapy. Psychooncology. 2007;16:980–4.

119. Monti DA, Peterson C, Kunkel EJ, et al. A randomized, controlled trial of mindfulness-based art therapy (MBAT) for women with cancer. Psychooncology. 2006;15:363–73.

120. Monti DA, Gomella L, Peterson C, Kunkel, E. Preliminary results from a novel psychosocial intervention for men with prostate cancer. Poster presented at ASCO Prostate Cancer Symposium, Orlando, Florida, February, 2007.

121. Cameron LD, Booth RJ, Schlatter M, Ziginskas D, Harman JE. Changes in emotion regulation and psychological adjustment following use of a group psychosocial support program for women recently diagnosed with breast cancer. Psycho-oncology. 2007;16(3):171–80.

122. Pelletier CL. The effect of music on decreasing arousal due to stress: a meta-analysis. J Music Ther. 2004;41(3):192–214.

123. Zaza C, Sellick SM, Hillier LM. Coping with cancer: what do patients do. J Psychosoc Oncol. 2005;23(1):55–73.

124. Cassileth BR, Vickers AJ, Magill LA. Music therapy for mood disturbance during hospitalization for autologous stem cell transplantation: a randomized controlled trial. Cancer. 2003;98(12):2723–9.

125. Clark M, Isaacks-Downton G, Wells N, Redlin-Frazier S, Eck C, Hepworth JT, Chakravarthy B. J Music Ther. 2006;43(3):247–65.

126. Hilliard RE. The effects of music therapy on the quality and length of life of people diagnosed with terminal cancer. J Music Ther. 2003;40(2): 113–37.

127. Monti DA, Stoner ME, et al. Short term correlates of the neuro emotional technique for cancer-related traumatic stress symptoms: a pilot case series. J Cancer Surviv. 2007;1:161–6.

128. Herzog H, Lele VR, Kuwert T, et al. Changed pattern of regional glucose metabolism during yoga meditative relaxation. Neuropsychobiology. 1990–1991;23:182–7.

129. Lou HC, Kjaer TW, Friberg L, et al. A 15O-H2O PET study of meditation and the resting state of normal consciousness. Human Brain Map. 1999;7:98–105.

130. Newberg AB, Alavi A, Baime M, et al. The measurement of regional cerebral blood flow during the complex cognitive task of meditation: a preliminary SPECT study. Psychiatr Res Neuroimag. 2001;106:113–22.

131. Lazar SW, Bush G, Gollub RL, et al. Functional brain mapping of the relaxation response and meditation. Neuroreport. 2000;11:1581–5.

132. Ingvar DH. The will of the brain: cerebral correlates of willful acts. J Theor Biol. 1994;171:7–12.

133. Frith CD, Friston K, Liddle PF, et al. Willed action and the prefrontal cortex in man. a study with PET. Proc R Soc Lond. 1991;244:241–6.

134. Posner MI, Petersen SE. The attention system of the human brain. Ann Rev Neurosci. 1990;13:25–42.

135. Pardo JV, Fox PT, Raichle ME. Localization of a human system for sustained attention by positron emission tomography. Nature. 1991;349:61–4.

136. Vogt BA, Finch DM, Olson CR. Functional heterogeneity in cingulate cortex: the anterior executive and posterior evaluative regions. Cereb Cortex. 1992;2:435–43.

137. Elias AN, Guich S, Wilson AF. Ketosis with enhanced GABAergic tone promotes physiological changes in transcendental meditation. Med Hypotheses. 2000;54:660–2.

138. Kjaer TW, Bertelsen C, Piccini P, Brooks D, Alving J, Lou HC. Increased dopamine tone during meditation-induced change of consciousness. Brain Res Cogn Brain Res. 2002;13(2):255–9.

139. Fish DR, Gloor P, Quesney FL, et al. Clinical responses to electrical brain stimulation of the temporal and frontal lobes in patients with epilepsy. Brain. 1993;116:397–414.

140. Saver JL, Rabin J. The neural substrates of religious experience. J Neuropsychiatr Clin Neurosci. 1997;9:498–510.

141. Lieberman MD, et al. Putting feelings into words: affect labeling disrupts amygdale activity in response to affective stimuli. Psychol Sci. 2007;18:421–8.

142. Creswell JD, Way BM, et al. Neural correlates of dispositional mindfulness during affect labeling. Psychosom Med. 2007;69:560–5.

143. Davis M. The role of the amygdala in fear and anxiety. Ann Rev Neurosci. 1992;15:353–75.

144. Jevning R, Wallace RK, Beidebach M. The physiology of meditation: a review. A wakeful hypometabolic integrated response. Neurosci Biobeh Rev. 1992;16:415–24.

145. Peterson J, Loizzo J, Charlson M. A program in contemplative self-healing: stress, allostasis, and learning in the Indo-Tibetan tradition. Ann N Y Acad Sci. 2009;1172:123–47.

146. Peng CK, Mietus JE, Liu Y, et al. Exaggerates heart rate oscillations during two meditation techniques. Intern J Cardiol. 1999;70:101–7.

End-of-Life Communication in Cancer Care

Wen-ying Sylvia Chou, Karley Abramson, and Lee Ellington

The Context of End-of-Life Communication in the USA

While advances in treatment have extended cancer survival rate in recent years, cancer continues to be the second most common cause of death in the USA, accounting for 1 of every 4 deaths in this country [1]. In 2011, about 569,490 Americans are expected to die of cancer, more than 1,500 people a day. Consequently, enabling optimal end-of-life care and effective communication represents a key priority in cancer care in all levels and settings, including family communication, clinical care, and public health.

A book chapter for Psychological *Aspects of Cancer: A Guide to Emotional and Psychological Consequences of Cancer, Their Causes and Their Management*, edited by Brian I. Carr and Jennifer L. Steele.

W.-y.S. Chou, Ph.D., M.P.H. (✉)
Health Communication and Informatics Research Branch, Division of Cancer Control and Population Sciences, National Cancer Institute, National Institutes of Health, 6130 Executive Blvd. EPN 4046, Bethesda, MD 20892, USA
e-mail: chouws@mail.nih.gov

K. Abramson, M.P.H
National Cancer Institute, Bethesda, MD, USA

University of Michigan School of Law, Ann Arbor, MI, USA

L. Ellington, Ph.D.
University of Utah, Salt Lake City, UT, USA

Communication about the end of life has been fraught with barriers and challenges even in current times. With the myths and taboos surrounding death and dying, medicine's predominant focus on curative and life-prolonging treatments over palliative care, and barriers to care coordination and transition, it was not until recent decades that concerted efforts have been made to improve communication and alleviate burden and suffering at the end of life for cancer patients and their families [2, 3]. This chapter will review key advances in end-of-life communication research in cancer care, identify important domains of end-of-life communication, describe key intervention efforts to date in various areas of care, and highlight remaining research questions and future directions.

To understand current issues in end-of-life communication research and practice, it is necessary to trace the history of the hospice movement. Hospice and palliative medicine, pioneered in the late 1960s by Cicely Saunders in the UK and Elizabeth Kübler-Ross in the USA, has made significant progress in demystifying and improving communication and about end-of-life decisions and care [4, 5]. The hospice philosophy stresses the role of communication in all domains of care [6]. In public discourse, the language of hospice distinguishes itself from cure-based medicine with positive framing of the end of life (e.g., "moving towards the end of life" and "letting go," as opposed to "losing to cancer" or "giving up"). In the context of patient-provider communication, there is a heavy emphasis placed on patient-centered discussions and shared decision-making about end-of-life options (e.g., on treatment, palliation, and whether and when to go home) as well as patient's families and social networks, personal priorities and existential topics [7]. Hospice also promotes an open and frank communication dynamic for patients, family, and all those affected by the diagnosis [3]. Moreover, optimal end-of-life care requires a multidisciplinary team [8]. This means that communication occurs around many individuals with different roles in the care of a patient, including the physicians, social workers, chaplains, nurses, medical assistants, family members, and friends. Finally, it is important to note that the hospice approach to care has implications for communication at all phases of the cancer care spectrum.

For the past several decades, new and emerging fields including psycho-oncology have placed greater emphasis on quality of life, which focused attention to communication as well as emotional and psychosocial aspects of patients and their families' experiences [9]. Among research aimed at documenting barriers to end-of-life care, communication problems are among the most frequently identified factors associated with poor care [3, 10–12]. Common communication challenges noted include delayed discussions about the end of life (e.g., DNR status), mismatched understanding of the diagnosis and prognosis, and inadequate attention to patients' emotions and preferences [13]. On the other hand, patient-centered communication has been associated with better cancer care [14, 15]. Specifically, effective communication has been shown to correlate with better pain management, improved quality of life, better patient satisfaction, and notably, length of survival [16–18].

In clinical practice, medical curriculum and training have demonstrated continuing emphasis on communication throughout the cancer care continuum. Efforts began with teaching clinicians and medical trainees communication skills in interacting with patients and families [19]. One area of focus across different communication skills training approaches is how to break bad news (e.g., diagnosis or prognosis) to patients and families [20–22]; these efforts are pertinent to end-of-life communication where the focus of

discussion has moved from curative and life-prolonging options to palliation and patients' priorities. Moreover, while early efforts in communication skills training suggested a unidirectional communication, where information is delivered from the provider to the patient, recent work has emphasized shared/joint decision-making and patient-centered communication [23–25]. In terms of the overall training curriculum and standardized exams, beginning in the 1990s, communication skills are integrated into medical school curriculums throughout the USA and required in the National Board of Medical Examiners and the Federation of State Medical Boards and residency programs [26, 27]. Other health care disciplines, such as nursing, pharmacy, and genetic counseling, are beginning to follow graduate medical educators' lead in expanding curriculum to include communication.

Domains of End-of-Life Communication

Key communication tasks surrounding cancer care (including palliative care) have been identified in several earlier publications [3, 14]. To briefly summarize, Epstein and Street identified five communication tasks of physicians: eliciting patient's symptoms, communicating prognosis while maintaining hope, making end-of-life decisions, responding to emotions, and helping the patient navigate the transition to hospice care [14]. Similarly, de Haes' review of the palliative care literature lists the following communication goals for the providers: patient-provide relationship building, information exchange, decision making, giving advice, and addressing emotions [3]. In this chapter, we will not expand on these previously discussed domains except to highlight two concepts across the domains of end-of-life communication. These are emerging areas where additional research and innovative practice are most needed in the end-of-life context. The first is agency for patients (sometimes referred to as control or autonomy), and the second is the role of family and informal caregivers [28, 29].

Outside of palliative care, respecting and enabling patient agency has been a priority concept in major movements towards improving clinical care. For example, the framework of patient-centered cancer care emphasizes the patient's perspective and preference in decision-making and self-management [14]. In addition, the model of shared decision-making stresses the patient's autonomy and involvement in all phases of decision-making about the care [30].

However, to date, research on patient agency has primarily been focused on decision-making about treatment options; therefore the majority of data on the topic comes from oncology encounters. In the case of end-of-life care, when curative or life-prolonging treatment may no longer be available, a sense of agency continues to be essential to many patients as they stop making treatment decisions. An ethnographic study of seriously ill cancer patients revealed a number of crucial communication domains where patient agency takes on an important role in the care, and bares implications for clinicians and patient support team [28]. In particular, in in-depth patient interviews and clinical interactions, patients referred to their pre-diagnosis life identities (in Mishler's terms, "voices of the lifeworld," as opposed to "voices of medicine") and spiritual values and make sense of their end-of-life experience through these priority domains [28, 31]. From a providers' perspective, understanding, listening to, and respecting the ways patients establish agency/control would promote true patient-centered communication and care, beyond moments of medical decision-making. Incorporating the concept into interventions, particularly those targeting providers, has the potential to promote patient-centered care and humane medicine.

In addition to promoting patient agency, another area gaining attention in end-of-life care and research is the importance of supporting and facilitating informal caregivers. As patient care has become increasingly dependent on informal caregivers, providing optimal support and education for caregivers has become an important priority. In contrast, our current understanding of how best to communicate with caregivers in regards to their physically and emotionally demanding role lags behind the trend in health care. Indeed, even though health care providers are highly skilled in providing direct care, they have had minimal training in how to teach skills and build confidence and competence in lay care providers. One important conduit for empowering caregivers is through the use of advanced clinician communication skills. Managing end-of-life care typically requires lay caregivers to assess symptom severity, administer medication, provide treatments and physically lift and turn the patient, and be amenable to the constantly changing care requirements common with patients in the advance stages of disease [32–35]. Furthermore, because of the demanding nature of caregiving responsibilities, lay caregivers may neglect their own self-care and this may compromise their own health. Family caregivers report multiple unmet needs, including insufficient education and skills to competently care for the patient, and a lack of spiritual and emotional support [36–39]. Effective communication between palliative care clinicians and family caregivers is critical to patient symptom management, and has the potential reduce caregiver distress, and even improve bereavement adjustment [40].

Major Interventions Research Aiming to Improve EOL Communication

Over the last decades, large and small intervention efforts with different approaches have been developed and tested with the goal to improve end-of-life communication for cancer patients and families. Interventions and clinical practices can be generally categorized into three broad approaches. The first and most common type of intervention is communication training programs aimed at teaching providers how to effectively and compassionately communicate with patients and families [19]. This effort is reflected in the current medical curriculum and continuing medical education for palliative care, primary care, oncology, nursing providers, social workers, and chaplains.

The second type of intervention targets patients and caregivers, aiming to increase patient engagement, self efficacy, and health literacy, and creating a easier and more effective navigation of the clinical system, with the broader goal of improving communication and promoting comfort and dignity for seriously ill patients and their caregivers. Examples of this type of efforts are patient navigation programs, counseling therapies, and community-based end-of-life education programs.

Finally, a third type of intervention is implemented within the broader health care system and affects patients and providers on multiple levels, for example, in timely reporting of symptoms, coordinating communication with providers, and providing social and emotional support for patients and caregivers. Quality improvement efforts in health care systems represent examples of this type of intervention. We will separately describe the intervention efforts and highlight exemplary programs and projects within each type of interventions.

Provider-Oriented Communication Interventions: Clinical Skills Training

Providers' communication skills training programs are the most common and well-tested form of end-of-life communication interventions to date. These training efforts are most commonly part of the medical core curriculum in the USA and many parts of the world and typically focus on improving provider-patient communication and relationship [12, 41]. These programs are most commonly developed for attending physicians, residents, and medical students. For example, a train-the-trainer program for attending oncologists was developed to improve communication skills, particularly how to promote shared decision-making. This intervention demonstrated improvement in the providers' communication skills following the training [24].

Within the practice of palliative care, several controlled trials have been conducted with residents to assess their ability in delivering bad news and in eliciting patient preferences [42, 43]. In terms of the content of the training, topics most commonly covered include the delivery and discussion of "bad news" or prognosis, responses to

patient's emotions, and advanced care planning (e.g., DNR discussion) [43]. In summary, intervention programs have generally reported improvement in specific provider communication behaviors for the short-term. To date, the evaluation efforts have mostly been conducted shortly after the interventions and rarely assess the long-term impact of patient outcomes. Therefore, major gaps in the field include the lack of systematic evaluation on the sustainability and long-term effect of these provider-based training programs and the important impact of these programs on patient outcomes.

In addition to targeting MD providers, several communication interventions for other health professionals both in and outside of end-of-life care have also been developed and reported. The majority of programs we reviewed have focused on nurses. The 10-year SUPPORT study was the largest and well-known longitudinal intervention effort, using trained nurses to improve communication, in areas including eliciting preferences, improving understanding of outcomes, encouraging attention to pain control, and facilitating advance care planning and patient–physician communication [44]. The intervention failed to demonstrate improvement in targeted outcomes, including patient-provider communication, DNR order timing, number of days on ICU, or level of reported pain. In a subsequent qualitative study based on interviews with the study's nurse participants, a central theme that emerged was the importance of facilitating "effective communication" and the provision of emotional support for patients and caregivers, domains not measured in the original study [45].

After the conclusion of the SUPPORT study, comprehensive curriculum to support crucial cancer nurses, such as the ELNEC, which has modules devoted to communication skills, has been found to improve nursing education and subsequently clinical outcomes [46, 47]. In addition to comprehensive education programs, interventions focusing on techniques of emotional self-control and coping strategies have demonstrated success in improving communication skills of nurses in caring for seriously ill patients [48]. For example, a training program in a hospital in

Madrid incorporated muscular relaxation and cognitive restructuring to improve communication skills, particularly in listening, empathizing, not interrupting, and coping with emotions [48]. Extending into chronic care, brief training interventions targeted at nurses have been shown to improve communication skills [49]. For instance, dementia care is an area where nurse communication training has been implemented and positively evaluated, with specific outcomes including promoting patient participation in decisions and activities [50].

Patient/Caregiver-Oriented Communication Interventions: Psychosocial and Communication Support, Navigation, and Community-based Programs

In addition to provider-based communication programs, interventions targeting patient and caregivers have also been shown to improve communication and care at the end of life [51]. Most of the existing interventions emphasize psychosocial and spiritual aspects of end-of-life communication and coping [52]. For instance, the "Outlook" program guides patient participants through discussions of end-of-life preparation, addressing patients' spiritual and emotional concerns through semi-structured, one-on-one interview sessions, where patients are encouraged to discuss life stories, forgiveness, and their heritage and legacy [53]. This strategy for discussing life completion has been shown to improve health outcomes. Specifically, participants showed improvements in anxiety, depression, preparation, and functional status [51]. Another patient intervention, Project ENABLE, involved nurse-administered, telephone-based coaching in problem solving, advance care planning, family and health care team communication strategies, symptom management, crisis prevention, and referrals to palliative care resources for patients [17]. This program was found to facilitate patient activation and self-management and improve quality of life, though improvement of symptoms and utilization of resources were not observed in

this particular study [17]. Finally, another example of patient-oriented intervention is the Dignity Therapy, a psychotherapy intervention aimed at addressing the feelings among seriously ill patients of a loss of dignity [54]. An analysis of therapy sessions found that a patient's value system makes up a significant aspect of their narratives and was a integral part of their perceptions of end of life [55].

The key role of family/informal caregivers in optimal end-of-life care has been well documented. Recent reviews of caregiver need identified significant lack of foundational information on home-based care [56, 57]. The informational needs, given the complexity of the caregiver role and the daunting medical tasks, have prompted interventions to improve communication, education and training for caregivers. To date, promising communication interventions for caregivers range from prompt lists to cue question asking during medical visits [58], psycho-educational group format [59], to multi-component interventions. The largest study on end-of-life caregiving is the COPE trial which involved a nurse intervention with home hospice cancer caregivers [60]. Patient/family caregiver dyads were randomly assigned to one of three study arms: standard hospice care, standard care plus three emotionally supportive nurse visits, or standard care plus three visits during which the nurse taught coping skills. Compared to the two other conditions, the caregivers assigned to the coping skills condition reported significantly better quality of life, reduced burden due to patient symptoms and to caregiving tasks at 1 month follow-up. While the COPE intervention was not specifically a communication intervention, the study demonstrated the unique problem solving skills and cognitive restructuring a clinical needed to foster in lay caregivers to manage their personal burden and distress in caring for a dying cancer patient. Empowering caregivers in this way require advanced communication training skills training on the part of clinicians.

Other caregiver-oriented communication interventions have focused on initiating end-of-life discussions and bereavement support. For example, one communication intervention proposed a proactive communication strategy in family end-of-life conferences and provided support on grieving and bereavement. Compared to customary practice, the intervention was shown to have increased mutual support in decision-making, fostered expression of emotions, helped families accept realistic goals of care, and lessened bereavement burden and PTSD-related systems [61].

Outside of the clinical system, state- and community-based programs have demonstrated success in educating patients and caregivers about communication and decision-making at the end of life. For example, the Coalition for Compassionate Care in California is a statewide partnership of organizations, agencies, and individuals working together to promote high-quality, compassionate end-of-life care through multi-level efforts such as patient education, provider training, policy and legislative activities [62]. In response to increasing cultural and linguistic diversity in the USA, grassroots organizations serving specific ethnic/cultural communities have also been promoting and educating about end-of-life communication. For instance, the Chinese–American Coalition for Compassionate Care exemplifies efforts rooted from within the community/ethnic enclave to educate patients and providers and bridge the gap between mainstream end-of-life education efforts with specific and distinct needs of a community [63]. A key part of its program is a multi-level efforts aimed at promoting open communication about end-of-life options within the family and in the health care system, including advance directives and communicating preferences and priorities among family members.

Systems-Level Communication Interventions: Palliative Care and Internet-based Programs

Despite reported successes in small-scale interventions targeting individual patients, caregivers and providers, clinicians and researchers are increasingly questioning the sustainability and lim-

ited long-term positive impact from individual-level interventions.. "System-level innovation(s) and quality improvement in routine care" have been suggested as "more powerful opportunities for improvement" [64]. Unlike more didactic training or education programs, while these larger efforts are not explicitly stated as communication interventions, communications at all levels (e.g., communication between patient and provider, among the multidisciplinary health care team, within the family) are integral in system-based approaches to end-of-life care. Here we discuss system-based interventions in two areas, including systematic studies of the impact of integrated palliative care as opposed to usual oncology care, and health information technology implementation to facilitate communication and support for patients and caregivers.

A recent widely publicized randomized trial study documents the benefits of palliative care: the intervention group (receiving palliative care early) demonstrated better patient-reported quality of life, less depressive symptoms, and had higher median survival rate despite lower use of aggressive treatment, the intervention group [16]. While not explicitly framed as a communication intervention, the palliative care protocol in this study placed heavy emphasis on communication across all levels of care, namely in better symptom assessments, jointly establishing goals of care and assisting with decision making and care coordination [16]. In this way, such system-level intervention takes into account the multiple communication points throughout the end of life.

Finally, responding to the growth of health information technologies, current system-based communication interventions commonly take the form of Web-based information and navigation systems for patients and caregivers. For example, the Web-based Interactive Health Communication System (IHCS) is under development with the goal to bridge communication gaps (such as decision-making) for patients with advanced lung cancer and their families [65]. One case example of IHCS is the Comprehensive Health Enhancement Support System (CHESS), a user-driven system designed to provide disease-specific information and symptoms-tracking system and interactive coaching resources for those facing a health crisis such as cancer. These systems have been found to facilitate shared decision-making, increase social support, improve patients' quality of life, and enable more efficient health serve use [65–67].

Future Research Areas and Clinical Priorities

Palliative care and end-of-life communication is still in its early stages and there are several areas in which further research is needed. First, based on findings to date. The field must respond to the growing cultural, ethnic and socioeconomic diversity in the US [68]. Differences in attitudes, beliefs, and involvement of family members vary widely by cultural and socioeconomic groups, and require an increased understanding and flexibility in clinician communication skills. Currently, there is scant research documenting the end-of-life communication needs of underserved and vulnerable populations in the USA; nor are there intervention studies focusing on unique socio-economic contexts. Second and related to this priority area is the need for broader inclusion of study participants. It is widely acknowledged that conducting research at end-of-life is fraught with difficulties in recruitment, concern over participant burden, and destined for high rates of attrition. Only with better documentation of reasons for non-participation and attrition will future research be able to design studies to meet the unique needs of this population [52].

Third, expansion of end-of-life communication measures is needed, particularly in developing matrices and measures to assess the long-term and sustainable clinical impact of palliative care and communication interventions [69]. When research funding is limited, researchers may be tempted to forego costly longitudinal studies with multi-measurement components (e.g., observational, self-report, electronic, and biophysical). However, end-of-life research is at a critical junction in which rigorous longitudinal, multi-site, multi-measure studies will truly advance knowledge and

clinical care. With the current emphasis on team science, hopefully researchers and funding agencies will recognize the importance of addressing both the big and small questions facing current end-of-life care practices and the need for solid evidence. Fourth, as patient care is increasingly moving into the home and with many families preferring a home death, strategies to effectively prepare and transition a family to end-of-life care at home [70]. Furthermore, nearly all of end-of-life communication research has been conducted in hospital and clinic settings, whereas, little is known about the communication needs of home-based patients and their caregivers. The home setting provides a unique context where the clinician is the guest and faces multiple challenges, including travel, limited access to other health care provider opinions, limited access to medical supplies and equipment, and increasing dependence on the family for proxy information on patient status.

Finally, in the era of rapid advances in Internet technologies, all contexts of communication need to document the influence of and opportunities for new communication technologies on patient care. We have evidence that cancer survivors are increasingly engaging in health-related Internet use, including participation in online support groups, emailing their providers, and seeking cancer information online [71]. In the end-of-life context, opportunities exist to examine how Web 2.0 technologies (social media, blogs, and mobile devices) may provide social support as well as timely and useful information for patients and caregivers. In the clinical setting, with the implementation of electronic medical records and patient portals, work remains in how to effectively integrate education and support for seriously ill patients and their caregivers into exiting Web-based communication systems. Additionally, the use and role of technology in supporting communication for home-based palliative care is a virtual black box. It is crucial that any electronic system enhance patient-provider communication and relationship-building, rather than replace face-to-face communication, which is of critical importance during the difficult and highly emotional period facing death.

In terms of the clinical priorities, there is increasing evidence for improved cancer care through the introduction and expansion of communication on end-of-life care. Recent findings demonstrate the multifold benefits of integrating palliative and end-of-life communication throughout the care continuum to ensure continuity of care and improve transitions from curative to palliative care [16]. Conversations about end-of-life care must involve both the patient and the informal caregiver (and often multiple informal caregivers) When all are well informed and supported, not only is the patient likely to receive positive benefits, but the caregivers' stress and burden will potentially be reduced. End-of-life communication skills curriculum needs to advance and expand quickly to prepare clinicians to responsibly handle the complexities of palliative care. Clinicians need to develop advanced skills to communicate with multiple health care disciplines and with the patient and family, and to also be proficient in the discussion of a wide range of palliative care domains (e.g., physical, psychosocial, spiritual, ethical), while being emotional responsive.

Conclusions

The outcomes from end-of-life intervention research, communication skills training, patient and caregiver navigation, and clinical applications demonstrate the importance of effective communication for optimal patient care. Said simply, "more is better": in order to enable comfort and dignity for patients and caregivers, we need more skilled communication by clinicians, more informed conversations about end-of-life decisions throughout the cancer care continuum, and more research to advance the promising field of end-of-life science. Yet, the acceptance of the importance of end-of-life communication by researchers and clinicians is not enough. The promising impact of all forms of end-of-life communication must be disseminated in such a way to change the social-cultural dialogue about death and health care policies that impact cancer patients and their families.

References

1. ACS. Facts and figures. Atlanta: American Cancer Society; 2008.
2. Han PK, Rayson D. The coordination of primary and oncology specialty care at the end of life. J Natl Cancer Inst Monogr. 2010;2010(40):31–7.
3. de Haes H, Teunissen S. Communication in palliative care: a review of recent literature. Curr Opin Oncol. 2005;17(4):345–50.
4. Kübler-Ross E. On death and dying, vol. viii. New York: Macmillan; 1969. 260 p.
5. Saunders CM, Kastenbaum R. Hospice care on the international scene. The Springer series on death and suicide, vol. xii. New York: Springer Pub. Co; 1997. 303 p.
6. Lynn J. Perspectives on care at the close of life. Serving patients who may die soon and their families: the role of hospice and other services. JAMA. 2001;285(7):925–32.
7. Covinsky KE, Fuller JD, Yaffe K, Johnston CB, Hamel MB, Lynn J, et al. Communication and decision-making in seriously ill patients: findings of the SUPPORT project. The study to understand prognoses and preferences for outcomes and risks of treatments. J Am Geriatr Soc. 2000;48(5 Suppl):S187–S93.
8. Improving End-of-Life Care. NIH Consens State Sci Statements. 2004;Dec 6-8;21(3):1–28. http://consensus.nih.gov/2004/2004EndOfLifeCareSOs024PDF.pdf
9. Holland JC, Lewis S. The human side of cancer: living with hope, coping with uncertainty, vol. xii. 1st ed. New York: HarperCollins; 2000. 340 p.
10. Yabroff KR, Mandelblatt JS, Ingham J. The quality of medical care at the end-of-life in the USA: existing barriers and examples of process and outcome measures. Palliat Med. 2004;18(3):202–16.
11. Hack TF, Degner LF, Parker PA. The communication goals and needs of cancer patients: a review. Psychooncology. 2005;14(10):831–45. discussion 846–7.
12. Stiefel F, Barth J, Bensing J, Fallowfield L, Jost L, Razavi D, et al. Communication skills training in oncology: a position paper based on a consensus meeting among European experts in 2009. Ann Oncol. 2010;21(2):204–7.
13. Jenkins V, Fallowfield L, Saul J. Information needs of patients with cancer: results from a large study in UK cancer centers. Br J Cancer. 2001;84(1):48–51.
14. Epstein RM, Street RLJ. Patient-centered communication in cancer care: promoting healing and reducing suffering in NIH publication. Bethesda: National Institutes of Health; 2007.
15. Arora NK, Street Jr RL, Epstein RM, Butow PN. Facilitating patient-centered cancer communication: a road map. Patient Educ Couns. 2009;77(3):319–21.
16. Temel JS, Greer JA, Muzikansky A, Gallagher ER, Admane S, Jackson VA, et al. Early palliative care for patients with metastatic non-small-cell lung cancer. N Engl J Med. 2010;363(8):733–42.

17. Bakitas M, Lyons KD, Hegel MT, Balan S, Brokaw FC, Seville J, et al. Effects of a palliative care intervention on clinical outcomes in patients with advanced cancer: the Project ENABLE II randomized controlled trial. JAMA. 2009;302(7):741–9.

18. Connor SR, Pyenson B, Fitch K, Spence C, Iwasaki K. Comparing hospice and nonhospice patient survival among patients who die within a three-year window. J Pain Symptom Manage. 2007;33(3):238–46.

19. Lipkin M, Putnam SM, Lazare A. The medical interview: clinical care, education, and research. Frontiers of primary care, vol. xxii. New York: Springer; 1995. 643 p.

20. Girgis A, Sanson-Fisher RW. Breaking bad news: consensus guidelines for medical practitioners. J Clin Oncol. 1995;13(9):2449–56.

21. Buckman R, Kason Y. How to break bad news: a guide for health care professionals, vol. x. Baltimore: Johns Hopkins University Press; 1992. 223 p.

22. Garg A, Buckman R, Kason Y. Teaching medical students how to break bad news. CMAJ. 1997;156(8):1159–64.

23. Siminoff LA, Step MM. A communication model of shared decision making: accounting for cancer treatment decisions. Health Psychol. 2005;24(4 Suppl):S99–S105.

24. Bylund CL, Brown R, Gueguen JA, Diamond C, Bianculli J, Kissane DW. The implementation and assessment of a comprehensive communication skills training curriculum for oncologists. Psychooncology. 2010;19(6):583–93.

25. Weiner JS, Cole SA. ACare: a communication training program for shared decision making along a life-limiting illness. Palliat Support Care. 2004;2(3):231–41.

26. Teutsch C. Patient–doctor communication. Med Clin North Am. 2003;87(5):1115–45.

27. Hauser J, Makoul G. Medical student training in communication skills. In: Kissane DW, Barry DB, Phyllis MB, Finlay IG, editors. Handbook of communication in oncology and palliative care. Oxford: Oxford University Press; 2011.

28. Chou WS. End-of-life discourse: an analysis of agency, coherence, and questions. Washington, DC: Linguistics Department, Georgetown University; 2004.

29. DuBenske LL, Chih MY, Gustafson DH, Dinauer S, Cleary JF. Caregivers' participation in the oncology clinic visit mediates the relationship between their information competence and their need fulfillment and clinic visit satisfaction. Patient Educ Couns. 2010;81(Suppl):S94–S9.

30. Brown RF, Butow PN, Juraskova I, Ribi K, Gerber D, Bernhard J, et al. Sharing decisions in breast cancer care: development of the decision analysis system for oncology (DAS-O) to identify shared decision making during treatment consultations. Health Expect. 2011;14(1):29–37.

31. Mishler EG. The discourse of medicine: dialectics of medical interviews, vol. xii. Norwood: Ablex Pub. Corp; 1984. 211 p.

32. Hester NO, Miller KL, Foster RL, Vojir CP. Symptom management outcomes. Do they reflect variations in care delivery systems? Med Care. 1997;35 (11 Suppl):NS69–83.

33. Patrick DL, Ferketich SL, Frame PS, Harris JJ, Hendricks CB, Levin B, et al. National Institutes of Health State-of-the-Science Conference Statement: Symptom management in cancer: pain, depression, and fatigue, July 15–17, 2002. J Natl Cancer Inst. 2003;95(15):1110–7.

34. Given B, Wyatt G, Given C, Sherwood P, Gift A, DeVoss D, et al. Burden and depression among caregivers of patients with cancer at the end of life. Oncol Nurs Forum. 2004;31(6):1105–17.

35. Weitzner MA, Haley WE, Chen H. The family caregiver of the older cancer patient. Hematol Oncol Clin North Am. 2000;14(1):269–81.

36. Doorenbos AZ, Given B, Given CW, Wyatt G, Gift A, Rahbar M, et al. The influence of end-of-life cancer care on caregivers. Res Nurs Health. 2007;30(3):270–81.

37. Proot IM, Abu-Saad HH, Crebolder HF, Goldsteen M, Luker KA, Widdershoven GA. Vulnerability of family caregivers in terminal palliative care at home; balancing between burden and capacity. Scand J Caring Sci. 2003;17(2):113–21.

38. Sharpe L, Butow P, Smith C, McConnell D, Clarke S. The relationship between available support, unmet needs and caregiver burden in patients with advanced cancer and their carers. Psychooncology. 2005;14(2):102–14.

39. Gaston-Johansson F, Lachica EM, Fall-Dickson JM, Kennedy MJ. Psychological distress, fatigue, burden of care, and quality of life in primary caregivers of patients with breast cancer undergoing autologous bone marrow transplantation. Oncol Nurs Forum. 2004;31(6):1161–9.

40. Stroebe M, Schut H, Stroebe W. Health outcomes of bereavement. Lancet. 2007;370:1960–73.

41. Williams DM, Fisicaro T, Veloski JJ, Berg D. Development and evaluation of a program to strengthen first year residents' proficiency in leading end-of-life discussions. Am J Hosp Palliat Care. 2011;28(5):328–34.

42. Alexander SC, Keitz SA, Sloane R, Tulsky JA. A controlled trial of a short course to improve residents' communication with patients at the end of life. Acad Med. 2006;81(11):1008–12.

43. Szmuilowicz E, el-Jawahri A, Chiappetta L, Kamdar M, Block S. Improving residents' end-of-life communication skills with a short retreat: a randomized controlled trial. J Palliat Med. 2010;13(4):439–52.

44. The SUPPORT Principal Investigators. A controlled trial to improve care for seriously ill hospitalized patients: The study to understand prognoses and preferences for outcomes and risks of treatments (SUPPORT). JAMA 1995;274(20):1591–8.

45. Murphy PA, Price DM, Stevens M, Lynn J, Kathryn E. Under the radar: contributions of the SUPPORT nurses. Nurs Outlook. 2001;49(5):238–42.

46. Jacobs HH, Ferrell B, Virani R, Malloy P. Appraisal of the pediatric end-of-life nursing education consortium training program. J Pediatr Nurs. 2009;24(3):216–21.

47. Ferrell B, Virani R, Paice JA, Coyle N, Coyne P. Evaluation of palliative care nursing education seminars. Eur J Oncol Nurs. 2010;14(1):74–9.

48. de Garcia Lucio L, Garcia Lopez FJ, Marin Lopez MT, Mas Hesse B, Caamano Vaz MD. Training programme in techniques of self-control and communication skills to improve nurses' relationships with relatives of seriously ill patients: a randomized controlled study. J Adv Nurs. 2000;32(2):425–31.

49. Boscart VM. A communication intervention for nursing staff in chronic care. J Adv Nurs. 2009;65(9):1823–32.

50. Kihlgren M, Kuremyr D, Norberg A, Brane G, Karlson I, Engstrom B, et al. Nurse-patient interaction after training in integrity promoting care at a long-term ward: analysis of video-recorded morning care sessions. Int J Nurs Stud. 1993;30(1):1–13.

51. Steinhauser KE, Alexander SC, Byock IR, George LK, Olsen MK, Tulsky JA. Do preparation and life completion discussions improve functioning and quality of life in seriously ill patients? Pilot randomized control trial. J Palliat Med. 2008;11(9):1234–40.

52. Schildmann EK, Higginson IJ. Evaluating psycho-educational interventions for informal carers of patients receiving cancer care or palliative care: strengths and limitations of different study designs. Palliat Med. 2011;25(4):345–56.

53. Steinhauser KE, Alexander SC, Byock IR, George LK, Tulsky JA. Seriously ill patients' discussions of preparation and life completion: an intervention to assist with transition at the end of life. Palliat Support Care. 2009;7(4):393–404.

54. Hall S, Edmonds P, Harding R, Chochinov H, Higginson IJ. Assessing the feasibility, acceptability and potential effectiveness of Dignity Therapy for people with advanced cancer referred to a hospital-based palliative care team: Study protocol. BMC Palliat Care. 2009;8:5.

55. Hack TF, McClement SE, Chochinov HM, Cann BJ, Hassard TH, Kristjanson LJ, et al. Learning from dying patients during their final days: life reflections gleaned from dignity therapy. Palliat Med. 2010;24(7):715–23.

56. Bee PE, Barnes P, Luker KA. A systematic review of informal caregivers' needs in providing home-based end-of-life care to people with cancer. J Clin Nurs. 2009;18(10):1379–93.

57. Steinhauser KE, Christakis NA, Clipp EC, McNeilly M, McIntyre L, Tulsky JA. Factors considered important at the end of life by patients, family, physicians, and other care providers. JAMA. 2000;284(19):2476–82.

58. Clayton JM, Butow PN, Tattersall MH, Devine RJ, Simpson JM, Aggarwal G, et al. Randomized controlled trial of a prompt list to help advanced cancer patients and their caregivers to ask questions about prognosis and end-of-life care. J Clin Oncol. 2007;25(6):715–23.

59. Hudson P, Quinn K, Kristjanson L, Thomas T, Braithwaite M, Fisher J, et al. Evaluation of a psycho-educational group programme for family caregivers in home-based palliative care. Palliat Med. 2008;22(3):270–80.

60. McMillan SC, Small BJ. Using the COPE intervention for family caregivers to improve symptoms of hospice homecare patients: a clinical trial. Oncol Nurs Forum. 2007;34(2):313–21.

61. Lautrette A, Darmon M, Megarbane B, Joly LM, Chevret S, Adrie C, et al. A communication strategy and brochure for relatives of patients dying in the ICU. N Engl J Med. 2007;356(5):469–78.

62. Hill TE, Ginsburg M, Citko J, Cadogan M. Improving end-of-life care in nursing facilities: the Community State Partnership to Improve End-of-Life Care–California. J Palliat Med. 2005;8(2):300–12.

63. Chou WS, Stokes SC, Citko J, Davies B. Improving end-of-life care through community-based grassroots collaboration: developing of Chinese–American coalition for Compassionate Care. J Palliat Care. 2008;24(1):31–40.

64. Lynn J, Nolan K, Kabcenell A, Weissman D, Milne C, Berwick DM. Reforming care for persons near the end of life: the promise of quality improvement. Ann Intern Med. 2002;137(2):117–22.

65. DuBenske LL, Gustafson DH, Shaw BR, Cleary JF. Web-based cancer communication and decision making systems: connecting patients, caregivers, and clinicians for improved health outcomes. Med Decis Making. 2010;30(6):732–44.

66. Dubenske LL, Chih MY, Dinauer S, Gustafson DH, Cleary JF. Development and implementation of a clinician reporting system for advanced stage cancer: initial lessons learned. J Am Med Inform Assoc. 2008;15(5):679–86.

67. Kim E, Han JY, Moon TJ, Shaw B, Shah DV, McTavish FM, et al. The process and effect of supportive message expression and reception in online breast cancer support groups. Psychooncology. 2012;21(5):531–40.

68. Northouse LL, Katapodi MC, Song L, Zhang L, Mood DW. Interventions with family caregivers of cancer patients: meta-analysis of randomized trials. CA Cancer J Clin. 2010;60(5):317–39.

69. Weissman DE, Morrison RS, Meier DE. Center to Advance Palliative Care palliative care clinical care and customer satisfaction metrics consensus recommendations. J Palliat Med. 2010;13(2):179–84.

70. McCorkle R, Pasacreta JV. Enhancing caregiver outcomes in palliative care. Cancer Control. 2001;8(1):36–45.

71. Chou WY, Liu B, Post S, Hesse B. Health-related internet use among cancer survivors: data from the Health Information National Trends Survey, 2003–2008. J Cancer Surviv. 2011;5(3):263–70.

Further Reading

1. Kissane DW, et al. Handbook of communication in oncology and palliative care. Oxford: Oxford University Press; 2010.

The Intersection Between Cancer and Caregiver Survivorship

22

Jennifer Steel, Amanda M. Midboe, and Maureen L. Carney

Death and Dying

Despite the pervasiveness of death in our lives, preparing for our own or a loved one's death is often extremely challenging. Our cultural background as well as early childhood experiences with death greatly influences our later responses [1]. In times past, the family would assist with all aspects of caring for the sick and dying, making sure that they were as comfortable as possible until their death and then preparing the body and burying the deceased. The accepted duration of mourning by a family member lasted much longer than what is expected today. For example, the

J. Steel, Ph.D. (✉)
Division of Hepatobiliary and Pancreatic
Surgery and Transplantation, Department of Surgery,
Center for Excellence in Behavioral Medicine,
University of Pittsburgh School of Medicine,
3459 Fifth Avenue; Montefiore 7S,
Pittsburgh, PA 15213, USA
e-mail: steeljl@upmc.edu

A.M. Midboe, Ph.D.
Department of Psychiatry, Center for Health
Care Evaluation, VA Palo Alto Healthcare System,
Palo Alto, CA, USA

Department of Psychiatry and Behavioral Sciences,
Center for Health Care Evaluation, VA Palo Alto
Healthcare System, Stanford University School
of Medicine, Stanford, CA, USA

M.L. Carney, M.D., M.B.A.
Kaiser Permanente, Sunnybrook Medical Office,
Clackamas, OR, USA

generally accepted amount of paid leave from work today is 3 days after the loss of a family member in Western countries [1]. The mourning family members and friends are often expected to return to normal functioning within 6 months, an arbitrary time period. However, if an individual returns to normal functioning too early, or begins to have intimate relationships soon after a spouse's death, society looks upon this as an abnormal adjustment to the death even if it has been a prolonged caregiving period lasting years when a spouse has not had any form of intimacy or a functional relationship with his or her loved one (e.g., Alzheimer's disease or brain cancer).

Advances in medicine have changed the dynamics associated with the illness process—prolonging life while distancing loved ones from death. The end-of-life process has become much less personal and many individuals have limited exposure to the death and dying experience. In Western cultures the medical community is much more involved in an individual's care from the onset of illness to his or her death. Furthermore, after a person has died, s/he is often prepared and buried by professionals rather than family as in the past [2].

The Role of Health Care Professionals in End-of-Life Care

The health care professional's (HCP) own experiences and philosophy regarding death influences how they care for patients and families which may not be consistent with the patient's or family's

B.I. Carr and J. Steel (eds.), *Psychological Aspects of Cancer*,
DOI 10.1007/978-1-4614-4866-2_22, © Springer Science+Business Media, LLC 2013

ideas about end-of-life decisions. The HCPs often have little training or the emotional connection to the patient to provide culturally appropriate support and/or compassionate care to the person who is ill or to his or her family members, making communication and joint decisions regarding end of life challenging [2].

Communication and decisions about the end of life are further complicated by variation in preferences of patients or family members about how much they want to know about the details of the diagnosis and prognosis. The patient and/or family member may believe that they cannot cope with such information and therefore choose not to ask questions or avoid such conversations. Even when HCPs do discuss end-of-life issues with patients and families, the patients and their loved ones may not hear or remember information communicated by the provider. Many patients and family members need time to process information about the diagnosis and prognosis and may be emotionally overwhelmed at the time of the discussion. It is now recommended that physicians facilitating end-of-life discussions do so over the course of several meetings as a process rather than a one-time discussion [3]. However, the constraints of our health care system make putting this into practice challenging.

When a loved one is diagnosed with cancer, this may be the first time the patient or the family caregiver has considered death. Unlike other traumatic events that take a person's life immediately, cancer often allows the patient and family time to prepare, some more than others. The quality of that time depends on several factors, such as the symptoms of cancer, side effects of treatment, patient's and caregiver's personality and relationship, prior experience with loss, support from family and friends, spirituality, prior psychological functioning, and interactions with HCPs.

We know that details regarding the goals of care, life-sustaining options, where and how a person will spend his or her final days of life, and funeral arrangements are infrequently discussed until the final months or weeks of life. Wright and colleagues found that only 37% of patients had discussed end-of-life preferences with their physician [4]. Of those who did, the quality of life (QOL) was better and cost of health care less when compared to those who did not have the discussion with their medical team [4]. Another study demonstrated that discussions with physicians regarding end-of-life care resulted in earlier referral to hospice, less aggressive care, and better QOL [5].

When curative treatment is no longer an option, symptom management becomes critical to maintain the best QOL. The most common symptoms experienced at the end of life include pain, delirium, dyspnea, fever, and hemorrhage [4, 6, 7]. The most feared symptom reported by patients is unmanaged pain. Pain management is often difficult secondary to fears of addiction by the patient, family, or health care providers. However, close monitoring of opioid prescriptions by physicians or specialists in pain management can result in a better QOL for patients. In the final months of life, particularly if a patient enters hospice, management of pain with opioids becomes more acceptable by patients, families, and HCPs. At that point the primary concern may be that pain management could hasten death; however there is little evidence supporting this fear [8, 9].

As noted above, when an individual is dying, several issues should be discussed including nutrition, symptom management, the location where the individual would like to die, and circumstances under which the person would like to be resuscitated. Resuscitation often includes all interventions that provide cardiovascular, respiratory, and metabolic support necessary to maintain and sustain the life. Both the patient and family need to understand the advantages and disadvantages of resuscitation in order to make the most appropriate decision. Unfortunately, many dying patients have not made choices in advance or communicated their wishes to their families or health care team. As a result the families are left with difficult decisions. Often aggressive treatment is performed due to this lack of communication between patient and family. These aggressive treatments have been associated with poorer QOL for the patient and worse post-loss adjustment for the surviving loved ones [4, 7].

Few reports or studies have been conducted regarding the use of palliative sedation for psychosocial symptoms (e.g., anxiety, psychotic symptoms). Four palliative care programs in Israel, South Africa, and Spain reported the use of palliative sedation [10–13]. In addition, a retrospective study of 1,207 patients admitted to the palliative care unit at MD Anderson found that palliative sedation was used in 15% of patients. The most common indications were delirium (82%) and dyspnea (6%). Sedation in these circumstances is often used on a temporary basis and was reversible in 23% of these patients [13].

Palliative Care and Hospice

Palliative care may be used for a number of illnesses, including cancer, and is particularly beneficial at the end of life. According to the World Health Organization, palliative care may be defined as "an approach that improves the quality of life of patients and their families facing the problems associated with life-threatening illness, through the prevention and relief of suffering by means of early identification and treatment of pain and other problems, physical, psychosocial and spiritual" [14]. Palliative care has several goals: (1) provides relief from pain and other distressing symptoms; (2) affirms life and regards dying as a normal process; (3) intends neither to hasten nor to postpone death; (4) integrates the psychological and spiritual aspects of patient care; (5) offers a support system to help patients live as actively as possible until death; (6) offers a support system to help the family cope during the patients' illness and in their own bereavement; (7) uses a team approach to address the needs of patients and their families, including bereavement counseling, if indicated; (8) enhances QOL, and tries to positively influence the course of illness; and (9) is best applied early in the course of illness, in conjunction with other therapies that are intended to prolong life, such as chemotherapy or radiation therapy, and includes those investigations needed to better understand and manage distressing clinical complications.

Hospice refers to programs that provide special care for people who are near the end of life and for their families, at home, in freestanding facilities, or within hospitals. Although palliative care may also include care in a hospice setting, a referral to hospice occurs when the medical team has determined that a patient may no longer benefit from traditional medical treatments and the patient is expected to have less than 6 months of life. Hospice is interdisciplinary and targets physical, emotional, social, and spiritual discomfort during the last phase of life. In 2007, people with cancer made up approximately 43% of these admissions to hospice [15]. The duration in hospice is often quite short with a median length of stay in hospice of just 21.3 days [15]. Although the reasons for late referrals are not known, it is thought that advanced care discussions between the patient and health care provider are not being initiated by patients, families, or HCPs early enough.

Care During the Final Hours

As death bias become more institutionalized, signs of approaching death may appear obvious to HCPs, family members often lack that knowledge. Many family members may have never observed the death of a loved one. Educating family members about the signs of approaching death can help them understand changes in their loved one. For example, in the final days to hours of life, patients often experience a decreased desire to eat or drink, as evidenced by clenched teeth or turning away from offered food and fluids [14]. This behavior may be difficult for family members to accept because of the meaning of food in our society and the inference that the patient is "starving." Family members should be advised that forcing food or fluids can lead to aspiration. Reframing would include teaching the family to provide ice chips or a moistened oral applicator to keep a patient's mouth and lips moist [14]. The sensitivity and communication of the health care providers with the patient and family are critical in the final weeks and days of life. Poor relationships and conflict between patients and families and the health care providers can lead to short- and long-term psychological and health consequences for the grieving family members who misinterpret the apparent indifference of the health team to nutritional issues.

It is important for HCPs to explore with families any fears associated with the time of death and any cultural or religious rituals that may be important to them [16]. Such rituals might include placement of the body (e.g., the head of the bed facing Mecca for an Islamic patient) or having only same-sex caregivers or family members wash the body (as practiced in many orthodox religions) [16]. When death occurs, expressions of grief by those at the bedside vary greatly, dictated in part by culture and in part by their preparation for the death. Chaplains or other religious or spiritual leaders should be consulted as early as possible if the patient and family are interested in this type of assistance [16]. However, previous discussions with the patient and/or family are critical as prior conflict with the church and/or religious leaders may result in increased distress for the patient.

Grief and Bereavement of the Family Caregiver

The patient's QOL during the end of life and the medical team's communication and behaviors can have lasting effects on the family caregiver. If the relationship between the patient and/or family and medical team is poor, then early cessation of treatment, lack of access to hospice care, and conflict regarding end-of-life decisions (e.g., DNR) may result. The guilt that caregivers may develop can be long-lasting if s/he decides to stop life support before they have exhausted all options. HCPs who have more experience with end-of-life circumstances may not always understand the family's perspective when they know that the chances for extending life are minimal. The health care team has a responsibility to offer respect for the decisions of the patient and family. Patients and families also have the responsibility to discuss issues such as power of attorney and living wills prior to death or before the patient is unable to make decisions due to mental status changes that may occur in the final weeks of days of life.

A substantial body of research exists regarding the possible consequences of caregiving and bereavement on psychological well-being and health of family members. Caregiver stress or burden has been demonstrated to be associated with increased risk of depression, perceived stress, poorer QOL, and increased risk of health conditions including cardiovascular disease, obesity, hypertension, diabetes, high cholesterol, and even mortality [2–4, 7, 10–15, 17].

Only two studies to our knowledge has compared cancer caregivers to age-matched controls during the caregiving period and found that caregivers reported higher levels of emotional distress than controls [16]. Furthermore, the prevalence of medical comorbidities such as hypertension and heart disease was reported to be higher in cancer caregivers when compared to an age-matched control group during the caregiving period [16]. The second study, reported that cancer caregivers were at increased risk of coronary heart disease when compared to controls who were not caregiving. However, the control participants were not matched on any key variables (e.g., age, medical history; [18]). Caregivers of advanced cancer patients, when compared to caregivers of those patients at earlier stages in their disease, were at the greatest risk for cardiovascular disease and mortality highlighting the importance of studing caregivers of those with advanced cancer as proposed [18]. After adjusting for age, gender, income, and the care recipient's cancer severity, the caregiver's health morbidity at 5 years after the relative's cancer diagnosis was significantly related to levels of caregiving stress reported 3 years earlier [16]. However, no study has followed caregivers through the caregiving and bereavement period to determine the independent contribution of caregiving us bereavement on health.

If the prevalence of psychological morbidity of *cancer* caregivers is as high as caregivers of those diagnosed with dementia during caregiving and bereavement (approximately 50%), it is estimated that over six million current cancer caregivers may be at risk for increased psychological and health morbidity and possibly mortality. Stress, depression, and prolonged grief are all treatable conditions; therefore the ability to reduce these symptoms, improve QOL, and decrease health morbidity and mortality could be significant.

It appears that caregiving in general may affect psychological functioning and health but that there are differences across caregivers. The groundbreaking research by Schulz and colleagues (1999) found in a cohort of individuals providing care for loved ones with dementia that, at the 4-year follow-up, those who reported high levels of strain during caregiving had an increased mortality risk that was 63% higher than their non-caregiving controls [19]. Since this seminal paper, Christakis and colleagues (2006) have also found an increased risk of mortality after the hospitalization of a spouse (which may reflect increased perceived stress) [20].

In contrast, some researchers have not found evidence for this link between psychological morbidity during caregiving and mortality. In a recent study, the risk of mortality was found to be *lower* in caregivers of those with osteoporosis fractures when compared to non-caregivers at the 3-year follow-up [21]. Interestingly, those participants who reported higher levels of perceived stress had increased risk of mortality, independent of their role as a caregiver [21]. Furthermore, another study which compared caregivers to non-caregivers also found that as age increased, the risk of health problems became similar to that of non-caregiving controls [21]. As a result, further research is warranted to determine if the psychological consequences of caregiving are associated with increased risk of health morbidity and mortality in the context of cancer caregiving.

It appears that the type of caregiving (e.g., dementia vs. fracture) as well as other difficulties with post-loss adjustment are critical factors that may affect the association between psychological morbidity during caregiving and mortality [19–21]. Furthermore, several methodological problems exist with prior research that attemps to link caregiving with mortality including problems with recruitment and retention of both caregivers and controls (e.g., 10–20% of those approached for participation enrolled). In addition, there is a great disconnect between the caregiving and bereavement literatures, making it difficult to interpret the link between caregiving and long-term health consequences and mortality without understanding how psychological morbidity during the bereavement period (or prior to the loss) may affect the long-term health of caregivers.

The few studies that support the link between psychological morbidity and mortality may be secondary to the time frame of assessment. Generally psychological symptoms are assessed only cross-sectionally or for a short period of follow-up. Furthermore, inconsistent findings have been reported with post-loss adjustment of caregivers of care recipients diagnosed with dementia. High levels of stress, burden, and competing responsibilities during caregiving have also been associated with negative post-loss psychological outcomes [22, 23]. Conversely, other studies have found that caregivers who spent more time caregiving and had higher levels of distress experienced significant declines in depressive symptoms at 3 months and 1 year after the loss of their loved ones [22, 23].

Decades of research by Bonnano and his colleagues have resulted in four patterns of loss: (1) Resilience: the ability of adults in otherwise normal circumstances who are exposed to an isolated and potentially highly disruptive event, such as the death of a close relation or a violent or life-threatening situation, to maintain relatively stable, healthy levels of psychological and physical functioning as well as the capacity for generative experiences and positive emotions; (2) Recovery: when normal functioning temporarily gives way to threshold or subthreshold psychopathology, usually for a period of at least several months, and then gradually returns to pre-event levels; (3) Chronic dysfunction: prolonged suffering and inability to function, usually lasting several years or longer; and (4) Delayed grief or trauma: when adjustment seems normal but then distress and symptoms increase months later [24]. Although Bonnano's theory can guide the research concerning caregivers of those diagnosed with cancer, Bonnano's research has focused on sudden and traumatic loss and has not included the period prior to the loss of the loved one (caregiving) [24].

Bernard has applied trajectory analyses to the study of psychological functioning after the loss of a loved one diagnosed with cancer and has included both the caregiving and bereavement period [7]. The results of his work found that two trajectories emerged: (1) Relief Model, which predicts that caregiver stress or strain will abate and ease the bereavement process, and (2) Complicated Bereavement Model, which suggests that caregiver stress diminishes the psychological resources needed to cope during the bereavement process [27]. Interestingly, these trajectories were supported in spousal caregivers, but not in adult female children of breast cancer patients who were caregiving [7]. Furthermore, Bernard only followed the caregivers for 90 days after the loss of their loved ones; therefore other trajectory groups, particularly those associated with prolonged or delayed grief syndrome, may have not emerged [19].

Much of the previous research concerning predictors of caregiver outcomes has been conducted with those caring for loved ones diagnosed with dementia. Predictors of psychological morbidity during caregiving have included cognitive impairment, lack of anticipatory grief, younger age, female gender, lower education, poorer physical health, greater interference with life, and lower levels of caregiver mastery, poorer patient functional status, lower perceived control, greater number of hours spent caregiving, care recipient behavioral disturbances, and poorer quality of the patient–caregiver relationship [12, 25]. In regard to post-loss adjustment, prior research has found that caregivers with higher levels of pre-loss depressive symptoms and burden, a positive caregiving experience, and a cognitively impaired care recipient were more likely to report clinical levels of complicated grief.

Of the studies that have been conducted concerning *cancer* caregivers, similar findings were reported as those found in dementia caregivers. Predictors of depression during caregiving included high levels of caregiver burden, longer duration of caregiving and impact on other activities, mastery of caregiving tasks and neuroticism, previous health problems, lower levels of social support, avoidant coping, anxious attachment, and marital dissatisfaction [19–30]. Predictors of post-loss depressive symptoms in cancer caregivers have been found to include pessimism, pre-bereavement depressive symptoms, low levels of social support; and longer duration of caregiving.

Caregiving, Bereavement, and Health: Potential Biobehavioral Mediators

The two biobehavioral mediators that have been hypothesized to be one potential pathway linking caregiver stress and/or depression with mortality are health behaviors and/or immune system dysregulation. They may result in the worsening of preexisting illnesses or increase vulnerability to new health problems, including cardiovascular disease, some types of cancer (e.g., head and neck, pancreatic, stomach, lung), and diabetes. These diseases not only are considered some of the leading causes of death but may also be preventable [31].

Family members caring for loved ones with dementia have previously reported sleeping less, engaging in less regular exercise, and gaining weight when compared to their pre-caregiving behavior [32]. Caregivers report engaging less in preventative health care, such as mammograms or prostate exams, while providing care for a loved one [32]. Furthermore, caregivers have been found to use a greater amount of substances including alcohol and tobacco, and consume foods high in saturated fat than non-caregiving controls [33–36].

In regard to health care utilization, Schulz and colleagues reported that caregivers engage in fewer preventative health behaviors during the caregiving period [19]. The National Alliance for Caregiving found that 72% of caregivers reported that they had not gone to the doctor as often when compared to before they were caregiving. Fifty-five percent of caregivers reported that they had missed doctors appointments while caregiving [37]. Rural caregivers have reported even lower rates of physician visits during caregiving [37]. Finally, caregivers are less likely to fill prescriptions than non-caregivers [37].

In contrast, other studies have found that caregivers of dementia care recipients utilized more health services than their non-caregiver counterparts. These dementia caregivers demonstrated an increased number of physician visits, increased prescription drug use, and a higher incidence of inpatient hospitalizations [37]. Schubert and colleagues found that higher health care utilization was associated with depressive symptoms while others have reported that a greater number of stressors were associated with more frequent use of health care services [38]. Finally, the role of health care utilization in care recipients at the end of life has been found to be critical for the caregiver's health. A recent study found that higher rates of mortality were observed in those caregivers whose loved ones did not utilize hospice care [39]. Gender differences in survival were observed in wives who used hospice support whereas only a trend was observed in male spouses [39].

The second pathway that has been hypothesized linking psychological factors and health morbidity has been immune system dysregulation. As early as the 1990s, a meta-analysis was performed and confirmed the role of stress on immune system functioning [40]. Two other meta-analyses followed with the same conclusions [41, 42]. A series of papers has provided evidence for the link between stress and immunity specifically in caregivers [43–45]. Lasting effects of caregiver stress on immune system dysregulation have been reported up to one year after the end of caregiving [45]. A plethora of studies have also demonstrated that depressive symptoms are associated with immune system dysregulation and increased risk of mortality in those with chronic disease as well as in the general population [46–51]. Prolonged grief syndrome has also been associated with long-term immune system dysregulation and increased risk of mortality [52–55].

The link between immune system dysregulation and health is well documented. A plethora of studies have demonstrated an association between elevations in pro-inflammatory cytokines (e.g., IL-1α, IL-6, and TNF-α) and the development of cardiovascular disease [54, 55]. Similarly, development of diabetes and kidney disease has also been found to be associated with elevations in pro-inflammatory cytokines such as IL-6 and TNF-α [56, 57]. Dranoff has explained the importance of cytokines in cancer pathogenesis [58]. High levels of IL-6 and IL-10 in serum have been associated with poorer prognoses across cancer types [59, 60]. Respiratory diseases, such as allergies and asthma, rheumatoid arthritis, alcohol dependence, and hyper- and hypothyroidism, have also long been associated with changes in cytokines, particularly IL-1-β, TNF-α, and IL-6 [61, 62].

Despite decades of research regarding the link between psychological factors and immunity and a separate literature that has demonstrated the link between immunity and health outcomes, little evidence exists for the *mediation* of immune system dysregulation linking these psychological pathways with health outcomes. Possible explanations for this inability to link all three of these factors may be the following: (1) chronic levels of psychological morbidity were not assessed and analyzed, which is what is likely to have a profound effect on health, and (2) immune system markers that have been found to be associated with these psychological factors were in the normal range (when compared to controls) and as a result may not have an impact on health.

Due to the chronic levels of stress which caregiving has the potential to impose, strategies to reduce this stress, prevent depression, and decrease short- and long-term effects on health are warranted. Interventions have begun to be developed and tested to improve QOL at the end of life for patients, which can reduce caregiver stress and long-term health consequences. These interventions have begun to address the patient and caregiver as a unit. Interventions designed for the dyad that may have a significant impact on psychological functioning and health.

Interventions to Improve Quality of Life at the End of Life

With advances in modern medicine, it can be easy to focus on the eradication of disease and lose sight of the patient's experience of the illness.

However, the patients' QOL as they cope with the disease process, especially at the end of life, is an important focus of care. QOL is understood to be multifaceted, and includes physical, emotional, social, spiritual, and material domains [63, 64]. As such, assessment of disease-related QOL has been designed to reflect its multidimensional nature [e.g., European Organization for Research and Treatment of Cancer-Quality of Life Questionnaire (EOTRC-QLQ), Functional Assessment of Cancer Therapy (FACT)]. In earlier QOL work, however, some researchers assessed QOL in a more restricted manner, assessing primarily emotional functioning (e.g., depression, anxiety). Thus, earlier studies discussed will have less comprehensive measures of QOL, whereas later studies will include assessments of QOL measuring multiple domains.

A growing body of research has focused on understanding ways to enhance QOL, particularly at the end of life. Several of these interventions have been primarily psychosocial and administered by mental health professionals (e.g., social workers, psychologist, nurses with psychological training); however, several interventions have also been administered by physicians and/or nurses and focused on physical symptoms (e.g., Jordhøy et al. 2000, 85). Those interventions targeted on physical symptoms have resulted in little impact on QOL. Therefore, the primary focus of this discussion will be on interventions with a significant psychosocial focus.

In the first randomized controlled trial reported in the literature, a 2-week intervention, which was intended primarily to educate newly diagnosed advanced cancer patients, was compared to a no-treatment control group [65]. The intervention had a positive impact on patient's self-concept, hospital adjustment, and knowledge about cancer from pretreatment to immediately following the intervention.

Shortly thereafter, Spiegel and colleagues published results from a longitudinal study examining the effect of their group interventions on various aspects of functioning in women with metastatic breast cancer [66, 67]. Women participated for up to 3 years in a weekly supportive intervention. Those who received the intervention exhibited significantly less distress, fatigue, maladaptive coping responses, as well as reduced pain sensation and suffering over time than those in the control group. However, a later replication of this intervention, which included a multidimensional measure of Qo (EORTC QLQ-C30), found no effect of the intervention on QOL [68] but mood was improved and perception of pain was decreased [69]. In a similar study, comparing supportive-expressive group therapy to a control group receiving relaxation therapy, some benefit was observed. Participants in the intervention experienced less hopelessness, improved social functioning, and reduced intrusive and depressive symptoms [70].

Linn and colleagues conducted a randomized controlled trial with stage IV, primarily lung cancer patients, to test an intervention that was delivered over the course of multiple brief sessions per week by a therapist with expertise in death and dying [71]. Although no differences were found at 1-month follow-up, the treatment group was found to have lower levels of depression and alienation as well as more self-esteem and life satisfaction than the control group at 3–12 months. At 9–12 months, participants in the treatment group reported a greater internal locus of control.

As research in interventions to improve QoL in end-of-life cancer patients has grown, the interventions have become more multidimensional, which may be in part because of a recognition of the diverse nature of QoL. In a randomized controlled trial of lung cancer patients by McCorkle and colleagues [72], two specialized home care groups (i.e., visits by a member of an interdisciplinary team or visits by an oncology nurse with advanced training) had a 6-week delay in the amount of distress and dependence they experienced, in comparison to a standard office care control group [73]. A more recent randomized controlled trial examining the effects of a relatively brief intervention designed to target the multidimensional nature of QOL across eight sessions found that the treatment provided a buffer for advanced cancer patients. The treatment group did not experience a decrease in QOL experienced by the control group [73].

In a randomized controlled trial comparing the use of psychopharmacology alone to combined psychopharmacology treatments—one with social support provided by volunteers and one with structured psychotherapy [74]—the researchers found that patients receiving the combined treatment did not have a worsening of QOL over time, as measured by the Functional Living Index-Cancer (FLIC) and experienced decreased depression and anxiety. In contrast, the patients receiving psychopharmacology alone did worse with one exception (i.e., they experienced a reduction in anticipatory and posttreatment nausea and emesis).

These findings reflect unique challenges of conducting intervention research with patients at the end of life, and questions remain about how to design optimal interventions to improve QOL. The interventions have varied considerably in their content, fecilitators, and length of intervention. The early QOL findings of Spiegel and colleagues [66, 67] with women with metastatic breast cancer were not supported by later clinical trials [68, 70]. The multidimensional interventions show some promise in improving QOL, and brief interventions may have a positive impact [73].

Future research in this area would likely benefit from exploring whether briefer interventions have benefit. Many patients at the end of life view time as precious and focus on spending time with loved ones, potentially making lengthy interventions less practical and too burdensome. These patients may benefit from more flexible interventions that are tailored to their preferences and allow greater options for how treatment is delivered (e.g., telephone calls instead of face-to-face visits, Web based).

Interventions Targeting Caregiver Quality of Life

Although patients at the end of life face several unique challenges, the caregivers can experience a myriad of concerns, which include determining how to provide emotional and instrumental support as well as coping with the anticipated loss of a loved one. In addition to patients having significant concerns about their family's adjustment [75], caregivers can experience increased levels of psychological distress, such as anxiety and depression [76, 77], especially when they are unable to balance their caregiving responsibilities with engaging in activities [78]. Perhaps even more troubling is that some caregivers are reluctant to seek support from loved ones or professionals [79].

A large amount of research has examined caregiver interventions with only a small proportion of studies focused on *end-of-life* caregiving [80]. Although researchers have assessed the utility of various interventions (e.g., psychoeducational, skills based, supportive), none of the interventions has had a consistent impact on caregiver and patient outcomes, making it difficult to determine the type of intervention to best suit their needs. A discussion of these different interventions as well as associated outcomes follows. The focus will initially be on single modality interventions (e.g., supportive care), followed by multimodal treatments, which are designed to target symptom management as well as various psychosocial concerns (e.g., effective coping, social support).

One of the first randomized controlled trials with caregivers of patients at the end of life examined the effect of a weekly supportive treatment for caregivers, which occurred over 6 months and found no advantage of the treatment group over the control group [81]. Subsequent supportive interventions have had a limited impact as well. A randomized controlled trial comparing hospice care plus three supportive visits to as usual and hospice care combined with coping skills sessions found no benefit for the supportive intervention on caregiver outcomes [82]. Only participants in the third group had significantly improved caregiver QOL, reduced burden of patient symptoms, and reduced caregiver burden when compared to the other two groups.

The only study to show any benefit of a single modality, was a study examining family-focused grief therapy, which began during palliative care and continued into bereavement [105]. They found that caregivers experienced a reduction in distress at 13 months after the patient's death but only for the families who were highly distressed at initiation of the study. In another randomized controlled trial comparing standard home-based palliative care (SHPC) plus two-session psychoeducation to SHPC alone, a more positive caregiver experience over the long term in the psychoeducation group was found [83]. However perceived competence, self-efficacy, and anxiety did not differ between groups.

Multimodal interventions, which often have some degree of psychoeducational emphasis, have also been developed. In a study by McCorkle and colleagues [84], a weekly psychoeducational home care intervention was compared to the same type of treatment but with the inclusion of skills training as well as an office care control group. They found only a slight advantage for the group that included skills training (i.e., less depression and paranoid ideation) and did not find a significant group by time interaction [82].

In another study examining the impact of a supportive, psychoeducational family intervention, a decrease in psychological distress in both patients and caregivers in the intervention group was observed but only for a short period of time [85]. An examination of the influence of a brief, three-session skills training plus psychoeducational intervention found that caregivers experienced an increase in self-efficacy for helping the patient manage pain; however, there was no effect of the treatment on patients' pain [86]. A more recent randomized controlled trial comparing psychoeducation with a secondary supportive focus to usual care found no difference in caregiver outcomes between groups [87].

Couples Therapy at the End of Life

Research examining the effectiveness of couple's interventions targeting the spouses or significant others of cancer patients at the end of life is relatively new. Mohr and colleagues [88] conducted one of the first studies examining the impact of couple's therapy on nine couples. In this small sample, they found significant reductions in the patient's worry about dying as well as the partner's worry about the patients' demise [89]. They also found an improvement in relationship quality. Another intervention, Emotionally Focused Couple Therapy, has also shown some promise for improving marital function and decreasing symptoms of depression in both caregivers and patients [89].

In summary, caregivers of patients with cancer who are at the end of life are at risk for psychological distress, and it is not clear how to best support them. Neither single- nor multimodal interventions offer clear advantages. Research on couple's therapy, however, indicates that this type of intervention shows some promise in improving psychosocial outcomes. Future work in this area is desperately needed and should be theory driven and include outcome measures that are relevant to end of life in both patients and caregivers, such as QOL, pain management, and psychological distress.

Summary

The intersection between the end of life in the context of cancer and caregiver survivorship is beginning to receive the attention of researchers. There is an increasing focus on the psychological and health consequences that families can experience as a result of caregiving and/or bereavement. Research concerning predictors of the short- and long-term consequence have been studied extensively in caregivers of dementia; however, there is a relative paucity of research concerning cancer caregivers. Much work needs to be done to determine which medical and psychological interventions improve QOL for patients at the end of life and their surviving family members. Some work indicates that the patients and caregivers cannot always be treated separately and interventions developed for the dyad may be most effective; however, research in this area is still greatly needed to better understand the effects of the patient and caregiver functioning on one another particularly at the end of life (e.g., actor–partner independence).

Additionally, training of HCPs who interface with patients and families could be enhanced and practice guidelines across medical disciplines could be developed that include recommendations for appropriate and timely referral to palliative care and hospice where both the patient and caregiven may be supported. Clinicians and researchers may also want to consider the economic toll on society that caregiving and/or problems with bereavement may have on a large percentage of the population.

References

1. Despelder A, Strickland AL. The last dance: encountering death and dying. 6th ed. Whitby: McGraw-Hill Higher Education; 2001.
2. Ury WA, Berkman CS, Weber CM, Pignotti MG, Leipzig RM. Assessing medical students' training in end-of-life communication: a survey of interns at one urban teaching hospital. Acad Med. 2003;78(5):530–7.
3. Casarett DJ, Quill TE. "I'm not ready for hospice": strategies for timely and effective hospice discussions. Ann Intern Med. 2007;146:443–9.
4. Wright AA, Zhang B, Ray A, et al. Associations between end-of-life discussions, patient mental health, medical care near death, and caregiver bereavement adjustment. JAMA. 2008;300(14):1665–73.
5. NHPCO facts and figures: Hospice care in America. 2010 edition. Alexandria: National Hospice and Palliative Care Organization. 2010.
6. Byock I. Dying well: the prospect for growth at the end of life. New York: Riverhead Books; 1997.
7. Zhang B, Wright AA, Huskamp HA, et al. Health care costs in the last week of life: associations with end-of-life conversations. Arch Intern Med. 2009;169(5):480–8.
8. Fohr SA. The double effect of pain medication: separating myth from reality. J Palliat Med. 1998;1(4):315–28.
9. Walsh TD. Opiates and respiratory function in advanced cancer. Recent Results Cancer Res. 1984;41(89):115–7.
10. Fainsinger RL, Waller A, Bercovici M, et al. A multicentre international study of sedation for uncontrolled symptoms in terminally ill patients. Palliat Med. 2000;14(4):257–65.
11. Morita T, Chinone Y, Ikenaga M, et al. Ethical validity of palliative sedation therapy: a multicenter, prospective, observational study conducted on specialized palliative care units in Japan. J Pain Symptom Manage. 2005;30(4):308–19.
12. Morita T, Chinone Y, Ikenaga M, et al. Efficacy and safety of palliative sedation therapy: a multicenter, prospective, observational study conducted on specialized palliative care units in Japan. J Pain Symptom Manage. 2005;30(4):320–8.
13. Elsayem A, Curry Iii E, Boohene J, et al. Use of palliative sedation for intractable symptoms in the palliative care unit of a comprehensive cancer center. Support Care Cancer. 2009;17(1):53–9.
14. World Health Organizaiton. Palliative care: symptom management and of life. 2004
15. Caffrey C, Sengupta M, Moss A, Harris-Kojetin L, Valverde R. Home health care and discharged hospice care patients: United States, 2000 and 2007. National health statistics reports; no 38. Hyattsville: National Center for Health Statistics; 2011.
16. Lichter I, Hunt E. The last 48 hours of life. J Palliat Care. 1990;6(4):7–15.
17. Reid D, Field D, Payne S, Relf M. Adult bereavement in five English hospices: types of support. Int J Palliat Nurs. 2006;12(9):430–7.
18. Jianguang J, Bengrt Z, Sundquist K, Sundquist J. Increased risks of coronary heart disease and stroke among spousal caregivers of cancer patients. Circulation. 2012;125:1723–42.
19. Schulz R, Beach SR. Caregiving as a risk factor for mortality: the Caregiver Health Effects Study. JAMA. 1999;282:2215–9.
20. Christakis NA, Allison PD. Mortality after the hospitalization of a spouse. N Engl J Med. 2006;354:719–30.
21. Fredman L, Cauley JA, Hochberg M, Ensrud KE, Doros G. Mortality associated with caregiving, general stress, and caregiving-related stress in elderly women: results of caregiver-study of osteoporotic fractures. J Am Geriatr Soc. 2010;58(5):937–43.
22. Gallup. Gallup-healthways well-being index. Gallop Poll 2010.
23. Bodnar J, Kiecolt-Glaser JK. Caregiver depression after bereavement: chronic stress isn't over when it's over. Psychol Aging. 1994;9:372–80.
24. Bonanno GA. The other side of sadness: what the new science of bereavement tells us about life after loss Philadelphia basic books. 2009.
25. Aggarwal B, Liao M, Christian A, Mosca L. Influence of caregiving on lifestyle and psychosocial risk factors among family members of patients hospitalized with cardiovascular disease. J Gen Intern Med. 2009;24:93–8.
26. Schulz R, Boerner K, Shear K, Zhang S, Gitlin LN. Predictors of complicated grief among dementia caregivers: a prospective study of bereavement. Am J Geriatr Psychiatry. 2006;14:650–8.
27. Bernard LL, Guarnaccia CA. Two models of caregiver strain and bereavement adjustment: a comparison of husband and daughter caregivers of breast cancer hospice patients. Gerontologist. 2003;43:808–16.
28. Aggar C, Ronaldson S, Cameron ID. Reactions to caregiving of frail, older persons predict depression. Int J Ment Health Nurs. 2010;19:409–15.
29. Covinsky KE, Newcomer R, Fox P, Wood J, Sands L, Dane K, Yaffe K. Patient and caregiver characteristics associated with depression in caregivers of patients with dementia. J Gen Intern Med. 2003; 18:1006–14.

30. Byrnes D, Antoni MH, Goodkin K, Efantis-Potter J, Asthana D, Simon T, Munajj J, Ironson G, Fletcher MA. Stressful events, pessimism, natural killer cell cytotoxicity, and cytotoxic/suppressor T cells in HIV+black women at risk for cervical cancer. Psychosom Med. 1998;60:714–22.

31. Burton AM, Haley WE, Small BJ, Finley MR, Dillinger-Vasille M, Schonwetter R. Predictors of well-being in bereaved former hospice caregivers: the role of caregiving stressors, appraisals, and social resources. Palliat Support Care. 2008;6:149–58.

32. Vitaliano PP, Zhang J, Scanlan JM. Is caregiving hazardous to one's physical health? A meta-analysis. Psychol Bull. 2003;129:946–72.

33. Andre K, Schraub S, Mercier M, Bontemps P. Role of alcohol and tobacco in the aetiology of head and neck cancer: a case-control study in the Doubs region of France. Eur J Cancer B Oral Oncol. 1995; 31B:301–9.

34. Johansen D, Borgstrom A, Lindkvist B, et al. Different markers of alcohol consumption, smoking and body mass index in relation to risk of pancreatic cancer. A prospective cohort study within the Malmo Preventive Project. Pancreatology. 2009;9:677–86.

35. Lynch SM, Vrieling A, Lubin JH, et al. Cigarette smoking and pancreatic cancer: a pooled analysis from the pancreatic cancer cohort consortium. Am J Epidemiol. 2009;170:403–13.

36. Chao A, Thun MJ, Henley SJ, et al. Cigarette smoking, use of other tobacco products and stomach cancer mortality in US adults: The Cancer Prevention Study II. Int J Cancer. 2002;101:380–9.

37. National Alliance for Caregiving and Evercare. Evercare (R) study of caregivers in decline: a close-up look at the health risks of caring for a loved one. Bethesda: National Alliance for Caregiving and Minnetonka, MN: Evercare; 2006.

38. Evercare study of caregivers. A closeup look at the health risks of caring for a loved one. National Alliance for Caregiving and Evercare. 2006.

39. Ahrens J. The positive impact of hospice care on the surviving spouse. Home Healthc Nurse. 2005;23: 53–5.

40. Gouin JP, Hantsoo L, Kiecolt-Glaser JK. Immune dysregulation and chronic stress among older adults: a review. Neuroimmunomodulation. 2008;15:251–9.

41. Schneiderman N, Ironson G, Siegel SD. Stress and health: psychological, behavioral, and biological determinants. Annu Rev Clin Psychol. 2005;1: 607–28.

42. Herbert TB, Cohen S. Stress and immunity in humans: a meta-analytic review. Psychosom Med. 1993;55:364–79.

43. Kiecolt-Glaser JK, Dura JR, Speicher CE, Trask OJ, Glaser R. Spousal caregivers of dementia victims: longitudinal changes in immunity and health. Psychosom Med. 1991;53:345–62.

44. Kiecolt-Glaser JK, Glaser R, Shuttleworth EC, Dyer CS, Ogrocki P, Speicher CE. Chronic stress and immunity in family caregivers of Alzheimer's disease victims. Psychosom Med. 1987;49:523–35.

45. Cacioppo JT, Poehlmann KM, Kiecolt-Glaser JK, et al. Cellular immune responses to acute stress in female caregivers of dementia patients and matched controls. Health Psychol. 1998;17:182–9.

46. Steel JL, Geller DA, Gamblin TC, Olek MC, Carr BI. Depression, immunity, and survival in patients with hepatobiliary carcinoma. J Clin Oncol. 2007;25:2397–405.

47. Simonsick EM, Wallace RB, Blazer DG, Berkman LF. Depressive symptomatology and hypertension-associated morbidity and mortality in older adults. [see comment]. Psychosom Med. 1995;57: 427–35.

48. Yaffe K, Edwards ER, Covinsky KE, Lui LY, Eng C. Depressive symptoms and risk of mortality in frail, community-living elderly persons. Am J Geriatr Psychiatry. 2003;11:561–7.

49. Harris EC, Barraclough B. Excess mortality of mental disorder. Br J Psychiatry. 1998;173:11–53.

50. Orsi AJ, McCorkle R, Tax AW, Barsevick A. The relationship between depressive symptoms and immune status phenotypes in patients undergoing surgery for colorectal cancer. Psychooncology. 1996;5:311–9.

51. Sachs G, Rasoul-Rockenschaub S, Aschauer H, et al. Lytic effector cell activity and major depressive disorder in patients with breast cancer: a prospective study. J Neuroimmunol. 1995;59:83–9.

52. Siegel K, Karus DG, Raveis VH, Christ GH, Mesagno FP. Depressive distress among the spouses of terminally ill cancer patients. Cancer Pract. 1996;4:25–30.

53. Hebert RS, Dang Q, Schulz R, Hebert RS, Dang Q, Schulz R. Religious beliefs and practices are associated with better mental health in family caregivers of patients with dementia: findings from the REACH study. Am J Geriatr Psychiatry. 2007;15:292–300.

54. Latham AE, Prigerson HG. Suicidality and bereavement: complicated grief as psychiatric disorder presenting greatest risk for suicidality. Suicide Life Threat Behav. 2004;34:350–62.

55. Volpato S, Guralnik JM, Ferrucci L, Balfour J, Chaves P, Fried LP, Harris TB. Cardiovascular disease, interleukin-6, and risk of mortality in older women. Circulation. 2001;103:947.

56. Spranger J, Kroke A, Mohlig M, et al. Inflammatory cytokines and the risk to develop type 2 diabetes: results of the prospective population-based European Prospective Investigation into Cancer and Nutrition (EPIC)-Potsdam Study. Diabetes. 2003;52:812–7.

57. Liu S, Tinker L, Song Y, Rifai N, Bonds DE, Cook NR, Heiss G, Howard BV, Hotamisligil GS, Hu FB, Kuller LH, Manson JE. A prospective study of inflammatory cytokines and diabetes mellitus in a multiethnic cohort of postmenopausal women. Arch Intern Med. 2007;167:1676–85.

58. Dranoff G. Cytokines in cancer pathogenesis and cancer therapy. Nat Rev Cancer. 2004;4:11–22.

59. Brower V. Researchers attempting to define role of cytokines in cancer risk. J Natl Cancer Inst. 2005;97:1175–7.

60. Berger FG. The interleukin-6 gene: a susceptibility factor that may contribute to racial and ethnic disparities in breast cancer mortality. Breast Cancer Res Treat. 2004;88:281–5.
61. Karanikas G, John P, Wahl K, Schuetz M, Dudczak R, Willheim M. T-lymphocyte cytokine production patterns in nonimmune severe hypothyroid state and after thyroid hormone replacement therapy. Thyroid. 2004;14:488–92.
62. Irwin M, Hauger R, Patterson TL, Semple S, Ziegler M, Grant I. Alzheimer caregiver stress: basal natural killer cell activity, pituitary-adrenal cortical function, and sympathetic tone. Ann Behav Med. 1997;19:83–90.
63. Felce D, Perry J. Quality of life: its definition and measurement. Res Dev Disabil. 1995;16:51–74.
64. Steinhauser KE, Christakis NA, Clipp EC, McNeilly M, McIntyre L, Tulsky JA. Factors considered important at the end of life by patients, family, physicians, and other care providers. J Am Med Assoc. 2000;284:2476–82.
65. Ferlic M, Goldman A, Kennedy BJ. Group counseling in adult patients with advanced cancer. Cancer. 1979;43:760–6.
66. Spiegel D, Bloom JR. Group therapy and hypnosis reduce metastatic breast carcinoma pain. Psychosom Med. 1983;45:333–9.
67. Spiegel D, Bloom JR, Yalom I. Group support for patients with metastatic cancer: a randomized prospective outcome study. Arch Gen Psychiatry. 1981;38:527–33.
68. Bordeleau L, Szalai JP, Ennis M, et al. Quality of life in a randomized trial of group psychosocial support in metastatic breast cancer: overall effects of the intervention and an exploration of missing data. J Clin Oncol. 2003;21:1944–51.
69. Goodwin PJ, Leszc ZM, Ennis M, Koopmans V, Vincent L, Guther H, Drysdale F, Hundleny M, Chochina HM, Naramo M, Speed M, Hunter J. The effect of group psychosocial support on survival in matastatic breast cancer. NEJM, 2001;345(24): 1719–26.
70. Kissane DW, Crabsch B, clorance, Love AW, Bloch S, Snyder RD, Liy JV. Supportive-expressive group therapy for women with metastatic breast cancer: survival and psychosocial outcome from a randomized controlledtnal. Psychooncology, 2007;16(4): 277–86.
71. Linn MW, Linn BS, Harris R. Effects of counseling for late stage cancer patients. Cancer. 1982;49:1048–55.
72. McCorkle R, Benloliel JQ, Donaldson G, et al. A randomized clinical trial of home nursing care for lung cancer patients. Cancer. 1989;64:1375–82.
73. Rummans TA, Clark MM, Sloan JA, et al. Impacting quality of life for patients with advanced cancer with a structured multidisciplinary intervention: a randomized controlled trial. J Clin Oncol. 2006;24:635–42.
74. Mantovani G, Astara G, Lampis B, et al. Evaluation by multidimensional instruments of health-related quality of life of elderly cancer patients undergoing three different "psychosocial" treatment approaches:

a randomized clinical trial. Support Care Cancer. 1996;4:129–40.
75. Brown JE, Brown RF, Miller RM, et al. Coping with metastatic melanoma: the last year of life. Psychooncology. 2000;9:283–92.
76. Chentsova-Dutton Y, Shucter S, Hutchin S, Strause L, et al. Depression and grief reactions in hospice caregivers: from pre-death to 1 year afterwards. J Affect Disord. 2002;69:53–60.
77. Grunfeld E, Coyle D, Whelan T, et al. Family caregiver burden: results of a longitudinal study of breast cancer patients and their principal caregivers. CMAJ. 2004;170:1795–801.
78. Cameron JI, Franche R-L, Cheung AM, Stewart DE. Lifestyle interference and emotional distress in family caregivers of advanced cancer patients. Cancer. 2002;94:521–7.
79. Glasdam S, Jensen AB, Madsen EL, Rose C. Anxiety and depression in cancer patients' spouses. Psychooncology. 1996;5:23–9.
80. Northouse LL, Katapodi MC, Song L, Zhang L, Mood DW. Interventions with family caregivers of cancer patients: a meta-analysis of randomized trials. CA Cancer J Clin. 2010;60:317–39.
81. Goldberg RJ, Wool MS. Psychotherapy for the spouses of lung cancer patients: assessment of an intervention. Psychother Psychosom. 1985;43:141–50.
82. McMillan SC, Small BJ, Weitzner M, et al. Impact of coping skills intervention with family caregivers of hospice patients with cancer: a randomized clinical trial. Cancer. 2006;106:214–22.
83. Hudson PL, Aranda S, Hayman-White K. A psychoeducational intervention for family caregivers of patients receiving palliative care: a randomized controlled trial. J Pain Symptom Manage. 2005;30:329–41.
84. McCorkle R, Robinson L, Nuamah I, Lev E, Benoliel JQ. The effects of home nursing care for patients during terminal illness on the bereaved's psychological distress. Nurs Res. 1998;47:2–11.
85. Northouse LL, Kershaw T, Mood D, Schafenacker A. Effects of a family intervention on the quality of life of women with recurrent breast cancer and their family caregivers. Psychooncology. 2005;14: 478–91.
86. Keefe FJ, Ahles TA, Sutton L, et al. Partner-guided pain management at the end of life: a preliminary study. J Pain Symptom Manage. 2005;29:263–72.
87. Walsh K, Jones L, Tookman A, et al. Reducing emotional distress in people caring for patients receiving specialist palliative care: randomised trial. Br J Psychiatry. 2007;190:142–7.
88. Mohr DC, Moran PJ, Kohn C, et al. Couples therapy at end of life. Psychooncology. 2003;12:620–7.
89. McClean LM, Jones JM, Rydall AC, et al. A couple's intervention for patients facing advanced cancer and their spouse caregivers: outcomes of a pilot study. Psychooncology. 2008;17:1152–6.
90. Morita T, Tsunoda J, Inoue S, et al. Contributing factors to physical symptoms in terminally-ill cancer patients. J Pain Symptom Manage. 1999;18(5): 338–46.

91. Balboni TA, Vanderwerker LC, Block SD, et al. Religiousness and spiritual support among advanced cancer patients and associations with end-of-life treatment preferences and quality of life. J Clin Oncol. 2007;25(5):555–60.

92. Cancer survivors in the United States morbidity and mortality weekly report, 60:269-72.

93. Alspaugh MEL, Stephens MAP, Townsend AL, Zarit SH, Greene R. Longitudinal patterns of risk for depression in dementia caregivers: objective and subjective primary stress as predictors. Psychol Aging. 1999;14:34–43.

94. Ho A, Collins SR, David K, Doty M. A look at working-age caregivers roles, health concerns, and need for support. Issue Brief (Commonw Fund) 2005;(854):1–12.

95. Kim Y, Spillers RL, Hall DL. Quality of life of family caregivers 5 years after a relative's cancer diagnosis: follow-up of the national quality of life survey for caregivers. Psychooncology. 2012;21:273–81.

96. Schulz. Caregiving and bereavement. In: Handbook of bereavement research and practice: 21st century perspectives. Washington DC: American Psychological Association Press; 2008. p. 265–85.

97. Hebert RS, Dang Q, Schulz R, Hebert RS, Dang Q, Schulz R. Preparedness for the death of a loved one and mental health in bereaved caregivers of patients with dementia: findings from the REACH study. [see comment]. J Palliat Med. 2006;9:683–93.

98. Boerner K, Schulz R, Horowitz A, Boerner K, Schulz R, Horowitz A. Positive aspects of caregiving and adaptation to bereavement. Psychol Aging. 2004;19:668–75.

99. Mahony R, Regan C, Katona C, Livingston G. Anxiety and depression in family caregivers of people with Alzheimer disease: the LASER-AD Study. Am J Geriatr Psychiatry. 2005;13:795–801.

100. Braun M, Mikulincer M, Rydall A, Walsh A, Rodin G. Hidden morbidity in cancer: spouse caregivers. J Clin Oncol. 2007;25:4829–34.

101. Teel CS, Press AN. Fatigue among elders in caregiving and noncaregiving roles. West J Nurs Res. 1999;21:498–514. discussion -20.

102. Tanner SJ, Johnson AD, Townsend-Rocchiccioli J. The health status of rural caregivers. J Gerontol Nurs. 2005;31:25–31.

103. Jordhøy MS, Fayers P, Loge JH, Ahlner-Elmqvist M, Kaasa S. Quality of life in palliative cancer care: results from a cluster randomized trial. J Clin Oncol. 2001;19:3884–94.

104. Wong GY, Schroeder DR, Carns PE, et al. Effect of neurolytic celiac plexus block on pain relief, quality of life, and survival in patients with unresectable pancreatic cancer: a randomized controlled trial. J Am Med Assoc. 2004;291:1092–9.

105. Kissane DW, McKenzie M, Bloch S, Moskowitz C, McKenzie DP, O'Neill I. Family focused grief therapy: a randomized controlled trial in palliative care and bereavement. Am J Psychiatry. 2006;163:1208–18.

Carolyn Messner

Setting the Stage

A little help, rationally directed and purposefully focused at a strategic time is more effective than more extensive help given at a period of less emotional accessibility.

(Rapoport, L, 1962)

In cancer care, the goal of all intervention is to help individuals maximize their existing resources, strengths, and strategies as well as acquire any needed additions so that they experience the greatest sense of well-being of which they are capable. When they are able to do so to the degree that they can experience a sense of calm and strength in the midst of threat, they have achieved a still point.

(Jevne, RF, 1987)

The Art and Science of Resource Referral

A few weeks ago, Norma, a 70-year old, single woman called in crisis, not knowing what to do and where to turn. Norma is a member of a

C. Messner, D.S.W., M.S.W., B.C.D., A.C.S.W., F.N.A.P., L.C.S.W.-R. (✉)
CancerCare, 275 Seventh Avenue, New York, NY 10001, USA

Association of Oncology Social Work, 100 North 20th St., Suite 400, Philadelphia, PA 19103, USA

Social Work Academy, National Academies of Practice, Cleveland, OH, USA
e-mail: cmessner@cancercare.org

weekly, patient support group. She has attended this group for 2 years. She is a Holocaust survivor and had been a teacher until her cancer recurrence 4 years ago. She is a wise and courageous woman who values life and has undergone radical surgeries and treatments so that she could live. Her first encounter with cancer was at the age of 40, when she was diagnosed with breast cancer. At that time, she had a radical mastectomy followed by extensive radiation treatments. A side effect of her radiation treatments was severe damage to the skin in her chest area. Although this was a common occurrence at that time, current radiation treatments no longer have these side effects. The skin in Norma's chest area is paper thin and scarred. Four years ago, Norma developed metastatic breast cancer in her other breast and had a mastectomy, followed by chemotherapy.

Norma's current crisis was precipitated by a visit she made to a free local skin cancer screening clinic. She had a mole on her hand that "looked suspicious" and she had wanted to have it checked by a dermatologist for possible skin cancer. Although she was relieved to learn that the mole was not cancer, the dermatologist had examined Norma's body for possible skin cancers. The dermatologist had expressed concern about the radiated skin on her chest. He felt that she might have extensive skin cancer in this area and wanted to do a biopsy of the skin tissue to determine if Norma had skin cancer. Norma was terrified of having a biopsy since the skin tissue in that area of her chest was so thin and would probably not heal. She was also frightened that if she did nothing, she would then have an extensive area of skin cancer in her chest area which could not be surgically removed, because the skin no longer had the capacity to heal.

When she called for help, she was clearly in a state of crisis. She anticipated that the cancer would spread, if untreated, and could eventually be life threatening. Her balance of coping had been disrupted. She described her inability to think logically and coherently about what to do. Her health care professional suggested an immediate second opinion consultation with a leading cancer center in her city. Since her income is fixed, she was concerned about the cost. The oncology social worker offered to call the cancer center and clarify the cost. In the process, she learned that the office accepted Medicare assignment and that, if Norma wished, she could have an appointment the following day.

The social worker called Norma and told her what she had learned. Norma felt that a second opinion would be helpful to her and proceeded to call and secure the appointment for the following day. She then called back, much relieved. She talked with her social worker about some of the possible options and together, they made a list of the questions she needed to have answered. Her oncology social worker wondered about her going alone to such an important appointment. Norma realized that she had a close friend who could accompany her. Norma and her social worker again reviewed the possibilities and that if this dermatologist was not helpful, they would work together to find another doctor, until she felt satisfied. As she talked, Norma sounded calmer and more in control. Her social worker suggested that Norma and her friend go out after the appointment for some coffee so that she could process the appointment with her friend.

Norma called the following day after her appointment. She no longer felt in crisis. The dermatologist said that Norma did not have skin cancer. He felt that she might develop skin cancer in the future due to the extensive radiation treatments. He did not recommend a biopsy but rather wished to follow her every 3 months. He carefully told her how to care for the skin on her chest and also described the treatment he would recommend, should she ever develop skin cancer. He answered all her questions and spent time in alleviating her distress. She felt able to cope with the possibilities and more in control and had arranged to see the dermatologist again in 3 months. After the appointment, she and her friend had gone out to dinner to relax and celebrate the good news and Norma's renewed sense of mastery.

Norma is the archetypal cancer patient—scarred by her cancer but not overpowered, and wanting to find moments of solace, tranquility, and joy in her life. Her scars are not visible to the passerby as her cancer surgeries are covered by her clothing.

A possibility of recurrence can create a crisis for a cancer patient. Oncology health care professionals who work with cancer patients need a thorough understanding of the crisis intervention approach and the challenges people impacted by cancer face in order to be effective in service delivery and resource referrals for this population.

Types of Resources

Helping Our Patients and Their Loved Ones Utilize Resources

The majority of oncology patients and their caregivers who contact health care professionals or our institutions for resource information, like Norma, feel overwhelmed, anxious, and are often in a state of crisis. They turn to their health care professional for solutions to their particular problems. The problem often has many components and it is the art and science of the practitioner [17] to assess the level of distress [8] and come up with a resource outcome treatment plan. The Institute of Medicine Report, *Cancer Care For The Whole Patient: Meeting Psychosocial Health Needs* (2008) clearly raised the bar of expectations that treatment of cancer patients includes the full range of psychosocial health services. The following are the types of resources which those living with cancer and survivors often require:

- Information on specific-type of cancer, treatment decisions, side effect and pain management, survivorship care plans, palliative care and hospice.
- Practical help, financial and co-payment assistance, legal support, transportation, home care, child care, elder care, housing/lodging, wigs, prostheses.
- Psychosocial and psycho spiritual support and counseling, support groups, methods to cope with the anxiety, uncertainty and distress of cancer, mind/body techniques.
- Facts about the workplace and cancer, reasonable accommodation, Family and Medical Leave Act (FMLA), Americans with Disability Act (ADA), COBRA.
- Health insurance—private and government, including Medicare and Medicaid.
- Disability updates—short-term disability (STD), long-term disability (LTD), social security disability insurance (SSD).
- Government programs, federal, local, and state assistance, Supplemental Security Income (SSI), Medicaid and Veteran's benefits.
- End-of-life planning, including living will, health care proxy, advance directives, power of attorney, will, permanency planning for children, funeral arrangements, spiritual issues.

This extensive typology requires specialized knowledge of resources by health care professionals and how to access strategic information that our patients and their loved ones require [1–7, 11, 14, 16, 18]. The skill of the health care professional in communicating to patients and their caregivers about needed resources impacts their follow-up. Sometimes our referrals are reactive to a patient situation, but increasingly our referrals are proactive based on team assessment prior to crisis. Information and resource referrals are provided upfront to patients to empower and facilitate their coping [21].

Health care professionals have considerable expertise but their compassionate communication skills significantly impact patients' successful utilization and access to resources [9]. As in the case of Norma, follow-up with patients on a resource referral suggested is essential to insure the efficacy of the patient's benefit from a referral. Many of us spend our careers gathering resource information on how to connect our patients to needed resources. Patients depend upon their practitioners' network, guidance, roadmaps, and social capital to help them navigate their cancer experience and reduce cancer health disparities in accessing needed help [7, 19, 20].

Resource Guide

This section of the article includes a suggested compendium guide of useful resources for cancer patients. It would take many volumes to compile all the resources currently available. This resource roadmap is intended as a point of access for health care professionals as well as patients of free resources to address the myriad of problems patients and survivors confront. It is by no means exhaustive. Each organization listed is able to provide specific services. However, their staff of health care professionals will tailor additional resources to fit the patient, survivor, caregiver, or bereaved person's particular needs. The listing does not include the many nonprofit cancer-specific organizations that focus upon a particular type of cancer. The organizations listed are able to provide additional resources for all cancer types.

As you become familiar with these resources and their particular focus, it will facilitate matching each specific resource to the need or problem presented. For those who do not have Internet access in their homes, local libraries can be of assistance in providing access to information to websites listed. Many of these organizations have toll-free numbers staffed by information specialists to answer questions, guide patients, serve as patient navigators, and mail educational materials.

Collaboration brings together the strengths of each organization and profession to make the best use of their resources. When institutions and their staff partner together successfully, patients and families benefit due to their increased access to a broader range of resources, services, and programs [19]. Working together and pooling resources can energize people and result in innovative ways of tackling problems that might have seemed unsolvable. Interprofessional commitment and partnerships may also serve to counteract compassion fatigue of practitioners and enable novel help for patients [13].

Resources

AMERICAN CANCER SOCIETY combines an unyielding passion with nearly a century of experience to save lives and end suffering from cancer. As a global grassroots force of more than three million volunteers, we fight for every birthday threatened by every cancer in every community. We save lives by helping people stay well by preventing cancer or detecting it early; helping people get well by being there for them during and after a cancer diagnosis; by finding cures through investment in groundbreaking discovery; by fighting back by rallying lawmakers to pass laws to defeat cancer; and by rallying communities worldwide to join the fight. As the nation's largest nongovernmental investor in cancer research, contributing more than $3.5 billion since 1946, we turn what we know about cancer into what we do. As a result, more than 11 million people in America who have had cancer and countless more who have avoided it will be celebrating birthdays this year. To learn more about us or to get help, call us anytime, day or night, at 1-800-227-2345 or visit www.cancer.org.

AMERICAN PAIN FOUNDATION is an independent nonprofit organization serving people with pain through information, advocacy, and support. Its mission is to improve the quality of life for people with pain by raising public awareness, providing practical information, and advocating to remove barriers and increase access to effective pain management. All services are provided free of charge. For more information, visit our web site: www.painfoundation.org; Online Support Groups: http://painaid.painfoundation.org; Toll-Free Automated Information & Order Line: 1-888-615-PAIN (7246); or E-mail Service: info@painfoundation.org.

AMERICAN PSYCHOSOCIAL ONCOLOGY SOCIETY (APOS) is a nonprofit 501(c)(3) professional membership organization that provides a connection point for the professionals and patient advocates that support people affected by cancer. APOS members include physicians, mental health professionals, social workers, nurses, and clergy, among many others, dedicated to treating the human side of cancer. Our mission is to advance the science and practice of psychosocial oncology so that all people with cancer and their loved ones have access to psychosocial services as a part of quality cancer care. Among the programs offered is the APOS Toll-Free Helpline, which assists cancer patients and their caregivers to obtain a local referral to help manage distress: 1-866-APOS-4-HELP (1-866-276-7443). APOS also offers online education in psychosocial oncology and distress management, as well as two practical handbooks on adult and pediatric psychosocial care. Please visit www.apos-society.org.

AMERICAN SOCIETY OF CLINICAL ONCOLOGY (ASCO) is the world's leading professional organization representing physicians of all oncology subspecialties who care for people with cancer. ASCO's more than 20,000 members from the USA and abroad set the standard for patient care worldwide and lead the fight for more effective cancer treatments, increased funding for clinical and translational research, and, ultimately, cures for the many different types of cancer that strike an estimated ten million people worldwide each year. ASCO publishes the *Journal of Clinical Oncology (JCO)*, the preeminent, peer-reviewed, medical journal on clinical cancer research, and produces Cancer.Net, an award-winning website providing oncologist-vetted cancer information to help patients and families make informed health care decisions. For more information about ASCO patient resources, please visit www.cancer.net or call 1-888-651-3038.

ASSOCIATION OF CLINICIANS FOR THE UNDERSERVED (ACU) is a nonprofit, transdisciplinary organization whose vital mission is to improve the health of underserved populations and to enhance the development and support of the health care clinicians serving these communities. Membership in ACU is open to any person or organization in support of its mission. Our members are united by their common dedication for improving access to high quality medical, behavioral, pharmaceutical, and oral health care for our nation's underserved communities. Learn more at www.clinicians.org. Or call 1-703-442-5318.

ASSOCIATION OF ONCOLOGY SOCIAL WORK (AOSW) is a nonprofit, international organization dedicated to the enhancement of psychosocial services to people with cancer and their families. Created in 1984 by social workers and other professionals interested in oncology and by existing national cancer organizations, AOSW is an expanding force of psychosocial oncology professionals. For more information contact: AOSW, 100 North 20th Street, 4th Floor, Philadelphia, PA, 19103; phone: 215-599-6093; fax: 215-564-2175; E-mail: info@aosw.org; web site: www.aosw.org.

BLACK WOMEN'S HEALTH IMPERATIVE is a not-for-profit, education, advocacy, research, and leadership development organization that focuses on health issues that disproportionately affect Black women. It is the only national organization devoted solely to ensuring optimum health for Black women across their life span— physically, mentally, and spiritually. For more information about the Imperative, please visit www.BlackWomensHealth.org or call (202) 548-4000.

CANCERCARE is a national nonprofit, 501(c)(3) organization that provides free, professional support services to anyone affected by cancer: people with cancer, caregivers, children, loved ones, and the bereaved. CancerCare programs—including counseling and support groups, education, financial assistance, and practical help—are provided by professional oncology social workers and are completely free of charge.

For more information, visit www.cancercare.org or call 1-800-813-HOPE (4673).

CANCER FINANCIAL ASSISTANCE COALITION (CFAC) is a coalition of financial assistance organizations joining forces to help cancer patients experience better health and well-being by limiting financial challenges, through facilitating communication and collaboration among member organizations; educating patients and providers about existing resources and linking to other organizations that can disseminate information about the collective resources of the member organizations; and advocating on behalf of cancer patients who continue to bear financial burdens associated with the costs of cancer treatment and care. CFAC is a coalition of organizations and cannot respond to individual requests for financial assistance. To find out if financial help is available, please search the CFAC database at www.cancerfac.org. You may also contact each CFAC member organization individually for guidance and possible financial assistance (http://www.cancerfac.org/members.php).

CANCERCARE CO-PAYMENT ASSISTANCE FOUNDATION is a not-for-profit organization established in 2007 to address the needs of individuals who cannot afford their insurance co-payments to cover the cost of medications for treating cancer. The Foundation is proud to be affiliated with CancerCare, a national not-for-profit organization that has provided free professional support services including counseling, education, financial assistance, and practical help to people with cancer and their loved ones since 1944. For more information, visit www.cancercarecopay.org, or call 1-866-55-COPAY (866-552-6729).

CANCER PATIENT EDUCATION NETWORK (CPEN) is comprised of health care professionals who share experiences and best practices in all aspects of cancer patient education. The organization's overall mission is to promote and provide models of excellence in the areas of patient, family, and community education across the continuum of care. CPEN works in collaboration with the National Cancer Institute's Office of Education and Special Initiatives. For additional information, visit www.cancerpatienteducation.org.

CANCER SUPPORT COMMUNITY Backed by evidence that the best cancer care includes emotional and social support, the Cancer Support Community offers these services to all people affected by cancer. Likely the largest professionally-led network of cancer support worldwide, the organization delivers a comprehensive menu of personalized and essential services. Because no cancer care plan is complete without emotional and social support, the Cancer Support Community has a vibrant network of community-based centers and online services run by trained and licensed professionals. For more information, visit www.cancersupportcommunity.org, or call 1-888-793-9355.

EDUCATION NETWORK TO ADVANCE CANCER CLINICAL TRIALS (ENACCT) is a 501(c)(3) organization whose mission is to identify, implement, and validate innovative approaches to cancer clinical trials education, outreach, and recruitment to improve outcomes for all. Our key strategies are to: provide services that enhance the capacity of organizations conducting clinical trials outreach, education, and recruitment; support organizations in their efforts to reduce specific structural barriers to clinical trial recruitment; support the development of programs that enhance community literacy about clinical trials; and serve as a national clearinghouse for effective clinical trials education practices. For further information, visit our website at: www.enacct.org or call 1-240-482-4730.

INTERCULTURAL CANCER COUNCIL (ICC) promotes policies, programs, partnerships, and research to eliminate the unequal burden of cancer among racial and ethnic minorities and medically underserved populations in the USA and its associated territories. The ICC provides forums to identify shared problems and develop collabora-

tive solutions; promotes new partnerships to address the cancer crisis in our communities; convenes the National Biennial Symposium Series on Minorities, the Medically Underserved and Cancer; facilitates issue advocacy; and offers electronic networking and cancer education. For more information about ICC, call **713.798.4614** or visit our web site at www.iccnetwork.org.

JOE'S HOUSE is a nonprofit organization that provides an online nation-wide accommodation directory that helps cancer patients and their families find lodging near treatment centers. The website, www.joeshouse.org lists over 1,400 places to stay across the country that cater to patients. Lodging options include hospitality houses, hotels, motels, apartments, private homes, and more. All lodging facilities listed on the site are near hospitals and cancer treatment centers and offer some type of medical discount. Users of the site may search by city or by proximity to a hospital. Information about each lodging facility includes how to make a reservation, rate information, amenities, distance to the hospital, and more. Some facilities offer online booking capabilities. Website: www.joeshouse.org. Toll free line: 877 563 7468 (877 JOESHOU).

THE LGBT CANCER PROJECT is our country's first and leading Lesbian, Gay, Bisexual, and Transgendered cancer survivor support and advocacy nonprofit organization. The LGBT Cancer Project is committed to improving the health of LGBT cancer survivors through direct and support service, patient navigation, education, and advocacy. The LGBT Cancer Project volunteers include oncologists, social workers, and psychologists. Many of us are cancer survivors or family members of cancer survivors. All of us are united with you in our fight against cancer and in support of equal and appropriate access to health care for our LGBT community. For more information, visit our website at www.lgbtcancer.org, or E-mail us at info@lgbtcancer.org.

LIVESTRONG Founded in 1997 by cancer survivor and champion cyclist Lance Armstrong and based in Austin, Texas, **LIVESTRONG** fights for the 28 million people around the world living with cancer today. **LIVESTRONG** connects individuals to the support they need, leverages funding and resources to spur innovation, and engages communities and leaders to drive social change. Known for the iconic yellow wristband, **LIVESTRONG**'s mission is to inspire and empower anyone affected by cancer. For more information call 1-855-220-7777, or visit **LIVESTRONG**.org.

MEDICARE RIGHTS CENTER (MRC) is the largest independent source of health care information and assistance in the USA for people with Medicare. Founded in 1989, MRC helps older adults and people with disabilities get good, affordable health care. MRC provides counseling to individuals who need answers to Medicare-related questions or help getting care. Hotline counselors are available Monday through Friday, 9:00 AM–1:00 PM EST by calling 800-333-4114. MRC also operates a Medicare Part D hotline for nonprofit professionals serving the Medicare population. Call 877-794-3570 from 10 AM to 6 PM EST to speak to a counselor.

MULTINATIONAL ASSOCIATION OF SUPPORTIVE CARE IN CANCER (MASCC) is an international, multidisciplinary organization with over 750 members from 60 countries and 6 continents. It operates in collaboration with the International Society for Oral Oncology. Founded in 1990, this group is dedicated to research and education in all measures of supportive care for patients with cancer, regardless of the stage of the disease. MASCC aims to promote professional expertise of supportive care through research and international scientific exchange of ideas. Significant advances in cancer treatment in the last two decades have been made possible by strides in supportive care. The **MASCC Oral Agent Teaching Tool (MOATT)** was developed to assist health care providers in the assessment and education of patients receiving oral agents. To find out more information about MASCC, visit our web site: www.mascc.org.

NATIONAL ALLIANCE FOR CAREGIVING (NAC) is a nonprofit joint coalition of 40 national organizations focusing on issues of family caregiving. The Alliance conducts research and policy analysis, develops projects to support caregivers, and maintains an Internet clearinghouse of consumer materials. For more information contact: The National Alliance for Caregiving, 4720 Montgomery Lane, 5th Floor, Bethesda, MD 20814. Web site: www.caregiving.org. E-mail: **info@caregiving.org**.

NATIONAL CANCER INSTITUTE (NCI) is a component of the National Institutes of Health (NIH), one of eight agencies that compose the Public Health Service (PHS) in the Department of Health and Human Services (DHHS). The NCI is the Federal Government's principal agency for cancer research and training. The National Cancer Institute coordinates the National Cancer Program, which conducts and supports research, training, health information dissemination, and other programs with respect to the cause, diagnosis, prevention, and treatment of cancer, rehabilitation from cancer, and the continuing care of cancer patients and the families of cancer patients. To find out more about NCI, call **1-800-4-CANCER** (1-800-422-6237) or visit our website at www.cancer.gov.

NATIONAL CENTER FOR FRONTIER COMMUNITIES (NCFC) is the only national organization dedicated to the smallest and most geographically isolated communities in the USA. These communities generally have the fewest health services available, great distances to other services and the next level of care, and little or no public transportation. We advocate for local access to essential services and greater flexibility for frontier providers and facilities so that they can meet community needs. Projects of NCFC focus primarily on health services, community-based economics, education, and transportation. The work of the Center reflects its commitment to the "healthy communities" approach, which defines health holistically to include physical, emotional, economic, educational, environmental, and spiritual wellness. The real experts are the people living in frontier communities and we welcome learning from them. Our e-newsletter keeps hundreds of subscribers up to date on frontier issues. Visit us at www.frontierus.org or call 1-575-534-0101.

NATIONAL COALITION FOR CANCER SURVIVORSHIP (NCCS) advocates for quality cancer care for all Americans and provides tools that empower people affected by cancer to advocate for themselves. Founded by and for cancer survivors in 1986, NCCS created the widely accepted definition of survivorship and considers someone a cancer survivor from the time of diagnosis through the balance of life. Its free publications and resources include the award-winning **Cancer Survival Toolbox**®, a self-learning audio program created by leading cancer organizations to help people develop essential skills to meet the challenges of their illness. For more information about NCCS, its advocacy and patient materials, please visit www.canceradvocacy.org or call **1-888-650-9127**.

NATIONAL FAMILY CAREGIVERS ASSOCIATION (NFCA) supports, empowers, educates, and speaks up for the more than 50 million Americans who care for a chronically ill, aged, or disabled loved one. NFCA reaches across the boundaries of different diagnoses, different relationships, and different life stages to address the common needs and concerns of all family caregivers. Contact NFCA at 10400 Connecticut Avenue, Suite 500, Kensington, MD 20895; phone: (301) 942-6430 and 800-896-3650; fax: (301) 942-2302; website: www.thefamilycaregiver.org.

NATIONAL ORGANIZATION FOR RARE DISORDERS (NORD) is a federation of individuals and organizations representing the 25 million Americans with rare disorders. It was established in 1983 by patients and patient organizations working together to get the *Orphan Drug Act* passed by Congress and signed into law. Today, NORD provides information about rare disorders, referrals to support groups and other sources of help, assistance to the uninsured or under-insured in obtaining certain medications, research grants and fellowships, advocacy on public policy issues of interest to people with rare diseases, an annual patient/family confer-

ence, networking, and technical assistance to leaders of patient organizations or those attempting to start an organization. Contact NORD at (800) 999-NORD or orphan@rarediseases.org. Its web site is at www.rarediseases.org.

MARJORIE E. KORFF PACT PROGRAM is built on a fundamental belief that parents are experts on the strengths and needs of their own children. Together, a parent and child have negotiated countless challenges throughout the child's life. At the same time, PACT staff clinicians are fully trained child psychiatrists and child psychologists who have years of education and experience. We bring training in child development, temperament, personality, family dynamics, and effective parenting techniques to each parent consultation. We are also familiar with common reactions to a serious illness in the family and can explain what parents might expect from their children, when to feel comfortable that a child is handling the situation well, and when to worry. We work hand-in-hand with parents, combining our collective knowledge and experience to develop a plan for parents to support a child's continued healthy development. We strive to provide expert and compassionate guidance and education to parents that reinforces their own competence and confidence as they continue to love, nurture, and support their children. For more information, visit www.mghpact.org; E-mail moreinfo@mghpact.org, or call 617-724-7272.

PATIENT ACCESS NETWORK (PAN) FOUNDATION is an independent, nonprofit, charitable organization that provides assistance to under-insured patients with chronic or life-threatening illness to help them meet their out-of-pocket expenses for medications. PAN is dedicated to overcoming financial barriers to treatment and works efficiently and collaboratively with health care providers and specialty pharmacies to help patients receive prescribed treatments and the care that best meets their needs. Since 2004, PAN has provided more than $173 million in assistance for out-of-pocket expenses to more than 125,000 patients in need. For more information on Patient Access Network, please visit our website at www.PANFoundation.org or call us at 202-347-9272.

RESEARCH ADVOCACY NETWORK was founded in 2003 to bring together participants in the research process. Our mission is to develop a network of advocates and researchers who can influence medical research from concept to patient care through education, support, and collaborations. The patient advocacy movement has changed the face of research. Through their efforts, research advocates have begun to help shape the design, conduct, and dissemination of medical research. As the involvement of advocates in research grows, there is a need to educate more advocates and integrate them fully into the research community. Our services include advocate training, both onsite and online, patient education materials, tools for advocates, and models of patient advocate involvement in research activities. For more information call **877.276.2187** or visit our website at www.researchadvocacy.org.

SUPERSIBS! is a nonprofit organization that provides services to help brothers and sisters of children with cancer "survive and thrive" through and beyond this challenging life experience. Through ongoing, age-appropriate Comfort and Care mailings, Online Support (for siblings, parents, and others in the lives of these brothers and sisters), Sibling Scholarships and Outreach and Education, *SuperSibs!* services are entirely free of charge. Since 2003, *SuperSibs!* has provided direct program support to over 15,000 siblings (ages 4–18) and their families from across the USA and Canada. **For more information, visit** www.supersibs.org **(see *The Sib Spot* and *For You*) or call toll free: 1-888-417-4704.**

VITAL OPTIONS is an international cancer communications organization whose mission is *to facilitate a global cancer dialogue.* Founded 25 years ago as the first organization for young adults with cancer, Vital Options has expanded to include people of all ages and cancer types with its innovative programs such as *The Group Room®*, a weekly cancer talk radio show. Using creative multimedia technology, Vital Options enables patients and their loved ones to interact and speak directly with noted oncology medical professionals and researchers in the USA and Europe, and supports the efforts of the advocacy community. For more information or to listen to archived shows, go to www.vitaloptions.org or call 1-800 GRP-ROOM (1-800-477-7666).

Conclusion: Lessons Learned

It is always prudent to call a resource before referring a patient to check that their number or website has not changed and the resource can assist the person you are referring. Patients, survivors, caregivers, and the bereaved always appreciate our taking this extra step when making a referral as well as our follow-up with them to see if the needed service was received or there is still a need for additional help. Key components of successful usage of the many cancer resources available include: maintaining frank and open communication; establishing realistic and achievable expectations and goals; keeping at your finger tips a network of resources and interprofessional colleagues to contact for help; and guiding your patients on how best to work with the resource referral you have made.

Given the changing needs of cancer patients, it is the innovative health care professional and institution that will be able to meet the future needs of this population by increasing access to cancer resources [12]. It takes a village to meet their needs. We cannot do this work alone—it is our collaborative work together, interprofessional practice, partnerships, and evolving understanding of resources that enables us to stay the course and provide the highest quality care.

References

1. Adler NE, Page AEK. Cancer care for the whole patient: meeting psychosocial health needs. Washington, DC: The National Academies Press; 2008.
2. Altilio T, Otis-Green S. Oxford textbook of palliative social work. New York: Oxford University Press; 2011.

3. Berzoff J, Silverman PR. Living with dying: a handbook for end-of-life healthcare practitioners. New York: Columbia University Press; 2004.
4. Fleishman SB. Learn to live through cancer: what you need to know and do. New York: Demos Medical Publishing; 2011.
5. Garssen B, Lee M. Problems addressed during psycho-oncological therapy: a pilot study. J Psychosoc Oncol. 2011;29(6):657–63.
6. Herman JF. Cancer support groups. Atlanta: The American Cancer Society; 2002.
7. Hoffman B, Mullan F. A cancer survivor's almanac: charting your journey. Minneapolis: Chronimed Publishing; 1996.
8. Holland JC, Breitbart WS, et al. Psycho-oncology. New York: Oxford University Press; 2010.
9. Holland J, Lewis S. The human side of cancer. New York: Harper Collins Publisher; 2000.
10. Jevne RF. Creating still points: beyond a rational approach to counseling cancer patients. J Psychosoc Oncol. 1987;5(3):1–15.
11. Marbach TJ, Griffie J. Patient preferences concerning treatment plans, survivorship care plans, education and support services. Oncol Nurs Forum. 2011;38(3):335–42.
12. Messner C. Quiet heroes: stories of innovation in oncology social work. Ann Arbor: UMI ProQuest; 2004.
13. Nouwen H. The wounded healer. Garden City: Image Books; 1979.
14. Poirier P. The impact of fatigue on role functioning during radiation therapy. Oncol Nurs Forum. 2011;38(1):457–65.
15. Rapoport L. The state of crisis: some theoretical considerations. Soc Serv Rev. 1962;26(6):211–7.
16. van Ryn M, et al. Objective burden, resources, and other stressors among informal cancer caregivers: a hidden quality issue? Psychooncology. 2011;20(1):44–52.
17. Schon DA. The reflective practitioner: how professionals think in action. New York: Basic Books, Inc.; 1983.
18. Shin J, Casarett D. Facilitating hospice discussions: a six-step roadmap. J Support Oncol. 2011;9(3):97–102.
19. Torrence WA, et al. Evaluating coalition capacity to strengthen community-academic partnerships addressing cancer disparities. J Cancer Educ. 2011;26(4):658–63.
20. Wells KJ, et al. Innovative approaches to reducing cancer health disparities. J Cancer Educ. 2011;26(4):649–57.
21. Zabora J. Development of proactive model of health care versus a reactive system of referrals. In: Roberts A, editor. Social workers' desk reference. New York: Oxford University Press; 2009.

Bringing It All Together

Brian I. Carr

Introduction

The preceding essays address many of the ongoing areas of research and development of ideas and treatments relating to the cancer patient and his/her human environment and are presented in seven groups: (a) biological basis, explains the possible mediators for a mind–body interaction, which in itself may be bi-directional; (b) prevention and decision-making, discusses some genetic predispositions to cancer and preventive actions to be taken, as well as how the decisions for screening and preventive actions can be influenced; (c) theory in psychosocial oncology, discusses several aspects of hope and coping and how ideas of world-view, religiosity, spirituality, and philosophy form a background to patient fears and attitudes, as well as a review of some controversial aspects of patient support; (d) the social context, emphasizes that patients do not exist without a social context of partners and families and the consequences of this; (e) patient support, examines some of the methodologies in evaluating quality of life, as well as some new ideas (exercise, hallucinogens, and complementary

B.I. Carr, M.D., F.R.C.P., Ph.D. (✉)
IRCCS S. de Bellis, National Institute for Digestive Diseases, Via Turi 27, 70013, Castellana Grotte, BA, Italy

Department of Medical Oncology, Thomas Jefferson University, Philadelphia, PA, USA
e-mail: brianicarr@hotmail.com

techniques) and concepts (placebo, long-term post-treatment emotional distress) in the management of patient stress during the cancer continuum; (f) advanced cancer, discusses approaches to both the patient near the end-of-life and associate partner and family, and the bereavement issues and coping of those who are left behind after the death of the patient; and (g) reviews all the essays and presents a useful list of patient and caregiver resources.

Psychological Symptoms and Tumor Biology

Dr. Fagundes and colleagues examine the feedback loops and underlying mechanisms involved in the effects of stress, depression, and bodily function, including effects on cancer. They describe the effects of stress on dysregulation of the immune system, which in turn can impact fatigue and depressive symptoms. They report a meta-analysis of 165 studies linking stress-related psychosocial factors with cancer incidence among those who were initially healthy. For example, women who experienced stressful life events such as divorce, death of a husband, death of a relative, or close friend during a 5-year baseline period were more likely to be diagnosed with breast cancer during the next 15 years than those who did not experience these events. There is even stronger evidence that psychological factors play an important role in cancer progression and mortality. They also report that women with breast cancer who were more depressed were more likely to die within 5 years compared to those who were less depressed. A recent meta-analysis of 25 studies revealed that mortality rates are 39 % higher among breast cancer patients diagnosed with major or minor depression compared to those not depressed. Dr. Steel and I showed that hepatobiliary carcinoma patients who had higher levels of depressive symptoms at diagnosis had 6–9 months shorter survival than those who were less depressed [1–4]. Stress dysregulates immune function and enhances inflammation. It alters the function of the autonomic nervous system and the hypothalamo–pituitary–adrenal axis. Together, the affect levels of immune-mediator cells, norepinephrine, epinephrine, and catecholamines, which in turn can alter tumor cell growth and tumor angiogenesis, either directly on tumor cells, or via catecholamine modulation of vascular endothelial growth factor (VEGF) levels, which are important in tumor angiogenesis and thus in tumor growth. Psychological factors can also modulate VEGF, and colon cancer patients who were lonelier and/or depressed had higher levels of serum VEGF than those who were less lonely and/or depressed. VEGF also activates endothelial cells to produce matrix metalloproteinase (MMPs) enzymes, a family of matrix-degrading enzymes that contribute to metastasis. Higher levels of stress and depression were reported to be associated with elevated MMP-9 among women with ovarian cancer. A study showed that higher levels of depression and lower social support were associated with the up-regulation of over 200 gene transcripts involved in tumor growth and progression. Many interventions have been developed to reduce cancer-related distress. Given that depression and stress impact cancer biology, psychosocial interventions may impact cancer-related outcomes. However, at this time there are inconsistent results in the literature, as explained in the Controversies chapter.

Drs. Feridey Carr and Elizabeth Sosa point out that chronic inflammation has been linked with specific types of cancer, particularly those associated with viral infection or an inflammatory response, and that chronic inflammation is likely involved in cancer development. Chronic bron-

chitis in smokers is epidemiologically linked to subsequent lung cancer development, as is chronic hepatitis to hepatocellular carcinoma (HCC) development and inflammatory bowel disease (IBD) to risk of later colon cancer and chronic human papilloma virus infection predisposes to subsequent cancer of the cervix uteri. There is an increasing body of literature indicating that psychosocial factors directly contribute to the development and maintenance of chronic inflammation. Inflammation involves the presence of inflammatory cells and mediators, which include chemokines and cytokines in tumor tissues. Several pro-inflammatory cytokines have been related to tumor growth, including IL-1, IL-6, IL-8, and IL-18. Interleukins (ILs) are involved in different steps of tumor initiation and growth. A key molecular link between inflammation and tumor progression is transcription factor NF- κB, which regulates tumor necrosis factor (TNF), interleukins, and several chemokines. The relationship between the brain and the peripheral organs, often referred to as the "mind–body" connection, is based on alterations in the endocrine and immune systems that lead to the chemical changes that occur in clinical depression. Pro-inflammatory cytokines, particularly IL-6 (interleukin-6), have been found to occur in greater quantities in depressed patients. It has been shown that symptoms of fatigue and decreased appetite can be triggered by pro-inflammatory cytokines. These cytokines are responsible for developing the body's inflammatory response. There is thus a two-way process in which the mind can influence inflammatory processes and they in turn can influence the mind. It has been suspected that IL-6 could be related to colon cancer through its role in affecting the low-grade inflammation status of the intestine. Thus, mood and depression can modulate IL-6, an inflammatory mediator and IBD predisposes to bowel cancer.

There are psychotherapeutic implications of these lines of research. Higher serotonin levels are associated with lower levels of inflammatory mediators, and vice versa, suggesting that serotonin levels and thus mood in general can influence inflammation. Several anti-depressive agents (selective serotonin re-uptake inhibitors) can cause significant decrease in IL-1, IL-6, and TNF-alpha. Thus, clinical treatment of depression could result in both amelioration of depressive symptoms and decreased inflammation in the general population.

This biological framework provides a basis for proposing that treatment of depression might result in lower inflammation, and thus decrease the incidence of cancers that result in such predisposed people. Even more intriguing is the possibility that such psychological interventions could affect the course of established cancers that are associated with inflammation.

Cancer Prevention and Decision-Making

The chapter by Dr. Aspinwall and colleagues reminds us that while most cancers are sporadic, about 5 % occur due to an inherited cancer predisposition syndrome. Families with hereditary cancer syndromes are generally characterized by multiple occurrences of cancer on the same side of the family, individuals with multiple primary cancers, and an earlier than average age of cancer onset. Hereditary breast and ovarian cancer (HBOC) and Lynch syndrome (formerly referred to as hereditary non-polyposis colorectal cancer, HNPCC) are the two most common and well-studied conditions. A major problem for families being counseled, with factors predisposing to breast cancer is that while risk-reducing mastectomy (RRM) significantly reduces the risk for developing breast cancer by 90 %, the survival benefit in choosing RRM over annual breast screening is small. In addition, reports suggest that sustained psychological distress following hereditary cancer risk counseling and testing is rare. A framework is provided that situates hereditary cancer risk counseling and testing as tools to be used by patients and their families in an ongoing process of managing familial cancer risk and psychological concerns arising from awareness of this risk. It is shown that hereditary cancer risk counseling and testing have a powerful impact on screening adherence, other risk-reducing behaviors such as prophylactic

surgery, and in the case of hereditary melanoma, primary prevention behaviors.

Dr. Howard and colleagues review the issues concerning women who are found to carry a *BRCA1/2* mutation, bestowing a markedly increased probability of developing breast cancer and the management of their 45–87 % lifetime risk of breast cancer. *BRCA1/2* carriers have the option of ongoing breast cancer screening (RRM), prior to the development of cancer, generally offered with the option of reconstructive surgery. This reduces risk of developing breast cancer by 95 %. Although some women choose to do nothing, the majority of *BRCA1/2* carriers face choosing between ongoing breast cancer screening and RRM. She points out that a woman's decision about RRM is much more complex than interpreting the statistical risk of developing breast cancer. Decisions appear to be grounded in broader social and cultural contexts and vary regarding when decisions are made. Emotional distress and self-identity also factors in the decision-making. Thus, to maximize health outcomes, not only must we personalize health care services based on patient genetic profiles, but we must also personalize health care services based on patient psychosocial profiles. Dr. Leigl describes some aids to help patients in decision-making. She reminds us that the delicate balance between palliative goals of therapy, understanding prognosis, and preserving hope in the face of incurable malignancy is difficult to achieve. Decision aids are important tools to facilitate more informed decision-making for patients, to ensure that palliative treatment decisions are consistent with patient values for length and quality of life. Treatment decisions when the goal is not cure are increasingly complex, with a growing number of potential palliative treatment options, with uncertain and often modest benefits, while at least some toxicity from treatment is almost guaranteed. The majority of patients do wish to discuss prognosis in advanced disease and they wish to be active participants in decision-making about their treatments, although this varies in the literature from 40 to 73 % desiring shared decision-making with their physician. However, many patients are not well-equipped to make informed decisions about their care. Informed consent to treatment requires certain elements that include a discussion of prognosis with and without treatment, a review of risks and benefits, and of alternative options. Decision aids (DAs) are designed to help people make specific and difficult choices among options by providing information on the options and outcomes relevant to the person's health status and they help patients in clarifying their values for those different health outcomes and treatment options, to facilitate decision-making. They have been developed mainly for cancer screening, adjuvant therapy, and primary treatments in the setting of curable cancer. The chapter points out that balancing the potential benefits and toxicities of palliative therapy is complex, particularly when patients and families are unwilling to accept the limited goals of palliative therapy and that many patients get upset by the prognostic information. Accelerating the transfer of knowledge about limited prognosis and treatment benefit remains a major challenge in decision-making in advanced cancer, in order to minimize false hope and unrealistic expectations, while preserving reasonable hopes of modest improvements or symptom control at the end-of-life.

Theory Related to the Practice of Psychosocial Oncology

Dr. Cohen discusses various aspects of cancer fatalism, including its prevalence in different population groups and the correlates of fatalism with socio-demographic variables. Fatalism is a belief that events are pre-determined and that humans are unable to change their outcomes. She reviews the role of fatalism in screening behaviors and in delay in seeking help. Studies have shown that fatalistic beliefs are related to lower adherence to medical examinations and lifestyle regimens needed in the management of chronic diseases and to smoking and screening for the early detection of several types of cancer. Fatalism is incompatible with free will. Fatalism may or may not be based on belief in God. Believers tend to accept that God has control over every detail of life, while non-religious fatalism may be

expressed in the belief that things happen by chance or luck. It thus has negative connotations in our modern society. A study reported from the USA suggested that individuals with high fatalistic beliefs lead less healthy lifestyles: they perform less regular exercise, are less likely to eat fruits and vegetables and smoke more. Some longitudinal studies in cancer patients reported that patients who responded with a fighting spirit or with denial were more likely to be alive and free of recurrence at 5, 10, and 15 years after diagnosis than patients with fatalistic or helpless responses. The most important impact of fatalism is when it results in delays in seeking medical help after the first appearance of symptoms, as well as in the non-participation in screening programs or change to healthier lifestyles, on the basis that our fates are anyway pre-ordained. This is especially true of patients with genetic cancer predisposition genes, such as BRCA1 or 2, which can confer a sense of inevitability in some patients. In others, however, such knowledge about themselves leads to pro-active treatment or lifestyle choices.

Dr. Park describes "meaning-making" processes, spirituality, and stress-related growth in her chapter regarding positive psychology. A diagnosis of cancer can shatter aspects of a patient's extant global meaning. Thus, most people hold views of the world as benign, predictable, and fair and their own lives as safe and controllable. A cancer diagnosis is typically experienced as being at extreme odds with such beliefs, resulting in processes of distress and changes in meaning-making that ultimately lead to changes in survivors' situational and global meaning. The meanings that survivors assign to their cancer experience predict not only their coping and subsequent adjustment but also their treatment-related decisions and their well-being. In a breast cancer study, patients seeing their cancer as a challenge at diagnosis had less anxiety at follow-up than those who perceived it as the enemy. However, patients with various cancers who appraised with uncontrolled cancer had higher levels of stress. A longitudinal study of survivors of various cancers found that the extent to which the cancer was appraised as violating their beliefs in a just world was inversely related to their psychological well-being across the year of the study. Beliefs in a loving God may also be violated. Further, having cancer almost invariably violates individuals' goals for their current lives and their plans for the future and calls into question their existential philosophy, such as living a healthy lifestyle protects people from illness. At diagnosis, individuals' pre-cancer spirituality may influence the situational meaning they assign to their cancer. Those with higher religious beliefs had a higher sense of efficacy in coping with their cancer, which was related to higher levels of well-being. Another study found that women diagnosed with breast cancer who viewed God as benevolent and involved in their lives appraised their cancer as more of a challenge and an opportunity to grow. Stress-related growth describes the positive life changes that people report that they experience following stressful events, including a diagnosis of cancer, and has garnered increasing research interest in recent years. Myriad studies of survivors of many types of cancer have established that a majority of survivors report experiencing stress-related (post-traumatic) growth as a result of their experience with cancer. Researchers have posited that meaning-making efforts are essential to adjustment to cancer by helping survivors either assimilate the cancer experience into their pre-cancer global meaning or helping them to change their global meaning to accommodate it. It has been proposed, therefore, that meaning-making is critical to successfully navigate these changes. However, there are thus far few studies with controls to validate these ideas in clinical oncology practice.

Dr. Folkman points out that hope and psychological stress share a number of formal properties: both are contextual, meaning-based, and dynamic, and both affect well-being in difficult circumstances. The relationship between hope and coping is dynamic and reciprocal; each in turn supports and is supported by the other and are involved in managing uncertainty and a changing reality. Conversely, hopelessness is a dire state that gives rise to despair, depression, and ultimately loss of will to live. Stress and coping theory originally posited two kinds of coping:

problem-focused coping and emotion-focused coping. She reminds us that maintaining and restoring hope is seen as an important function of the physician. Coping with uncertainty, and especially the process of personalizing odds, can involve distortion of reality. Statements about odds, and the range of possibilities they imply, invite hope. Hope increases when the odds of a good outcome are favorable. She suggests that when odds are unfavorable, people initiate a re-appraisal process of their own personal odds that improves them and thus gives them hope. This coping strategy not only creates a toehold for hope, but it also reduces threat. In this process, patients identify reasons why the odds don't apply to their situation, or search for information that contradicts the odds that were given. Hope has a very special quality that is especially important in managing uncertainty over time: it allows us to hold conflicting expectations simultaneously. She points out that individuals who rate high on hope as a trait have the advantage of approaching situations with a hopeful bias that is protective; they show diminished stress reactivity and more effective emotional-recovery than those low in dispositional hope.

Dr. Thune-Boyle tells us that studies have reported that religious coping is one of the most commonly used coping strategies in cancer patients in the USA cancer patients, where up to 85 % of women with breast cancer indicate that religion helped them cope with their illness. However, there is potential confusion between religious coping cognitions versus religious service attendance, where an effect could be caused by perceived social support from the religious community rather than religious coping. Although many cancer patients experience clinical levels of distress and dysfunction including anxiety, depression and some may even suffer from post-traumatic stress disorder, many patients are able to find meaning in their illness such as experiencing profound positive changes in themselves, in their relationships, and in other life domains after cancer. Finding meaning in the cancer experience in the form of positive benefits is a common occurrence. This is described as positive psychological growth or post-traumatic growth. She points out that there is evidence that a higher level of faith/ religiousness is linked to greater levels of perceived cancer-related growth and benefit finding and that having respect for patients' spirituality as an important resource for their coping with illness. In the USA, between 58 and 77 % of hospitalized patients want physicians to consider their spiritual needs. However, religious/spiritual beliefs and practices are very different across cultures and these findings may therefore not generalize to cancer patients outside the USA.

Dr. Stefanek describes four controversies in the field of psycho-oncology: (1) the benefit of screening for distress among cancer patients; (2) the effectiveness of psychological interventions among cancer patients; (3) the role of "positive psychology" (optimism, benefit finding) in cancer care; and (4) the benefit of group therapy in extending survival among cancer patients. Depression, anxiety, and distress are common following the diagnosis of cancer, with overall prevalence in unselected cancer patients greater than 30 %. It appears that screening, while offering a seemingly simple solution for early successful treatment of emotional distress, has yet to demonstrate a clear benefit over standard approaches such as simply offering patients the chance to discuss their concerns, regardless of formal screening programs. He tells us that though the distress, anxiety, and depression accompanying a cancer diagnosis impact quality of life, and even satisfaction with and adherence to treatment regimens, there is not yet an unqualified answer to the question of whether interventions work, what interventions, and with whom. In addition, he points out that studies to date in cancer have not warranted the seemingly strong belief that optimism does indeed make a difference in health outcomes related to cancer. Regarding psychosocial interventions and their impact on survival, no randomized trial designed with survival as a primary endpoint and in which psychotherapy was not confounded with medical care has yielded a positive effect. A meta-analysis supported no overall treatment effect by psychosocial interventions on survival, by randomized or non-randomized trials. Chronic depression, social support, and chronic stress may influence multiple aspects of

tumor growth and metastasis through neuroendocrine regulation. Work in this area may highlight how behavioral or pharmacological interventions might impact neuroendocrine effects on tumors and slow progression or increase survival, as noted in the first two chapters of this book. In addition, psychological factors seem to have an influence in apoptosis, which is considered on important in the balance between cell life and death in cancer development. However, both quality of life and psychological stress are important and achievable endpoints in their own right in cancer patient care and clinical trials of psychological-based interventions.

The Social Context

Dr. Badr and colleagues remind us that for most individuals diagnosed with cancer, their psychological adjustment depends strongly on their interpersonal relationships. Cancer patients identify their spouses or intimate partners as their most important sources of practical and emotional support and coping with cancer treatment can also challenge a couple's established communication patterns, roles and responsibilities, either in a positive or negative sense. A supportive spouse can serve as a resource for the patient in terms of providing assistance in cognitive processing, but other spouses can serve as a barrier to effective processing if unavailable or unsupportive. Physical intimacy is vital to maintaining satisfying relationships and may reduce emotional distress. Virtually, all cancers and their treatments (i.e., surgery, radiation therapy, chemotherapy, and hormone therapy) affect patients' sexual function. Despite this, the vast majority of studies addressing sexual problems in cancer patients have been confined to problems that affect the reproductive and sexual organs. Common cancer symptoms or treatment side effects include fatigue, pain, nausea, decreased sexual desire, and vaginal dryness and dyspareunia in women and erectile dysfunction in men. Cancer thus takes a toll on both patients and their partners.

The impact of cancer on an individual's sexuality is enormous and overwhelmingly negative in most cases, and Dr. Susan Carr tells us that this occurs in more than 50 % of cancer patients. Women with cancer can experience disruption to sexual arousal, lubrication, orgasm, and develop pain on intercourse, particularly if they have experienced menopause as a result of chemotherapy or surgery. This functional disruption leads to lack of pleasure in sex and can result in total loss of libido, or sexual interest. Commonest symptoms include loss of libido in males and females. In females-anorgasmia, vaginismus, and dyspareunia. In males, erectile dysfunction and premature ejaculation. Cognitive behavioral therapy is useful in female sexual dysfunction. Body image and sexual self-confidence are intrinsically linked. Cancer and its therapies can cause major alterations in body image which in turn can have negative impact on sexuality and sexual satisfaction. Physical changes in cancer patients include baldness following chemotherapy, weight fluctuations, body shape changes such as loss of breast, stoma onto the skin, lymphedema, or some disfiguring features following head and neck cancer. Changes in body self-perception, however, need not necessarily stem from outward change, and for a lot of young women, loss of fertility can greatly lower their feelings of femininity. Symptoms such as shortness of breath due to lung involvement, or severe pain are also major physical inhibitors of sex. None of this fails to have an emotional impact on the patient and their partner. In addition, lowering of self-esteem and feelings of being subsumed by the cancer, take their emotional toll. In relation to sexuality, a partner will almost invariably be also affected. Clinicians often avoid emotional issues by focusing on physical and physiological signs and symptoms. The standard clinician consultation does not always allow the patient opportunity to express sensitive or deeper sexual or emotional issues. Allowing silence and space in questioning allows the patient better opportunity to disclose sexual issues to the treating oncologist or psychologist.

The chapter by Dr. Kim focusses on the stresses of the caregiver, who is usually the spouse or another family member. This role includes providing the patient with cognitive/ informational, emotional, and spiritual support, as well as facilitating communication with medical professionals and other family members and assisting in the maintenance of social relationships. These aspects of caregiving can contribute to caregivers' stress when they perceive it difficult to mobilize their personal and social resources to carry out each of the caregiving-related tasks. Studies have also reported caregivers improved sense of self-worth, and increased personal satisfaction and the degree to which family caregivers have negative and positive experiences in caregiving may affect their ability to care for the survivor. Spousal caregivers, who are the majority, can have a poorer quality of life, particularly when involved in long-term cancer care. Overall, caregiving burden during the advanced stages of the patient's cancer, is the strongest predictor of caregiver *psychological* distress during this phase of caregiver ship, even more than the patient's physical and emotional status. Although survivorship ends at the death of the person with the disease, the caregivership continues. The death of a close family member is one of the most stressful of life events.

Patient Support

Drs. Benedict and Pinedo report that a significant number of cancer survivors report psychological responses that range from normal feelings of vulnerability, sadness, and fear to problems that can become disabling, such as clinical levels of depression, anxiety and panic disorder/attacks, interpersonal dysfunction, sexual dysfunction, social isolation and existential, or spiritual crisis. Distress may be experienced as a reaction to the disease or to its treatment, as well as disruption in quality of life. Not all psychological reactions are negative and many cancer survivors report finding some benefit in their cancer experience, such as a new appreciation of life and improved self-esteem and sense of mastery. Psychosocial distress associated with cancer exists on a continuum ranging from normal adjustment issues to clinically significant symptoms of mental disorder. Up to 47 % of cancer survivors indicated clinically significant psychiatric disorders. Among patients receiving palliative care, estimates are that around 20 % meet diagnostic criteria for depression. However, the majority of cancer survivors adjust relatively well. Though the initial reaction to a cancer diagnosis may be that of alarm and distress and coping with treatment-related side effects may be difficult, most never have the diagnostic criteria for a mental health disorder. A number of common psychosocial factors have been shown to predict adjustment and well-being, including availability of inter- and intrapersonal resources, optimism and active coping styles, and higher levels of social support from partners, family members, and loved ones. Conversely, avoidance of cancer-related discussions have been associated with worse emotional well-being and quality of life. Psychosocial interventions for cancer survivors generally aim to reduce emotional distress, enhance coping skills, and improve quality of life. Many different types of interventions have been conducted among individuals, couples, and families, including supportive–expressive group therapy, psycho-educational interventions, and multimodal intervention approaches. The initial diagnosis of cancer is often a traumatic and distressing experience. Emotional reactions often include feelings of disbelief, denial, and despair. The spectrum of emotional reactions ranges from depressive symptoms, such as normal sadness, to clinically significant symptoms of adjustment disorder or major depressive disorder. Individuals must adjust to the idea of being diagnosed with a devastating illness that may be life threatening and often struggle with feelings of uncertainty and fear for the future. Although distressing, the initial emotional response to a diagnosis of cancer is often brief, extending over days to weeks. Psychological interventions are tailored to the pre-treatment decision and preparation period, active cancer treatment period, the treatment period of advanced or progressive cancer associated with the greatest level of psychological stress, and to the post-treatment survival period. Psychological interventions typically aim to improve adjustment and well-being by: promoting adaptive coping strategies, improving support-seeking behaviors, and

reducing social isolation and by addressing maladaptive cognitions related to disease- or treatment-related outcomes. Many different types of interventions are described, typically involving an emotionally supportive context to address fears and anxieties, information about the disease and its treatment, and cognitive and behavioral coping strategies, including stress management and relaxation training, in an individual, couples or group setting, usually in person, but sometimes via the telephone or the Web. Several studies have also examined the effects of psychological interventions on patient survival, with conflicting results. In a meta-analysis of the effect of psychosocial interventions on survival time in cancer, neither randomized nor non-randomized studies indicated a significant effect on survival in studies performed thus far. However, several psychosocial factors have been linked to the development and progression of cancer and have been shown to be important considerations in cancer care, including helplessness/hopelessness, coping styles, and social isolation.

Dr. Salsman and colleagues review health-related quality of life (HRQOL) issues. Weighing survival versus quality of life benefits is a critical part of medical decision-making for cancer patients and *quality* of life has proven to be a recent and meaningful subjective complement to survival benefits derived from treatments, as the overall 5-year survival rate has increased to over 65 % of patients. Physical, emotional, social, functional, and in some cases, spiritual domains are studied. An essential consideration in symptom assessment is that patient ratings of symptom importance are subjective and may differ from those of oncology professionals. However, treating oncologists can often have a good sense of their patient symptoms and HRQOL [5]. Furthermore, since around 30 % of US households have a member giving caregiver support, caregiver HRQOL is receiving the increased attention that its importance requires. Dr. Mustian reviews the literature on the use of exercise in improving some of the most prevalent side effects experienced by cancer patients and increasing HRQOL before, during, and after cancer treatments. Cancer patients report cancer-related fatigue throughout the entire cancer experience from the point of diagnosis, throughout treatments and in many cases for years after treatments are complete and it is one of the most frequent and troublesome of cancer patient symptoms. Over 2/3 of survivors report this symptom long after therapies have stopped and there are few remedies. Exercise can be performed using a variety of modes, such as aerobic exercise, resistance training, and mindfulness-based exercise, all of which have been found to reduce various side effects from cancer and its treatment, as well as aerobic, resistance, and mindfulness exercise (Tai Chi and Yoga). Preliminary evidence consistently suggests that physical activity is not only safe but advantageous for cancer survivors in managing multiple side effects associated with cancer and cancer treatments.

Dr. Grob et al. report on the psycho-spiritual distress and demoralization that often accompanies a life-threatening cancer diagnosis, and the potential of a treatment approach that uses the hallucinogen psilocybin from mushrooms, a novel psychoactive drug, to ameliorate these symptoms. It is metabolized to psilocin, which is a highly potent agonist at serotonin 5-HT-2A and 5-HT-2C receptors and produces an altered state of consciousness that is characterized by changes in perception, cognition, and mood in the presence of an otherwise clear sensorium. Advanced stage and terminal cancer patients have been reported to have significant improvements of their psycho-spiritual status on psilocybin treatment. A growing body of research has shown that higher levels of spiritual well-being are correlated with lower levels of emotional distress and serve as a buffer against depression, desire for hastened death, loss of will to live, and hopelessness.

Drs. Schuricht and Nestoriuc explain that understanding the placebo and nocebo effect will help us to gain new insights in the interaction of psychological and physiological processes in health and disease. Placebos are often used in a no-treatment arm of clinical trials. The placebo effect raises the question of how something that is thought to be inert can actually cause desired effects. *Placebo response* refers to the psy-

chophysiological processes attributed to the context of treatment. Nocebo refers to the administration of an inert substance (i.e., placebo) along with the suggestion or expectation to get worse and about 25 % of patients in a placebo group report adverse side effects (i.e., nocebo effects). Discontinuation rates due to adverse effects have been shown to be equally high in drug and placebo groups. Nocebo (non-specific) side effects often appear as generalized and diffuse symptoms such as fatigue, difficulties in concentrating, headache, or insomnia, they occur mostly dose independent. Two placebo-controlled treatment trials showed high rates of both improvements and side-effects in the placebo arms. The placebo benefit effect has been observed in clinical trials for cancer-related fatigue, pain, and for chemotherapy-induced nausea and emesis. A randomized controlled trial examined innovative nonpharmacological approaches to cancer pain management. The effectiveness of transcutaneous electrical nerve stimulation (TENS), transcutaneous spinal electro analgesia (TSE), and a sham TSE (placebo) was compared, in 41 women with chronic pain following breast cancer treatment. TENS and TSE devices both used electricity to ease pain. The placebo devices had disabled wires but apart from that were identical to the active machines. The researchers found improved worst and average pain scores in all the three intervention groups throughout a 3-week trial. Furthermore, patients exhibited significantly lower anxiety scores after TENS and placebo use. The finding that improvements in pain were significantly more likely for patients in the placebo groups than in the best supportive care groups suggests that receiving a specific treatment, regardless whether it is active or placebo, rather than receiving regular care, promotes analgesic effects. Ten to sixty percent of patients in placebo conditions experienced distressing symptoms that were quite similar among trials, including nausea and vomiting, abdominal pain, lethargy, dry mouth, and diarrhea. An association could be found between the incidence and type of negative effects in the placebo groups and side effects in the treatment groups, thus pointing to the potential role of specific expectations about adverse symptom profiles in the development of nocebo effects. Recent neuro-imaging research indicates that placebo treatments have broad effects on opioid activity in cortical and subcortical regions as well as on their functional connectivity. These results point to the profound effects of patient expectations on symptomatology.

The chapter on psychological experiences in post-cancer treatment survivors by Dr. Beckjord and colleagues reports that emotional and psychological concerns are exceedingly common in this group that now numbers around 12 million in the USA, with less than 50 % getting help that they need. Although most of them have insufficient distress to disrupt their lives, a significant minority have distress that is cause for concern. For many patients with breast cancer who are treated with chemotherapy, the associated psychological distress tends to subside within 2 years, with or without psychological intervention. For other patients, psychological concerns can be long-lasting. Associations with better psychological outcomes in the post-treatment period include having a spouse or partner or adequate social support, higher socioeconomic status evidenced by level of education attained and annual income and an optimistic personality. Emotion concerns include fear of recurrence, sadness and depression, grief and identity concerns, and concerns about family member risk for cancer. Thus, while emotional concerns were common, they were usually not accompanied by high levels of functional impairment. Younger age, female gender, and reporting more physical concerns were associated with reporting more emotional concerns. Emotional and physical concerns were strongly associated.

Complementary and alternative medicine (CAM) refers to a range of modalities and practices that are not part of the conventional and encompasses whole medical systems such as homeopathy and ayurveda; mind–body medicine such as meditation and art therapy; biologically-based practices such as herbs and dietary supplements; manipulative and body-based practices such as chiropractic and massage; and energy medicine such as biofield therapies and magnets. At least 30 % people are thought to use these treatments in addition to conventional medical care. Many patients do not let their physicians know this. Motivations for CAM use in oncology include improvement of quality of life, enhancement of immune function, coping with pain, and control of anxiety and other psychological symptoms. Mind–body therapies are chosen because several have at least some positive supportive data and many target stress reduction, which is a tangible endpoint that is associated with improved quality of life. Moreover, such interventions generally are not practiced as an alternative to regular oncological care; hence, they can be integrated into the overall cancer survivorship treatment plan. The CAM chapter reviews the most commonly used and available procedures.

Advanced Cancer

In the chapter on end-of-life communication, it is reported that currently over 500,000 people annually die of cancer in the USA. Optimal end-of-life care and effective communication represents a key priority in cancer care in all levels and settings, including family communication, clinical care, and public health and requires a multidisciplinary team approach. Communication problems are among the most frequently identified factors associated with poor end-of-life care. These include delayed discussions about the end-of-life interventions such as ventilator use, mismatched understanding of the diagnosis and prognosis, and inadequate attention to patient emotions and preferences. While physicians have traditionally been trained to impart information and advice to patients, recent work has emphasized shared/joint decision-making between patient and health care professionals. In this context, five communication tasks of physicians have been identified: eliciting patient's symptoms, communicating prognosis while maintaining hope, responding to emotions, making end-of-life decisions, and helping the patient navigate the transition to hospice care. Nearly all of end-of-life communication research has been conducted in hospital and clinic settings, whereas little is known about the communication needs of home-based patients and their caregivers. However, many families are increasingly preferring a home death, and strategies to effectively prepare and transition a family to end-of-life care at home are needed. There is evidence that cancer survivors are increasingly engaging in health-related Internet use, including participation in online support groups, emailing their providers, and seeking cancer information online. In the end-of-life context, Dr. Chou relates that opportunities exist to examine how Web 2.0 technologies (social media, blogs, and mobile devices) may provide social support as well as timely and useful information for patients and caregivers. In the clinical setting, with the implementation of electronic medical records and patient portals, work remains in how to effectively integrate education and support for seriously-ill patients and their caregivers into evolving web-based communication systems. Recent findings demonstrate many benefits of integrating palliative and end-of-life communication throughout the care continuum to ensure continuity of care and improve transitions from curative to palliative care. The support from the medical team who cares for the patient often abruptly ends when treatment is discontinued and for the minority of patients diagnosed with cancer who are referred to hospice, bereavement support is offered but rarely utilized for the caregivers after the loss of their loved one. The final chapter is devoted to those caregivers.

Dr. Steel reports that caregivers of patients with cancer who are at the end-of-life are at risk for psychological distress, and it is not yet clear how to best support them. No current interventions offer clear advantages. When a loved one is diagnosed with cancer, this may be the first time the patient or family caregiver has considered death. Unlike traumatic events that take a person's life immediately, cancer often allows the patient and family time to prepare. The quality of that time depends on several factors, such as the cancer symptoms, side effects of treatment, patient and caregiver personality and relationship, prior experience with loss, support from family and friends, spirituality, prior psychological functioning, and interactions with health care professionals. One study found that only 37 % of patients had discussed end-of-life preferences with their physician. Another study demonstrated that discussions with physicians regarding end-

of-life care resulted in earlier referral to hospice, less aggressive care, and better quality of life. The most feared symptom reported by patients is unmanaged pain. Pain symptoms can also be associated with worse survival [6]. Palliative care aims to integrate support for the physical and psychological needs of the patient and offer support to help the family cope, including bereavement counseling. Patient HRQL during the end-of-life and the medical team's communication and behaviors can have lasting effects on the family and caregiver and has the potential for resulting in long-lasting remorse, guilt, or pain on the part of the family, without sensitive and careful discussions of terminal care decision-making. Caregiver stress has been reported to be associated with increased risk of depression, perceived stress, poorer HRQL, increased risk of health conditions and even mortality. Stress, depression, and prolonged grief are all treatable conditions. After the death of the patient, two different caregiver trajectories have been described. They are abatement of caregiver stress, or the opposite, with caregiver stress causing a diminishment of the psychological resources needed to cope during the bereavement process. Immune system dysregulation has been reported amongst caregivers during bereavement, possibly mediated by increased levels of inflammatory cytokines, with the potential to result in new health problems, including cardiovascular disease and some types of cancer. Given the large number of annual cancer deaths and thus grieving caregivers, these issues merit continued study and evaluation of potential clinical interventions.

Summary

This collection of essays describes a range of patient and caregiver needs and concerns over the cancer patient disease continuum, as well as many of the supportive and treatment approaches that are being used and evaluated. Given the staggering number of cancer patients and the increasing and large numbers of cancer survivors and the effects on their families, the psychological issues and care have become an important part of the total medical care of cancer patients. Evolving techniques, approaches, therapies, and advances in neuroscience, endocrinology, and molecular biology, as well as new molecular and neural imaging modalities, are underpinning a revolution in our approach to the mind–body relationship in general and in the cancer patient in particular. As we better understand the biochemical basis of mind and behavior and how these mediators also alter bodily function, new ideas about the mechanisms underlying these psychological processes should translate into new and more effective therapies.

The availability of several approaches to the treatment of anxiety and depression, gives hope for these to be used not only to benefit patient psychological reactions to cancer, but possibly to also alter the biology of the cancer itself and thus survival, since there is a likely bi-directionality to the mind–body relationship. There is greatly increased understanding of how cognitive and emotional influences might impact many of the known biochemical and molecular processes of cancer biology. Although it has long been known that psychological factors can influence biological pathways and even mortality, there are inconsistent findings with regard to whether interventions that reduce psychological morbidity can also

influence disease outcomes, especially survival. The ideas presented in this book give an indication of a flourishing and developing area of biobehavioral study in process of the healthy foment that characterizes new knowledge and change.

References

1. Steel JL, Eton DT, Cella D, Olek MC, Carr BI. Clinically meaningful changes in health-related quality of life in patients diagnosed with hepatobiliary carcinoma. Ann Oncol. 2006;17:304–12.
2. Steel JL, Chopra K, Olek MC, Carr BI. Health-related quality of life: Hepatocellular carcinoma, chronic liver disease, and the general population. Qual Life Res. 2007;16:203–15.
3. Steel JL, Nadeau K, Olek M, Carr BI. Preliminary results of an individually tailored psychosocial intervention for patients with advanced hepatobiliary carcinoma. J Psychosoc Oncol. 2007;25:19–42.
4. Steel JL, Dimartini A, Drew MA. Psychosocial issues in Hepatocellular Carcinoma in Hepatocellular Carcinoma. 2nd Ed (Carr BI-Ed). Humana press/ Springer Science, New York, NY) 2010;641–71.
5. Steel JL, Geller DA, Carr BI Proxy ratings of health related quality of life in patients with hepatocellular carcinoma. Quality of Life Research. 2005;14: 1025–33.
6. Carr BI, Pujol L Pain at presentation and survival in hepatocellular carcinoma. J Pain. 2010;11:988–93.

Index

A

ACU. *See* Association of Clinicians for the Underserved (ACU)
Adherence, cancer fatalism
  clinical breast, 87
  non-adherence, 83
Advanced cancer
  caregivers, 405
  DAs (*see* Decision aids (DAs))
  end-of-life communication, 404–405
  immune system dysregulation, 406
  unmanaged pain, 405
Aerobic exercise, 281–282
Affected family member, 32, 41, 44, 55, 58
African American respondents, 56, 57
American Cancer Society (ACS), 269, 279, 327, 388
American Pain Foundation, 388
American Psychosocial Oncology Society (APOS), 388
American Society of Clinical Oncology (ASCO), 388
ANS. *See* Autonomic nervous system (ANS)
Anxiety, 32, 34, 41–45, 49, 51, 53, 59
AOSW. *See* Association of Oncology Social Work (AOSW)
APOS. *See* American Psychosocial Oncology Society (APOS)
Art therapy, 352–353
ASCO. *See* American Society of Clinical Oncology (ASCO)
Association of Clinicians for the Underserved (ACU), 389
Association of Oncology Social Work (AOSW), 389
Autonomic nervous system (ANS), 2, 6

B

Behavior
  CanCOPE, 186
  cognitive therapy, 191–192
  marital therapy, 191–192
  psychosocial intervention
    couples coping, cancer, 180–183
    lifestyle behavioral change, 192–193
Benefit finding, 50–53, 59, 142
Bereavement, 43, 374–377
Biobehavioral mediators
  chronic levels of stress, 377

dementia, 376
depression, 376
health care utilization, 376–377
immunity, 377
pro-inflammatory cytokines, 377
psychological factors and health morbidity, 377
Black Women's Health Imperative, 389
BMI. *See* Body-mass index (BMI)
Body image, cancer
  body self-perception, changes, 204
  delayed ejaculation, 202–203
  description, 199
  different treatments, 204–205
  emotional aspects, sex, 205–206
  female sexual problems (*see* Female sexual problems)
  femininity, 204
  gender identity, 199
  hereditary breast and ovarian cancer, 45
  loss of libido, 203
  Lynch syndrome, 46
  male sexual problems, 202
  partners, 206–207
  physical changes, 204
  premature ejaculation, 202
  prevalence, 200–201
  prophylactic surgery, 50
  sex communication, 208
  sexual minority groups, 207–208
  sexual orientation, 199–200
  sexual problems, 201
  sexual response, 200
  stem, patient's, 204
  treatments, 203–204
Body-mass index (BMI), 19
Body-mind
  brain and peripheral organs, 396
  interaction, mediators, 395
  medicine, 404
  therapies, 404
Bone loss, 280
BRCA1/2, 34, 37, 38, 42–44, 48–51, 53, 55–57, 65–69
BRCA self-concept scale, 49
Breast
  cancer, mastectomy (*see* Women's decision-making)
  MRI, 35–36, 38

C

CABG. *See* Coronary artery bypass graft (CABG)
CAM. *See* Complementary and alternative medicine
    (CAM)
Cancer
    body image (*see* Body image, cancer)
    CARES, 258
    coping (*see* Religiousness and spirituality coping)
    couples coping (*see* Psychosocial interventions,
        couples coping)
    CPILS and IOCv2, 260
    disease-specific measures, 261
    EORTC QLQ-C30, 258–259
    exercise (*see* Exercise)
    FACT-G, FACIT and FLIC, 259
    fatalism (*see* Fatalism)
    fear, 49
    inflammation (*see* Inflammation and chronic disease)
    LTQL, 260–261
    MQOL and QLI-CV II, 259–260
    prevention, 44, 59
    prevention and decision-making, 397–398
    psychoneuroimmunology (*see*
        Psychoneuroimmunology and cancer)
    QLACS and QOL-CS, 261
    risk assessment, 33
    risk information, 32, 33
    screening, 32, 35, 37, 39, 41, 56, 58
    survivorship, 33, 52
    symptom and treatment, 261–262
Cancer Coping for Couples (CanCOPE), 186, 190, 193
Cancer Financial Assistance Coalition (CFAC), 389
Cancer Patient Education Network (CPEN), 389–390
Cancer patients, resources
    ACS, 388
    ACU and AOSW, 389
    American Pain Foundation, 388
    APOS and ASCO, 388
    Black Women's Health Imperative, 389
    CancerCare and CFAC, 389
    CancerCare Co-payment Assistance
        Foundation, 389
    Cancer Support Community, 390
    collaboration, 387–388
    CPEN, 389–390
    ENACCT and ICC, 390
    HCPs, 386–387
    The LGBT Cancer Project, 390
    LIVESTRONG, 390–391
    Marjorie E. Korff PACT Program, 392
    MRC, MASCC and NAC, 391
    NCCS, NFCA and NORD, 392
    NCI and NCFC, 391–392
    PAN Foundation, 392–393
    referral, 385–386
    Research Advocacy Network, 393
    SuperSibs!, 393
    Vital Options, 393
Cancer Problems in Living Scale (CPILS), 260
Cancer Rehabilitation Evaluation System
    (CARES), 258

Cancer-related fatigue (CRF)
    cardiotoxicity, 281
    exercise (*see* Exercise)
    placebo and nocebo effects, 312–313
    treatment, side effects, 280
Cancer Support Community, 390
Cancer survivors
    psychosocial responses
        active treatment, 225–226
        advanced-stage disease, 226–227
        aftereffects, 229–231
        diagnosis, 223–224
        long-term survivorship, 231–232
        posttreatment survivorship, 227–228
        short-term survivorship, 229
        transition period, 228–229
        treatment and pretreatment, 224
    quality of life and inflammation
        and depression, 6–7
        description, 4
        and fatigue, 5–6
        humans and animals, sickness behaviors, 4–5
        proinflammatory cytokines, 5
Cancer worry, 33, 41, 42, 49, 51–53, 55, 58, 59
CanCOPE. *See* Cancer Coping for Couples (CanCOPE)
Cardiopulmonary resuscitation (CPR), 22
Cardiotoxicity, 281
Caregiver bereavement
    caregiver stress, 374
    dementia, 374–375
    fracture *vs.* dementia, 375
    HCPs, 374
    hypertension and heart disease, 374
    patterns of loss, 375
    predictors, 376
    psychological symptoms, 375
    risk of mortality, 375
    trajectory analyses, 375–376
Caregiver HRQOL
    American Cancer Society consensus conference, 269
    anxiety and depression, 268
    groups, 268–269
    interest, population, 269
    survival rates, 268
Caregivership
    approaches, 219
    demographic correlation, 213–214
    family caregivers and survivors, 213
    illness trajectory, 214–216
    methodological concerns, 218
    personal and social resources, 213
    potential biobehavioral pathways, 216–217
    survivorship, 217–218
Caregiver survivorship
    biobehavioral mediators (*see* Biobehavioral
        mediators)
    couple's therapy, 380
    death and dying, 371
    final hours, care, 373–374
    grief and bereavement (*see* Caregiver bereavement)
    HCP, 371–373

palliative care and hospice, 373
QOL (*see* Quality of life (QOL))
CARES. *See* Cancer Rehabilitation Evaluation System (CARES)
Carriers
  breast self-examination and clinical breast, 37
  clinical total body skin examinations, 41
  colonoscopy, 39
  definition, 32, 34
  genetic test results, 42–43
  health behaviors, 38
  hereditary
    breast and ovarian cancer, 45
    melanoma, 46
  lynch syndrome, 45–46
  mammography, 37
  ovarian cancer, 37
  prophylactic
    mastectomy, 37–38
    oophorectomy, 38
  relief and positive experiences, 48
  skin self-examinations, 41
  testing-specific forms of distress, 44
  uncertain significance test results, 43–44
  uncertainty regarding cancer risk, 48
CAT tools. *See* Computerized adaptive testing (CAT) tools
CBSM. *See* Cognitive-behavioral stress management (CBSM)
CCK. *See* Cholecystokinin (CCK)
CD. *See* Crohn's disease (CD)
CDKN2A/p16 (p16), 35, 40
CFAC. *See* Cancer Financial Assistance Coalition (CFAC)
CHD. *See* Coronary heart disease (CHD)
Chemotherapy
  first-line, breast cancer, 77–78
  ovarian cancer, 77
  prostate cancer, first to fourth-line, 78
Chemotherapy-induced nausea and vomiting (CINV), 313
Childhood cancer prevention, 47, 57
Cholecystokinin (CCK), 320, 322
Chronic illness. *See* Inflammation and chronic disease
Chronic obstructive pulmonary disease (COPD)
  chronic inflammation, 20–21
  severity, 21
CINV. *See* Chemotherapy-induced nausea and vomiting (CINV)
Classical conditioning, 318
Clinical breast examinations, 34, 36, 37
Cognitive-behavioral interventions
  approaches, 235
  short-term effects, 241
  therapeutic techniques, 248
Cognitive-behavioral stress management (CBSM), 7
Collaboration
  CFAC, 389
  CPEN, 390

MASCC, 391
  organization and profession, 387–388
Colonoscopy, 35, 39, 40, 43, 51
Communication, sex and cancer, 208
Complementary and alternative medicine (CAM)
  cancer survivorship, 347
  categorization, 347
  mind-body therapies (*see* Mind-body therapies, CAM)
  modalities, 348
  motivations, 348
  potential advantages, 348
  psychosocial stress, 348–349
  self-regulation, 349–350
  survey, 347
Computerized adaptive testing (CAT) tools, 263, 264
Consolidated Standards of Reporting Trials (CONSORT), 163, 164
CONSORT. *See* Consolidated Standards of Reporting Trials (CONSORT)
Context
  cultural, 397
  end-of-life, 405
  social, 397, 400–401
  treatment, placebo response, 403
Controversies, psycho-oncology
  behavioral science, 157
  description, 158
  interventions, emotional distress
    "con" position, 162–163
    CONSORT, 163
    cumulative science, 164–165
    diagnosis, 161
    "pro" position, 163–164
    psychological intervention, 161–162
    significant resources, 165
  patient distress, 160
  politics/religion driven, 157
  positive psychology (*see* Positive psychology)
  screening, emotional distress, 158–160
  standard cancer care, 160
  support groups and survival
    assessment-only groups, 170
    control groups, 169
    individual variables m, 171
    malignant melanoma, 168–169
    meta-analysis, 169
    metastatic breast cancer patients, 168
    participation, 168
    psychological interventions, 171
    psychosocial intervention, 170
    tumor growth and metastasis, 171
COPD. *See* Chronic obstructive pulmonary disease (COPD)
Coping
  approach-oriented forms, 50
  colonoscopy, 43
  fatalism, cancer patients, 89
  religiousness and spirituality (*see* Religiousness and spirituality coping)

Coping and hope
    changing reality, 124–126
    interdependence, 121
    revival, 121
    situations, 121
    and uncertainty
        and distortion of reality, 122–123
        managing uncertainty over time, 123–124
        odds, 122
        process, 121
        psychological stress, 121
        rationales people, 122
Coping skills training (CST), 189
Coronary artery bypass graft (CABG), 23
Coronary heart disease (CHD), 22
Couples coping, cancer. *See* Psychosocial interventions, couples coping
CPEN. *See* Cancer Patient Education Network (CPEN)
CPILS. *See* Cancer Problems in Living Scale (CPILS)
CPR. *See* Cardiopulmonary resuscitation (CPR)
CRF. *See* Cancer-related fatigue (CRF)
Crisis, 385–386
Crohn's disease (CD), 7, 18
CST. *See* Coping skills training (CST)
Culturally tailored genetic counseling, 54, 56–57

D
Decision
    aids (*see* Decision aids (DAs))
    RRM, 397
    support and interventions, 69–70
    treatment, 397
Decision aids (DAs)
    advanced cancer
        breast cancer, 77–78
        decision-making, 76
        development, 76
        end-of-life planning, 79
        goals, 75
        informed consent, 75–76
        lung cancer, 77
        metastatic prostate cancer, 77
        ovarian cancer, 77
        pilot trial, 78
        randomized trials, 78–79
    RRM, 69
Decision-making
    active participants, 75
    DAs, 76, 78
Decliners of genetic testing, 37, 39, 55–56
Delay, cancer fatalism
    diagnosis, 87–88
    seeking medical help, 84
Delayed distress, 43
Depression, 6–7, 32, 41–44, 51, 53, 59, 328, 330, 334, 336
Desmoid tumors, 39
Diet, 38, 51, 53

Distress
    level assessment, 386
    management, 388
    patients, 190
    psychological, 186
Dyadic-level theories
    and communal coping, 187–188
    relationship intimacy model, 187–188

E
Early detection, 34, 41, 44, 51, 55, 57–59
Education Network to Advance Cancer Clinical Trials (ENACCT), 390
EGFR. *See* Epithelial growth factor receptor (EGFR)
Emotional concerns
    bivariate analyses, 336–337
    functional impairment, 341
    hypothesis, 343
    identification, distress, 342
    limitations, 343
    linear regression model, 337, 340
    LIVESTRONG survey (*see* LIVESTRONG survey)
    logistic regressions model
        chemotherapy, radiation and surgery, 337
        men *vs.* women, recurrence (fear of), 337
        receipt of care, 340, 341
        sociodemographic and medical characteristics, 337–339
    prevalence, 336
    vs. receipt of care, 342
    sample characteristics, 335
    SCPs, 342–343
    sociodemographic and medical variables, 342
ENACCT. *See* Education Network to Advance Cancer Clinical Trials (ENACCT)
End-of-life
    communication
        caregiver-oriented communication, 365–366
        clinical priorities, 357–358
        communication tasks, 362
        hospice and palliative care, 361–362
        medical curriculum and training, 362
        myths and taboos, 361
        patient agency, 363
        patient-provider communication, 364–365
        psycho-oncology, 362
        system-level interventions, 366–367
        type, interventions, 363–364
    couple's therapy, 381
    decision aids, 79
    HCPs, 371–373
    health care utilization, 376–377
    hospice, 373
    QOL, 377–379
Endometrial cancer, 259
EORTC QLQ-C30. *See* European Organization for Research and Treatment of Cancer Quality of Life Questionnaire-CORE 30 (EORTC QLQ-C30)

Epithelial growth factor receptor (EGFR), 20
Ethnic/racial minorities, 56–57
European Organization for Research and Treatment of
        Cancer Quality of Life Questionnaire-CORE
        30 (EORTC QLQ-C30), 258–259
Exercise
    aerobic, 281–282
    description, 281
    information, 284
    medical clearance and contraindications, 284
    prescriptions, 285–286
    professionals, 284–285
    resistance, 282–283
    Tai Chi and Yoga, 283–284
Existential distress
    enhanced spiritual
        depression and psychological distress, 297
        meaning-enhancing interventions, 297–298
        mystical experience, 298–299
        protection, 298
        SEGT and awareness, 298
        total pain, 298
    hallucinogens, 292–294
    prevalence, 295
    psilocybin (see Psilocybin)
    religion vs. spirituality, 296
    spiritual distress, palliative care, 296
    spiritual well-being and psychological distress,
        296–297

F
FACIT. See Functional Assessment of Chronic Illness
        Therapy (FACIT)
FACT-G. See Functional Assessment of Cacer Therapy-
        General, Version 4 (FACT-G)
FACT-Lung Symptom Index (FLSI), 265
Familial adenomatous polyposis (FAP), 31, 35, 38–40,
        42, 48–49, 52
Family caregivers
    employment benefits and health insurance, 214
    negative and positive experiences, 213–214
    relative's death, 217
    role, 218
    self-care and care, 215
Family communication, 44, 53
FAP. See Familial adenomatous polyposis (FAP)
Fatalism
    and cancer patients, 88–90
    definition, 83
    delay, diagnosis, 87–88
    diverse population groups
        African Americans, 85
        ethnic groups, 86
        existing empirical data, 86
        Jewish and Arab women, 85
        Latina and Caucasian women, 85
        Palestinian women, 86
        studies, 84–85
    ethnicity and socioeconomic status, 84
    genetic fatalism and cancer, 90–91

multidimensional construction
    conflicting, cause confusion and mistrust, 93
    consequences and possible outcomes, 91, 92
    dimensions, 91
    emotions, 94
    ethnic groups, 95
    external health locus, 94
    healthy participants, 95
    personal traits, 94
    psychological factors, 93
    religions, 92–93
    religious-related fatalism, 93
    tailoring interventions to overcome barriers,
        94–95
    Western countries, ethnic minority groups, 92
    perception, 83–84
    and screening, 86–87
Fatigue and cancer survivors, 5–6
Female sexual problems
    anorgasmia, 201
    primary vaginismus, 201
    secondary vaginismus and dyspareunia,
        201–202
Fertility and sexuality, 204
FLIC. See Functional Living Index-Cancer (FLIC)
FLSI. See FACT-Lung Symptom Index (FLSI)
Functional Assessment of Cacer Therapy-General,
        Version 4 (FACT-G), 259
Functional Assessment of Chronic Illness Therapy
        (FACIT), 259, 267
Functional Living Index-Cancer (FLIC), 259

G
Gender identity, 199
Generic quality of life (QOL)
    description, 256–257
    NHP and PAIS-SR, 257–258
    SF-36 and SF-12, 257
    SIP and QL-I, 258
Genetic determinism, 50–54
Genetic mutation, 32, 33, 38, 42
Genetic risk, 395, 397
Genetics
    cancer fatalism, 84, 90–91
    psychological aspects, 31–59
Genetic testing, 31–59
    for minors, 39, 47, 56, 57
    uptake, 34–39, 52, 54–57
Global health, 263–264
Group therapy, 169, 170
Guilt, 32, 33, 44–46, 58

H
Hallucinogen
    alkaloids, 292–293
    dosages, 293
    positive response, 293–294
    potential treatment applications, 293
    psychoactive plants, 292

HBOC. *See* Hereditary breast and ovarian cancer (HBOC)
HCC. *See* Hepatocellular carcinoma (HCC)
HCPs. *See* Health care professionals (HCPs)
HCRC. *See* Hereditary cancer risk counseling (HCRC)
Health care professionals (HCPs)
   cancer patients, resources, 386–387
   communication and decisions, 372
   death influence, 371–372
   diagnosis, cancer, 372
   palliative sedation, 373
   QOL, 372
   symptom management, 372
   training, 380
Health disparities, 56
Health-related quality of life (HRQOL)
   caregiver (*see* Caregiver HRQOL)
   development, 268
   dimensions, 256
   IRT and CAT tools, 263
   measurement, 256–263
   PROMIS, 263–264
   RCTs, 265–267
   symptom monitoring, 264–265
   symptoms and concerns, 267–268
Hepatoblastoma, 39
Hepatocellular carcinoma (HCC), 14, 19
Hereditary breast and ovarian cancer (HBOC),
    31, 32, 35, 42, 45, 46, 55–57
Hereditary cancer risk counseling (HCRC), 31–59
Hereditary cancer syndromes, 31–33, 35,
    39, 40, 52, 57–59
Hereditary colorectal cancer, 48
Hereditary melanoma, 31, 34, 35, 40–41, 45, 46, 52, 58
Hereditary nonpolyposis colorectal cancer
    (HNPCC), 32, 35, 38–39
HNPCC. *See* Hereditary nonpolyposis colorectal cancer
    (HNPCC)
Hope, 120–121
Hopelessness, 45
Hospice and palliative care, 361–362
HPA. *See* Hypothalamic-pituitary-adrenal (HPA)
HPVs. *See* Human papilloma viruses (HPVs)
Human papilloma viruses (HPVs), 4
Hypothalamic-pituitary-adrenal (HPA), 2, 5, 6

I
IBD. *See* Inflammatory bowel disease (IBD)
ICC. *See* Intercultural Cancer Council (ICC)
IHCS. *See* Interactive Health Communication System
    (IHCS)
Illness trajectory, cancer caregivership
   caregivers' stress, 214–215
   demographic factors, 215
   depressive symptoms, 216
   existential experience, 216
   gender, 215
   mental health, 215
   physical burden, 216

   status, spouse, 215
   stressor, acute type, 215–216
Immune
   function
     dysregulated, 1, 2
     neuroendocrine and cellular, 7
     psychosocial interventions, 7
   responses, cell-mediated, 4
   system
     cancer interacts, 7–8
     depression, 6
     fatigue, 5
     virus latency, 4
Impact of Cancer version 2 (IOCv2), 260
Individual differences, 43, 51, 52
Inflammation
   and depressive symptoms, 6
   induces macrophages, 3
   quality of life, cancer survivors (*see* Cancer
     survivors)
Inflammation and chronic disease
   behavioral factors, 23–24
   chronic inflammation, 13–14
   and depression, inter-relationship, 14–15
   gastrointestinal disease, 17–18
   obesity and type-2 diabetes, 18–20
   psychological distress and chronic disease, 24
   pulmonary and cardiovascular disease, 20–23
   rheumatic disease, 15–16
   treatment considerations, 23
Inflammatory bowel disease (IBD), 17–18
Informed consent, advanced cancer patients, 75–76
Institute of Medicine (IOM) report, 229–230
Insurance coverage, 40
Insurance discrimination, 32, 33, 38, 44, 51, 55
Intensive surveillance, 33, 49
Interactive Health Communication System (IHCS),
    366–367
Intercultural Cancer Council (ICC), 390
Interferon-α (IFN-α), 14
Interleukin 6 (IL-6)
   depressed patients, 14–15
   fatigued cancer survivors, 5
   post-vaccination levels, 6–7
   PPARG, 17
   proinflammatory cytokines, 3, 6
   RA, 15
   and TNF-α, 19, 23
   tumor initiation and growth, 14
Interventions, psychosocial. *See* Psychosocial
    interventions, couples coping
IOCv2. *See* Impact of Cancer version 2 (IOCv2)
IRT. *See* Item response theory (IRT)
Item response theory (IRT), 263, 264

L
Latino respondents, 57
Lesbian/gay/bisexual, 207
LFS. *See* Li–Fraumeni syndrome (LFS)

Li–Fraumeni syndrome (LFS), 36, 57–58
LIVESTRONG survey
　data analysis, 334–335
　fear of recurrence, 334
　functional impairment, 334
　limitations, 343, 344
　participants and procedures, 333
　post-treatment cancer survivors, 334
　receipt of care, 334
　SCPs, 342–343
　sociodemographic and medical variables, 334
　surveillance data, 333
Long Term Quality of Life Scale (LTQL), 260–261
Long-term survivorship, 232
LTQL. See Long Term Quality of Life Scale (LTQL)
Lynch syndrome, 31, 32, 35, 38–39, 42, 43, 45–46, 49,
　52, 56

M
Male sexual problems, 202
Mammography, 37, 38, 51
Marjorie E. Korff PACT Program, 392
MASCC. See Multinational Association of Supportive
　Care in Cancer (MASCC)
Mastery, 45, 48–51
Matrix metalloproteinase (MMPs), 2–3, 396
MBAT. See Mindfulness-based art therapy (MBAT)
MBSR. See Mindfulness-based stress reduction (MBSR)
McGill Quality of Life Questionnaire-Revised (MQOL),
　259–260
Measurement, HRQOL
　cancer (see Cancer)
　conceptual representation, 256–257
　generic (see Generic quality of life (QOL))
　pediatrics, 262
　selection, 262–263
Medical management, 31, 33, 34, 50, 53
Medical mistrust, 51, 56, 57
Medicare Rights Center (MRC), 391
Meditation
　MBSR, 351
　neuroimaging
　　biological effects, 353–354
　　brain imaging, 354
　　cortical-thalamic activity, 354
　　paraympathetic activity, 355
　　techniques, 354
　Qigong, 351
　Tai Chi, 351–352
　yoga, 350
Mental health, 280
MICRA. See Multidimensional impact of cancer risk
　assessment (MICRA)
MIDs. See Minimally important differences (MIDs)
Mind-body
　brain and peripheral organs, 396
　interaction, mediators, 395
　medicine, 404
　therapies, 404

Mind-body therapies, CAM
　art therapy, 352
　description, 350
　hypnosis, 350
　MBAT, 352–353
　meditation practices (see Meditation)
　music therapy, 353
　NET, 353
　self-regulation, neuroimaging
　　biological effects, 353–354
　　brain imaging, 354
　　cortical-thalamic activity, 354
　　paraympathetic activity, 355
　　techniques, 354
Mindfulness-based art therapy (MBAT), 352–353
Mindfulness-based stress reduction (MBSR), 351, 352
Minimally important differences (MIDs), 267
MMPs. See Matrix metalloproteinase (MMPs)
Monitoring, 35, 39, 51, 52
MQOL. See McGill Quality of Life Questionnaire-
　Revised (MQOL)
MRC. See Medicare Rights Center (MRC)
Multidimensional impact of cancer risk assessment
　(MICRA), 44, 48
Multinational Association of Supportive Care in Cancer
　(MASCC), 391
Muscle loss, 280
Music therapy, 353
Mystical experience, psilocybin
　characteristics, 300
　meaning and transcendence, 299
　perennial philosophy, 299
　self-experience, 299–300
　spirituality, 299
　transpersonal psychology, 299

N
NAC. See National Alliance for Caregiving (NAC)
National Alliance for Caregiving (NAC), 391
National Cancer Institute (NCI), 391
National Center for Frontier Communities (NCFC),
　391–392
National Coalition for Cancer Survivorship (NCCS), 392
National Family Caregivers Association (NFCA), 392
National Organization for Rare Disorders (NORD), 392
National Society of Genetic Counselors, 32
Natural killer (NK) cell, 3, 7
NCCS. See National Coalition for Cancer Survivorship
　(NCCS)
NCFC. See National Center for Frontier Communities
　(NCFC)
NCI. See National Cancer Institute (NCI)
Negative mood, 42
NET. See Neuroemotional technique (NET)
Neurobiological and immunological responses
　hormone secretion and suppressive effects, 319
　hyperalgesic effects, 320
　opioids and CCK, 320
　physiological correlates, 320–321

Neuroemotional technique (NET), 353
Neuroticism, 51
NFCA. *See* National Family Caregivers Association (NFCA)
NF-kB. *See* Nuclear factor-kappB (NF-kB)
NHP. *See* Nottingham Health Profile (NHP)
NK cell. *See* Natural killer (NK) cell
   Nocebo effect*See also* Placebo and nocebo effects, cancer treatmentdefinition, 310
   discontinuation rates, 311
   nocebo responses, 311
   non-specific side effects, 311
Noncarrier, 34, 37–40, 42, 44–48, 50, 52, 53, 58
NORD. *See* National Organization for Rare Disorders (NORD)
Nottingham Health Profile (NHP), 257–258
Nuclear factor-kappB (NF-kB), 14, 20

O
Oncology-distress management, 147
Oncology resources
   AOSW, 389
   APOS and ASCO, 388
   HCPs, 386–387
Optimism, 42, 51
Outcomes
   PROMIS, 263–264
   PROs, 255
   QOL-CS, 261
   SF-36 and SF-12, 257
Ovarian cancer screening
   CA-125, 37
   transvaginal ultrasound, 37

P
p53, 36, 57, 58
PAGIS. *See* Psychological adaptation to genetic information scale (PAGIS)
PAIS-SR. *See* Psychological Adjustment to Illness Scale—Self Report (PAIS-SR)
Palliative care and hospice, 373
Palliative care and internet-based programs, 366–367
Palliative care and psycho-oncology, psilocybin, 304–305
Palliative treatment
   advanced cancer, 75–76
   anticancer therapy, 79, 80
   chemotherapy, 77, 78
Pancreatic cancer, 35, 41
PAN Foundation. *See* Patient Access Network (PAN) Foundation
Partners in Coping Program (PICP), 188
Patient Access Network (PAN) Foundation, 392–393
Patient agency, end-of-life communication, 363
Patient-centered cancer care, 363
Patient expectations
   vs. classical conditioning, 319, 320
   negative and positive, 319

post chemotherapy nausea, 319
   self-regulation model, health, 318–319
Patient-provider communication
   clinical skills training, 364–365
   COPE trial, 365
   decision-making, 366
   Dignity Therapy, 365
   "Outlook" program, 365
   state-and community-based programs, 366
Patient-Reported Outcomes Measurement Information System (PROMIS), 263–264
Patient support
   CAM, 404
   distress, 401
   emotional reactions, 402
   HRQOL, 403
   palliative care, 401–402
   placebo and nocebo effects, 403–404
   post-cancer treatment survivors, 404
   psychological interventions, 402–403
Perceived advantages of genetic testing, 45
Perceived control, 31, 45–48, 51
Perceived disadvantages of genetic testing, 57
Perceived personal control measure (PPC), 48
Perceived risk, 51, 54, 55
Personal growth, 45, 46, 51, 53
Personalized medicine, 41, 59
Photoprotection, 40, 46, 47
Physical activity, 285, 286
Physician recommendation and referral, 33, 37
PICP. *See* Partners in Coping Program (PICP)
Placebo and nocebo effects, cancer treatment
   adverse events, 315
   anxiety and pain relief, 314
   chronic pain, 313
   CINV, 313
   classical conditioning, 318
   CRF, 312–313
   ethical dilemma, intervention, 323
   hypothesis, 314
   information and personal interaction
      media, 321
      positive and negative expectations, 321, 322
      side effects, 321–322
      SPIKES-Protocol, 322
      TENS *vs.* TSE, 321
      therapeutic benefit, 322–323
   neurobiological and immunological responses, 319–321
   objective measures, 315
   patient expectations, 318–319
   psychological and physiological processes, 309
   RCTs, patients' responses, 314
   recommendations, 323–324
   TENS/TSE treatment, 313–314
   tumor responses, 317
   vasomotor symptoms, 314–315
   weight gain and performance status, 316
Placebo effect*See also* Placebo and nocebo effects, cancer treatmentadministration, 310

"black box", clinical trials, 310, 311
definition, 309
placebo response, 310
therapeutic context, 310
Polyps, 35, 39, 40, 52
Positive mood, 42
Positive psychology
benefits, 167
cancer diagnosis
appraised meaning, 104–105
global meaning violation, 105–106
making meaning, experience, 106–107
meaning made, experience, 107–109
cancer survivorship, 101–102, 113
constructs, 165–166
description, 167
dispositional optimism, 166–167
hypothesis, 166
and interventions, cancer survivors, 112–113
meaning making model
components, 102, 103
global meaning, 102
meanings made, 104
situational meaning, 103
stress, global and situational meaning, 103–104
meta-analysis, 166
optimism, 166
physical health and optimism, association, 166
spirituality and cancer survivorship
and appraised meaning, 109–110
description, 109
meaning making, experience, 110
meanings made, experience, 110–111
stress-related growth and cancer, 111–112
"tossing of the baby", 167–168
"tyranny of optimism", 165
Posttraumatic growth, 50
Posttraumatic growth inventory (PTGI), 50
Post-traumatic stress disorder (PTSD), 328, 330
Post-treatment cancer survivorships
emotional concerns (see Emotional concerns)
psychological factors (see Psychological experience)
PPC. See Perceived personal control measure (PPC)
Prevalence of sexual problems, 200–201
Primary sclerosing cholangitis (PSC), 17
PROMIS. See Patient-Reported Outcomes Measurement
Information System (PROMIS)
Prophylactic surgery
colectomy, 35, 39, 51
prophylactic mastectomy, 34, 35, 37–38
prophylactic oophorectomy, 34, 38
Protective clothing, 40
PSC. See Primary sclerosing cholangitis (PSC)
Psilocybin
careful medical and laboratory evaluations, 292
clinical experiences, 302–304
Death Transcendence Scale, 302
hallucinogenic drugs, 300–301
Harbor-UCLA protocol, 294–295

hospice movement and palliative medicine, 294
living room-like session room, 300, 301
LSD, 292
metastatic ovarian cancer, 295
methylphenidate hydrochloride, 300
mystical (see Mystical experience, psilocybin)
palliative care and psycho-oncology, 304–305
psychoactive effects, 291
retrospective ratings, doses, 301–302
teonanacatl, 291
use, plant hallucinogens, 291
Psychological adaptation, 43
Psychological adaptation to genetic information scale
(PAGIS), 48
Psychological Adjustment to Illness Scale—Self Report
(PAIS-SR), 258
Psychological distress, 42–44, 55, 59
Psychological experience
breast cancer, 328
childhood cancers, 329
components, 328
description, 332–333
disease and sociodemographic factors
characteristics, 332
chemotherapy, 331
"emotional fallout", 332
framework's validity, 331
physical and emotional problems, 331
recovery, breast cancer survivors, 332
resources, 332
stem cell transplantation, 331
stress and burden, 331
emotional distress, 330
inquiry and clinical care, 329
levels, emotional distress, 329–330
NHL and HRQOL, 329
number of cancer survivors, 327–328
posttraumatic growth, 329
PTSD symptoms, 330
recurrence (fears of), 330–331
"war on cancer", 327
Psychological interventions, emotional distress
CONSORT, 163
cumulative science, 164–165
diagnosis, 161
meta-analyses, 162–163
"pro" position, 163–164
psychological intervention, 161–162
significant resources, 165
Psychological screening, emotional distress, 158–160
Psychological stress. See Inflammation and chronic
disease
Psychological symptoms and tumor biology
breast cancer, 395–396
chronic inflammation, 396
interleukins (ILs), 396
serotonin levels, 396–397
treatment, depression, 397
VEGF and MMPs, 396

Psychoneuroimmunology and cancer
  dysregulated immune function, 1
  psychological factors
    ANS and HPA axes, 2
    gene regulation, 3
    glucocorticoids, 3–4
    IL-6, 3
    incidence and progression, 1–2
    MMPs, 2–3
    NK, 3
    oncoviruses, 4
    pFAKy397, 3
    TAMs, 3
    VGEF, 2
  psychosocial interventions and biological outcomes, 7
  quality of life and inflammation
    and depression, 6–7
    description, 4
    and fatigue, 5–6
    humans and animals, sickness behaviors, 4–5
    proinflammatory cytokines, 5
  researchers, 7–8
Psycho-oncology
  and cancer survivorship
    and appraised meaning, 109–110
    description, 109
    meaning making, experience, 110
    meanings made, experience, 110–111
  making model
    components, 102, 103
    global meaning, 102
    meanings made, 104
    situational meaning, 103
    stress, global and situational meaning, 103–104
  stress-related, positive life changes, 111–112
Psychosexual medicine, 202, 203, 206, 207
Psychosocial
  interventions (see Psychosocial interventions)
  recovery, breast cancer, 332
  resources, 332
  SCPs, 342–343
Psychosocial interventions
  cancer continuum
    coping styles, 246
    emotional, physical well-being and quality
      of life, 241
    immune function, 241–242
    medical factors, 243
    mixed findings, 242–243
    perceived stress, 244
    personality traits, 245–246
    physical and emotional well-being, 244
    pretreatment, 239–241
    social support, 244
    sociodemographic factors, 243
    survival, 242
  cancer survivors, 221
  couples coping
    dyadic perspective, 193–194
    goals, 178

    lifestyle behavioral change, 192–193
    meta-analysis, 177–178
    modalities, 194–195
    multiple outcomes, 191
    significant number, 192
    spouses/partners, 177
    systematic reviews(see Systematic reviews)
    thematic review, 177
  couples interventions, 237–238
  delivery, 238–239
  diagnostic criteria, 222
  emotional reactions, 222
  group interventions, 236–237
  individual-and group-based, 248–249
  individual support and self-administered,
    235–236
  responses, cancer survivors (see Cancer survivors)
  sociodemographic factors, 249
  stepped care approach, 246–248
  stress, 223
  targets, 232–234
  types, 234–235
Psychosocial oncology
  breast cancer, 399–400
  cancer diagnosis, 398–399
  controversies, 400
  distress, anxiety and depression, 400
  fatalism, 398
  stress and coping theory, 399
Psychospiritual
  consciousness, 292
  distress, 300
  Harbor-UCLA protocol, 294
  total pain, 298
PTGI. See Posttraumatic growth inventory (PTGI)
PTSD. See Post-traumatic stress disorder (PTSD)
Pulmonary toxicity, 281

Q
QLACS. See Quality of Life in Adult Cancer Survivors
    (QLACS)
QL-I. See Quality of Life Index (QL-I)
QLI-CV III. See Quality of Life Index-Cancer Version III
    (QLI-CV III)
QOL. See Quality of life (QOL)
QOL-CS. See Quality of Life—Cancer Survivors
    (QOL-CS)
Qualitative research, 41
Quality of life (QOL)
  CAM, 404
  cancer caregivership, 213–219
  cancer survivors, 229
  caregiver
    anxiety and depression, 379
    family-focused grief therapy, 379
    psychoeducational emphasis, 380
    randomized controlled trials, 379
    SHPC, 379–380
    supportive care, 379

challenges, interventions, 379
decision aids (DAs), 397
definition, 255–256
depression anxiety, 377–378
depression, anxiety and distress, 400
description, 1
disease-specific, 189, 192, 238, 239
emotional and physical well-being, 241
emotional well-being, 234
evaluation, cancer, 255
health-related, 245, 248
HRQOL (*see* Health-related quality of life
    (HRQOL))
and inflammation, cancer survivors (*see* Cancer
    survivors)
lung cancer patients, 378
mental health professionals, 378
metastatic breast cancer, 378
patient outcomes, 184
primary and secondary goals, 178
PROs, 255
prostate cancer patients and partners, 189
psychopharmacology, 378–379
psychosocial interventions, 402
side effects (*see* Side effects)
significant impact, patients, 189
spousal caregivers, 401
symptom management, 372
Quality of Life—Cancer Survivors (QOL-CS), 261
Quality of Life in Adult Cancer Survivors (QLACS), 261
Quality of Life Index (QL-I), 258
Quality of Life Index-Cancer Version III
    (QLI-CV III), 260

R
RA. *See* Rheumatoid arthritis (RA)
Radio Resource Management (RRM). *See* Women's
    decision-making
Randomized controlled trials (RCTs)
    distribution methods, 267
    emotional symptoms, 265
    HRQOL instruments, 267
    industry and nonindustry sponsored trials, 267
    MIDs, 267
    psychological factors, 265
    symptom control, 266
Rare cancer syndromes, 39, 47, 54, 57–58
RCTs. *See* Randomized controlled trials (RCTs)
Receipt of care
    description, 334
    LIVESTRONG data, 343
    logistic regression modeling, 340, 341
    prevalence, 336
Recurrence (fear of)
    emotional concerns, 334, 336–339
    psychological experience, 330–331
Referral, cancer patients, 385–386

Regression
    linear, 337, 340
    logistic
        chemotherapy, radiation and surgery, 337
        men *vs.* women, recurrence (fear of), 337
        receipt of care, 340, 341
        sociodemographic and medical characteristics,
            337–339
Relationship satisfaction, 184
Relief, 33, 44–46, 48, 51
Religions, cancer fatalism, 92, 93
Religious and spiritual beliefs, 51, 52, 57
Religiousness and spirituality coping
    definition, 129–130
    illness adjustment
        efficacy, 139–140
        and growth, 142–143
        non-religious variables, 140–142
        relationship, 139
    measurement, 132–136
    nature, 130–132
    prevalence
        change, illness course, 137–138
        cultural and denominational differences,
            138–139
        German study, 137
        RCOPE, 136
        USA and UK, 136
    spiritual needs (*see* Spiritual needs)
    use, 130
Religious/spiritual coping strategies
    functions, 132
    instruments examination, 134
Research Advocacy Network, 393
Resistance exercise, 282–283
Rheumatoid arthritis (RA), 15–16

S
SCPMs. *See* Social cognitive processing models
    (SCPMs)
SCPs. *See* Survivorship care plans (SCPs)
Screening. *See* Fatalism
SDS. *See* Symptom Distress Scale (SDS)
SEGT. *See* Supportive-Expressive Group Therapy
    (SEGT)
Selective serotonin-reuptake inhibitors (SSRIs), 23
Self breast examinations, 37
Self-concept, 45, 48–50
Self-efficacy, 45, 48, 52, 58
Self-esteem, 42, 49–50
Sex friendly options for cancer treatment, 207
Sexual attractiveness, 49–50
Sexuality and cancer. *see* Body image, cancer
Sexual orientation, 199, 203, 207
Sexual response, 199, 200
SHPC. *See* Standard home-based palliative care (SHPC)
Sickness Impact Profile (SIP), 258

Side effects
    cardiopulmonary toxicity, 281
    CRF, 280
    description, 279
    exercise, 281
    mental health, 280
    muscle and bone loss, 280
Signal transducer activator of transcription-3
        (Stat3), 14, 17, 19
SIP. *See* Sickness Impact Profile (SIP)
Six-Step Protocol for Delivering Bad News
        (SPIKES-Protocol), 322
Skin self-examinations (SSEs), 40, 41, 51
SLE. *See* Systemic lupus erythematosus (SLE)
Smoking cessation, 38, 51
Social cognitive processing models (SCPMs),
        185, 186
Social context, 400–401
Social support, 32, 43, 51, 58
Sociodemographic factors, cancer survivors
    age, 243
    ethnicity and cultural backgrounds, 243
    socioeconomic status, 243
Socioeconomic factors, 33, 43
SPIKES-Protocol. *See* Six-Step Protocol for Delivering
        Bad News (SPIKES-Protocol)
Spiritual assessment, 144–146
Spiritual needs
    assessments, 144–146
    barriers, assessment and management, 148–149
    directions, 149–150
    spiritual distress management, 146–148
SSEs. *See* Skin self-examinations (SSEs)
SSRIs. *See* Selective serotonin-reuptake inhibitors
        (SSRIs)
Standard home-based palliative care (SHPC), 379
Stat3. *See* Signal transducer activator of transcription-3
        (Stat3)
Stepped care, 246–248
Stigma, 49–51
Stress and coping theory
    appraisal, 120
    meaning-focused coping, 120
    types, 120
Stress management training, 241
Sunscreen, 40, 47
SuperSibs, 393
Supportive care
    metastatic colorectal cancer, 78
    randomized trial, 78
Supportive-Expressive Group Therapy (SEGT), 298
Survey. *See* LIVESTRONG survey
Survivor guilt, 33, 45
Survivorship, 217–218
Survivorship care plans (SCPs), 342–343
SyMon-L. *See* Symptom Monitoring and reporting
        system for advanced Lung cancer
        (SyMon-L)
Symptom Distress Scale (SDS), 261, 265
Symptom management, 372, 379

Symptom monitoring
    assessment, HRQOL, 265
    cumulative graphs, 265, 266
    description, 264
    FLSI, 265
    health care provider and patient levels, 264
    potential benefits, 264–265
    SDS, 265
    SyMon-L system, 265
    treatment schedule, 265
Symptom Monitoring and reporting system
        for advanced Lung cancer (SyMon-L), 265
Systematic reviews
    designs, 178–184
    dyadic-level theories, 187–188
    electronic searches, 178
    EPPI-Reviewer 4.0 software, 178
    individual stress and coping models, 185
    interventions, explicit/implied theory
        CanCOPE, 190
        couples and sex therapy, 189–190
        CST, 189
        description, 189
        partner-guided pain management training, 189
        patient and partner attitudinal barriers, 190
        patient-only, 190
        problem-solving therapy, 190
        QOL and RCT, 189
        uncertainty management, 190
    participant characteristics, 184
    resource theories, 185–187
    theoretical frameworks, 185
Systemic lupus erythematosus (SLE), 15, 16

T
Tai Chi, 283
Tai chi, 351–352
TAMs. *See* Tumor associated macrophages (TAMs)
TBSEs. *See* Total body skin examinations (TBSEs)
TENS. *See* Transcutaneous electrical nerve stimulation
        (TENS)
TNF-α. *See* Tumor necrosis factor-α (TNF-α)
Total body skin examinations (TBSEs), 40, 41
Transcutaneous electrical nerve stimulation (TENS),
        313–314
Transcutaneous spinal electro analgesia (TSE), 313–314
Transpersonal dimension, 299–300
Treatments, sexuality, 203–204
Trier Social Stress Task (TSST), 5
TSE. *See* Transcutaneous spinal electro analgesia (TSE)
TSST. *See* Trier Social Stress Task (TSST)
Tumor associated macrophages (TAMs), 3
Tumor necrosis factor-α (TNF-α)
    adipose tissue, 19
    correlation, depression score, 21
    IBD patients, 17
    SSRIs, 23
    transcription factors, 14
Tumor responses, placebo and nocebo effects, 317

U
UC. *See* Ulcerative colitis (UC)
Ulcerative colitis (UC), 17–18
Ultraviolet radiation (UVR) exposure, 35, 40, 46, 52, 58
Unaffected family member, 32, 34, 41
Uncertainty, 31, 33, 41, 43–46, 48, 51, 55, 58
Uninformative genetic test result, 38
UVR exposure. *See* Ultraviolet radiation (UVR)
        exposure

V
Variant of uncertain significance, 32, 34, 38, 43–44
Vascular endothelial growth factor (VEGF),
        2, 396
Vasomotor symptoms, 314–315
VEGF. *See* Vascular endothelial growth factor (VEGF)
VHL. *See* Von Hippel–Lindau (VHL)
Vigilance, 46, 47, 52

Von Hippel–Lindau (VHL), 36, 57, 58
Vulnerability, 49–52

W
Weight gain and performance status, 316
Well-being, 119, 121, 123, 126
Women's decision-making
        diversity, uptake and timing, 65–66
        family matters, 68
        patient involvement, 68–69
        perceived risk, decisional conflict and uncertainty,
                66–67
        psychological considerations, RRM, 67
        support and interventions, 69–70

Y
Yoga, 283–284

Printed by Printforce, the Netherlands